Therapeutic Exercise

Techniques for Intervention

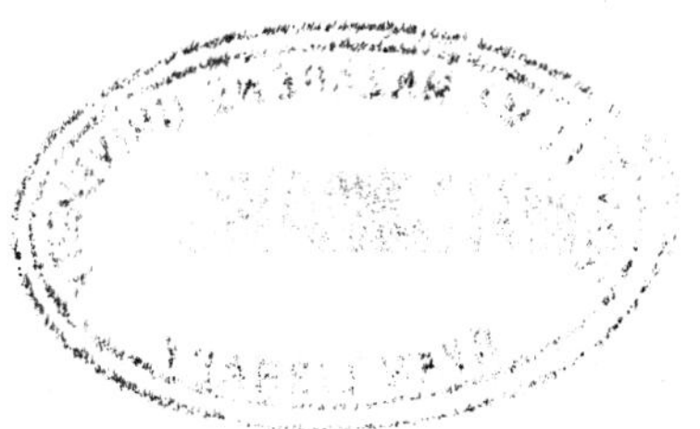

Therapeutic Exercise

Techniques for Intervention

William D. Bandy, PhD, PT, SCS, ATC
University of Central Arkansas
Department of Physical Therapy
Conway, Arkansas

Barbara Sanders, PhD, PT, SCS
Southwest Texas State University
Department of Physical Therapy
San Marcos, Texas

Photography by Michael A. Morris, FBCA
University of Arkansas for Medical Sciences

Editor: Pete Darcy
Managing Editor: Eric Branger
Marketing Manager: Christen DeMarco
Production Editor: Lisa JC Franko

351 West Camden Street
Baltimore, Maryland 21201-2436 USA

530 Walnut Street
Philadelphia, Pennsylvania 19106 USA

The publisher is not responsible (as a matter of product liability, negligence, or otherwise) for any injury resulting from any material contained herein. This publication contains information relating to general principles of medical care which should not be construed as specific instructions for individual patients. Manufacturers' product information and package inserts should be reviewed for current information, including contraindications, dosages, and precautions.

Printed in the United States of America

Library of Congress Cataloging-in-Publication Data
Therapeutic Exercise: Techniques for Intervention / [edited by] William D. Bandy, Barbara Sanders.
p. ;cm.
Includes bibliographical references and index.
ISBN 0-7817-2130-X
1. Musculoskeletal system—Diseases—Exercise therapy. I. Bandy, William D. II. Sanders, Barbara.
[DNLM: 1. Musculoskeletal Diseases—therapy. 2. Exercise Therapy—methods. WE 140 T398 2001]
RC925.5 .T48 2001
616.7'062—dc21 00-049325

The publishers have made every effort to trace the copyright holders for borrowed material. If they have inadvertently overlooked any, they will be pleased to make the necessary arrangements at the first opportunity.

To purchase additional copies of this book call our customer service department at (800) 638-3030 or fax orders to (301) 824-7390. International customers should call (301) 714-2324.

02 03
2 3 4 5 6 7 8 9 10

To Beth, Melissa, and Jamie for providing constant love, patience, and inspiration.
WDB

To Mike and Whitney whose love and support allow me to do the things I enjoy.
BS

PREFACE

Therapeutic exercise consists of a broad category of activities intended to improve a patient's function and health status. In today's health-care environment, passive modalities are no longer thought of as the core element in a rehabilitation program. The future health-care arena will rely more and more on therapeutic exercise for the rehabilitation of individuals with impairment.

The purpose of this textbook is to provide descriptions and rationale for use of a variety of therapeutic exercise techniques from which the clinician can choose the appropriate activities for the rehabilitation of an individual with impairment or for the prevention of potential problems. The primary audience for this textbook is individuals in physical therapy and athletic training educational programs. In addition, this text could serve as a reference for practitioners.

The basic assumption of this text is that the patient has been examined and the impairment has been identified. The focus of the text is on the implementation of the treatment plan and intervention using the appropriate therapeutic exercise. The emphasis is not on the examination, evaluation, diagnosis, and prognosis of the patient. In addition, the focus is on therapeutic exercise techniques. In-depth information on physiology, anatomy, kinesiology, and pathology have been omitted so that more detailed information could be presented on the actual therapeutic exercise activity.

A look at the Contents shows that the textbook is divided into three sections. Section I demonstrates exercises for increasing mobility by performing range of motion techniques (passive, active assistive, active), increasing flexibility of muscle by using a variety of stretching activities, and treating capsular adhesions through the use of mobilization. If a strict definition of therapeutic exercise is used, one might argue that mobilization is not truly a therapeutic exercise and is better categorized under manual therapy. However, to present a complete discussion of activities that increase mobility, mobilization is included here.

Section II presents information on activities for increasing strength and power, ranging from frequently used therapeutic exercise techniques (open-chain and closed-chain exercises) to more sophisticated and aggressive exercises (proprioceptive neuromuscular facilitation and plyometrics). In addition, the unique concepts of medical exercise training are presented along with information on aerobic endurance training.

Section III introduces the important therapeutic exercise concepts of balance and posture, body mechanics, and spinal stabilization. The section contains information concerning the broad possibilities of applications in which aquatic therapy can be used, including enhancing strength and endurance, facilitating balance, and increasing range of motion. The final two chapters integrate information from the previous chapters and progress the patient to the highest possible level. Thus, the first 13 chapters provide the reader with progressively more information until the final two chapters integrate the information and provide programs for progressing patients with upper extremity and lower extremity impairments.

The clinician must have an understanding of therapeutic exercise across the lifespan so that he or she is able to prescribe exercise for children and older adults. To this end, information specific to pediatric and geriatric clients is presented in boxes within each chapter. These Pediatric Perspectives and Geriatric Perspectives offer information that is vital for understanding the appropriate use of the specific therapeutic exercise for all ages.

Most chapters also include at least one case study to provide the reader with examples of how to use therapeutic exercise for actual patients. In addition, the case studies allow the reader to be exposed to the progression of an exercise program, from basic activities to more advanced techniques. Within each case study, exercises from other chapters are noted, and the reader should refer to those other chapters for more detailed information on a particular technique. In this way, the reader will gain a more integrated approach to all types of therapeutic exercise.

Each case study also contains links to the *Guide to Physical Therapist Practice* and the *Athletic Training Educational Competencies.* These documents suggest that therapeutic exercise is a core element for intervention of patients with dysfunction and for clients in need of preventative measures. These links provide additional information that will facilitate the integration of therapeutic exercise into a plan of care.

The final two chapters contain more than one case study, including at least one case study on a pediatric patient and one on a geriatric patient. These extra case studies help the reader integrate all the information presented in the text.

Therapeutic exercise can be considered a craft. As such, therapeutic exercise must be learned by doing, not by reading. This textbook provides ideas and techniques; however, to fully learn therapeutic exercise, the student must practice the techniques under the supervision of an experienced educator. To gain this practical experience, the student should begin by practicing on an individual who is free from dysfunction before trying the techniques on patients with impairments—and the student should always practice in a supervised environment.

Although written primarily for students, this textbook provides experienced clinicians with background and illustrations of specific exercise techniques. By reviewing each chapter, practicing clinicians will be able to add to their repertoire of therapeutic exercises used to effectively treat patients with a variety of impairments.

ACKNOWLEDGMENTS

The writing of a textbook is an enormous undertaking, a task that cannot be accomplished without a supporting cast of friends, family, and colleagues. We wish to acknowledge all the support provided by the editorial staff at Lippincott Williams & Wilkins. Your preparation, encouragement, and professional attitudes were greatly appreciated.

We are excited about the outstanding photographs that are included in this text. The photographs were made possible by Michael Morris, FBCA, who spent countless hours on land and underwater taking (and retaking) the shots to provide the exact pictures we desired. We would be remiss not to give our thanks to the individuals who acted as models for this book: Michael Adkins, Melissa Bandy, Rachel Cloud, Laura Cabrera, Neil Hattlestad, Renatto Hess, Jean Irion, and Trigg Ross. We need to give special thanks to Nancy Reese, who not only served as the model for the clinician but who also frequently made herself available to provide assistance and guidance in the preparation of this textbook.

Obviously, this book would not have been possible without the work and dedication of the contributing authors, who are listed by name in a separate section. Your willingness to share your expertise and to meet the deadlines is greatly appreciated. In addition, the assistance of graduate assistants Jenny Hood and Stacey Ihler, from the University of Central Arkansas, was invaluable. This book could not have been completed without your valuable assistance and patience.

Each of us believe that we are blessed to work with such an outstanding faculty and wish to acknowledge the support of the faculty members in the Departments of Physical Therapy at the University of Central Arkansas and Southwest Texas University. We are proud and honored to be considered a part of our respective faculty and truly enjoy coming to work each day.

Finally, the writing of a textbook takes time and energy away from family. We wish to thank our families for their love, patience, and support. We especially want to thank our spouses for taking up the slack we created and supporting our teenage girls while we were working on the textbook.

CONTRIBUTORS

William D. Bandy, PhD, PT, SCS, ATC
Professor
Department of Physical Therapy
University of Central Arkansas
Conway, Arkansas

Janet Bezner, PhD, PT
Assistant Professor
Department of Physical Therapy
Southwest Texas State University
San Marcos, Texas

James P. Fletcher, MS, PT, ATC
Clinical Instructor
Department of Physical Therapy
University of Central Arkansas
Conway, Arkansas

J. Allen Hardin, MS, PT, SCS, ATC
Therapy Fellow
Physical Therapist and Athletic Trainer
Department of Intercollegiate Athletics for Men
University of Texas at Austin
Austin, Texas

Clayton F. Holmes, EdD, PT, ATC
Assistant Professor
Department of Physical Therapy
University of Central Arkansas
Conway, Arkansas

Barbara Hoogenboom, PT, SCS, ATC
Assistant Professor
School of Health Professions
Grand Valley State University
Allendale, Michigan

Jean M. Irion, EdD, PT, SCS, ATC
Assistant Professor
Department of Physical Therapy
University of Central Arkansas
Conway, Arkansas

Ginny Keely, MS, PT
Instructor
Department of Physical Therapy
Southwest Texas State University
San Marcos, Texas

Michael M. Reinold, MS, PT
Sports Physical Therapy Fellow
Health South Rehabilitation
Birmingham, Alabama

Barbara Sanders, PhD, PT, SCS
Professor and Chair
Department of Physical Therapy
Southwest Texas State University
San Marcos, Texas

Michael Sanders, EdD
Director, Life Skills
Department of Intercollegiate Athletics for Men
University of Texas at Austin
Austin, Texas

Marcia H. Stalvey, PT, MS, NCS
Director of Physical Therapy
Edwin Shaw Hospital for Rehabilitation
Akron, Ohio

Steven R. Tippett, PhD, PT, SCS, ATC
Assistant Professor
Department of Physical Therapy
Bradley University
Peoria, Illinois

Michael L. Voight, DHSc, PT, OCS, SCS, ATC
Associate Professor
Department of Physical Therapy
Belmont University
Nashville, Tennessee

Bridgett Wallace, PT
Senior Vice President
VESTANT
Austin, Texas

Kevin E. Wilk, PT
National Director Research & Clinical Education
Health South Rehabilitation Corporation
Birmingham, Alabama
Adjunct Assistant Professor
Marquette University
Programs in Physical Therapy
Milwaukee, Wisconsin

Reta Zabel, PhD, PT, GCS
Assistant Professor
Department of Physical Therapy
University of Central Arkansas
Conway, Arkansas

CONTENTS

CHAPTER 1

Introduction

William D. Bandy, PhD, PT, SCS, ATC

The purpose of this chapter is to define therapeutic exercise. But before a detailed account and in-depth discussion on therapeutic exercise can be undertaken, terms that are commonly used in the practice arena must be defined so that clinicians from diverse backgrounds can understand not only this text but each other. Think about the last new patient you saw on the sidelines, in your clinic, or in your training room. What did the *interpretation* of the test results indicate? Did your *evaluation* indicate an individual with an anterior cruciate ligament–deficient knee or was your *assessment* that the patient had a meniscus injury? Or did you think that, based on your *examination*, the patient had damage to the medial collateral ligament? Regardless of what your clinical decision-making skills tell you about the patient's knee, do you realize that, based on the italicized words, we may not be even talking the same language! How do we understand each other when we do not use a language that is consistent among clinicians in the same treatment venue, much less among clinicians in different states or across different professions?

■ *Five Elements of Patient/Client Management*

The American Physical Therapy Association (APTA) defined key terms used in the field of patient rehabilitation and presented them as the "five elements of patient/client management."[1] The APTA's definitions serve as the operational definitions used throughout this text. Examination, evaluation, and establishment of a diagnosis and a prognosis are all part of the process that guides the clinician in determining the most appropriate intervention:

Examination. Required before any intervention (treatment); must be performed on all patients and clients; consists of three components.

History. Account of past and current health status; specific mechanism of injury, if available.

Systems review. Brief or limited examination that provides additional information about the general health of the patient/client; includes a review of the four systems: cardiopulmonary, integumentary, musculoskeletal, and neuromuscular.

Tests and measures. Special tests or tools that determine the cause of the problem (e.g., for a patient with knee dysfunction, may include a Lachman test, valgus and varus tests, and anterior and posterior drawer tests to the knee).

Evaluation. Thought process that accompanies each and every examination procedure; information gained from the outcome of a particular test (e.g., the actual performance of a valgus test to the knee is an examination procedure; because the patient's knee does not have a tight end feel and the knee gives, the clinician determines that the patient has a positive test—the evaluation).

Diagnosis. Encompasses a cluster of signs, symptoms, syndromes, and categories; the decision reached as a result of the evaluation of information obtained during the examination (e.g., after the examination and evaluation of the knee, the clinician determines that the cluster of signs—positive valgus test, negative Lachman test, negative anterior drawer and posterior drawer test, negative varus test—indicates a diagnosis of medial collateral ligament damage to the knee).

Prognosis. The predicted optimal level of improvement in function and amount of time needed to reach that level; at this point, the clinician establishes a plan of care, including goals (e.g., a patient with second-degree medial collateral ligament damage to the knee is expected to return to full, unrestricted activity within 3 to 6 weeks).

Intervention. The treatment or rehabilitation program, which may be performed at the clinic or independently; includes strength work, increasing range of motion, manual therapy, aerobic conditioning, appropriate sequence of exercise.

■ *The Disablement Model*

Before providing a definition for and beginning a discussion of therapeutic exercise, a few more terms need to be introduced.

Disablement refers to "the various impact(s) of chronic and acute conditions on the functioning of specific body systems, on basic human performance, and on people's functioning in necessary, usual, expected, and personally desired roles in society."[2] Several conceptual schemes or models for disablement exist, including those developed by Nagi,[3] the World Health Organization[4] (WHO), and the National Center for Medical Rehabilitation Research.[5] For a detailed comparison of these models, see Jette.[2] This textbook uses the Nagi model and definition.

In the Nagi classification model of the disablement process, clinicians provide services to patients and clients with impairment, functional limitation, and disability. *Impairment* is an abnormality or loss of an anatomic, physiologic, or psychological origin.[6] Examples of impairments are decreased range of motion, strength, and endurance; hypomobility of the joint; and pain.

Functional limitation is defined as a limitation in the ability of the individual to perform an activity in an efficient or competent manner.[1] Inability to take an object from an overhead shelf, to walk without a limp, and to sit without pain are examples of functional limitations.

Disabilities are restrictions to function within normal limits[6] and represent any inability to perform socially defined roles expected of an individual in a sociocultural and physical environment.[2] Examples of disabilities include inability to perform the normal duties associated with work, school, recreation, and personal care.

Two examples illustrate these definitions. First, consider a lawyer who has back pain (impairment). Because of the back pain, she is unable to sit in a chair for more than 10 min and cannot walk for more than 5 min (functional limitation). As a result of the pain and inability to sit or walk, she is not able to go to work (disability). One goal for intervention is to use therapeutic exercise—such as mobilization of the spine (see Chapter 4) and instruction in posture, body mechanics, and spinal stabilization (see Chapter 12)—to treat the impairment of pain, alleviating the functional limitation and disability.

Second, consider a college athlete who has undergone anterior cruciate ligament surgery. After surgery, the athlete has decreased range of motion and decreased strength in the quadriceps and hamstring muscles (impairments). Because of these impairments, he cannot run, cut, or jump (functional limitations). Therefore, he will not able to participate in his sport (disability). One goal for intervention is to use therapeutic exercise—such as passive range of motion (see Chapter 2), open and closed chain exercises (see Chapters 6 and 9), aquatic therapy (see Chapter 13), and functional progression (see Chapter 14)—to treat the impairments of motion and strength, alleviating the functional limitations and disability.

The presence of an impairment does not mean that a functional limitation must occur. Similarly, a disability does not automatically follow from a functional limitation. For example, an individual might present with an anterior cruciate–deficient knee, with hypermobility as the impairment. But the goals of this patient are to play racquetball, hike, and bike. She decides to avoid surgery and participate in a therapeutic exercise program. After the intervention, the patient finds that she is able to play racquetball if she wears a brace and is able to hike and bike without the brace. Therefore, this individual has an impairment (hypermobility); but through intervention, she is able to avoid any functional limitation (running and cutting) or disability (participation in recreational sports). According to the *Guide to Physical Therapist Practice:*[1] Impairments, functional limitations, and disabilities do not follow each other in lockstep. Through examination, evaluation, and diagnosis, the clinician determines the interrelationships among impairment, functional limitations, and disabilities for a specific diagnostic group.

After considering the examination, evaluation, and diagnosis, the clinician is challenged to provide intervention for a patient with any level of disablement, to provide services to an individual with a disability, to provide treatment for a client with a functional limitation, or to alleviate an impairment in a patient. Based on a consideration of the interrelationships among impairment, functional limitation, and disability, this textbook focuses on the alleviation of impairments through the creative and effective use of therapeutic exercise.

■ *Therapeutic Exercise*

HISTORICAL PERSPECTIVE

In a 1967 survey of more than 100 clinicians and faculty who were using or teaching therapeutic exercise, Bouman[7] collected 53 definitions of therapeutic exercise. Bouman[7] concluded, "I think we all know what therapeutic exercise is. It is just difficult to define."

Before providing an operational definition of therapeutic exercise, a brief discussion of the historical development of the field is presented. The following review of the significant highlights in the history of therapeutic exercise provides the reader with a perspective of how far clinicians have come. For an extensive history of the field, see Licht,[8] who defined therapeutic exercise as "motions of the body or its parts to relieve symptoms or to improve function."

The use of therapeutic exercise (referred to as medical gymnastics) was recorded as early as 800 b.c.e. in the *Atharva-Veda,* a medical manuscript from India. According to the manuscript, exercise and massage were recommended for chronic rheumatism. However, most historians in the field believe that therapeutic exercise first gained popularity and widespread use in ancient Greece. Herodicus is believed to be the first physician to write on the subject (ca. 480 b.c.e.) and is considered the Father of Therapeutic Exercise. Herodicus claimed to have used exercise to cure himself of an "incurable" disease and developed an elaborate system of exercises for athletes. Hippocrates, the most famous of Herodicus' students, wrote of the beneficial effects of exercise and its value in strengthening muscle, improving mental attitude, and decreasing obesity.

Galen, considered by some as the greatest physician in ancient Rome, wrote of exercise in the 2nd century c.e. He was appointed the physician for the gladiators and classified exercise according to intensity, duration, and frequency. In the 5th century c.e., another Roman physician, Aurelianus, recommended exercise during convalescence from surgery and advocated the use of weights and pulleys.

In 1553 in Spain, Mendez wrote *Libro Del Exercicio,* the first book on exercise. The book emphasized exercises to improve hygiene.

Therapeutic exercise in modern times appears to have originated in Sweden in the 19th century with a fencing instructor named Pehr Henri Ling. Ling believed that a good fencer should also be a good athlete, and he developed and taught a system of specific movements. His system of therapeutic exercise included dosage, counting, and detailed instruction for each exercise. He demonstrated that precise movements, if scientifically applied, could serve to remedy disease and dysfunction of the body.[9] In 1932, McMillan[10] wrote, "It is Peter Henry Ling and the Swedish systematical order that we owe much today in the field of medical gymnastics and therapeutic exercise."

About the same time that Ling developed his system, Swiss physician Frenkel[11] wrote a controversial paper (1889). Frenkel proposed an exercise program for ataxia that incorporated repetitive activities to improve damaged nerve cells. No weights or strengthening activities were used, and the program became very popular. Although Frenkel's program is not as popular as it once was, his greatest contribution to the development of therapeutic exercise is the insistence on repetition.

Several individuals made major contributions to the development of therapeutic exercise in the 20th century. In 1934, Codman[12] developed a series of exercises to alleviate pain in the shoulder; these exercises are now referred to as Codman's, or pendulum, exercises. One of the most important advances was the adaptation of progressive resistance exercises (PRE) by Delorme[13] in 1945. This exercise program was developed in a military hospital in an effort to rehabilitate patients after knee surgery. According to Licht,[8] PRE was adapted more widely and rapidly than any other concept of therapeutic exercise in the century, except for early ambulation.

Kabat[14] took therapeutic exercise out of the cardinal plane by introducing diagonal movement and the use of a variety of reflexes to facilitate muscle contraction. His work was further developed by Knott and Voss,[15] who published the textbook *Proprioceptive Neuromuscular Facilitation* in 1956.

Using the principles of vector analysis on the flexor and extensor muscles that control the spine, Williams[16] developed a series of postural exercises and strengthening activities to alleviate back pain and emphasize flexion. In 1971, McKenzie[17] introduced a program to treat patients with back pain that focused on extension to facilitate anterior movement of the disks.

Hislop and Perrine[18] introduced the concept of isokinetic exercise in 1967, which was quite popular in the 1970s and 1980s. Finally, the work of Maitland,[19] Mennell,[20] and Kaltenborn[21]—who introduced the basic concepts of arthrokinematics and the use of mobilization and manipulation to decrease pain and capsular stiffness—cannot be overlooked as an important contribution in the 20th century.

It is impossible to name all the accomplishments related to the area of therapeutic exercise, but some of the more important events and concepts were highlighted. This textbook was written by current experts in the field of therapeutic exercise. Each chapter focuses on a specialized field of therapeutic exercise and includes background information and references to the major researchers and scholars in that area. In addition, all the authors are clinicians and, therefore, have firsthand knowledge and understanding of the exercise techniques presented. When Licht's[8] history of therapeutic exercise is revised, it may well refer to the authors of the chapters of this textbook.

PHYSICAL THERAPY PERSPECTIVE: *GUIDE TO PHYSICAL THERAPIST PRACTICE*

In November 1997, the APTA first published the *Guide to Physical Therapist Practice.*[1] The *Guide* provides an outline of the body of knowledge for physical therapists and delineates preferred practice patterns. In addition, the *Guide* describes boundaries within which the physical therapist may select appropriate care. It represents the

TABLE 1-1 Procedural Interventions

Therapeutic Exercise

Therapeutic exercise is the systematic performance or execution of planned physical movements, postures, or activities intended to enable the patient/client to (1) remediate or prevent impairments, (2) enhance function, (3) reduce risk, (4) optimize overall health, and (5) enhance fitness and well-being. Therapeutic exercise may include aerobic and endurance conditioning and reconditioning; agility training; balance training, both static and dynamic; body mechanics training; breathing exercises; coordination exercises; developmental activities training; gait and locomotion training; motor training; muscle lengthening; movement pattern training; neuromotor development activities training; neuromuscular education or reeducation; perceptual training; postural stabilization and training; range-of-motion exercises and soft tissue stretching; relaxation exercises; and strength, power, and endurance exercises.

Physical therapists select, prescribe, and implement exercise activities when the examination findings, diagnosis, and prognosis indicate the use of therapeutic exercise to enhance bone density; enhance breathing; enhance or maintain physical performance; enhance performance in activities of daily living (ADL) and instrumental activities of daily living (IADL); improve safety; increase aerobic capacity/endurance; increase muscle strength, power, and endurance; enhance postural control and relaxation; increase sensory awareness; increase tolerance to activity; prevent or remediate impairments, functional limitations, or disabilities to improve physical function; enhance health, wellness, and fitness; reduce complications, pain, restriction, and swelling; or reduce risk and increase safety during activity performance.

Clinical Considerations

Examination findings that may direct the type and specificity of the procedural intervention may include:

- *Pathology/pathophysiology (disease, disorder, or condition), history (including risk factors) of medical/surgical conditions, or signs and symptoms (eg, pain, shortness of breath, stress) in the following systems:*
  - — cardiovascular
  - — endrocrine/metabolic
  - — genitourinary
  - — integumentary
  - — multiple systems
  - — musculoskeletal
  - — neuromuscular
  - — pulmonary
- *Impairments in the following catergories:*
  - — aerobic capacity/endurance (eg, decreased walk distance)
  - — anthropometric characteristics (eg, increased body mass index)
  - — arousal, attention, and cognition (eg. decreased motivation to participate in fitness activities)
  - — circulation (eg, abnormal elevation in heart rate with activity)
  - — cranial and peripheral nerve integrity (eg, difficulty with swallowing, risk of aspiration, positive neural provocation response)
  - — ergonomics and body mechanics (eg, inability to squat because of weakness in gluteus maximus and quadriceps femoris muscles)
  - — gait, locomotion, and balance (eg, inability to perform ankle dorisflexion)
  - — integumentary integrity (eg, limited finger flexion as a result of dorsal burn scar)
  - — joint integrity and mobility (eg, limited range of motion in the shoulder)
  - — motor function (eg, uncoordinated limb movements)
  - — muscle performance (eg, weakness of lumbar stabilizers)
  - — neuromotor development and sensory integration (eg, delayed development)
  - — posture (eg, forward head, kyphosis)
  - — range of motion (eg, increased laxity in patellofemoral joint)
  - — reflex integrity (eg, poor balance in standing)
  - — sensory integrity (eg, lack of position sense)
  - — ventilation and respiration/gas exchange (eg, abnormal breathing patterns)
- *Functional limitations in the ability to perform actions, tasks, and activities in the following categories:*
  - — self-care (eg, difficult with dressing, bathing)
  - — home management (eg, difficulty with raking, shoveling, making bed)
  - — work (job/school/play) (eg, difficulty with keyboarding, pushing, or pulling, difficulty with play activities)
  - — community/leisure (eg, inability to negotiate steps and curbs)
- *Disability—that is, the inability or restricted ability to perform actions, tasks, or activities of required roles within the individual's sociocultural context—in the following categories:*
  - — work (eg, inability to assume parenting role, inability to care for elderly relatives, inability to return to work as a police officer)
  - — community/leisure (eg, difficulty with jogging or playing golf, inability to attend religious services)
- *Risk reduction/prevention in the following areas:*
  - — risk factors (eg, need to decrease body fat composition)
  - — recurrence of condition (eg, need to increase mobility and postural control for work [job/school/play] actions, tasks and activities)
  - — secondary impairments (eg, need to improve strength and balance for fall risk reduction)
- *Health, wellness, and fitness needs:*
  - — fitness, including physical performance (eg, need to improve golf-swing timing, need to maximize gymnastic performance, need to maximize pelvic-floor muscle function)
  - — health and wellness (eg, need to improve balance for recreation, need to increase muscle strength to help maintain bone density)

(*continued*)

TABLE 1-1 (continued)

Interventions

Therapeutic exercise may include:

- Aerobic capacity/endurance conditioning or reconditioning
  - aquatic programs
  - gait and locomotion training
  - increased workload over time
  - movement efficiency and energy conservation training
  - walking and wheelchair propulsion programs
- Balance, coordination, and agility training
  - developmental activities training
  - motor function (motor control and motor learning) training or retraining
  - neuromuscular education or reeducation
  - perceptual training
  - posture awareness training
  - sensory training or retraining
  - standardized, programmatic, complementary exercise approaches
  - task-specific performance training
  - vestibular training
- Body mechanics and postural stabilization
  - body mechanics training
  - postural control training
  - postural stabilization activities
  - posture awareness training
- Flexibility exercises
  - muscle lengthening
  - range of motion
  - stretching
- Gait and locomotion training
  - developmental activities training
  - gait training
  - implement and device training
  - perceptual training
  - standardized, programmatic, complementary exercise approaches
  - wheelchair training
- Neuromotor development training
  - developmental activities training
  - motor training
  - movement pattern training
  - neuromuscular education or reeducation
- Relaxation
  - breathing strategies
  - movement strategies
  - relaxation techniques
  - standardized, programmatic, complementary exercise approaches
- Strength, power, and endurance training for head, neck, limb, pelvic-floor, trunk, and ventilatory muscles
  - active assistive, active, and resistive exercises (including concentric, dynamic/isotonic, eccentric, isokinetic, isometric, and plyometric
  - aquatic programs
  - standardized, programmatic, complementary exercise approaches
  - task-specific performance training

Anticipated Goals and Expected Outcomes

Anticipated goals and expected outcomes related to therapeutic exercises may include:

- Impact on pathology/pathophysiology (disease, disorder, or condition)
  - Atelectasis is decreased.
  - Joint swelling, inflammation, or restriction is reduced.
  - Nutrient delivery to tissue is increased.
  - Osteogenic effects of exercise are maximized.
  - Pain is decreased.
  - Physiological response to increased oxygen demand is improved.
  - Soft tissue swelling, inflammation, or restriction is reduced.
  - Symptoms associated with increased oxygen demand are decreased.
  - Tissue perfusion and oxygenation are enhanced.
- Impact on impairment
  - Aerovic capacity is increased.
  - Airway clearance is improved.
  - Balance is improved.
  - Endurance is increased.
  - Energy expenditure per unit of work is decreased.
  - Gait, locomotion, and balance are improved.
  - Integumentary integrity is improved.
  - Joint integrity and mobility are improved.
  - Motor function (motor control and motor learning) is improved.
  - Muscle performance (strength, power, and endurance) is increased.
  - Postural control is improved.
  - Quality and quantity of movement between and across body segments are improved.
  - Range of motion is improved.
  - Relaxation is increased.
  - Sensory awareness is increased.
  - Ventilation and respiratory/gas exchange are improved.
  - Weight-bearing status is improved.
  - Work of breathing is decreased.
- Impact on functional limitations
  - Ability to perform physical actions, tasks, or activities related to self-care, home management, work (job/school/ play), community, and leisure is improved.
  - Level of supervision required for task performance is decreased.
  - Performance of and independence in ADL and IADL with or without devices and equipment are increased.
  - Tolerance of positions and activities is increased.
- Impact on disabilities
  - Ability to assume or resume required self-care, home management, work (job/school/play), community, and leisure roles is improved.
- Risk reduction/prevention
  - Preoperative and postoperative complications are reduced.
  - Risk factors are reduced.
  - Risk or recurrence of condition is reduced.
  - Risk of secondary impairment is reduced.
  - Safety is improved.
  - Self-management of symptoms is improved.
- Impact on health, wellness, and fitness
  - Fitness is improved.
  - Health status is improved.
  - Physical capacity is increased.
  - Physical function is improved.
- Impact on societal resources
  - Utilization of physical therapy services is optimized.
  - Utilization of physical therapy services results in efficient use of health care dollars.
- Patient/client satisfaction
  - Access, availability, and services provided are acceptable to patient/client.
  - Administrative management of practice is acceptable to patient/client.
  - Clinical proficiency of physical therapist is acceptable to patient/client.
  - Coordination of care is acceptable to patient/client.
  - Cost of health care services is decreased.
  - Intensity of care is decreased.
  - Interpersonal skills of physical therapist are acceptable to patient/client, family, and significant others.
  - Sense of well-being is improved.
  - Stressors are decreased.

Source: Reprinted with permission from the American Physical Therapy Association. Journal of Physical Therapy 2001; 81(1):S104–S105.

TABLE 1-2 Athletic Training Clinical Proficiencies: Therapeutic Exercise

Teaching Objective

The student will demonstrate the ability to perform therapeutic exercises.

Specific Outcomes[a]

1. Exercise to improve joint range of motion. The student will demonstrate the ability to instruct the following exercises.

Upper Body	Lower Body	Trunk	Cervical
a. Codman's exercises	a. Wall slides	a. William's exercises	a. Flexion/extension
b. Backward C exercises	b. Heel slides	b. McKenzie's exercises	b. Lateral flexion
c. T exercises	c. CPM	c. Rotation	c. Rotation
d. PNF stretching	d. PNF stretching	d. Stabilization	d. Stabilization
e. CPM	e. Prone knee extension hang	e. AROM	e. AROM
f. AROM	f. AROM	f. PROM	f. PROM
g. PROM	g. PROM		

2. Exercise to improve muscle strength. The student will demonstrate the ability to instruct the following exercises using isometric and progressive resistance techniques.

Upper Body	Lower Body	Neck	Trunk
a. Shoulder abduction	a. Ankle dorsiflexion	a. Neck flexion	a. Trunk flexion
b. Shoulder adduction	b. Ankle eversion	b. Neck extension	b. Trunk extension
c. Shoulder flexion	c. Ankle inversion	c. Neck rotation	c. Trunk rotation
d. Shoulder extension	d. Ankle plantar flexion	d. Neck lateral flexion	d. Trunk lateral flexion
e. Shoulder internal rotation	e. Heel raises		
f. Shoulder external rotation	f. Toe extension		
g. Scaption	g. Toe flexion		
h. Shoulder horizontal	h. Hip abduction		
i. Shoulder horizontal flexion	i. Hip adduction		
j. Shoulder girdle elevation	j. Hip extension		
k. Shoulder girdle depression	k. Hip flexion		
l. Shoulder girdle protraction	l. Lower extremity PNF patterns		
m. Shoulder girdle retraction	m. Leg curls		
n. Upper extremity PNF patterns	n. Leg extensions		
o. Elbow flexion	o. Leg press		
p. Elbow extension	p. Quadriceps/hamstring co-contraction		
q. Radius/ulna pronation	q. Quadriceps setting		
r. Radius/ulna supination	r. Short arc quadriceps extensions		
s. Wrist flexion	s. Squats		
t. Wrist extension	t. Straight leg raises		
u. Wrist ulnar deviation (adduction)			
v. Wrist radial deviation (abduction)			
w. Thumb flexion			
x. Thumb extension			
y. Thumb abduction			
z. Thumb adduction			
aa. Finger flexion			
bb. Finger extension			
cc. Finger abduction			
dd. Finger adduction			

(*continued*)

TABLE 1-2 (continued)

3. Exercise to improve muscle endurance. The student will demonstrate the ability to instruct the following.

Upper Body	Lower Body
a. Swimming b. Upper body ergometer/ stationary bicycle c. Stair climber	a. Swimming b. Stationary bicycle c. Stair climber

4. Exercise to improve muscle speed. The student will demonstrate the ability to instruct the following.

Upper Body	Lower Body
a. Reaction drills	a. Reaction drills b. Sprint work c. Fartlek training

5. Exercise to improve muscle power. The student will demonstrate the ability to instruct plyometrics for the upper and lower body.
6. Exercise to improve neuromuscular control and coordination. The student will demonstrate the ability to instruct the following.

Upper Body	Lower Body	Neck	Trunk
a. PNF patterns b. Rhythmic stabilization c. Double and single arm balancing d. Wobble board or balance apparatus e. Weighted ball rebounding	a. PNF patterns b. Wobble board or balance apparatus c. Incline board	a. Stabilization	a. Stabilization

7. Exercise to improve agility. The student will demonstrate the ability to instruct the following.

Upper Body	Lower Body
a. Throwing	a. Carioca b. Crossover c. Figure eight

8. Exercise to improve cardiorespiratory endurance. The student will demonstrate the ability to instruct the following.

Upper Body	Lower Body
a. Upper body ergometer b. Stationary bicycle	a. Bicycle ergometer b. Treadmill c. Stair climber

9. Manual therapy techniques. The student will demonstrate the ability to select and perform appropriate joint mobilization for the following.

Upper Body	Lower Body
a. Distal traction of the head of the humerus b. Anterior/posterior glide of the head of the humerus c. Anterior/posterior glide of radius d. Distal traction of ulna e. Posterior glide of ulna f. Anterior/posterior glide of wrist g. Anterior/posterior glide of fingers	a. Tibiofemoral joint traction b. Posterior glide of the tibia on the femur c. Anterior glide of the tibia on the femur d. Patellofemoral joint distal glide e. Patellofemoral joint medial-lateral glide f. Anterior/posterior glide of the ankle

10. The students will demonstrate the ability to instruct and perform exercise to improve activity-specific skills.

Modified from National Athletic Trainers' Association. Athletic training educational competencies. 3rd ed. Dallas: NATA, 1999.
[a]*PNF*, proprioceptive neuromuscular facilitation; *CPM*, continuous passive motion.

best efforts of the physical therapy profession to define itself. The document was developed over 3 years and involved the expert consensus of more than 1000 members of the physical therapy community.

The *Guide* defines intervention as "the purposeful and skilled interaction of the physical therapist with the patient/client." According to the *Guide,* physical therapy intervention has the following three components, listed in order of importance:

Coordination, communication, and documentation
Patient/client-related instruction
Procedural interventions
- Therapeutic exercise
- Functional training in self-care and home management (activities of daily living, instrumental activities of daily living)
- Functional training in work (job, school, play) community, and leisure integration or reintegration
- Manual therapy
- Prescription, application, fabrication of devices and equipment
- Airway clearance techniques
- Integumentary repair and protective techniques
- Electrotherapeutic modalities
- Physical agents and mechanical mxodalities

Note that therapeutic exercise is considered the most important procedural intervention. Table 1-1 presents a definition of therapeutic exercise and a detailed account of the types of therapeutic exercises used in the practice of physical therapy. The operational definition of therapeutic exercise used in this textbook is the one given in table.

ATHLETIC TRAINING PERSPECTIVE: *ATHLETIC TRAINING EDUCATIONAL COMPETENCIES*

In 1999, the National Athletic Trainers' Association (NATA) revised its *Athletic Training Educational Competencies,*[22] which identifies the knowledge and skills to be mastered in an entry-level athletic-training educational program. The *Competencies* is also used by the Joint Review Committee—Athletic Training (JRC-AT) for curriculum development and education of students in accredited entry-level athletic training educational programs. Furthermore, the *Competencies* serves as a guide for certification of athletic trainers by the NATA Board of Certification (NATA-BOC).

NATA categorizes the required competencies into the following 12 content areas, listed in alphabetical order:

Acute care of injury and illness
Assessment and evaluation
General medical conditions and disabilities
Health care administration
Nutritional aspects of injury and illness
Pathology of injuries and illnesses
Pharmacology
Professional development and responsibilities
Psychosocial intervention and referral
Risk management and injury prevention
Therapeutic exercise
Therapeutic modalities

Within each of these content areas, the competencies are divided into four domains: cognitive (knowledge and intellectual skills), psychomotor (manipulative and motor skills), affective (attitudes and values), and clinical (decision making and skill application) proficiencies.

The *Competencies* defines therapeutic exercise as

> a collection of knowledge, skills, and values required of the entry-level certified athletic trainer to plan, implement, document, and evaluate the efficacy of therapeutic exercise programs for the rehabilitation/reconditioning of injuries to and illnesses of athletes and others involved in physical activity.

Within each domain, the *Competencies* includes a list of minimal proficiencies that serves as a guide for the subject matter in each accredited educational program. In other words, the proficiencies define the minimal set of skills each entry-level athletic trainer should possess. Although the topics covered in education programs are based on the lists of minimal proficiencies, these lists do not include all clinical skills taught (e.g., more advanced techniques may be taught). Table 1-2 presents the athletic training clinical proficiencies for therapeutic exercise listed in the *Competencies.*

■ *Summary*

- Both the *Guide* and the *Competencies* note that therapeutic exercise is a vital component of patient intervention and is a core element in the care of patients with dysfunctions and of clients who require preventative measures. This textbook emphasizes the specific techniques used in programs of care for individuals with dysfunction, as well as prevention of dysfunction.

REFERENCES

1. American Physical Therapy Association. Guide to physical therapist practice, second edition. Phys Ther 2001;81:1–768.
2. Jette AM. Physical disablement: concepts for physical therapy research and practice. Phys Ther 1994;74:380–387.

3. Nagi SA. Disability concepts revisted. In: A Pope, A Tarlov, eds. Disability in America: toward a national agenda for prevention. Washington, DC: National Academy Press.
4. World Health Organization. International classification of im pairments, disabilities, and handicaps. Geneva: WHO, 1980.
5. National Advisory Board on Medical Rehabilitation Research. Draft V: report and plan for medical rehabilitation research. Bethesda, MD: National Institutes of Health, 1992.
6. Schenkman M, Donavan J, Tsubota J, et al. Management of individuals with Parkinson's disease: rationale and case studies. Phys Ther 1989;69:944–955.
7. Bouman HD. Delineating the dilemma. Am J Phys Med 1967; 46: 26–41.
8. Licht S, ed. Therapeutic exercise. New Haven, CT: Licht, 1965.
9. Taylor GH. An exposition of the Swedish movement-cure. New York: Fowler & Wells, 1860.
10. McMillan M. Massage and therapeutic exercise. Philadelphia: Saunders, 1932.
11. Frenkel HS. The treatment of tabetic ataxia. Philadelphia: Blakeston, 1902.
12. Codman EA. The shoulder. Philadelphia: Harper & Row, 1934.
13. Delorme TL. Restoration of muscle power by heavy resistance exercises. J Bone Joint Surg Am 1945;27:645–650.
14. Kabat H. Studies in neuromuscular dysfunction XIII: new concepts and techniques of neuromuscular reeducation for paralysis. Perm Found Med Bull 1950;8:112–120.
15. Knott M, Voss DE. Proprioceptive neuromuscular facilitation. Philadelphia: Harper & Row, 1956.
16. Williams PC. Examination and conservative treatment for disc lesion of the lower spine. Clin Orthop 1955;5:28–39.
17. McKenzie RA. The lumbar spine: mechanical diagnosis and therapy. Upper Hutt, New Zealand: Spinal, 1971.
18. Hislop HJ, Perrine JA. The isokinetic concept of exercise. Phys Ther 1967;47:114–118.
19. Maitland GD. Vertebral manipulation. 4th ed. London: Butterworth, 1977.
20. Mennell JM. The musculoskeletal system: differential diagnosis from symptoms and physical signs. Gaithersburg, MD: Aspen, 1992.
21. Kaltenborn FM. The spine. 2nd ed. Oslo: Olaf Norris, 1993.
22. National Athletic Trainers' Association. Athletic training educational competencies. 3rd ed. Dallas: NATA, 1999.

SECTION

Mobility

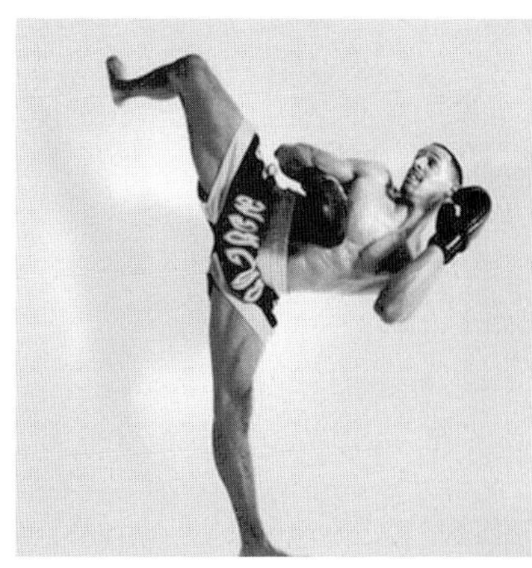

CHAPTER

Range of Motion

James P. Fletcher, MS, PT, ATC

The concept of range of motion specific to the human body brings many thoughts and ideas to the mind of the healthcare professional. Along with strength, endurance, power, balance, and coordination, range of motion plays a major role in physical ability and, therefore, contributes significantly to the overall quality of a person's physical functions.[1] This is obvious when one considers the negative effect a range of motion impairment can have on the quality and efficiency of human movement.

One broadly accepted notion is that range of motion occurs through the interdependent function of the musculoskeletal and synovial joint systems, enabling the human body to perform free and easy movement. The basic functional purpose and use of range of motion allow the effective movement of the extremities, head, and trunk in performing body positioning and mobility.[2] This chapter discusses range of motion primarily in the context of osteokinematic movement resulting from synovial joint movement. Issues of muscle length and joint arthrokinematics are presented in Chapters 3 and 4, respectively.

■ *Scientific Basis*

DEFINITIONS

Much like human anatomy, range of motion and its associated terminology are descriptive in nature. A brief introduction of several anatomic and kinesiologic terms is essential. The reader must have a working knowledge of the terminology associated with body planes (e.g., sagittal, frontal, horizontal), anatomic position (e.g., medial, lateral, proximal), and osteokinematic and arthrokinematic movement.[2–5]

The basic definition of range of motion (ROM) differs among published sources.[6–10] One of the clearest descriptions is that range of motion is the extent of osteokinematic motion available for movement activities, functional or otherwise, with or without assistance.[6] Osteokinematic motion is the movement of a whole bone resulting from rolling, sliding, or spinning movements (arthrokinematics) between the articulating bony surfaces making up a synovial joint.[3] The assistance in moving a body segment provided by the clinician, as well as effort generated by the patient, requires the division of range of motion into three levels of performance: active range of motion (AROM), active-assistive range of motion (AAROM), and passive range of motion (PROM).[6,9]

Active range of motion. Joint movement performed and controlled solely by the voluntary muscular efforts of the individual without the aid or resistance of an external force; the individual is independent in this activity.

Active-assistive range of motion. Joint movement performed and controlled, in large or small part, by the voluntary muscular efforts of the individual combined with the assistance of an external force (e.g., assistance from another body part, another person, or a mechanical device).

Passive range of motion. Joint movement performed and controlled solely by the efforts of an external force without the use of voluntary muscular contraction by the person.

Although gravity does act on the mass of the body segment, offering some assistance or resistance to the movement being performed, it is a variable that is controlled by the position of the body segment during the movement. External forces used in the assistance of a movement (AAROM or PROM) are considered nongravitational.

PHYSICAL AND PHYSIOLOGIC CONSIDERATIONS

The amount of ROM available at a synovial joint depends on many factors, both intrinsic and extrinsic. Intrinsic factors are related to the anatomic composition of the joint, such as shape and congruency of the articulating bony surfaces and pliability of the joint capsule, ligaments, and other collagenous tissues. In addition, the strength and flexibility of musculature acting on or crossing the joint are considered intrinsic factors.[2,3] One or more of these factors create anatomic limits to joint range of motion. For example, most osteokinematic motions at the glenohumeral and hip joints are limited by soft tissue extensibility rather than a bony restriction, except in cases of pathology (e.g., osteoarthritis). Conversely, the limitations to osteokinematic motion at the humeroulnar joint owe more to bony contact. This is not to say that joints with anatomic movement limitations related to bone shape, congruency, and approximation have less ROM than other synovial joints. Zachazewski[10] points out that, although the amount of joint range of motion is determined primarily by the shape and congruency of the articulating surfaces, the periarticular connective tissues are the limiting factors at the end of the range of motion. More detailed discussions of the intrinsic factors affecting joint ROM are available in the literature.[2,3,11]

Other factors affecting joint range of motion are extrinsic, which may have a direct effect on the intrinsic factors. One significant factor is age. Decreased pliability in contractile and noncontractile tissues caused by changes in tissue composition and tissue degeneration that occur with aging can decrease joint ROM.[1,3] Body segment size related to muscle or adipose tissue bulk is another extrinsic factor that may affect joint ROM; it often limits osteokinematic motions such as knee flexion and elbow flexion.[12]

Finally, the known effects of disease, injury, overuse, and immobilization on joint tissues and joint range of motion must be considered. The well-being of joint tissues depends on a certain amount of use of the joint and stress to the joint structures. For example, hyaline cartilage nutrition depends on the compression and decompression that occurs with joint movement. In addition, maintenance of ligament and capsule strength and pliability depends on a certain amount of tissue stress and strain associated with joint movement.

Common diseases affecting the joints include rheumatoid arthritis and osteoarthritis, which adversely affect the synovial membrane and hyaline cartilage, respectively. These diseases (along with traumatic injuries to ligament, capsule, or hyaline cartilage) result in pain, swelling, and loss of joint motion. Often, disease and traumatic injuries alter the biomechanics of the joint, leading to malalignment, abnormal motion, and joint tissue degeneration.

Microtrauma to joint tissues from overuse related to prolonged or repetitive work or athletic activities can lead to problems such as ligament and capsule lengthening and cartilage degeneration. The overall effects of microtrauma are similar to changes resulting from disease and joint tissue injury: pain, swelling, and loss of joint motion. The adverse effects of immobilization and joint disuse are commonly recognized and include regional osteoporosis, cartilage dehydration and degeneration, collagenous tissue fibrosis and adhesion, and muscle tissue contracture and atrophy.[3,13–15]

BENEFITS OF RANGE OF MOTION EXERCISE

When AROM, AAROM, or PROM is performed repetitively for the general purpose of maintaining current joint movement and preventing decreased pliability of tissue, the action is called a range of motion exercise. Range of motion exercise also offers a potential benefit to the mechanical properties of noncontractile tissue.[11] For example, performing a movement repetitively, actively or passively, through a full range of motion moves a joint into and out of the closed packed position (which is the position that a joint is in when the articulating surfaces are maximally approximated and the ligaments and capsule are tight).[4] Movement into and out of this position results in an intermittent compression and decompression of the articular cartilage, which is the natural mechanism used for nutrition and continuous remodeling of the tissue.[15]

The benefits of ROM exercise, beyond maintaining joint mobility and nutrition and preventing tissue adhesion and contracture, depend on the type of movement. To aid blood circulation, inhibit pain via stimulation of joint mechanoreceptors (gate control), and promote ligament and capsule remodeling, PROM exercises may be used.[16,17] In addition, AROM and AAROM exercises may increase blood circulation, prevent clot formation from venous stasis, increase proprioceptive input, maintain contractility, slow the rate of atrophy of contracting muscles, and improve coordination and motor control specific to the motion performed.[17] Furthermore, as low-level exercises that use gravity for resistance, AROM and AAROM may help reduce an individual's emotional or psychological stress and depression and improve psychological outlook while serving as a method of exercise in the early phases of rehabilitation for the client who is deconditioned secondary to illness, injury, or surgery.

Continuous passive motion (CPM) is essentially PROM exercise that is performed continuously to a joint by a mechanical device for hours at a time. After a surgical procedure, CPM is primarily used to decrease the effects of joint immobilization, help with pain management, and promote early recovery of range of motion.[16,18–20] Typically, the range, rate, and duration of the motion can be programmed, and specific recommendations are based on the surgeon's preference, the patient's response, and the surgical procedure. A variety of CPM devices are available on the market, and devices for almost all extremity joints exist.

■ Clinical Guidelines

A brief discussion of how the *Guide to Physical Therapist Practice*[21] portrays the role of ROM exercise for direct intervention will allow the reader to appreciate the broad range of applications that these exercises can offer the health-care professional. The *Guide* notes that the direct interventions of therapeutic exercise and manual therapy can improve range of motion. Specifically, the *Guide* categorizes AROM and AAROM as therapeutic exercise and PROM as manual therapy, which is broadly defined as a passive intervention in which the physical therapist uses his or her hands to administer a skilled movement.[21] Manual therapy also includes such interventions as therapeutic massage, joint mobilization, and joint manipulation. A review of the direct interventions listed in the *Guide* for practice patterns in the musculoskeletal, neuromuscular, cardiopulmonary, and integumentary domains reveals that some form of range of motion exercise is a potential method of treatment in the vast majority of practice patterns.

The health-care professional must carefully examine joint pathologies and ROM impairments to determine the source of the problem(s). Direct interventions such as muscular stretching (Chapter 3) and joint mobilization (Chapter 4) may be more effective than ROM exercise for improving the impairment of a joint's range of motion caused by capsule, ligament, or musculotendinous tissue restriction. However, ROM exercise is an appropriate adjunct or complement to these interventions. Range of motion exercise is a recommended component of the treatment program for postsurgical musculoskeletal conditions; pathologic conditions such as musculotendinous spasm, strain, inflammation, and contusion; and joint sprain, inflammation, degeneration, and contracture.[17,22]

Clinical decision making regarding the use of ROM exercises as a method of intervention is based on a knowledge of the needs of the client and the potential benefits, precautions, and limitations of the intervention. The primary precaution for performing ROM exercises has traditionally been the presence of acute injury. With the discovery of the benefits of early motion for preventing tissue shortening and degeneration and maintaining joint nutrition after trauma or surgery, ROM exercise in the acute phase of rehabilitation is recommended if performed with rigid adherence to specific precautions dictated by the nature of the tissue injury or surgical repair. The primary therapeutic limitations of AROM exercise are that it typically will not increase muscular strength or prevent atrophy. Passive range of motion exercise has the additional limitations of little to no potential for even slowing muscle atrophy or maintaining strength. Furthermore, PROM exercise is less effective than AROM exercise at increasing circulation, owing to the lack of voluntary muscle contraction.[16]

Once the health-care professional determines that range of motion exercise is an appropriate intervention for a given client, a decision must be made on the use of AROM, AAROM, or PROM. Passive range of motion exercises are typically used when the client is not able to perform an active joint movement because of pain, weakness, paralysis, or unresponsiveness. In the event that the client is not supposed to actively move a joint owing to injury, inflammation, or surgical repair, PROM exercises might be carefully performed with strict adherence to all motion precautions and avoidance of pain. In most other situations, AAROM or AROM exercise is preferred because of the added benefits and potential for more independent performance by the client. Tomberlin and Saunders[17] provide a general recommendation for progressing from PROM to AAROM and AROM exercises as part of an intervention program after traumatic injury and add specific precautions for avoiding muscle guarding and pain.

A session of ROM exercises should emphasize full range of movement within the client's tolerance. Each movement sequence has two phases: (1) beginning position to ending position and (2) reversal. The movements should be performed slowly and rhythmically. The specific number of sessions per day, repetitions within each session, and the inclusion or exclusion of a hold time at the end range depend on the goals of the exercise, the underlying pathology, and the client's response to treatment. Keep in mind that a patient's independent performance will be best if sessions and repetitions take only a few minutes to perform and use of equipment is kept to a minimum. Finally, establishing a regimen that ensures consistency and quality of independent performance by a client requires a committed effort to effective communication between the client and clinician.

■ *Techniques*

Range of motion exercise techniques are performed either in anatomic body planes with classic osteokinematic movements, in diagonal or combined joint patterns, or in functional patterns that simulate those used in a client's daily activities. The techniques presented in this chapter primarily emphasize passive, active-assistive, and active osteokinematic motions performed in anatomic body planes, both with and without equipment. The purposes of all these techniques are to maintain or increase joint mobility, joint nutrition, and tissue pliability. (Given that the purposes of all the exercises are the same, they will not be repeated for each technique.)

The clinician who provides assistance with PROM and AAROM exercise techniques should remember the key factors affecting the application and performance of the techniques. These factors include supportive handling of body segments, proper positioning of the client, and use of appropriate levels of force to avoid causing intense pain when performing the exercise.

SPINE AND EXTREMITIES

Figures 2-1 to 2-29 illustrate common techniques for ROM exercises. Figures 2-1 to 2-8 show frequently used techniques for the spine. Figures 2-9 to 2-29 show the techniques commonly used for the extremities.

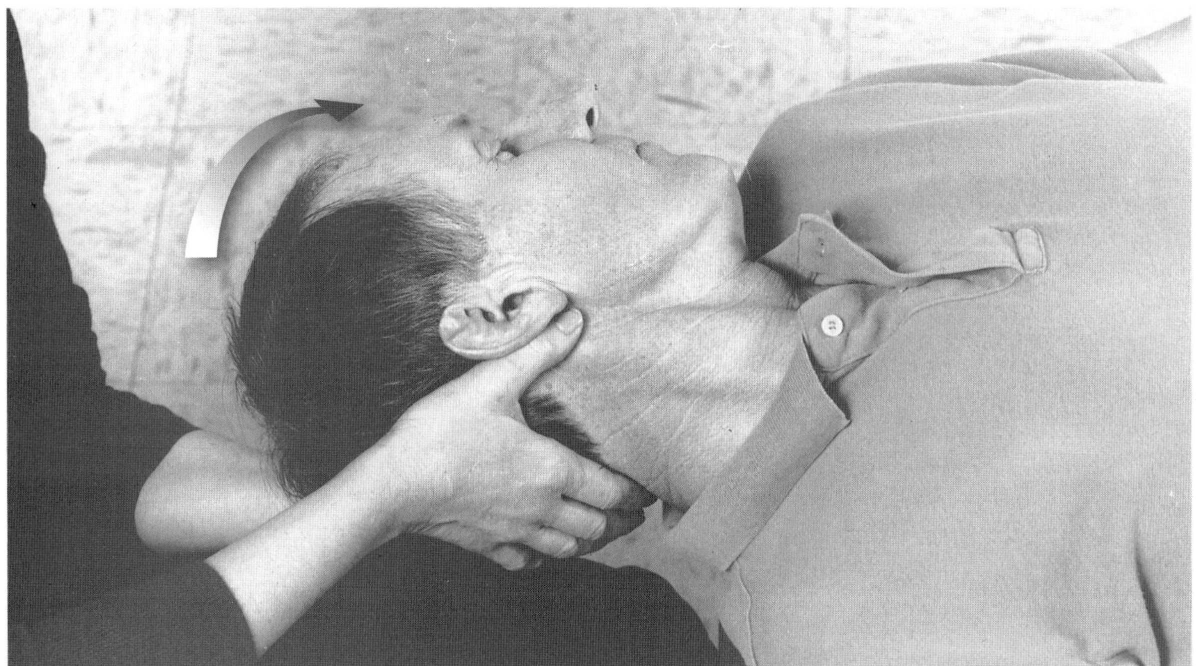

FIGURE 2-1 **Cervical rotation AAROM or PROM.**

POSITIONING: Client lying supine with head off stable surface. Clinician sitting or standing at end of stable surface, supporting client's head with his or her elbows at about 90°.

PROCEDURE: Clinician performs cervical rotation motion bilaterally with grasp and support applied to client's occipital region. Extension and lateral flexion motions are avoided.

NOTE: Similar positioning can be used for AAROM and PROM for cervical flexion, lateral flexion, and extension.

FIGURE 2-2 **Cervical rotation AROM.**

POSITIONING: Client sitting, standing, or lying supine.

PROCEDURE: Client performs active cervical rotation motion bilaterally; flexion, extension, and lateral flexion motion are avoided.

NOTE: Rotation motion can be self-assisted by client using one hand to support the mandible and assist with the motion. Similar positioning can be used for AROM for cervical flexion, lateral flexion, and extension.

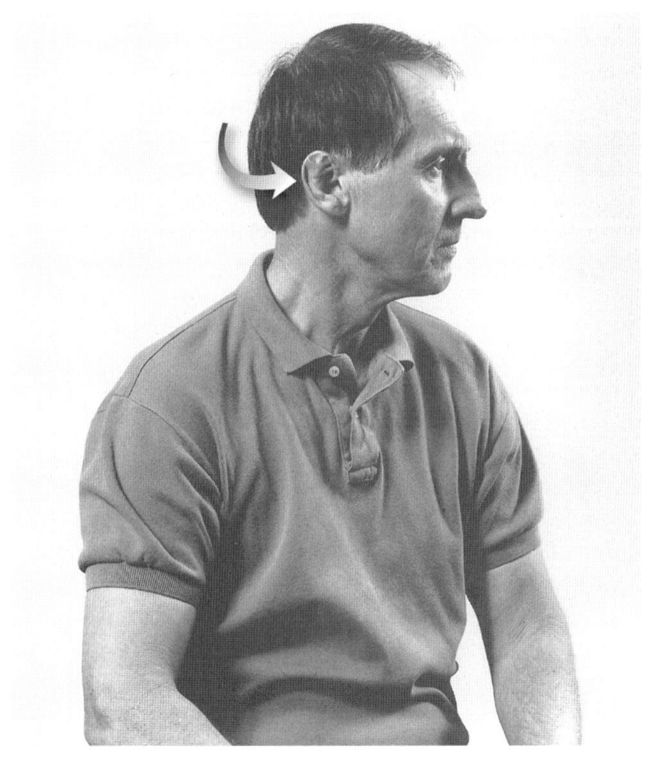

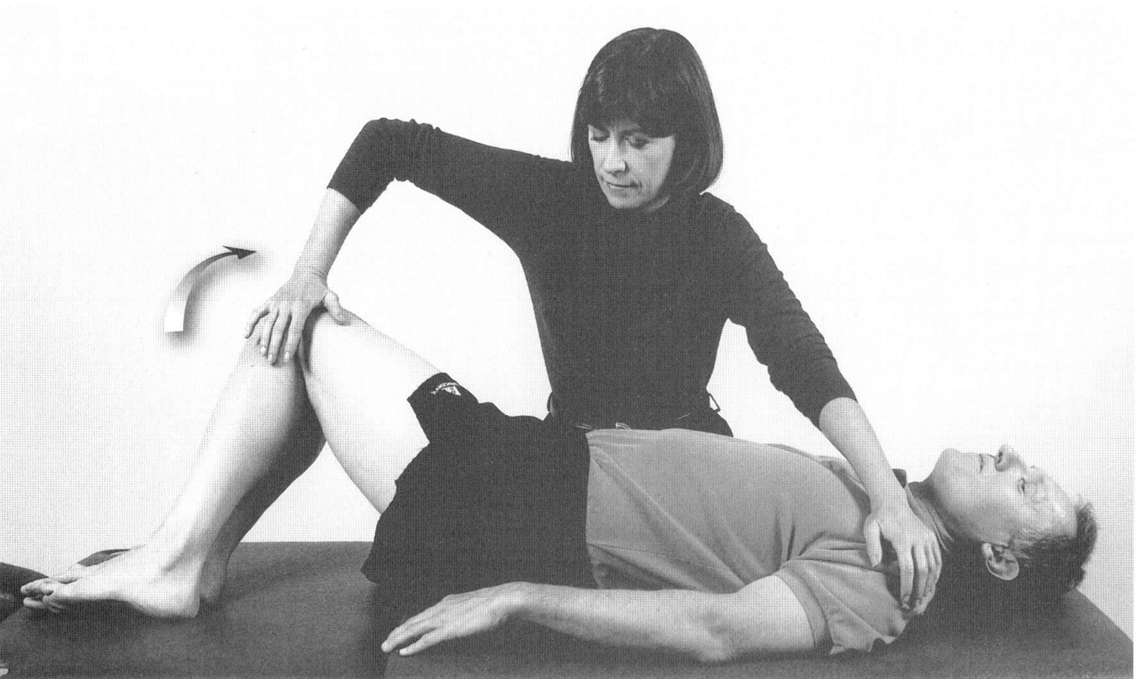

FIGURE 2-3 **Lumbar rotation AAROM or PROM.**

POSITIONING: Client lying supine with knees flexed, feet flat on stable surface, and arms relaxed at side (hook-lying). Clinician standing to one side of client and adjacent to lumbopelvic region.

PROCEDURE: Clinician performs lumbar rotation motion bilaterally by moving knees laterally with one hand and stabilizing thorax with other. Pelvis should raise off the stable surface on the opposite side during movement.

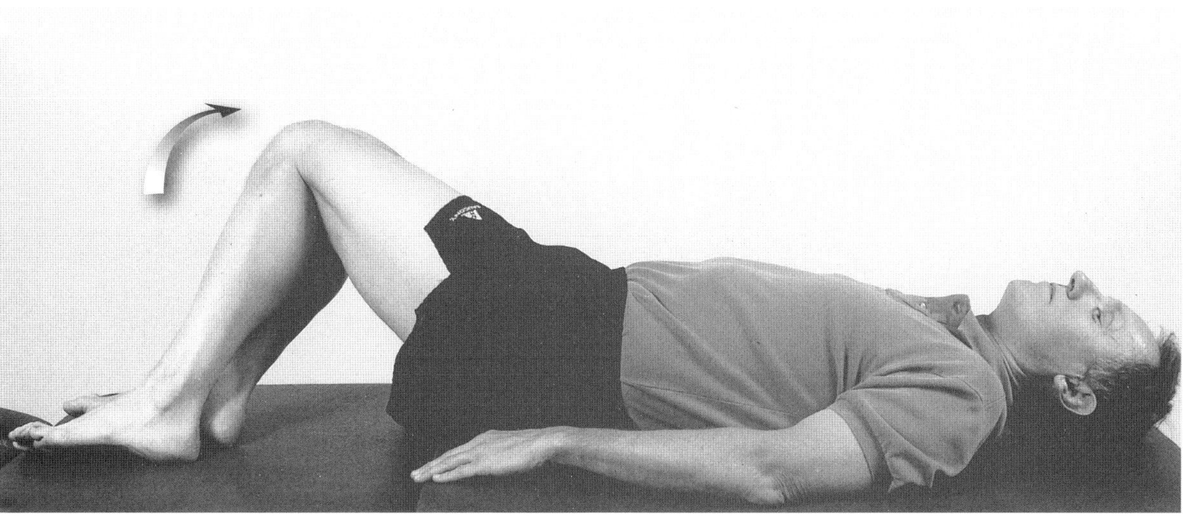

FIGURE 2-4 **Lumbar rotation AROM.**

POSITIONING: Client lying supine with knees flexed, feet flat on stable surface, and arms relaxed at side (hook lying).

PROCEDURE: Client performs active lumbar rotation motion bilaterally by moving knees laterally while keeping shoulder girdles and upper back flat on the stable surface. One side of pelvis should rise up off the stable surface during movement.

FIGURE 2-5 **Lumbar flexion AROM.**

POSITIONING: Client sitting upright in sturdy chair with feet flat on floor, pelvis in neutral, and hands in midline.

PROCEDURE: Client performs active lumbar flexion by slowly lowering head, upper extremities, and trunk toward floor while allowing pelvis to tilt posteriorly and then returns to upright position. Cervical spine should be kept in neutral position relative to flexion and extension.

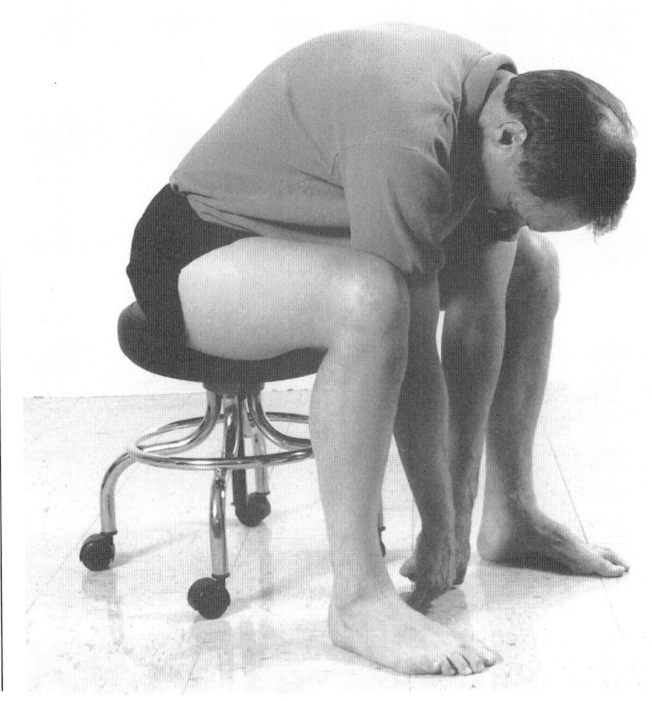

FIGURE 2-6 **Thoracic and lumbar extension AROM.**

POSITIONING: Client standing on stable, level surface with hands placed on iliac crests; pelvis in neutral.

PROCEDURE: Client performs active thoracic and lumbar extension by slowly leaning trunk backward and allowing pelvis to tilt anteriorly and then returns to upright position.

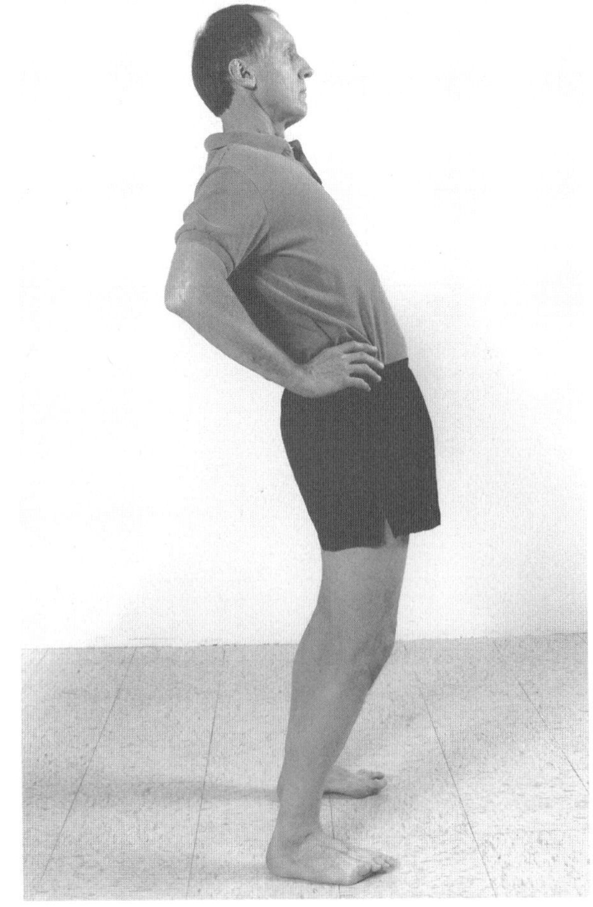

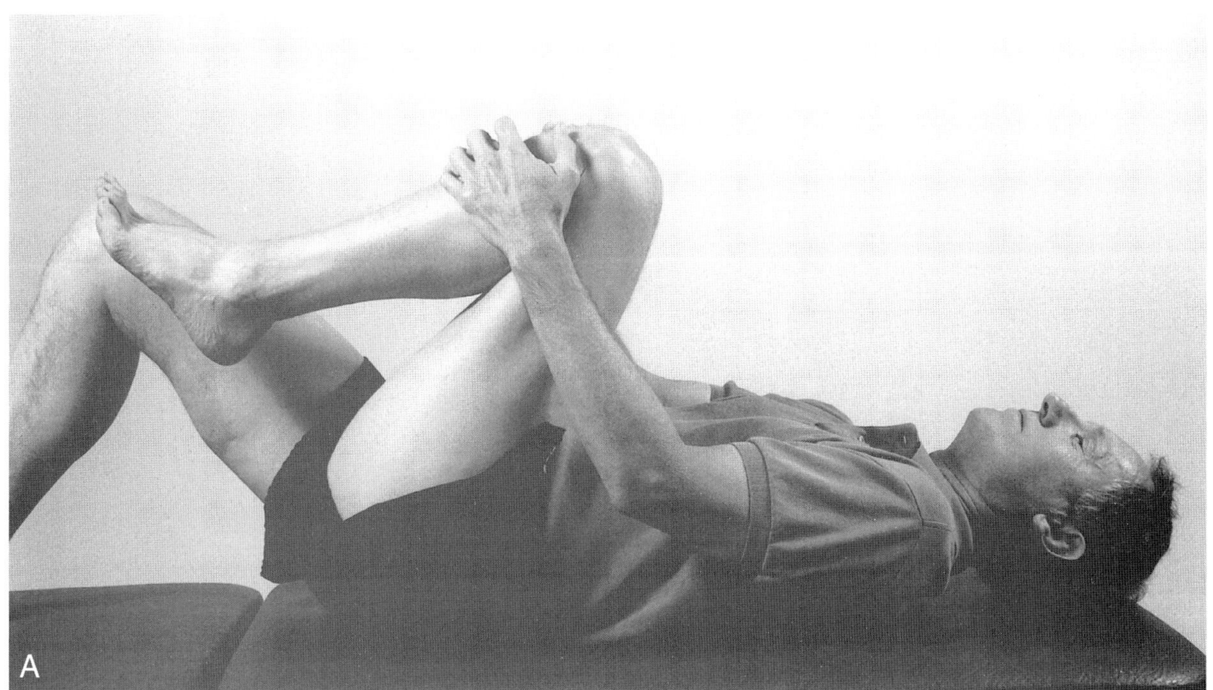

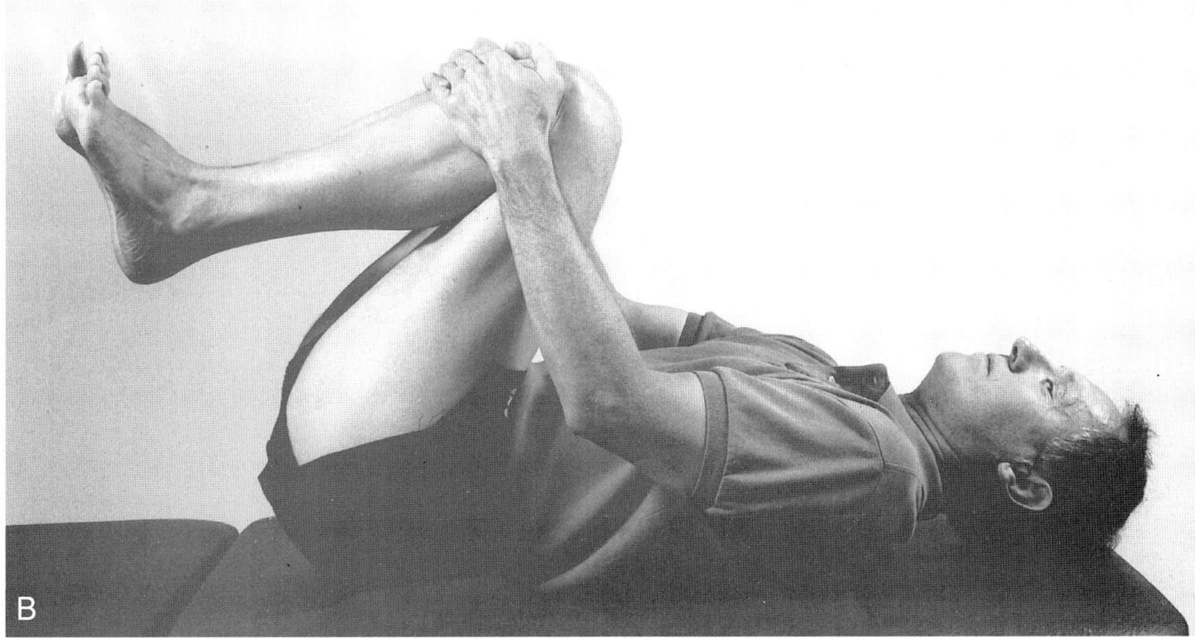

FIGURE 2-7 **Lumbar and hip flexion AAROM (self-assisted).**

POSITIONING: Client lying supine with knees flexed, feet flat on stable surface, and arms relaxed at side (hook lying).

PROCEDURE: (Panel A) Client performs self-assisted lumbar and bilateral hip flexion by grasping behind one knee and pulling the knee toward chest. (Panel B) For a slightly more difficult exercise, client grasps both knees and pulls knees toward chest.

NOTE: Allowing pelvis to tilt posteriorly during motion will result in greater range of lumbar flexion; stabilizing pelvis in neutral will result in greater range of hip flexion.

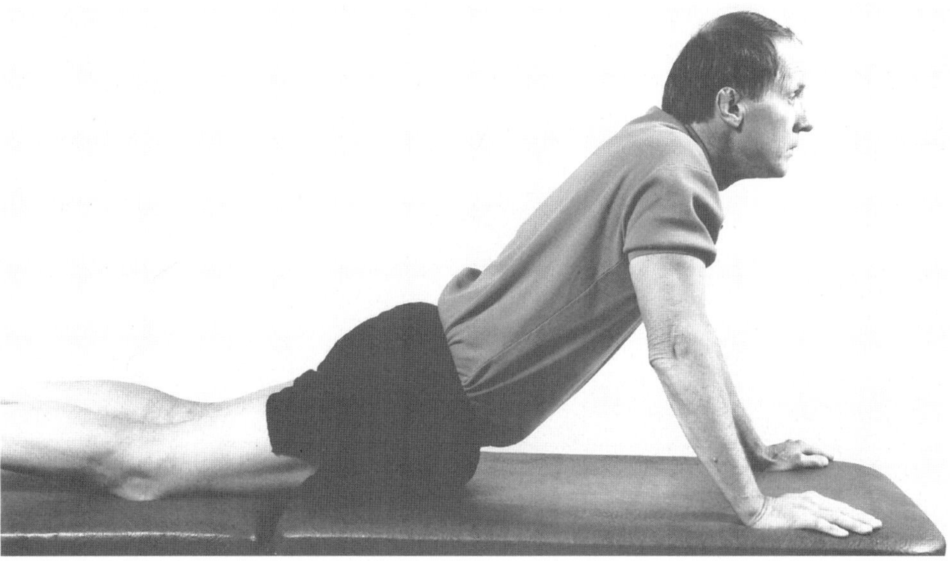

FIGURE 2-8 **Lumbar extension AAROM (self-assisted).**

POSITIONING: Client lying prone on stable surface with elbows flexed so that forearms and hands are under shoulder and upper arm.

PROCEDURE: Client performs self-assisted lumbar extension by raising head and upper back up off of surface. Force is provided by elbow extensors straightening elbows. Lumbar extensor muscles should remain relaxed during motion.

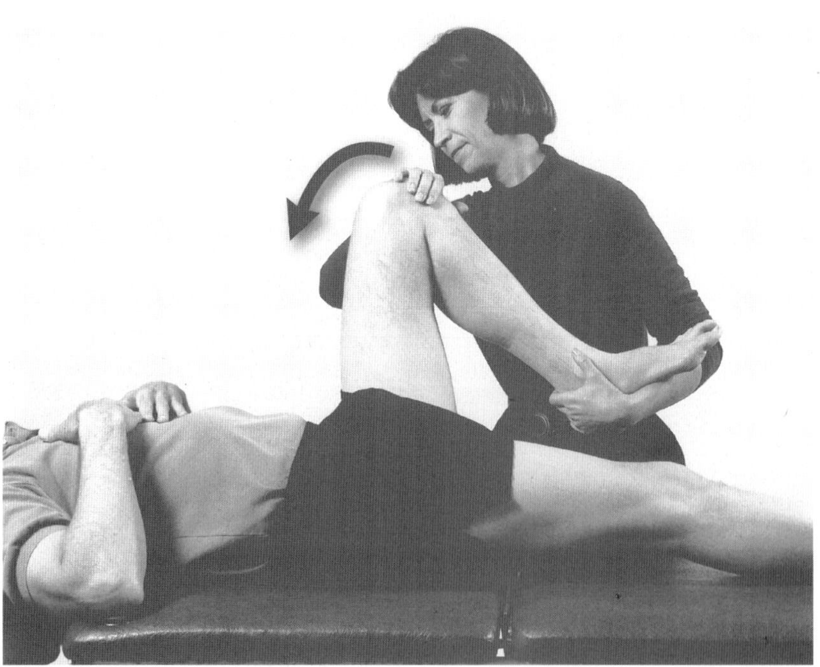

FIGURE 2-9 **Hip and knee flexion AAROM or PROM.**

POSITIONING: Client lying supine with one knee flexed and foot flat on stable surface. Clinician standing next to leg that is flexed.

PROCEDURE: Clinician performs unilateral flexion of hip and knee by grasping client's limb at knee and under heel and pushing knee toward client's shoulder on same side.

NOTE: Same positioning can be used for AROM hip flexion. Client actively flexes knee and hip on one side and brings knee toward shoulder. Motion can be performed with self-assistance by having client grasp on top of knee and pull hip and knee into flexion by pulling knee toward shoulder on same side.

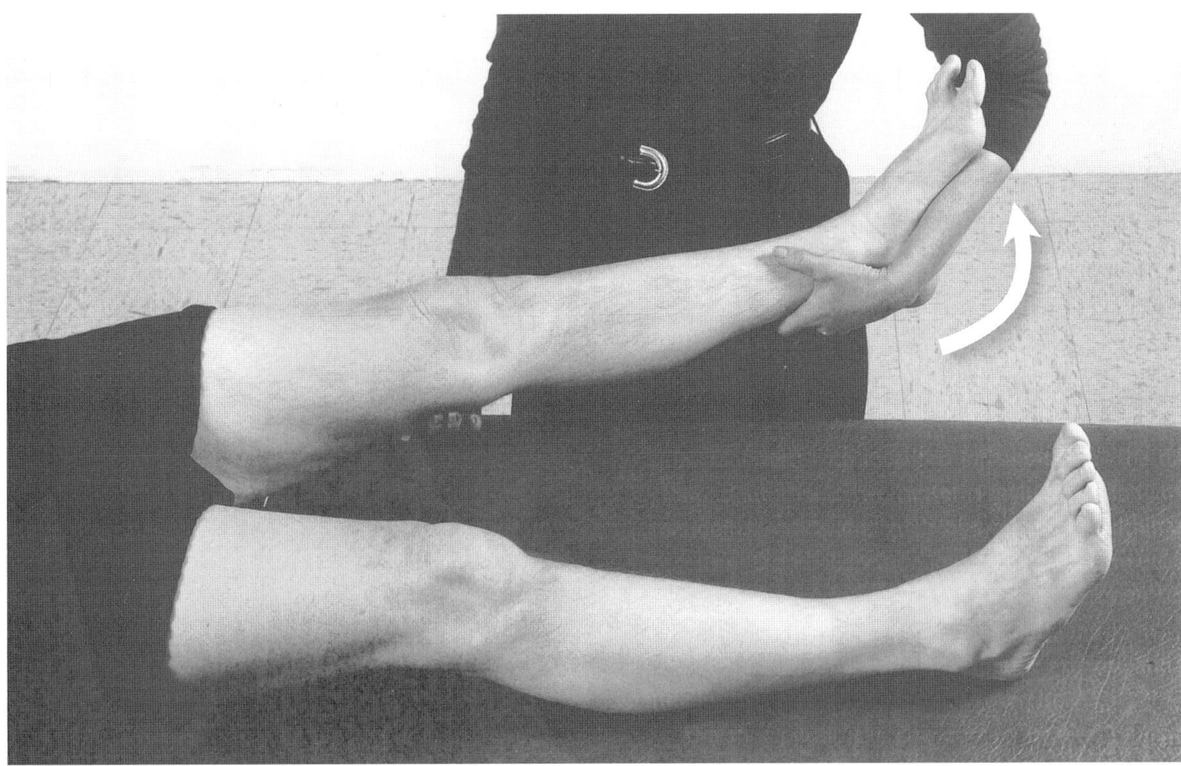

FIGURE 2-10 **Hip abduction and adduction AAROM or PROM.**

POSITIONING: Client lying supine on stable surface with both limbs extended and one limb positioned in slight hip abduction. Clinician standing adjacent to client's leg.

PROCEDURE: Clinician performs unilateral abduction and adduction by grasping client's leg under knee and ankle and moving extended, neutrally rotated limb into abduction and adduction.

NOTE: Same position can be used for AROM hip abduction and adduction. Client moves hip by sliding extended, neutrally rotated limb back and forth across surface.

FIGURE 2-11 **Hip rotation AAROM or PROM.**

POSITIONING: Client lying supine with one knee flexed and foot flat on stable surface. Clinician standing at side of flexed limb and adjacent to client's bent leg.

PROCEDURE: Clinician performs unilateral medial and lateral rotation of hip by first grasping client's limb at knee and heel and positioning client's limb in 90° of flexion at hip and knee. In this position, clinician stabilizes client's distal thigh, knee, and leg while rotating hip by performing a swinging motion of leg in a horizontal plane.

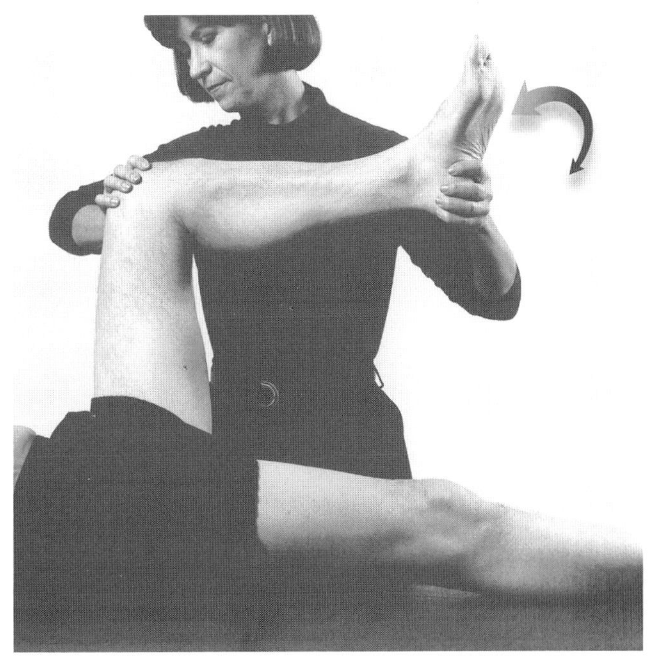

FIGURE 2-12 **Hip rotation AROM.**

POSITIONING: Client lying prone on stable surface with one knee flexed to 90°.

PROCEDURE: Client performs unilateral active medial and lateral rotation of hip by moving leg toward floor, keeping thigh and pelvis flat and knee neutral regarding flexion and extension.

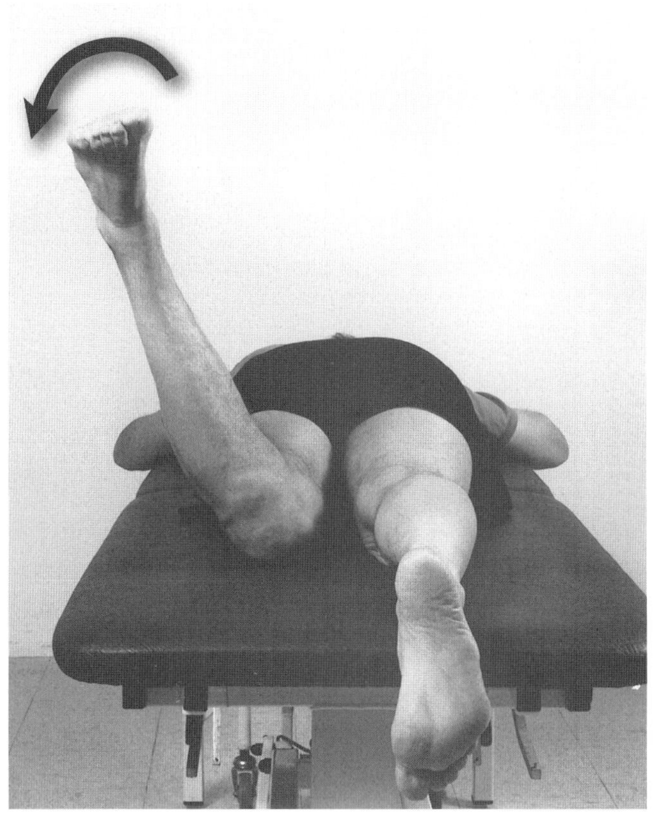

FIGURE 2-13 **Knee flexion and extension AROM.**

POSITIONING: Client lying prone on a stable surface with both legs extended.

PROCEDURE: Client performs unilateral active flexion and extension of knee by moving leg toward and away from hip in a sagittal plane, keeping thigh and pelvis flat.

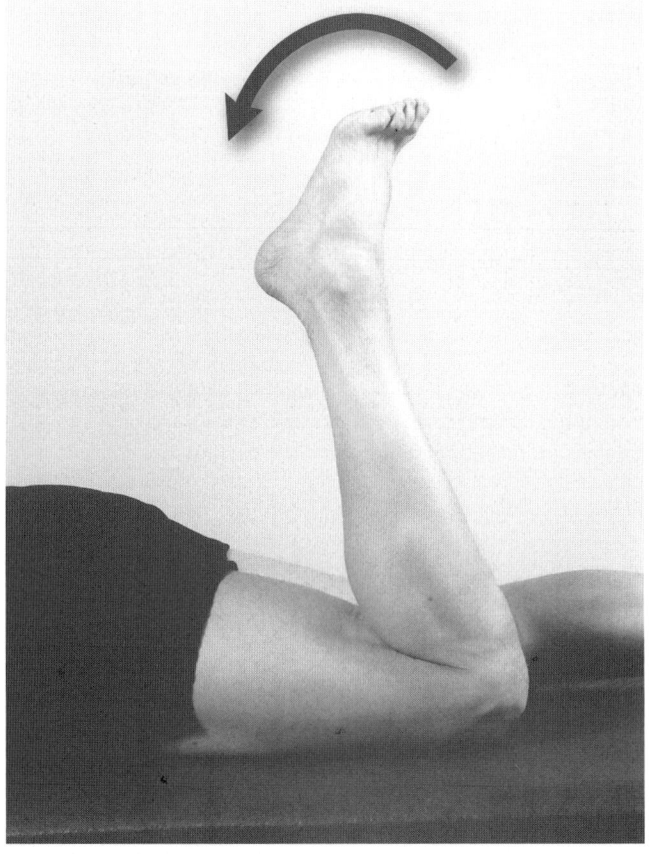

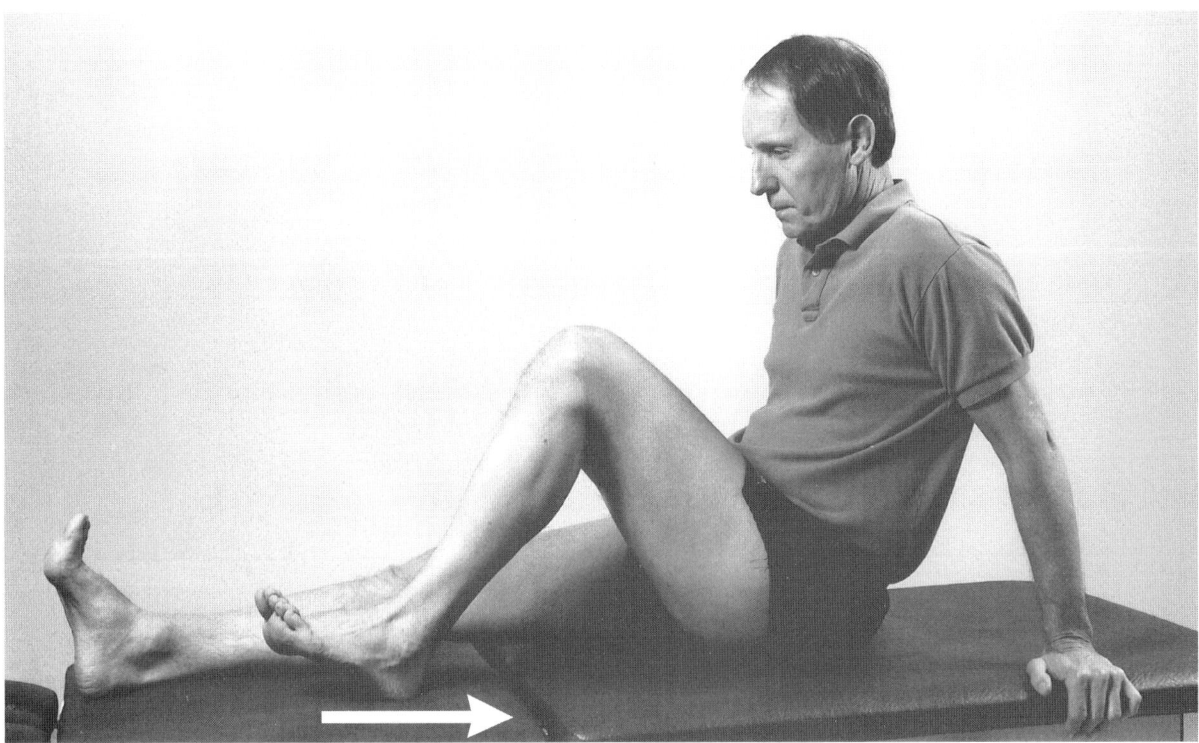

FIGURE 2-14 **Knee and hip flexion and extension AROM (heel slides).**

POSITIONING: Client sitting in long sitting position on stable surface with back supported or with client leaning back on extended arms (tripod sitting).

PROCEDURE: Client performs active unilateral flexion and extension of knee by moving heel of leg toward and away from hip in a sagittal plane, keeping pelvis in neutral position.

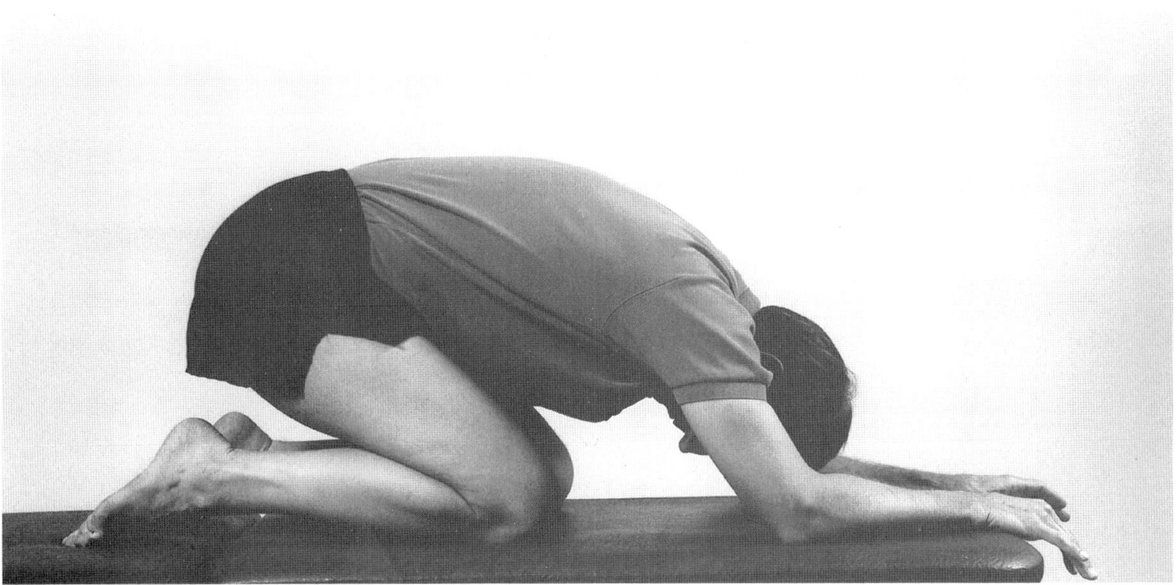

FIGURE 2-15 **Combined thoracic, lumbar, hip, and knee flexion.**

POSITIONING: Client kneeling on hands and knees (quadruped).

PROCEDURE: Client performs combined thoracic, lumbar, hip, and knee flexion by sitting back on heels, keeping hands forward, and lowering chest to surface. Pelvis tilts posteriorly, with cervical spine maintained in neutral regarding flexion and extension.

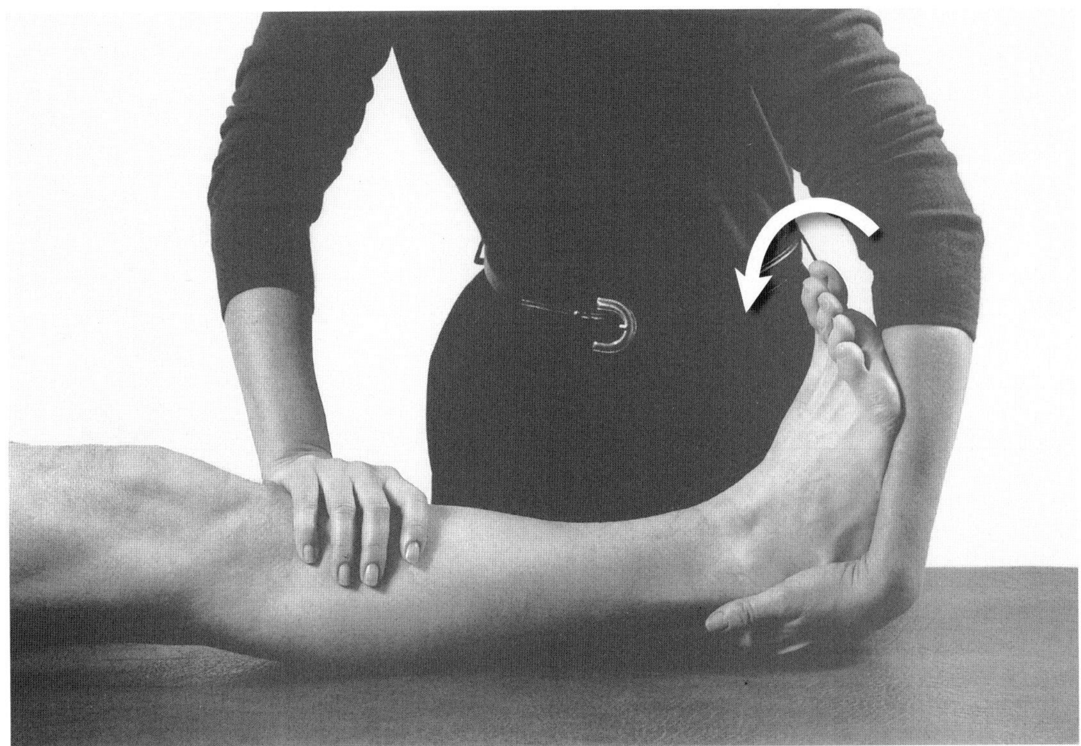

FIGURE 2-16 **Ankle plantarflexion and dorsiflexion AAROM or PROM.**

POSITIONING: Client sitting or lying supine on stable surface with limbs extended. Clinician standing to side of leg and adjacent to ankle and foot.

PROCEDURE: Clinician performs unilateral plantarflexion and dorsiflexion of ankle by stabilizing leg at proximal tibia and pulling foot up and down in a sagittal plane. Dorsiflexion motion should be performed by grasping heel while pushing plantar surface of forefoot with clinician's forearm. Dorsiflexion should be performed both with client's knee extended and with it slightly flexed. Plantarflexion motion should be performed by pushing on dorsal surface of midfoot and forefoot.

NOTE: Same position can be used for AROM of ankle. Client actively performs dorsiflexion and plantarflexion of the ankle, both with the knee extended and with it slightly flexed.

FIGURE 2-17 **Toe flexion and extension AAROM or PROM.**

POSITIONING: Client sitting or lying supine on stable surface with legs extended. Clinician standing to side of leg and adjacent to ankle and foot.

PROCEDURE: Clinician performs unilateral flexion and extension of one or more toes at metatarsophalangeal joints by grasping entire digit and moving it in a sagittal plane, while stabilizing metatarsal bones of forefoot.

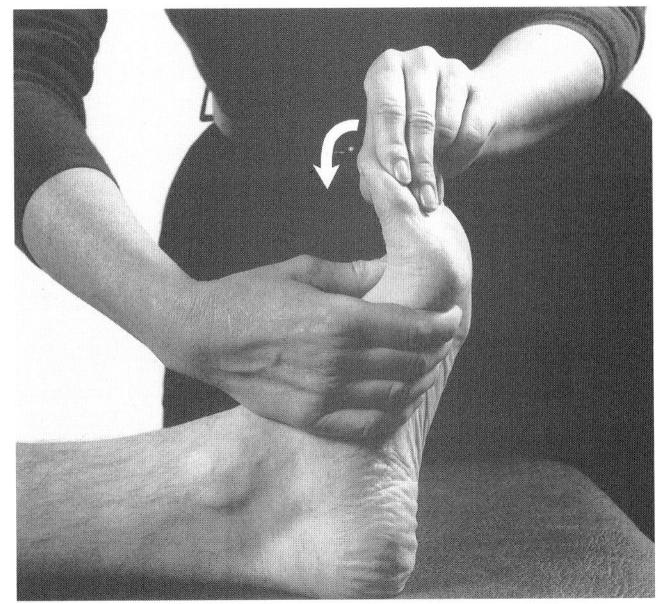

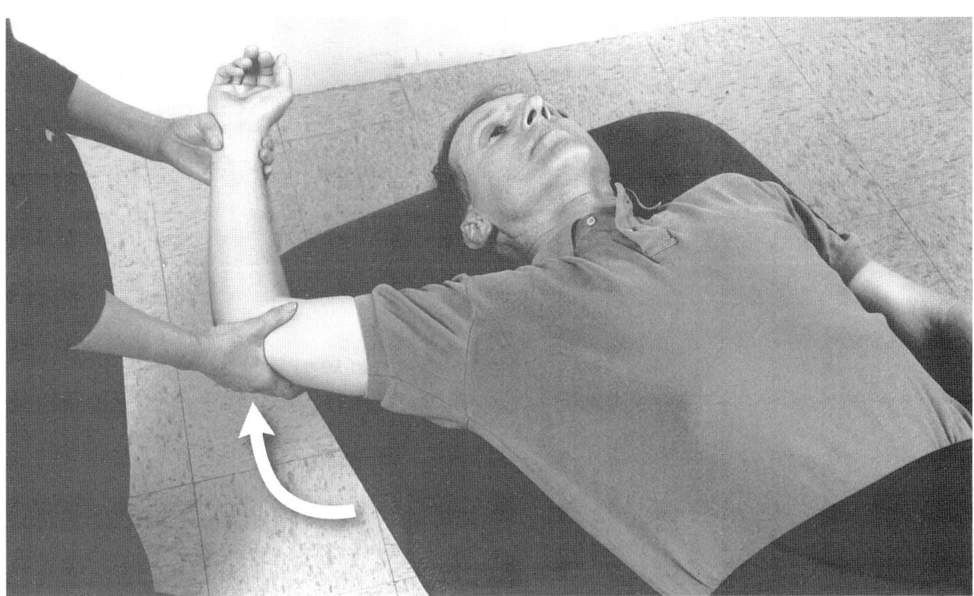

FIGURE 2-18 Shoulder abduction and adduction AAROM or PROM.

POSITIONING: Client lying supine on stable surface with one arm at side and shoulder in lateral rotation. Clinician standing at client's side and adjacent to shoulder.

PROCEDURE: Clinician performs unilateral abduction and adduction of shoulder by grasping client's limb under elbow and at wrist and hand and moving arm toward head and then back to client's side in a frontal plane. Elbow can be positioned in flexion or extension. Client's scapula should be allowed to move, and shoulder must be positioned in lateral rotation when moving arm overhead to minimize subacromial impingement.

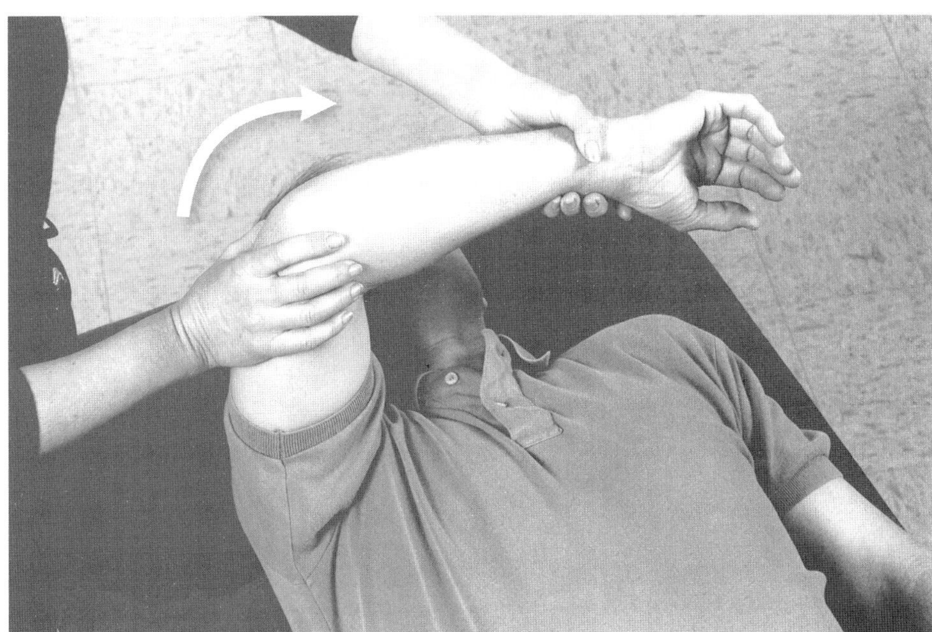

FIGURE 2-19 Shoulder horizontal abduction and adduction AAROM or PROM.

POSITIONING: Client lying supine on stable surface with one arm in 90° of flexion. Clinician is positioned at client's side adjacent to shoulder.

PROCEDURE: Clinician performs unilateral horizontal abduction and adduction of shoulder by grasping client's wrist and elbow and moving upper arm toward opposite shoulder and then back to starting position in a horizontal plane (relative to patient). Client's scapula should be allowed to move, and elbow can be positioned in flexion or extension.

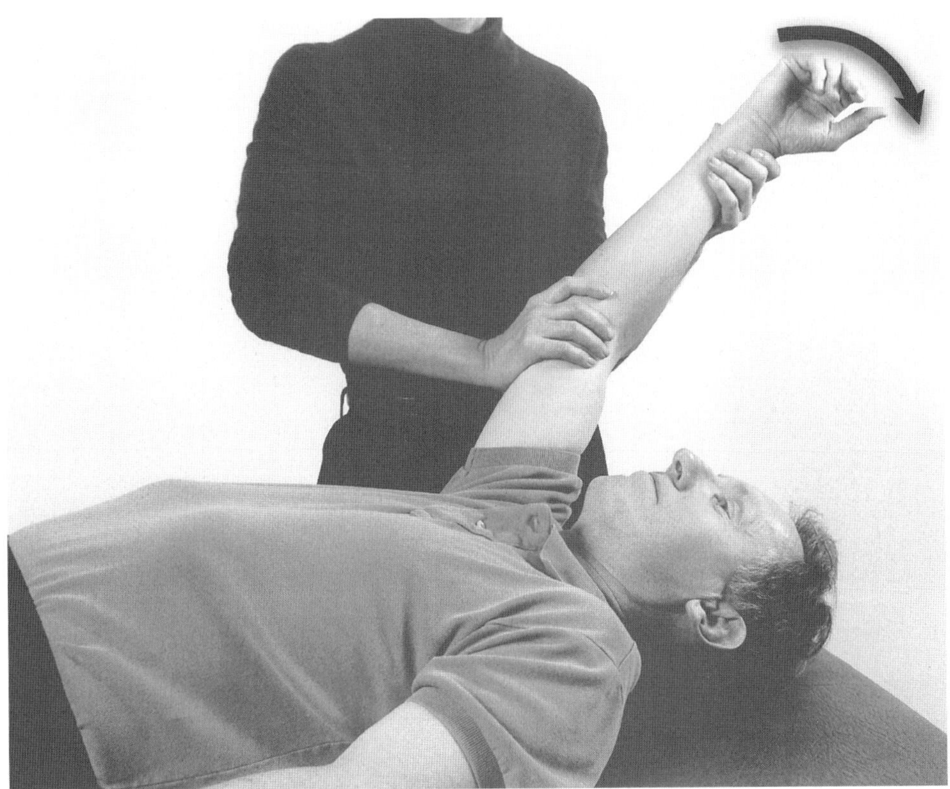

FIGURE 2-20 Shoulder flexion AAROM or PROM.

POSITIONING: Client lying supine on stable surface with one arm at side and with shoulder positioned in neutral relative to rotation. Clinician standing at client's side and adjacent to shoulder.

PROCEDURE: Clinician performs unilateral flexion of shoulder by grasping client's arm at elbow, crossing over to grasp client's wrist and hand, and moving arm toward head and then back to client's side in a sagittal plane. Elbow can be positioned in extension, and client's scapula should be allowed to move.

FIGURE 2-21 Shoulder abduction and adduction AROM.

POSITIONING: Client standing or sitting with upper extremities in anatomical position.

PROCEDURE: Client performs active shoulder abduction and adduction (unilateral or bilateral).

NOTE: Same position can be used for performing AROM for shoulder flexion, extension, horizontal abduction, and horizontal adduction.

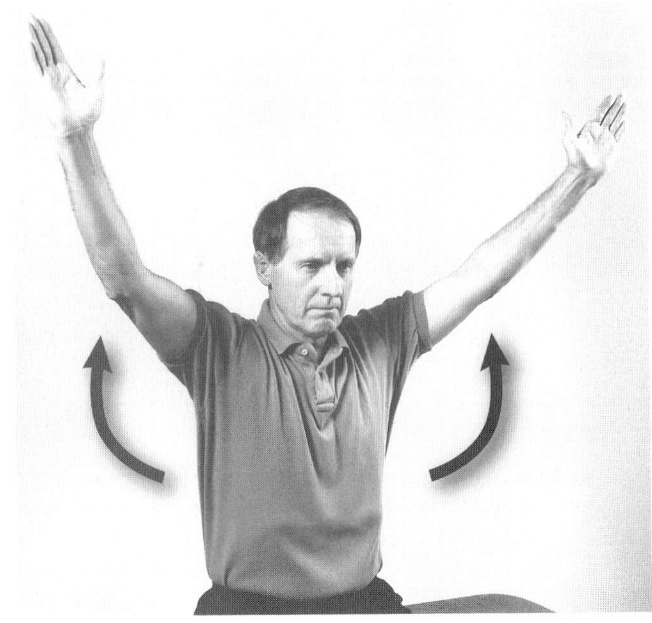

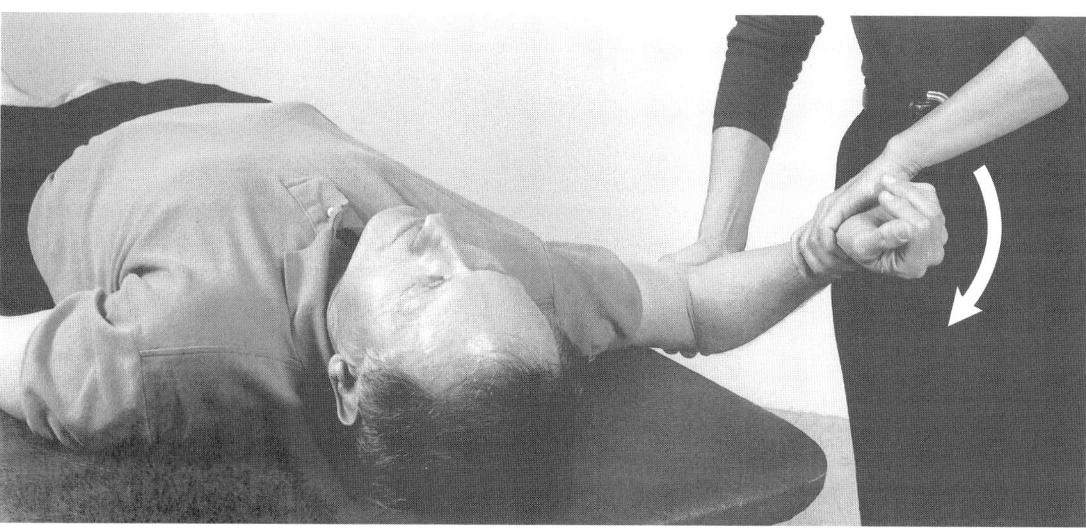

FIGURE 2-22 Shoulder rotation AAROM or PROM.

POSITIONING: Client lying supine on stable surface with one arm in 90° of shoulder abduction (neutral rotation) and 90° of elbow flexion. Clinician standing at client's side and adjacent to elbow.

PROCEDURE: Clinician performs unilateral medial and lateral rotation of shoulder by grasping client's distal forearm, stabilizing elbow, and moving forearm in a swinging motion toward floor in a sagittal plane (relative to patient).

NOTE: Rotation motion can also be performed with client's shoulder in less than 90° of abduction if necessary.

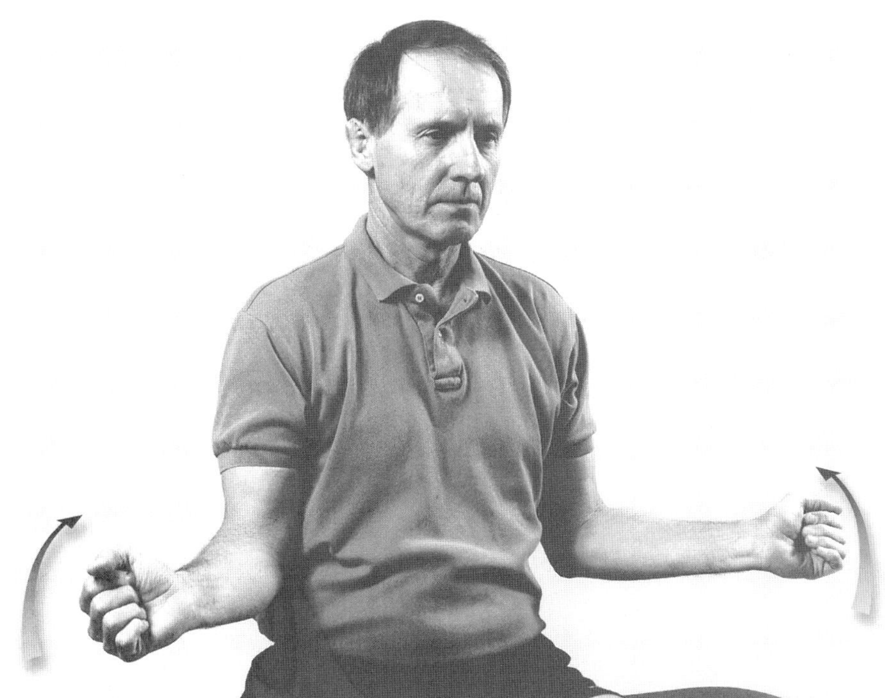

FIGURE 2-23 Shoulder rotation AROM.

POSITIONING: Client standing or sitting with elbows flexed at 90°.

PROCEDURE: Client performs active medial and lateral rotation of shoulder (unilateral or bilateral) by swinging forearms toward and away from abdomen in a horizontal plane while keeping upper arms against trunk.

FIGURE 2-24 **Combined shoulder flexion and lateral rotation AROM.**

POSITIONING: Client standing or sitting with arms at side.

PROCEDURE: Client performs active motion of combined shoulder flexion and lateral rotation at one shoulder by performing shoulder flexion with elbow flexed and reaching toward posterior portion of shoulder and scapula on same side.

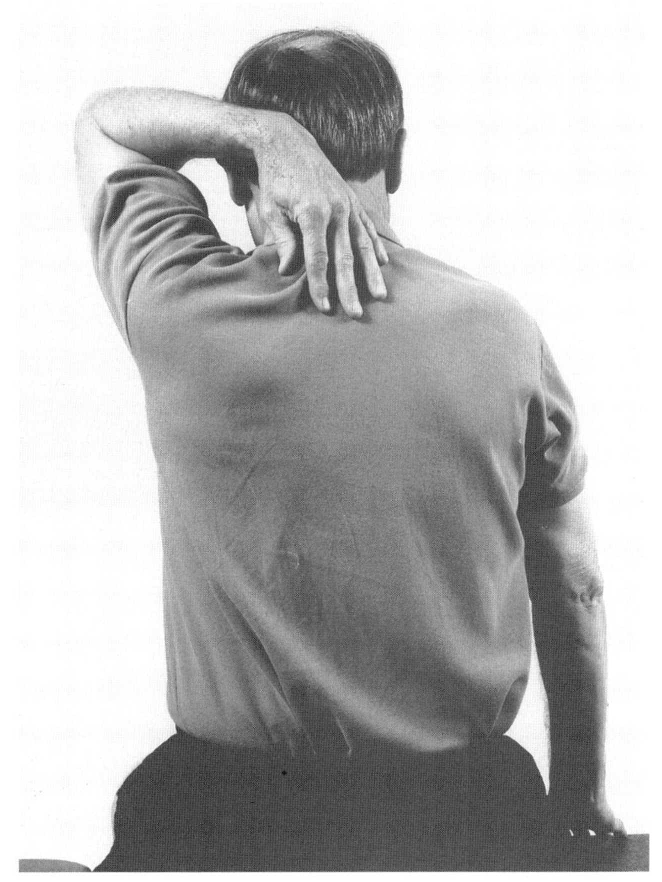

FIGURE 2-25 **Combined shoulder extension and internal rotation AROM.**

POSITIONING: Client standing or sitting with arms at side.

PROCEDURE: Client performs active motion of combined shoulder extension and medial rotation at one shoulder by performing shoulder extension with elbow flexed while reaching toward inferior angle of scapula on same side.

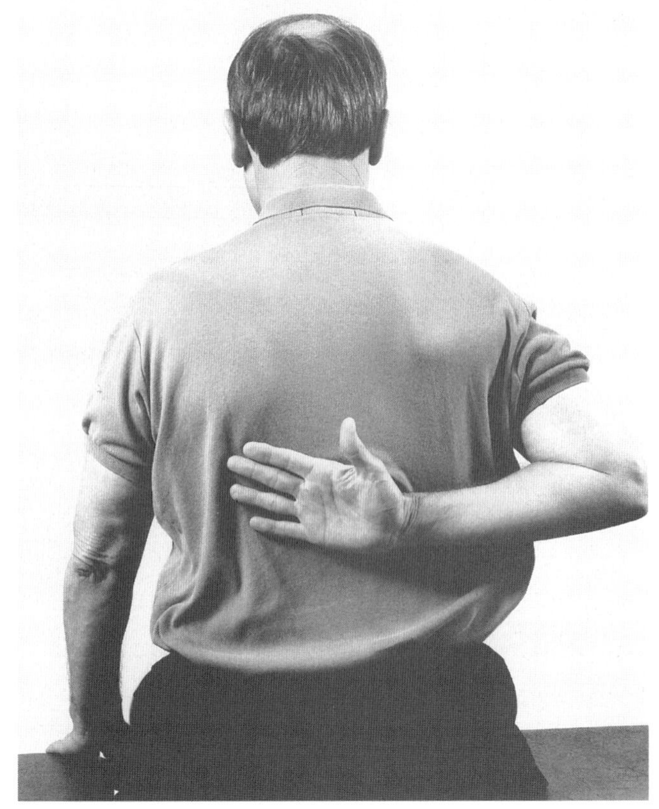

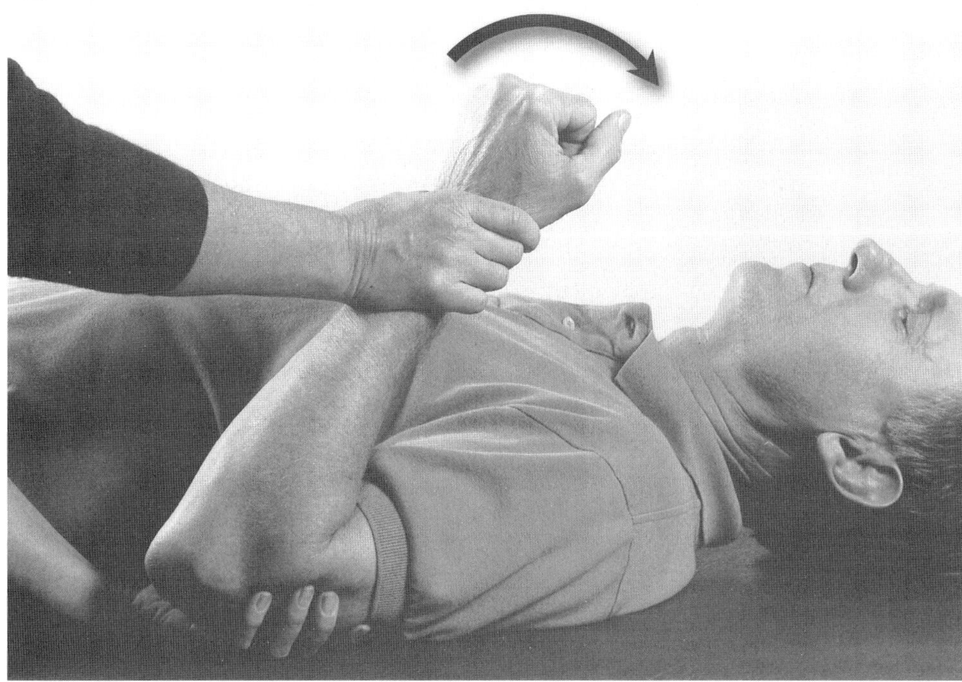

FIGURE 2-26 **Elbow flexion and extension AAROM or PROM.**

POSITIONING: Client lying supine on stable surface with arms at side. Clinician standing or sitting at side of client and adjacent to elbow and forearm.

PROCEDURE: Clinician performs unilateral elbow flexion and extension by grasping client's distal forearm, stabilizing elbow and upper arm, and moving forearm toward and away from upper arm in sagittal plane. Movement should be performed with client's forearm pronated and supinated.

NOTE: Same position can be used for AROM of elbow flexion and extension.

FIGURE 2-27 **Forearm pronation and supination AAROM or PROM.**

POSITIONING: Client lying supine on stable surface with one arm in 90° of elbow flexion. Clinician standing or sitting at client's side and adjacent to elbow.

PROCEDURE: Clinician performs unilateral forearm pronation and supination by grasping client's distal forearm, stabilizing elbow and upper arm, and rotating forearm toward and away from client a horizontal plane.

NOTE: Same position can be used for AROM of forearm pronation and supination. Client actively rotates forearm.

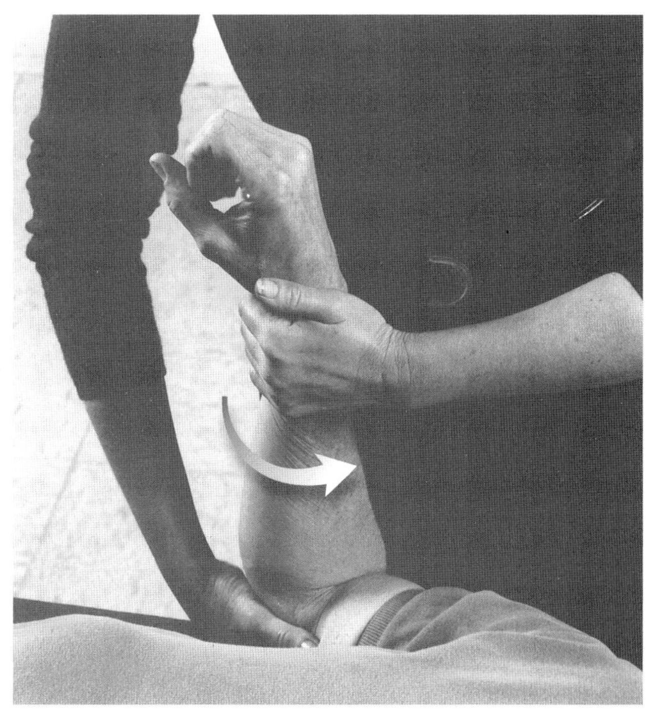

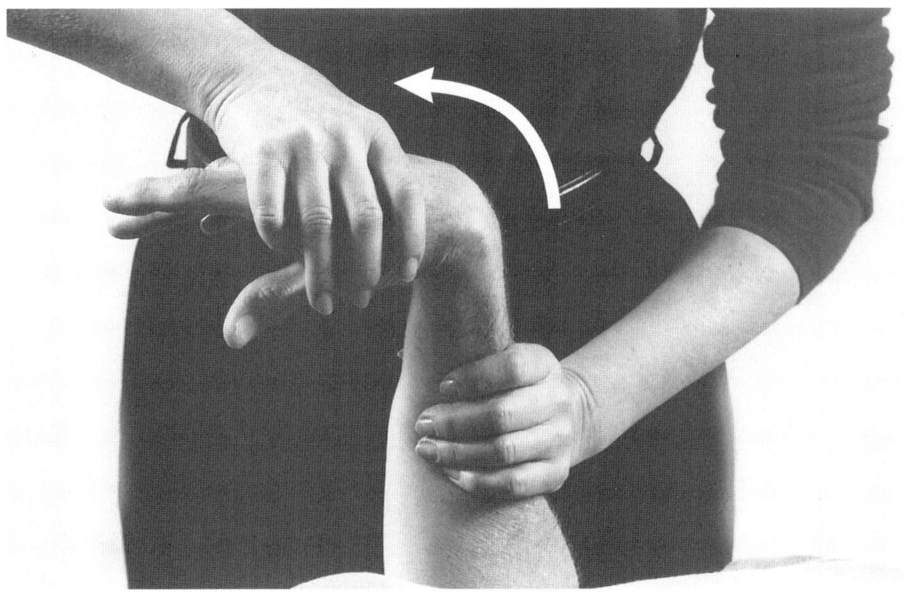

FIGURE 2-28 Wrist flexion, extension, and deviation AAROM or PROM.

POSITIONING: Client lying supine on stable surface with one arm in 90° of elbow flexion. Clinician standing or sitting at client's side and adjacent to forearm.

PROCEDURE: Clinician performs unilateral flexion, extension, and deviation of wrist by grasping client's hand; stabilizing distal forearm in neutral rotation; and moving wrist into flexion, extension, radial deviation, and ulnar deviation.

NOTE: Same position can be used for AROM at wrist. Client actively flexes, extends, and deviates wrist.

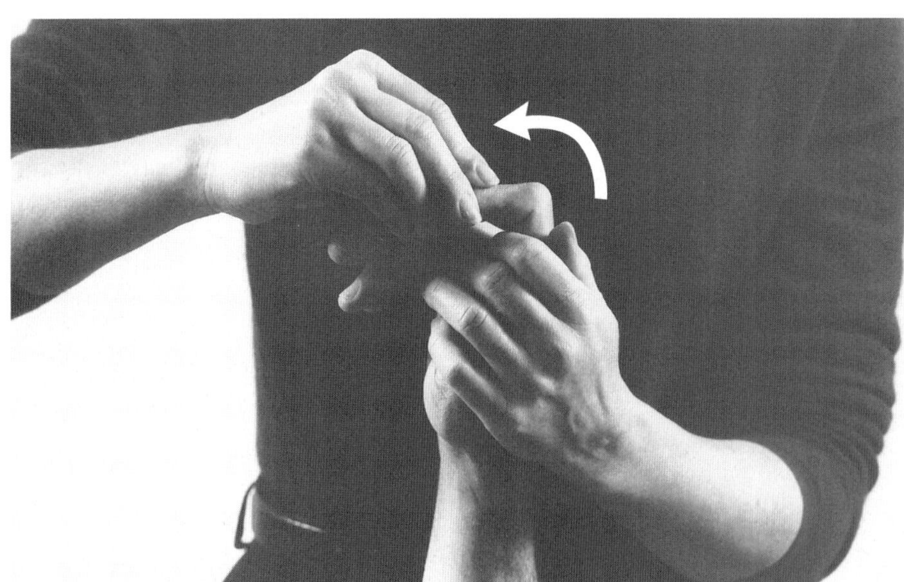

FIGURE 2-29 Finger flexion and extension AAROM or PROM.

POSITIONING: Client lying supine on stable surface or sitting in chair with one arm in 90° of elbow flexion. Clinician standing or sitting at client's side and adjacent to hand.

PROCEDURE: Clinician performs unilateral flexion and extension of one or more digits at metacarpophalangeal and interphalangeal joints by grasping segment distal to joint and moving it in a sagittal plane while stabilizing segment proximal to joint.

NOTE: Same position can be used for AROM at fingers. Client actively flexes and extends fingers.

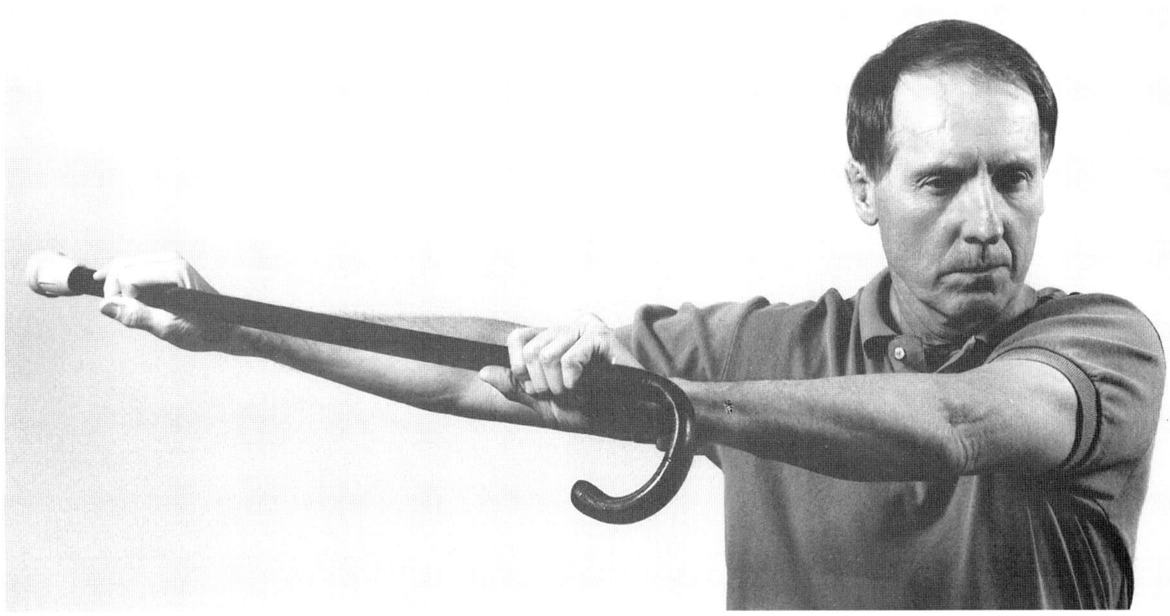

FIGURE 2-30 Shoulder horizontal adduction and abduction AAROM.

POSITIONING: Client lying supine on stable surface or standing with arms in 90° of shoulder flexion and elbows fairly extended and wand held in hands.

PROCEDURE: Client performs unilateral or bilateral horizontal abduction and adduction of shoulder by moving wand and arms back and forth across chest, keeping trunk stable.

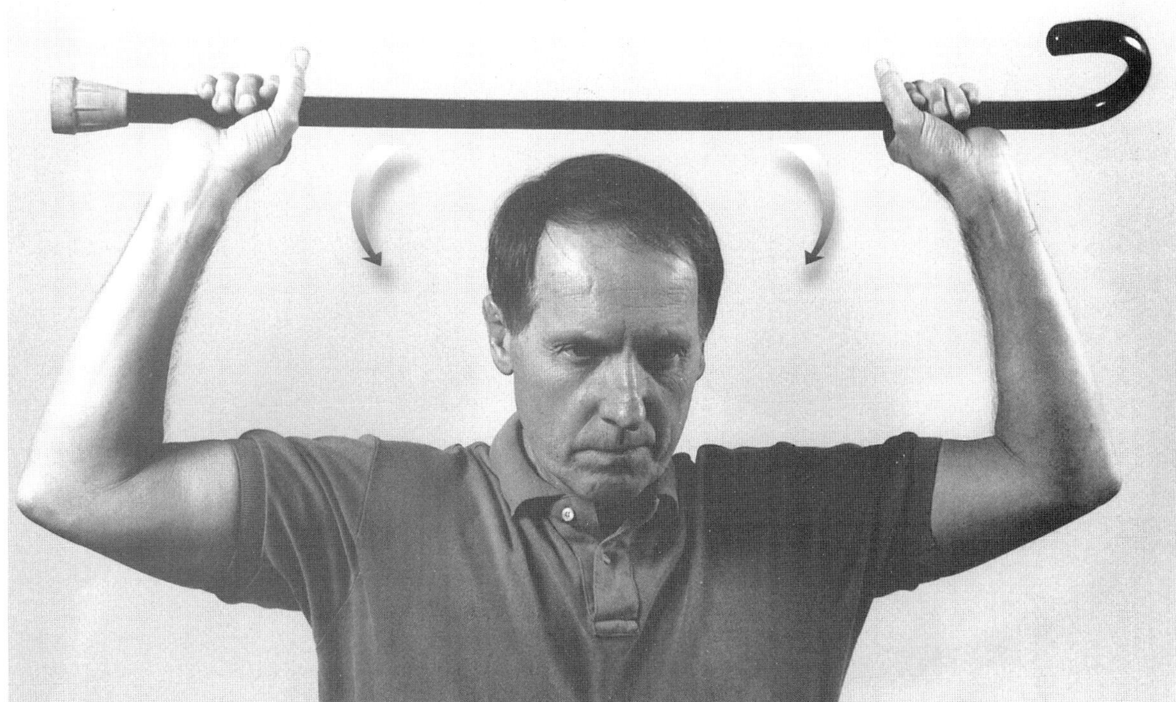

FIGURE 2-31 Shoulder rotation AAROM (standing or supine).

POSITIONING: Client lying supine on stable surface or standing with arms in 90° of shoulder abduction and 90° of elbow flexion and wand held in hands.

PROCEDURE: Client performs bilateral medial and lateral rotation of shoulders by moving wand and arms back and forth from abdomen to overhead while keeping shoulders and elbows at 90°.

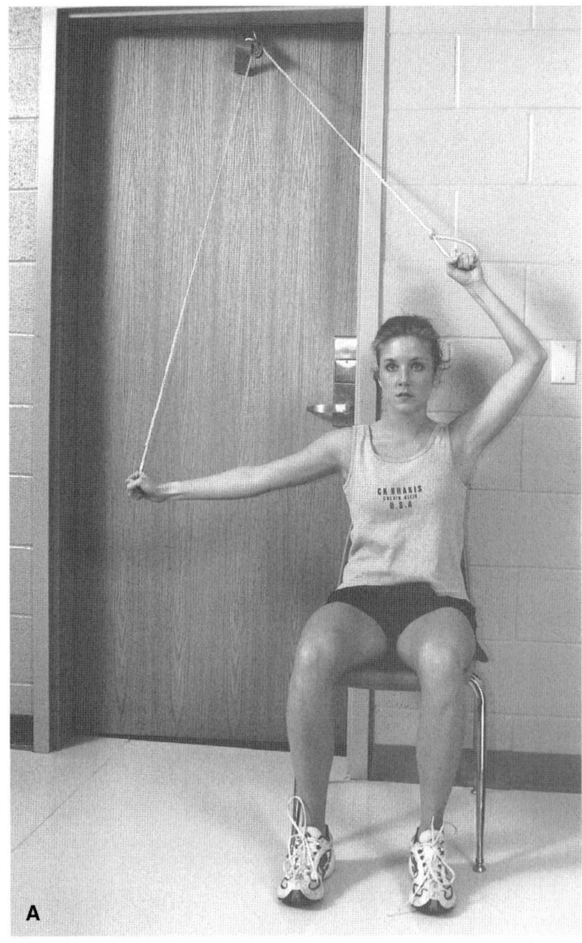

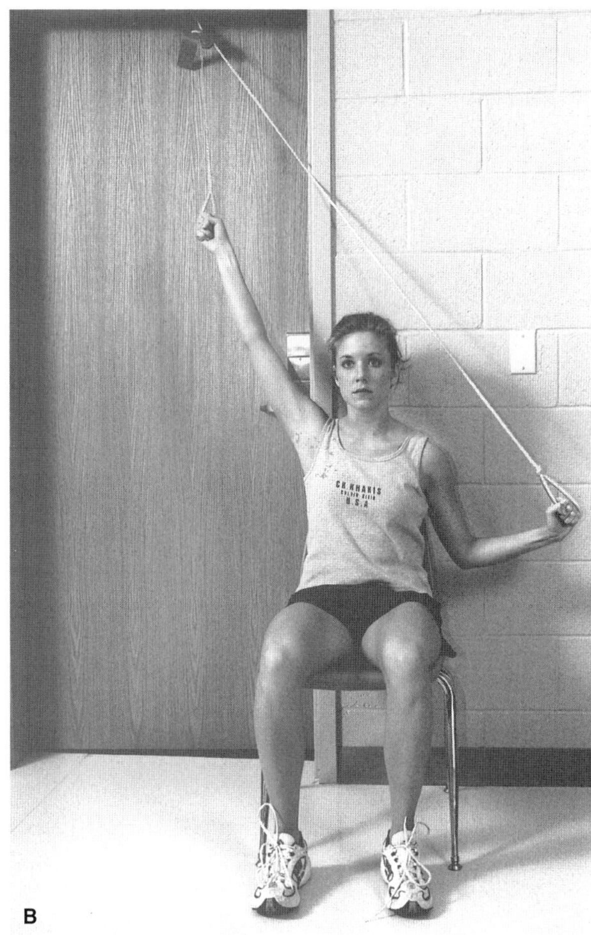

FIGURE 2-32 Shoulder abduction AAROM (with pulley).

POSITIONING: (Panel A) Client sitting and holding one handle of pulley system in each hand.

PROCEDURE: (Panel B) Client performs unilateral or bilateral abduction of shoulders by pulling rope down on one side, causing other arm to be lifted into abduction. Trunk should be kept stable, elbow extended on arm being lifted, and shoulder being lifted must be positioned in lateral rotation when moving arm overhead to minimize subacromial impingement.

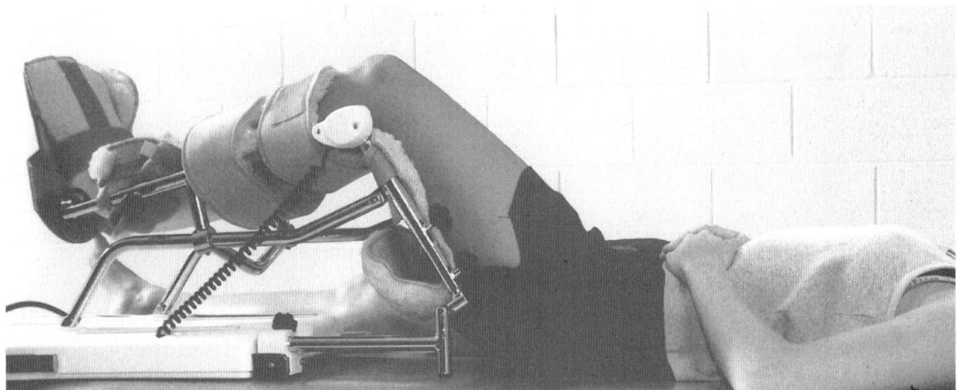

FIGURE 2-33 CPM for knee flexion and extension.

POSITIONING: Client lying supine in bed with involved lower extremity stabilized in CPM device (with straps, padding, and an underlying rigid frame). Movement hinge is aligned with knee joint.

PROCEDURE: Range, rate, and duration of motion are programmed. Unilateral flexion and extension of knee are performed continuously by device for hours at a time.

EQUIPMENT

Figures 2-30 to 2-33 illustrate a sampling of ROM exercise techniques that use equipment, including wands, pulleys, and CPM devices.

CASE STUDY

PATIENT INFORMATION

The patient was an 18-year-old female track-and-field athlete who reported an injury to the anterior portion of her right knee. The injury occurred while landing during a long jump competition. She stated that her coach applied ice to her knee; she sat out the remainder of the competition and rested her knee for 2 days. Over the following two weeks, she attempted to resume her training regimen, which was mostly running and jumping training; but she was experiencing sharp pain, swelling, and thigh muscle weakness.

Her first visit was 3 weeks after the injury. At that time, her complaints were anterior knee pain with ambulation, increased pain on stairs, pain when sitting down and standing up (sit–stand transferring), and inability to run or jump because of pain. The patient reported no previous history of injury to either lower extremity. Current treatment consisted of a nonprescriptive anti-inflammatory medication.

Relevant findings from the examination included painful and limited supine active knee flexion (105°); painful and limited prone active knee flexion (84°); painful and limited active knee extension against gravity (lacked the final 20° of extension); antalgic gait; and palpable tenderness, swelling, and crepitation over the midportion of the patellar tendon between the patella and tibial tuberosity. Because she was unable to extend her knee fully against gravity, quadriceps strength was given a manual muscle testing grade of fair minus (3−/5). The patient's condition was diagnosed as patellar tendon strain and tendonitis.

LINKS TO

Guide to Physical Therapist Practice* and *Athletic Training Educational Competencies

The diagnosis relates to patterns 4D and 4E in the musculoskeletal domain of the *Guide.*[21] Patterns 4D and 4E are described, respectively, as: "impaired joint mobility, motor function, muscle performance, and range of motion associated with connective tissue dysfunction" and "impaired joint mobility, motor function, muscle performance, and range of motion associated with localized inflammation." The disorders grouped into these two patterns include tendon strain and tendonitis. Anticipated goals of intervention within practice patterns 4D and 4E include improvement of the quality and quantity of movement between and across body segments and improvement of tissue extensibility and joint mobility through the use of specific therapeutic exercise and manual therapy techniques, such as ROM exercise.

The therapeutic exercise domain in the *Competencies*[23] refers to the treatment of athletes by using "passive, active, active assistive, and resistive exercises." Teaching objectives listed under the competencies of this domain include specific outcomes of exercise that increase joint range of motion by using CPM, AROM, and PROM for the upper body, lower body, and trunk.

INTERVENTION

Short-term goals centered around decreasing pain and inflammation and increasing ROM to improve ambulation and sit–stand transferring. Because the patient was in the off-season of her sport and did not need to train rigorously, no modifications or restrictions in her physical activity, other than limiting stair ambulation, were originally established. Initial treatment consisted of patellar mobilization (Fig. 4-27) to stress the tendon tissue appropriately, seated knee flexion AROM (Fig. 2-14) to increase range of motion and gently stretch the patellar tendon, quadriceps isometrics (quad sets) in full extension while avoiding increased pain, and ice massage. All of these activities were prescribed for the patient's daily home program.

PROGRESSION

One Week After Initial Examination

The patient reported that her pain had reduced about 20% with ambulation and sit–stand transferring but was unchanged with stair ambulation. Knee flexion AROM was 120° in supine (gain of 15° since initial examination) and 96° in prone (gain of 12°). Treatment continued to focus on meeting the short-term goals; but exercises were added to work toward the long-term goals of restoring strength and flexibility, resuming an active lifestyle, and participating in athletic activities. Prone knee flexion AAROM and AROM exercises (Fig. 2-13) and open kinematic chain knee extension against gravity, with the assistance of the left leg as needed, were added to the daily home program. Application of ice was continued, and quadriceps isometric exercise and patellar mobilization were discontinued.

Two Weeks After Initial Examination

The patient reported slow improvement in her pain with ambulation, sit–stand transfers, and stair ambulation. She stated that her symptoms had reduced by about 50% since her initial visit. Knee flexion AROM was 125° in supine (gain of 20° since initial examination) and 110° in prone (gain of 26°); anterior knee pain was the limiting factor. Active knee extension against gravity was not limited, and quadriceps manual muscle testing revealed a strength grade of good minus (4−/5). The tendonitis was slow to resolve, and inflammation continued to be the primary concern. Therefore, the therapeutic exercise portion of the treatment program was not progressed and continued to emphasize knee flexion and extension AAROM and AROM exercises.

Three and One-Half Weeks After Initial Examination

The patient indicated that she was pain free with ambulation, sit–stand transfers, and stair ambulation. She was employed in a food service position and was not having any major difficulty with her knee; but she did experience some discomfort when squatting and kneeling. The patient had been swimming at a fitness center for exercise and was having mild discomfort with aggressive kicking. Knee flexion ROM of the right knee was pain free and equal to the left in supine and prone. Manual muscle testing of the right quadriceps revealed mild pain and weakness (4+/5). The home treatment program was changed to prone quadriceps stretching (Fig. 3-9); open and closed kinematic chain resistance exercises for the quadriceps, hamstrings, hip musculature, and lower leg musculature; balance training; and application of ice after exercise. The patient was released and told to begin alternating jogging and biking for 20 min of aerobic exercise every other day and to progress to 30 min or more if no problems were experienced after 1 week.

OUTCOME

At the 5-week return visit, the patient reported independent performance of all activities without pain or difficulty. No abnormalities were discovered in the examination. The patient was instructed to continue her flexibility, strengthening, and aerobic exercise program; and she was discharged.

SUMMARY

- This chapter presented the benefits, applications, and techniques of various forms of ROM exercise as part of a rehabilitation program for the active individual. The three forms of range of motion exercise are passive, active-assistive, and active. All forms offer physiologic benefits such as maintenance of joint movement and nutrition, prevention of connective and muscle tissue shortening, increased circulation, pain inhibition, and promotion of connective tissue remodeling. AAROM and AROM exercises offer added benefits to muscle tissue, aiding motor function, movement performance, and coordination.
- A wide range of benefits are offered by ROM exercises; they play a useful role in the regimen of care for a multitude of pathologic conditions involving the musculoskeletal, neuromuscular, cardiopulmonary, and integumentary systems. Selection of the specific form of ROM exercise that is appropriate for the client depends on the diagnosis, impairment, and level of function. Performed gently and with caution, range of motion activities can be implemented quite early after trauma or surgery. Techniques of ROM exercise, regardless of the type, include motion in anatomic body planes, in diagonal or combined patterns, and in functional patterns that simulate those used in daily activities.
- External force used during PROM or AAROM exercises can be applied by another person or by the client. In addition, a wand, pulley, or mechanical device can be used as an external force to increase PROM or AAROM.

GERIATRIC *Perspectives*

- Joint ROM and flexibility (like strength) are lost gradually from approximately age 30 with greater losses after age 40.[1] The age-related changes affecting joint flexibility include increases in the viscosity of the synovium, calcification of articular cartilage, and stiffening of the soft tissue (particularly the joint capsule and ligaments).
- Joint movements that are often used in activities of daily living exhibit less decrease in ROM than less frequently used movements. For example, anterior trunk flexion range is less likely to be lost than backward extension, and upper extremities maintain ROM more than lower extremities. In addition, the ankle joint loses range of motion with aging. Women tend to lose more ankle range than men do. Between the ages of 55 and 85, women lose as much as 50% in ankle range, but men lose only 35%.[2] Occupational and leisure activities throughout the life may lead to osteokinematic limitations because of the development of bone spurs and degenerative changes in the articular surfaces.
- Normative data for ROM in older adults have not been adequately established. Range of motion for older adults has been found to differ from the general population.[3] Clinicians should consider these differences when examining older adults and setting goals for them.
- Functional ROM refers to the joint range used during performance of functional activities. An understanding of functional range of motion assists the clinician in establishing a plan of care that is based on functional need rather than an ideal or normal joint ROM.[4] Functional ranges for some activities of daily living have been established.[5]
- To maximize the benefits achieved through ROM exercises, the new motion should be incorporated into a functional activity or pattern. For example, a gain in shoulder flexion should be reinforced by passive, active-assistive, or active reaching tasks such as retrieving objects from overhead shelves. Research has shown that purposeful, task-oriented activity increases the physiologic gain for the patient.[6]

1. Spirduso WW. Physical dimensions of aging. Champaign, IL: Human Kinetics, 1995.
2. Vandervoort AA, Chesworth BM, Cunningham DA, et al. Age and sex effects on mobility of the human ankle. J Gerontol Med Sci 1992;47: M17–M21.
3. Walker JM, Sue D, Miles-Elkovsy N, et al. Active mobility of the extremities in older adults. Phys Ther 1984;64:919–923.
4. Goldstein TS. Functional rehabilitation in orthopaedics. Gaithersburg. MD: Aspen, 1995.
5. Young A. Exercise physiology in geriatric practice. Acta Med Scand 1986;711(suppl):227–232.
6. Gliner JA. Purposeful activity in motor learning theory: an event approach to motor skill acquisition. Am J Occup Ther 1985;39:28–34.

PEDIATRIC *Perspectives*

- The developing individual exhibits much greater mobility and flexibility than the adult.[1] Just as it is important to remember that ROM decreases with age secondary to collagen stiffening, clinicians must recognize that a wide range of normal mobility exists in children and adolescents. Because of immature bone and extremely flexible collagen, newborns exhibit patterns of extreme ROM, as evidenced by excessive dorsiflexion where the dorsum of the foot can be dorsiflexed to such a degree to make contact with the anterior tibia. This hypermobility decreases throughout childhood.
- Maintenance of ROM is essential for children with juvenile rheumatoid arthritis (JRA). Contractures involving both joint and muscle can be anticipated based on an understanding of typical patterns of restriction associated with JRA. Active range of motion exercises for management of morning stiffness in this population are essential. The soft tissue flexibility and hypermobility normally present in children suggest the need for intensive therapy for muscle and joint dysfunction in the young patient with JRA.[2] See Chapters 3 and 4 for more information on stretching and mobilization.

1. Kendall HO, Kendall FP, Boynton DA. Posture and pain. Melbourne, FL: Krieger, 1971.
2. Wright FV, Smith E. Physical therapy management of the child and adolescent with juvenile rheumatoid arthritis. In: JM Walker, A Helewa, eds. Physical therapy in arthritis. Philadelphia: Saunders, 1996:211–244.

REFERENCES

1. Cech D, Martin S. Functional movement development across the life span. Philadelphia: Saunders, 1995.
2. Rosse C, Gaddum-Rosse P. Hollinshead's Textbook of anatomy. 5th ed. Philadelphia: Lippincott-Raven, 1997.
3. Norkin CC, Levangie PK. Joint structure & function: a comprehensive analysis. 2nd ed. Philadelphia: Davis, 1992.
4. Prentice WE. Therapeutic modalities for allied health professionals. New York: McGraw-Hill, 1998.
5. Smith KL, Weiss EL, Lehmkuhl DL. Brunnstrom's clinical kinesiology. 5th ed. Philadelphia: 1983.
6. Blauvelt CT, Nelson FRT. A manual of orthopaedic terminology. 3rd ed. St. Louis: Mosby, 1985.
7. O'Toole M. Miller-Keane encyclopedia & dictionary of medicine, nursing, & allied health. 5th ed. Philadelphia: Saunders, 1992.
8. Norkin CC, White JD. Measurement of joint motion: a guide to goniometry. 2nd ed. Philadelphia: Davis, 1985.
9. Brown ME. Therapeutic recreation and exercise. Thorofare, NJ: Slack, 1990.
10. Zachazewski JE. Improving flexibility. In: RM Scully, MR Barnes, eds. Physical therapy. Philadelphia: Lippincott; 1989:698–738.
11. Cornwall MW. Biomechanics of noncontractile tissue. Phys Ther 1984;64:1869–1873.
12. Magee DJ. Orthopedic physical assessment. 3rd ed. Philadelphia: Saunders, 1997.
13. Akeson WH. Effects of immobilization on joints. Clin Orthop 1987;219:28–37.
14. Donatelli R, Owens-Burchhart H. Effects of immobilization on the extensibility of periarticular connective tissue. J Orthop Sports Phys Ther 1981;3:67–72.
15. Cummings GS, Tillman LJ. Remodeling of dense connective tissue in normal adult tissues. In: DP Currier, RM Nelson, eds. Dynamics of human biologic tissue. Philadelphia: Davis, 1992: 45–73.
16. Frank D. Physiology and therapeutic value of passive joint motion. Clin Orthop 1984;185:113–125.
17. Tomberlin JP, Saunders HD. Evaluation treatment and prevention of musculoskeletal disorders. 3rd ed. Chaska, MN: Saunders, 1994.
18. Salter RB. The physiologic basis of continuous passive motion for articular cartilage healing and regeneration. Hand Clin 1994;10: 211–219.
19. Salter RB. Textbook of disorders and injuries of the musculoskeletal system. 2nd ed. Baltimore: Williams & Wilkins. 1983.
20. Salter RB. Clinical application of basic research on continuous passive motion for disorders and injuries of synovial joints. J Orthop Res 1984;1:325–333.
21. American Physical Therapy Association. Guide to physical therapist practice, second edition. Phys Ther 2001;81:1–768.
22. Noyes FR, Barber-Westin SD. Reconstruction of the anterior and posterior cruciate ligaments after knee dislocation: use of early protected postoperative motion to decrease arthrofibrosis. Am J Sports Med 1997;25:769–778.

CHAPTER

Stretching Activities for Increasing Muscle Flexibility

William D. Bandy, PhD, PT, SCS, ATC

Muscle flexibility has been defined as "the ability of a muscle to lengthen, allowing one joint (or more than one joint in a series) to move through a range of motion."[1] Loss of flexibility is "a decrease in the ability of the muscle to deform,"[1] resulting in decreased range of motion about a joint. Studies have documented the importance of muscle flexibility for normal muscle function and for the prevention of injury. Such studies[1–4] suggest that the achievement of ideal flexibility can prevent injury, enhance athletic performance, and assist in rehabilitation after musculoskeletal injury.

The goal of a flexibility program is to improve the range of motion (ROM) at a given joint by altering the extensibility of the muscles that produce movement at that joint. Exercises that stretch these muscles over a period of time increase the range of motion around the given joint. To increase flexibility, three types of stretching exercises have been described in the literature: ballistic stretching, proprioceptive neuromuscular facilitation (PNF), and static stretching.

■ Scientific Basis

NEUROPHYSIOLOGIC PROPERTIES OF MUSCLE

To effectively stretch a muscle, the clinician must understand the neurophysiologic properties of muscle that can affect its ability to gain increased flexibility. Two sensory organs in the muscle are defined (muscle spindle and Golgi tendon organ) and two important neurophysiologic phenomena are described (autogenic inhibition and reciprocal inhibition).

Muscle Spindle

The muscle spindle is a specialized receptor consisting of unique muscle fibers, sensory endings, and motor endings that are located within muscles (Fig. 3-1). Inside the muscle spindle are specialized fibers called intrafusal muscle fibers, which are distinct from ordinary skeletal muscle fibers (extrafusal fibers).[5–7]

The sensory endings of the spindle respond to changes in the length of the muscle and the velocity at which the length changes. The ends of the intrafusal fibers connect to the extrafusal fibers; thus stretching the muscle stretches the intrafusal fibers. Afferent sensory nerves arise from the intrafusal fibers. Type Ia afferent sensory nerves respond to quick and tonic stretch of the muscle, and type II nerves monitor tonic stretch.[5–7]

When the muscle is stretched, the type Ia and type II afferent sensory nerves of the intrafusal fibers of the muscle spindle are activated. This activation causes the muscle being stretched to contract, thereby, resisting the stretch. For example, if a clinician applies a quick stretch to the hamstring muscles of a patient, the intrafusal muscle fibers within the muscle spindle react by sending impulses (via type Ia nerve fibers) to the spinal cord to inform the central nervous system (CNS) that the hamstring muscles are being stretched. Nerve impulses return from the CNS to the muscle (specifically, to the extrafusal muscle fibers via α motor neurons) to contract the hamstring muscles reflexively, essentially resisting the attempt of the hamstring muscle to elongate.[5–7]

Golgi Tendon Organ

Golgi tendon organs (GTOs) are encapsulated structures attached in series to the fibers of the tendons at the junction of extrafusal muscle fibers and tendons (Fig. 3-1). Within the capsule, sensory nerve afferent fibers (type Ib) are attached to small bundles of the tendon. The GTO is sensitive to slight changes in the tendon's tension and responds to added tension by both passive stretch of a muscle (especially at the lengthened range) and active muscle contraction.[5–7]

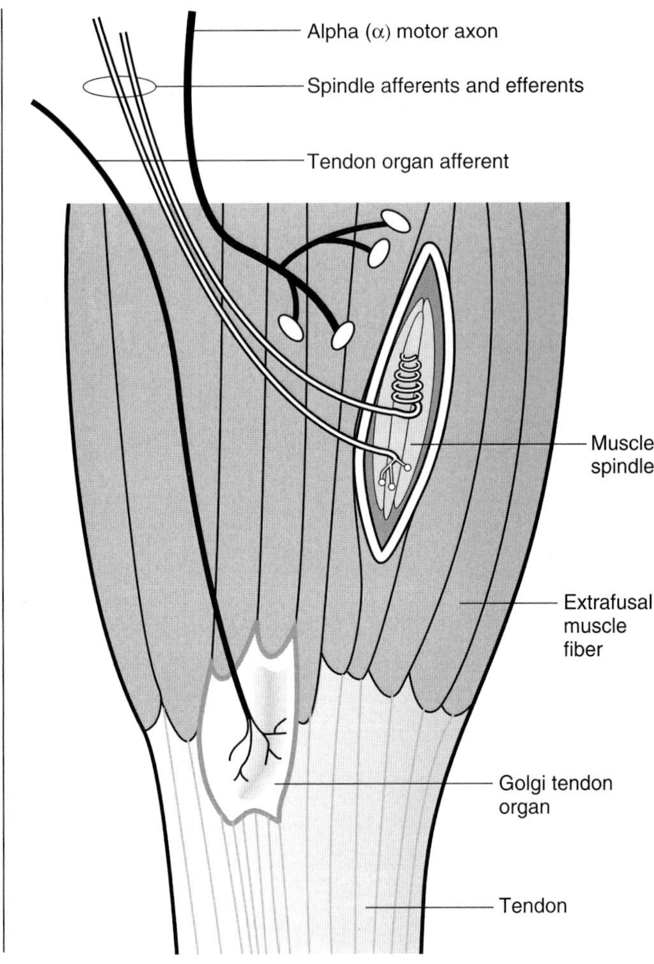

FIGURE 3-1 Muscle spindle and Golgi tendon organ.

(Reprinted with permission from Kandel ER, Schwartz JH, Jessell TM. Principles of neural science. 3rd ed. New York: Elsevier, 1991.)

The role of the GTO is to prevent overactivity of the nerve fibers innervating the extrafusal muscle (α motor neurons). In other words, if the muscle is stretched for a prolonged period of time or if an isometric contraction occurs, the GTO fires (via type Ib afferent nerve fibers) and inhibits the tension in that same muscle, allowing the muscle to elongate. For example, if the hamstring muscles are stretched for 15 to 30 sec in the lengthened range, tension is created in the tendon. The GTO responds to the tension via type Ib nerve fibers. These nerve fibers have the ability to override the impulses coming from the muscle spindle, allowing the hamstring muscles to relax reflexively. Therefore, the hamstring muscles relax and are allowed to elongate.[5–7]

Autogenic Inhibition

Stimulation of a muscle that causes its neurologic relaxation is called autogenic inhibition. Autogenic inhibition can occur when the GTO is activated. For example, a maximal isometric contraction of the hamstring muscles causes an increase in tension of the GTO. Impulses from the GTO protect the hamstring muscles by inhibiting α motor neuron activity, causing the muscles to relax.[5–7] Autogenic inhibition serves as the basis for the PNF stretching technique called contract–relax (discussed later in this chapter).

Reciprocal Inhibition

Reciprocal inhibition is an important neurologic mechanism that inhibits the antagonist muscle as the agonist muscle (the prime mover) moves a limb through the range of motion. In any synergistic muscle group, a contraction of the agonist causes a reflexive relaxation of the antagonist muscle. For example, during active flexion of the hip, reciprocal inhibition relaxes the hamstring muscles. This relaxation ensures that the hip flexors are able to move through the ROM without being influenced by contracting hamstring muscles.[5–7] Reciprocal inhibition serves as the basis for the PNF stretching technique called hold–relax (discussed later in this chapter).

BALLISTIC STRETCHING

Definition

Ballistic stretching imposes repetitive bouncing or jerking movements on the muscles to be stretched.[1,8] An example of a ballistic stretch is the sitting toe touch. The individual sits on the ground with the legs straight out in front (long sitting) and reaches the hands forward as far down the legs as possible. Leaning forward by contracting the abdominal muscles, the individual quickly reaches toward the ankles (or, if possible, past the feet) and immediately returns to the original long sitting position. This movement is repeated 10 to 15 times, with each bounce extending the arms a bit farther.

Although research indicates that ballistic stretching increases muscle flexibility, some clinicians are concerned that the bouncing activity has the potential to cause injury, especially when a previous injury has occurred in the muscle. Theoretically, the quick, jerking ballistic motion can exceed the limits of muscle extensibility in an uncontrolled manner and result in injury.[1,8]

In addition, the quick bouncing of the muscle stretches the muscle spindle. As noted earlier, activation of the muscle spindle sends sensory impulses to the spinal cord via type Ia afferent nerves, informing the CNS that the muscle is being stretched. Impulses returning to the muscle via α motor neurons cause the muscle to contract, thereby, resisting the stretch.[5–7] Concern exists that the facilitation of the muscle spindle that occurs during ballistic activities may cause microtrauma in the muscle owing to the tension created when the muscle is stretched.

Thus ballistic stretching has generally fallen out of favor among most clinicians because of the possibility of injury caused by uncontrolled jerking and bouncing motions and because the activation of the afferent nerve fibers of the muscle spindle causes a contraction of the same muscle that is being stretched.[1,8]

Alternative Perspective

Zachazewski[1] questions whether static stretching has been overemphasized in athletes at the expense of ballistic stretching. He argues that the dynamic actions required for high-performance athletic movements require ballistic-type activities (Fig. 3-2). If used appropriately, ballistic stretching may play a vital role in the training of an athlete, because so much of athletic activities are ballistic in nature.

Zachazewski proposes a "progressive velocity flexibility program," in which the athlete is taken through a series of ballistic stretching activities (Fig. 3-3). The program varies the velocity (slow, fast) and range of motion (end range, full range) of the ballistic stretch. He emphasizes that the individual must first perform static stretches (Fig. 3-3). After an unspecified period of training using static stretches, the athletes progress from slow, controlled stretching at the end of the ROM to high-velocity ballistic stretching through the full ROM.

As indicated in Figure 3-3, after a period of performing static stretches (SS), the next step in the progression is slow short end-range (SSER) activities. This portion of the stretching program incorporates ballistic stretches in a slow, controlled manner with small oscillations at the end of the range. Once the athlete is comfortable with performing the slow oscillations, the program is progressed to slow full-range (SFR) activities, which are slow ballistic stretches through a much greater range of the length of the muscle. As the program advances over weeks to months, the athlete performs a high-velocity ballistic stretch in a small range of motion at the end of the ROM, called fast short end-range (FSER) activities. Finally, a high-velocity ballistic stretch is performed by the athlete through the entire length of the muscle, called fast full-range (FFR) activities.

Zachazewski emphasizes that two important concepts should be considered before incorporating ballistic activities into a stretching program. First, because sedentary individuals and most geriatric individuals do not frequently

FIGURE 3-2

Dynamic activities such as gymnastics may be appropriately trained using ballistic stretching.

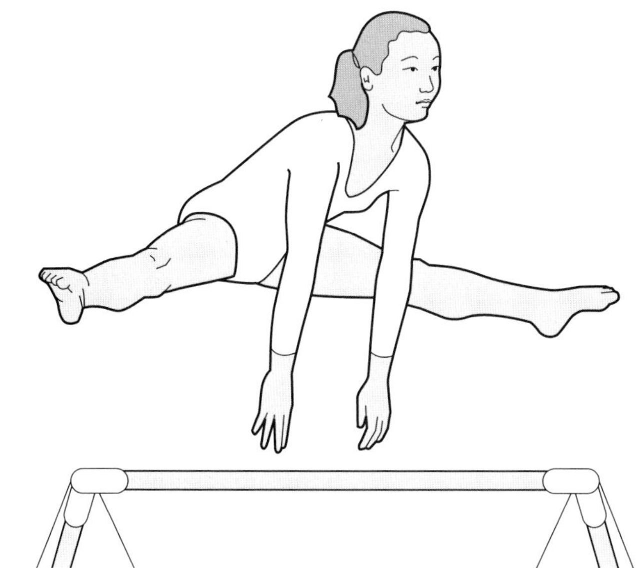

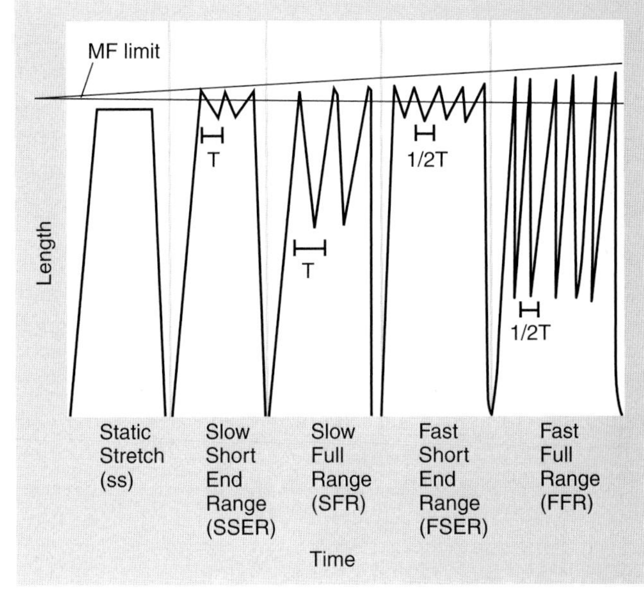

FIGURE 3-3 **Progressive velocity flexibility program.**

(Reprinted with permission from Zachazewski J. Flexibility for sports. In: B Sanders, ed. Sports physical therapy. Norwalk, CT: Appleton & Lange, 1990:201–238.)

use high-velocity, dynamic activities in their daily lives, ballistic stretching may not be appropriate for them. Static stretching appears to be the appropriate means of increasing flexibility of muscle in the nonathletic population. Second, before beginning a ballistic stretching program, the athlete should be properly and extensively trained in static stretching. The proportion of ballistic to static stretching should then be gradually increased as the athletic level of conditioning progresses.

To date, no research has been performed on Zachazewski's progressive velocity flexibility program. Therefore, initiation of the program should be carefully monitored by the clinician to ensure that the athlete is not being overaggressive, creating pain in or damage to the muscle being stretched. In addition, given the aggressive nature of ballistic stretching, it is not appropriate for an injured muscle.

PROPRIOCEPTIVE NEUROMUSCULAR FACILITATION

According to Knott and Voss,[9] PNF techniques are methods "of promoting or hastening the response of a neuromuscular mechanism through stimulation of the proprioceptor." Based on these concepts of influencing muscle response, the techniques of PNF can be used to strengthen and increase flexibility of muscle. This chapter focuses on the use of PNF to increase flexibility; Chapter 8 emphasizes the use of PNF to strengthen muscle.

Brief contraction before a brief static stretch of the muscle is the mainstay of the PNF techniques for increasing flexibility of the muscle. The terminology used to describe PNF stretching activities has varied widely, including the use of the following terms: contract–relax, hold–relax, slow reversal hold–relax, agonist contraction, contract–relax with agonist contraction, and hold–relax with agonist contraction. Furthermore, sometimes the same term is used for different PNF stretching techniques. For example, Etnyre and Lee[10] describe contract–relax as involving an isometric contraction, whereas the American Academy of Orthopaedic Surgeons (AAOS)[11] describes contract–relax as using a concentric contraction.

Part of the confusion in the terminology is that in their original description of PNF stretching techniques, Knott and Voss[9] specified diagonal patterns for performing the stretching activity. Today, most clinicians do not perform the techniques using the original diagonal patterns, rather they recommend moving in straight planes. Proprioceptive neuromuscular facilitation terminology cannot be transferred exactly from diagonal to straight-plane techniques. Thus, there is no consistency in the terminology used to describe PNF stretching techniques.

Three PNF stretching techniques will be defined in this chapter: hold–relax, contract–relax, and slow reversal hold–relax. The definitions presented are based on a review of literature[10–14] and on clinical experience.

Hold–Relax

1. The clinician passively moves the limb to be stretched to the end of the ROM. For example, if the hamstring muscles are to be stretched, the lower extremity (with knee extended) is passively flexed by the clinician to full hip flexion (Fig. 3-4).

2. Once the end range of motion of the muscle is attained, the client applies a 10-sec isometric force against the clinician, thereby, contracting the muscle. For example, the client contracts the hamstring muscles by extending the hip against the clinician (Fig 3-5). The isometric contraction of the muscle being stretched (ham-

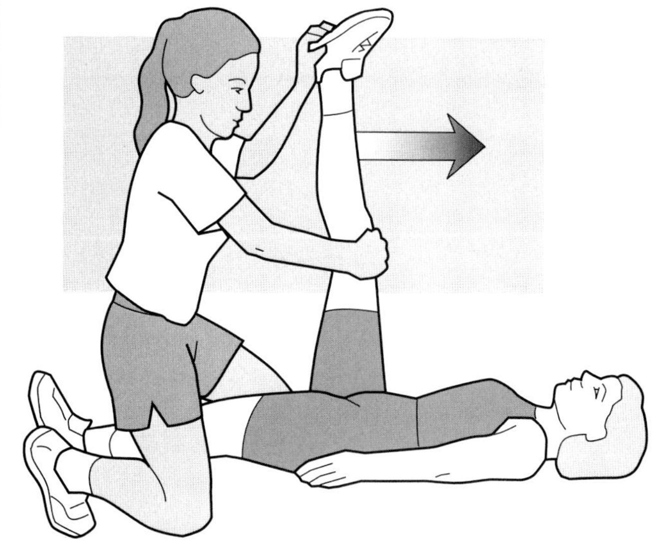

FIGURE 3-4

The lower extremity is passively flexed by the clinician to full hip flexion.

string muscles) causes an increase in tension in that muscle, which stimulates the GTO. The GTO then causes a reflexive relaxation of the muscle (autogenic inhibition) before the muscle is moved to a new stretch position and passively stretched (next step).

3. After the isometric contraction, the client is instructed to relax, and the limb is moved by the clinician to a new stretch position beyond the original starting point. The client's leg is then held in the new position for 10 to 15 sec. For example, the clinician passively and gently moves the leg into more hip flexion, maintaining the position for 10 to 15 sec (Fig. 3-6),

4. Without lowering the leg, the process (steps 2 and 3) may be repeated three to five times. After the last sequence is performed, the leg is lowered.

Contract–Relax

1. The clinician passively moves the limb to be stretched to the end of the ROM. For example, if the hamstring muscles are to be stretched, the lower extremity (with knee extended) is passively flexed by the clinician to full hip flexion (Fig. 3-4).

2. Once the end range of motion is attained, the clinician asks the client to attempt to perform a concentric contraction of the opposite muscle to the muscle being stretched, causing more of a stretch. For example, the

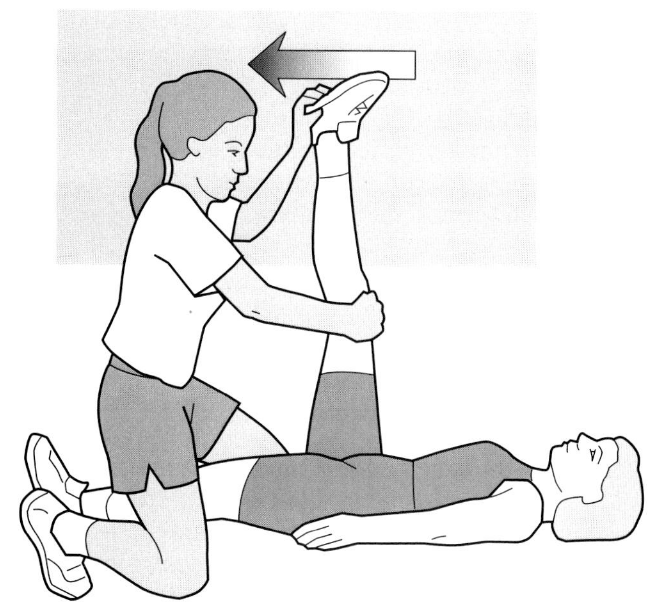

FIGURE 3-5

By isometrically extending the hip against the clinician, the hamstring muscles are contracted.

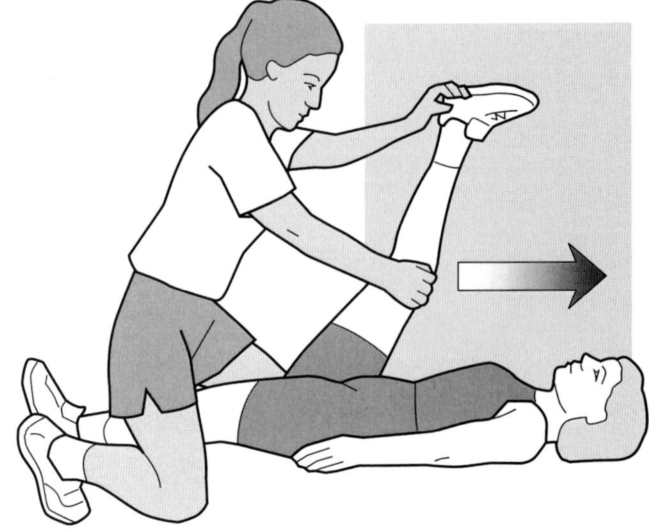

FIGURE 3-6

The clinician passively and gently moves the leg into more hip flexion.

client is asked to actively flex the hip farther to increase the stretch of the hamstring muscles. This activity is similar to that shown in Figure 3-6, except the increase in hip flexion ROM is not obtained passively by the clinician pushing but is obtained actively by the client contracting the hip flexors. As described earlier, in any synergistic muscle group, a contraction of the agonist (hip flexor) causes a reflexive relaxation of the antagonist muscle (hamstring), allowing the antagonist muscle to relax for a more effective stretch (reciprocal inhibition).

3. As the client performs the concentric contraction, causing more of a stretch, the clinician takes up the slack into any ROM that was gained. Keeping the limb in the new stretch position, the clinician asks the client to relax and holds the position for 10 to 15 sec. For example, as the client actively flexes the hip, the clinician maintains hands on the leg and moves with the leg into the hip flexion range of motion that is gained and then holds the leg there for 10 to 15 sec.

4. Without lowering the leg, the process (steps 2 and 3) may be repeated three to five times. After the last sequence is performed, the leg is lowered.

Slow Reversal Hold–Relax

1. The clinician passively moves the limb to be stretched to the end of the ROM. For example, if the hamstring muscles are to be stretched, the lower extremity (with knee extended) is passively flexed by the clinician to full hip flexion (Fig. 3-4).

2. Once the end range of motion of the muscle is attained, the client applies a 10-sec isometric force against the clinician, thereby contracting the muscle to be stretched (autogenic inhibition). For example, the client contracts the hamstrings by extending the hip against the clinician (Fig. 3-5).

3. After the isometric contraction of the muscle is performed, the clinician asks the client to attempt to perform a concentric contraction of the opposite muscle, causing more of a stretch (reciprocal inhibition). For example, after the isometric contraction of the hamstring muscles, the client is asked to actively flex the hip farther.

4. As the client performs the concentric contraction, causing more of a stretch, the clinician takes up the slack into any ROM that was gained. Keeping the limb in the new stretch position, the clinician asks the client to relax and holds the position for 10 to 15 sec. For example, as the client actively flexes the hip, the clinician maintains hands on the leg and moves with the leg into the hip flexion ROM that is gained and then holds the leg there for 10 to 15 sec.

5. Without lowering the leg, the process (steps 2 to 4) may be repeated three to five times. After the last sequence is performed, the leg is lowered.

Research has indicated that PNF stretching techniques are effective in increasing flexibility of muscle. To date, however, no consensus exists as to which single PNF technique is the most effective.[10,13,14]

STATIC STRETCHING

Definition

Static stretching is a method by which the muscle is slowly elongated to tolerance (a comfortable stretch, short of pain) and the position is held with the muscle in this greatest tolerated length. In this lengthened position, a mild tension should be felt in the muscle that is being stretched, and pain and discomfort should be avoided.[2,8]

A slow, prolonged stretch is used to reduce the reflex contraction from the muscle spindle. More specifically, if the static stretch is held long enough, any effect of the type

Ia and II afferent fibers from the muscle spindle may be minimized. In addition, because the static stretch in the lengthened position places tension on the tendon, the GTO may be facilitated to protect the muscle being stretched. This facilitation of the GTO fires type Ib nerve fibers, which inhibit and relax the muscle being stretched (autogenic inhibition). Therefore, the combined neurologic effects that occur during the static stretch are minimizing the influence of the muscle spindle and facilitating the effect of the GTO. This will ultimately allow the muscle being stretched to elongate, increasing muscle flexibility.[5–7]

Most literature documenting the effectiveness of static stretching has been performed on muscles of the lower extremities, and little research has been performed on the spine and upper extremities. Gajdosik[15] indicates that using a slow static stretch increases the flexibility of the hamstring muscles, Madding et al.[16] report gains in hip abduction ROM after passive stretching, and two studies by Bandy et al.[17,18] indicate static stretching is effective for increasing flexibility of the hamstring muscles.

Duration

Recommendations for the optimum duration of holding the static stretch vary from as little as 15 sec to as long as 60 sec.[15–18] Unfortunately, some authors have collected data before and after only one bout of stretching on one day and have not provided evidence for the most effective duration for stretching activities that take place for more than one day (e.g., weeks).

Bandy et al.[17,18] examined different durations of static stretching that were performed 5 days per week for 6 weeks. They examined the effects of hamstring muscle stretching across a variety of durations, including comparing groups that stretched for 15, 30, and 60 sec to a control group that did not stretch. The results indicate that 30 and 60 sec of static stretching were more effective at increasing hamstring muscle flexibility than stretching for 15 sec or not stretching at all. No difference was found between 30 and 60 sec of stretching, indicating that the two durations had equal effect on flexibility.

■ *Clinical Guidelines*

Although several investigations have studied the efficiency of one type of stretching over another, no absolute recommendation for the most appropriate type of stretching activity for increasing the flexibility of muscle has been made. Research indicates that ballistic stretching, PNF, and static stretching all increase flexibility of muscle.[1,2,8] But the greatest potential for trauma appears to be from ballistic stretching, because of its jerking motions. In addition, even those who advocate ballistic stretching for advanced training recommend a solid base of static stretching before incorporating ballistic movements into a flexibility program.

Techniques for PNF not only require the most expertise of the three types of stretching but also require a second individual to perform the techniques. The need for an experienced practitioner makes PNF somewhat cumbersome. The easiest and most common method of stretching used to increase flexibility of muscle appears to be static stretching. Therefore, the rest of this chapter emphasizes the static stretch.

Proper static stretching slowly elongates the muscles to a point at which a mild pull or tension is felt by the client. This elongated position should be held for 30 sec, during which time the client should not feel any discomfort. If during the 30-sec stretch the mild tension subsides, the client should change his or her position to achieve a more aggressive stretch of the muscle and to feel a mild pull or tension (but no discomfort or pain). If during the stretch, the tension grows in intensity and the client feels discomfort or pain, he or she should be instructed to ease off the stretch into a more comfortable position while maintaining mild tension. Each stretching activity should be performed at least once per day.[17,18]

If possible, attempts should be made to integrate the stretching activity into the client's daily activities. Holding a stretch for 30 sec can be boring. If the stretch can be performed at the office while talking on the phone, in the car while stopped in traffic at a stoplight, or at home while watching television, the client is more likely to be compliant with the stretching program than if the movements must be performed in a specific place at a specific time. Obviously, not all the techniques presented in this chapter can be performed in all work environments, but the creative clinician can be a great asset to clients who complain that they do not have time to practice a stretching program.

Ideally, stretching to increase flexibility should be performed after a general warmup. The warmup may be a 3- to 5-min repetitive activity such as walking, slow jogging, stationary bicycling, or active arm exercises. But inability or unwillingness to warm up should not preclude an individual from performing the stretching program. In fact, many stretching programs have failed because of this requirement to start with a warmup. If a warmup is not possible (for what ever reason), following the recommendation of performing the stretch to the point of mild tension should be strictly adhered to.[1,2]

If possible, the muscle to be stretched should be isolated, and the individual should be encouraged to focus on the muscle region that is pulling the body part into the stretch position. Isolating the muscle to be stretched is more effective than performing a general stretch that works two or three muscles (such as bending over and touching the toes). Generally, a stretching technique is appropriate if the client feels a mild pull in the muscle that he or she is trying to stretch.

Finally, one point must be reiterated. As noted, the client should feel only mild tension and no discomfort when stretching. In other words, the client should not stretch to the point that pain is felt in the muscle or joint. If the client stretches aggressively and into the painful range of motion, the muscle will actually tighten. Aggressive stretching while the muscles are being contracted and tightened may lead to microscopic tears, which in turn may lead to the formation of nonelastic scar tissue. Such scar tissue will not adapt to the normal demands made on the muscle, leading to injury caused by the lack of blood supply and disturbed afferent input.

Techniques

As noted, most of the techniques described in this chapter focus on the static stretch. In addition, for each technique presented, the suggested duration of stretch is 30 sec, unless otherwise noted.

EXTREMITIES

Figures 3-7 to 3-18 describe common static stretching activities for specific muscles of the lower extremities. Stretching techniques for the upper extremities are more general (i.e., not usually specific to any one muscle) and are presented in Figures 3-19 to 3-25.

SPINE

When stretching the cervical region, specific muscles can be identified and worked. These static stretches are presented in Figures 3-26 to 3-28. Muscles of the lumbar spine are usually stretched in a general manner, similar to

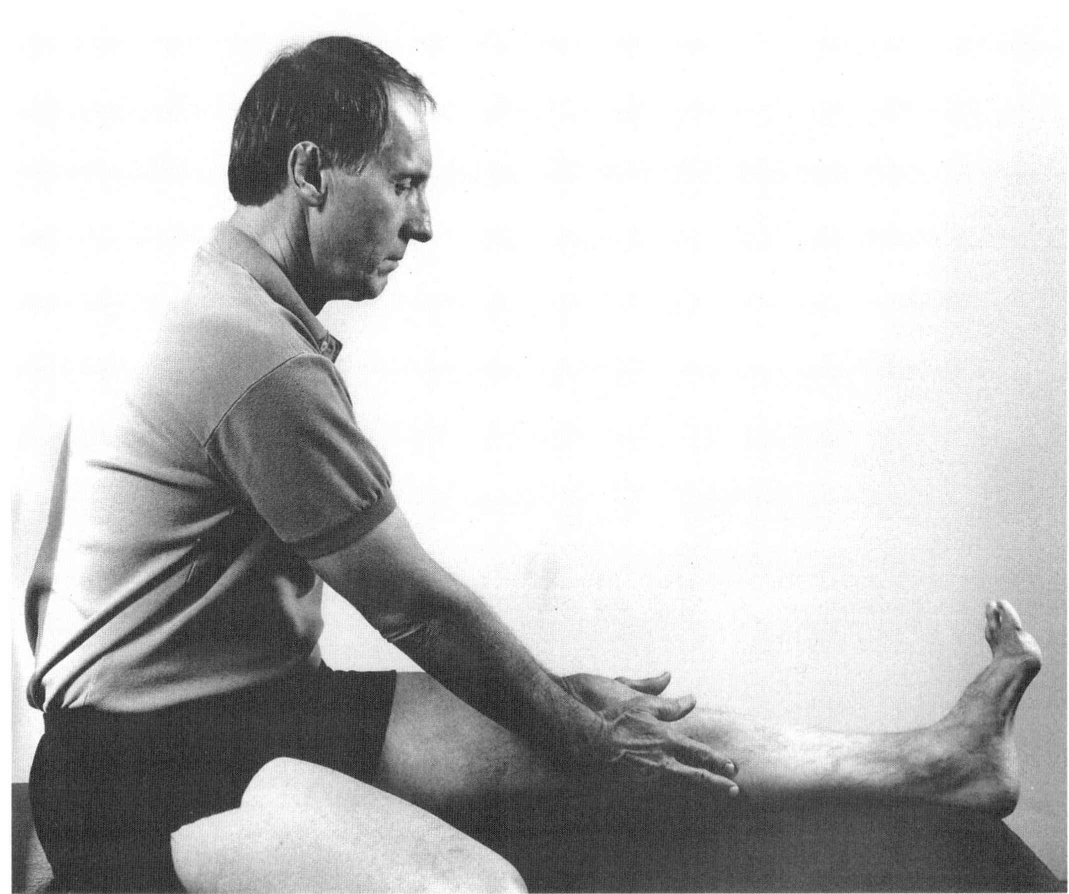

FIGURE 3-7 **Sitting hamstring muscle stretch.**

PURPOSE: Increase flexibility of the hamstring muscles.

POSITION: Client sitting with leg to be stretched straight out in front of body with the knee fully extended.

PROCEDURE: While maintaining the neutral position of the spine and flexing at the hips, the client reaches forward with both hands as far as possible down the leg until a mild tension is felt in the posterior thigh. Client should lean forward by bringing the chest forward. Flexion of the lumbar spine should be minimal.

FIGURE 3-8 **Standing hamstring muscle stretch.**

PURPOSE: Increase flexibility of the hamstring muscles.

POSITION: Client standing erect with one foot on floor and pointing straight ahead with no rotation of the hip. The heel of the leg to be stretched is placed on an elevated surface with the knee fully extended, toes pointed to ceiling, and no rotation of the hip. The elevated surface should be high enough to cause a gentle stretch in the posterior thigh when the client leans forward.

NOTE: It is vital that the foot position is maintained. If the weight-bearing foot is allowed to externally rotate, the hamstring muscle will not be effectively stretched.

PROCEDURE: While maintaining a neutral position of the spine and flexion from the hips, the client leans forward by bringing the chest forward until a mild tension is felt in the posterior thigh. Flexion of the lumbar spine should be minimal.

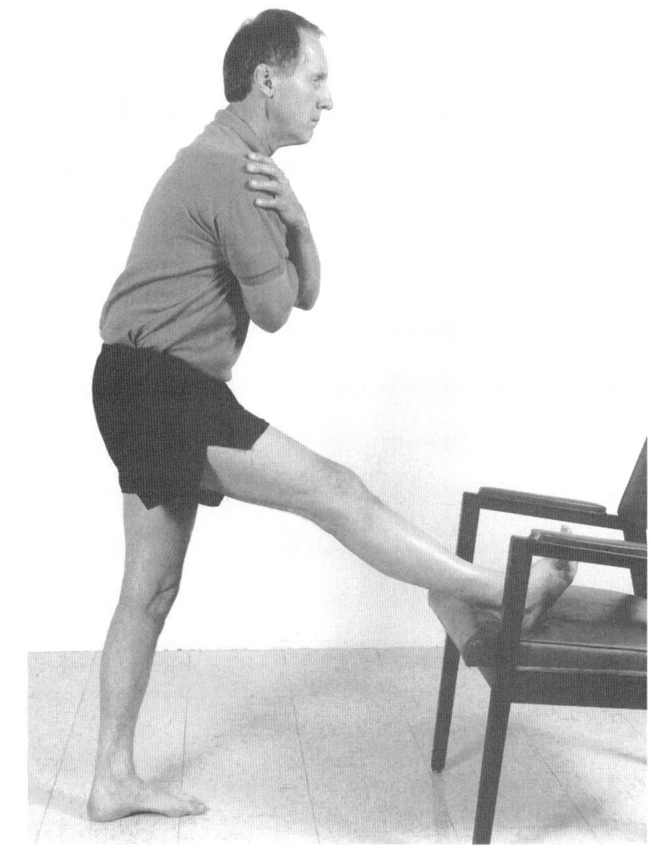

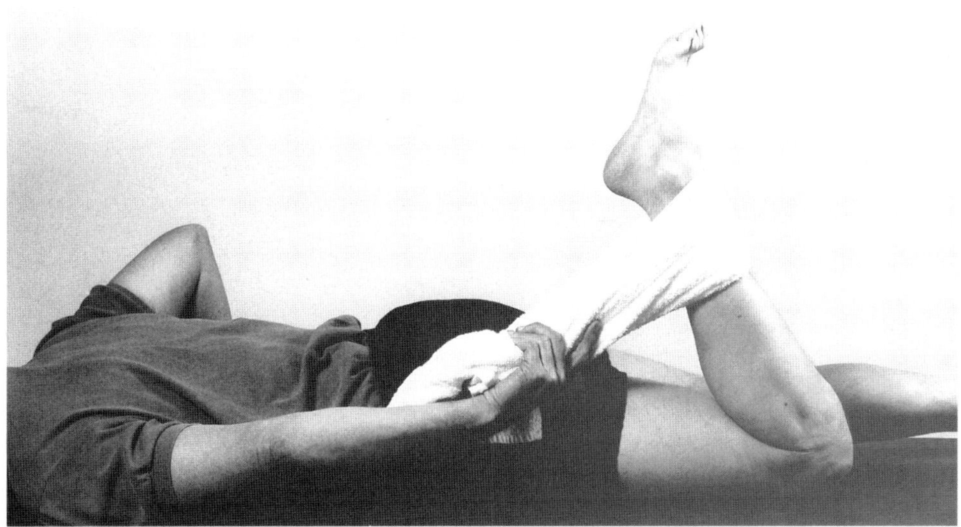

FIGURE 3-9 **Prone quadriceps muscle stretch.**

PURPOSE: Increase flexibility of the quadriceps muscles.

POSITION: Client lying prone. Hips should be placed in neutral and not abducted.

PROCEDURE: Client reaches back with one hand, grasps the foot, and moves the heel toward the buttock. By pulling on the foot, the client flexes the knee until a mild tension is felt in the anterior thigh.

NOTE: The figure demonstrates the use of a towel for a client who cannot reach the foot owing to lack of flexibility in the quadriceps muscle. The client pulls the towel, which is draped around the foot to flex the knee.

FIGURE 3-10 Standing quadriceps muscle stretch.

PURPOSE: Increase flexibility of the quadriceps muscles.

POSITION: Client standing and holding on to a chair for support, if necessary. Hip remains in neutral and not abducted or flexed.

PROCEDURE: Client reaches back with hand, grasps the foot, and moves the heel toward the buttock. By pulling on the foot, the client flexes the knee until a mild tension is felt in the anterior thigh. It is important not to let the hip abduct or flex during the stretch.

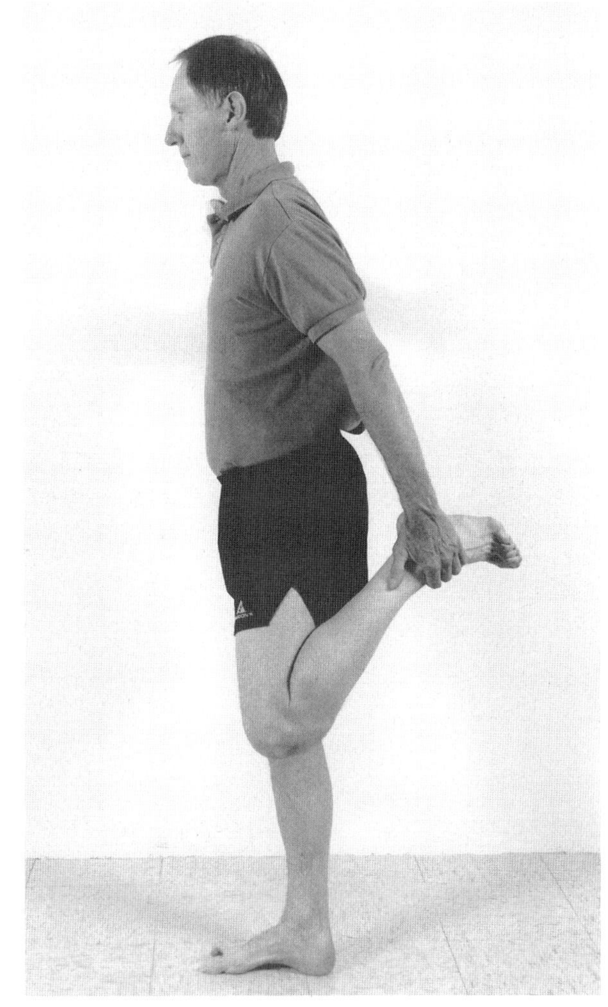

FIGURE 3-11 Modified lotus position.

PURPOSE: Increase flexibility of the adductor muscles.

POSITION: Client sitting, bending knees, and placing soles of feet together while maintaining neutral position of the spine. The client grasps both feet with hands.

PROCEDURE: Client slowly pulls self forward with hands and allows the knees to drop to the floor until a mild tension is felt in the groin. Client bends forward from the hips, maintaining neutral position of the spine. For increased stretch, the client can gently push the legs into more abduction by pushing down with the forearms.

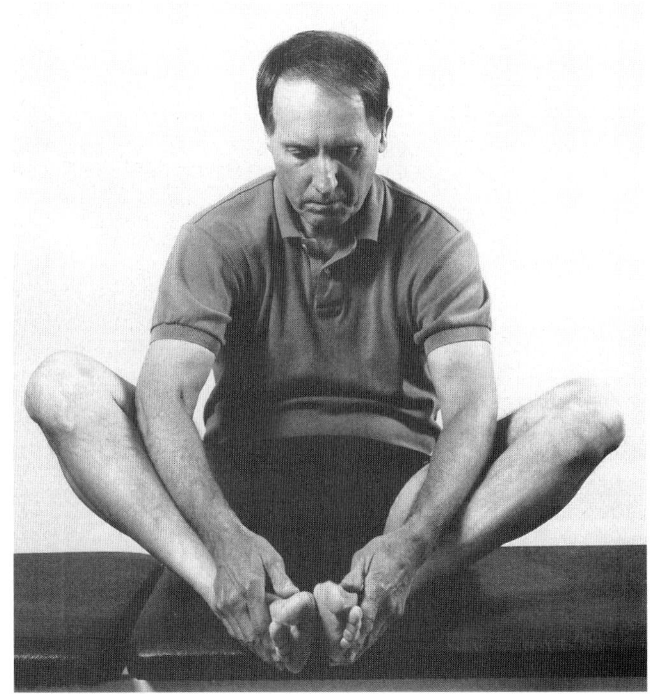

FIGURE 3-12 **Forward straddle.**

PURPOSE: Increase flexibility of the adductor muscles.

POSITION: Client sitting with knees extended and legs fully spread into abduction.

PROCEDURE: Maintaining neutral position of the spine, client bends forward from the hips. While bending forward, the hands slide forward in front of the client until a mild tension is felt in the groin bilaterally.

NOTE: The stretch can be modified by bending the trunk to the left or right and sliding the hands down the leg until a mild tension is felt in the groin unilaterally.

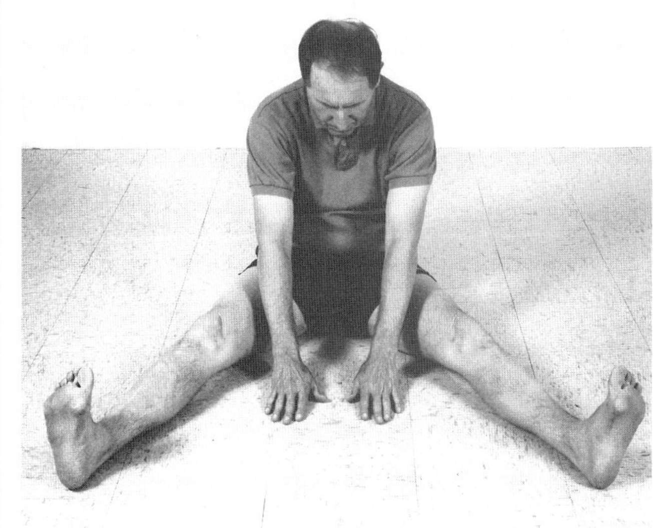

FIGURE 3-13 **Lunge.**

PURPOSE: Increase flexibility of the hip flexor muscles.

POSITION: Client standing with one leg forward, similar to taking a giant step.

PROCEDURE: Keeping a neutral spine, client moves forward into the lunge position until the forward leg is directly over the ankle. The knee of the opposite leg should be resting on the floor. Client should assume an upright position that allows a mild tension to be felt in the anterior hip of the trailing leg.

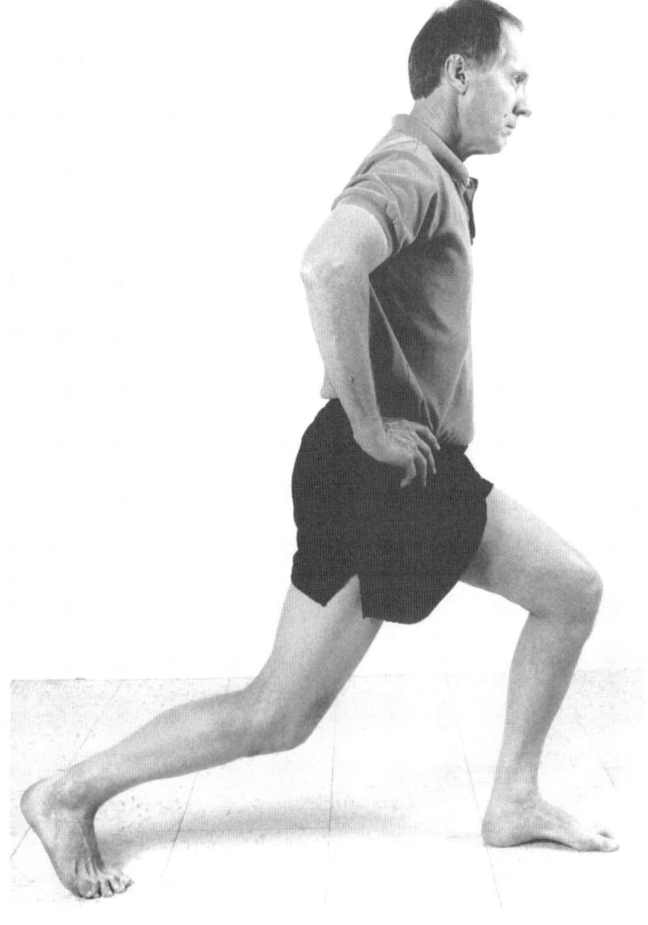

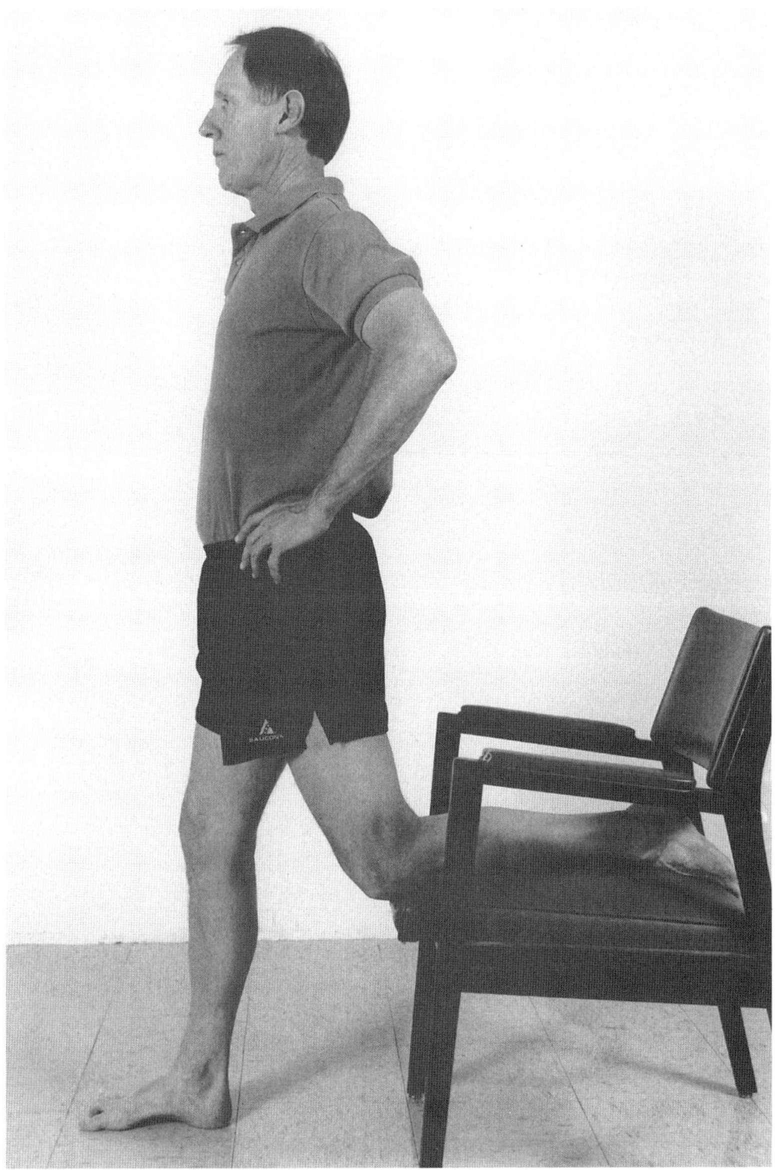

FIGURE 3-14 Hip flexor stretch using assistance of chair.

PURPOSE: Increase flexibility of the hip flexor muscles.

POSITION: Client standing and holding on to a chair for support, if necessary. One leg is firmly planted on the ground and other leg is placed on a chair behind client.

PROCEDURE: Standing upright, client carefully moves the leg on the ground forward by taking small hops. Once client finds a position in which a mild tension is felt in the anterior hip of the non-weight-bearing leg, the position is maintained.

the upper extremities (i.e., the techniques are not specific to any one muscle group). Static stretching techniques for the lumbar spine are presented in Figures 3-29 to 3-32.

PNF: CONTRACT–RELAX

The procedures of PNF contract–relax can be used for most static stretching procedures identified in Figures 3-7 to 3-32 by having a clinician add a contraction of the stretched muscle at the end of the ROM before the static stretch. Three types of PNF techniques for stretching the hamstring muscles were described earlier in this chapter. Using those basic principles, the clinician should be able to transform most of the static stretching techniques into PNF stretching techniques.

FIGURE 3-15 **Standing iliotibial band stretch.**

PURPOSE: Increase flexibility of the iliotibial band.

POSITION: Client standing approximately 3 feet away from wall and leaning on wall. Client places one leg on the ground in front leaving the other leg straight and behind. Client internally rotates the hip of the back leg.

PROCEDURE: Client protrudes the hip of the leg that is back out to the side, as the shoulders are leaned in the opposite direction. Mild tension should be felt at the lateral hip and thigh.

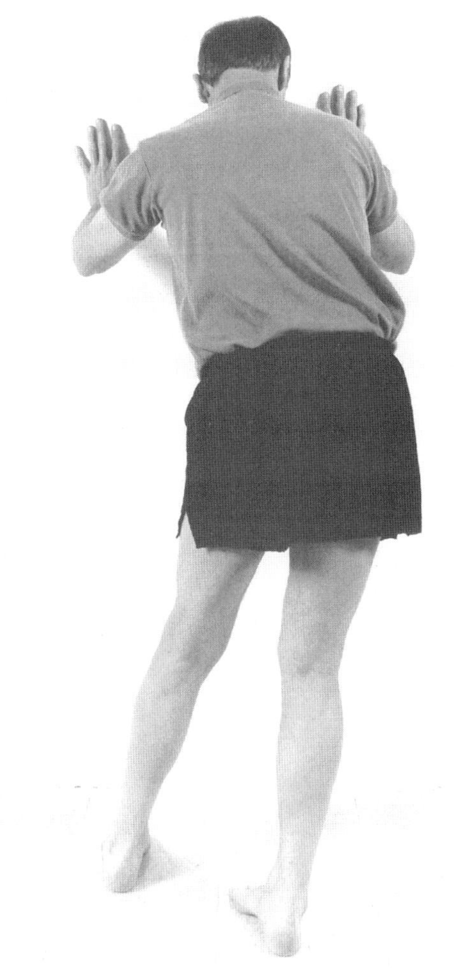

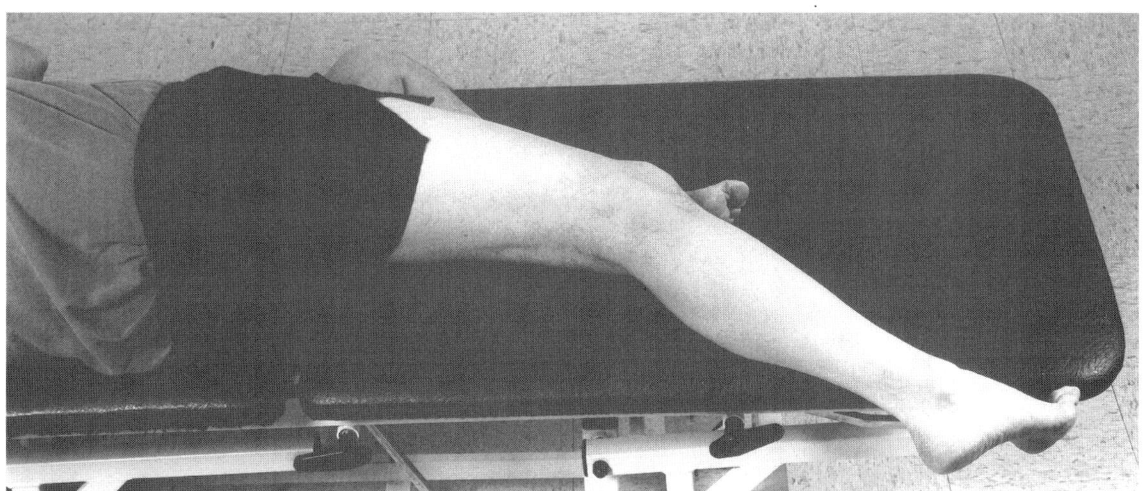

FIGURE 3-16 **Side-lying iliotibial band stretch.**

PURPOSE: Increase flexibility of the iliotibial band.

POSITION: Client side lying. Lower extremity on support surface (iliotibial band not being stretched) flexed to 45° hip and knee flexion.

PROCEDURE: Lower extremity to be stretched (iliotibial band not on support surface) is extended in line with the trunk and allowed to passively adduct toward the support surface. A mild tension should be felt in the lateral thigh.

FIGURE 3-17 **Gastrocnemius muscle stretch.**

PURPOSE: Increase flexibility of the gastrocnemius muscle.

POSITION: Client standing with feet shoulder-width apart approximately 3 feet from wall with hips internally rotated (toes of feet pointed inward). Knees are extended.

PROCEDURE: Client leans forward on the wall providing support with forearms. While leaning forward, the pelvis should be held in and not protruded. The heels should not come off the floor. A mild tension should be felt in the calf area. If it is not felt, client should stand farther away from the wall before leaning forward. If discomfort or pain are felt, client should move closer to the wall before leaning forward.

NOTE: During the procedure, it is important to maintain the original internally rotated position of the hips and flexion of the knees.

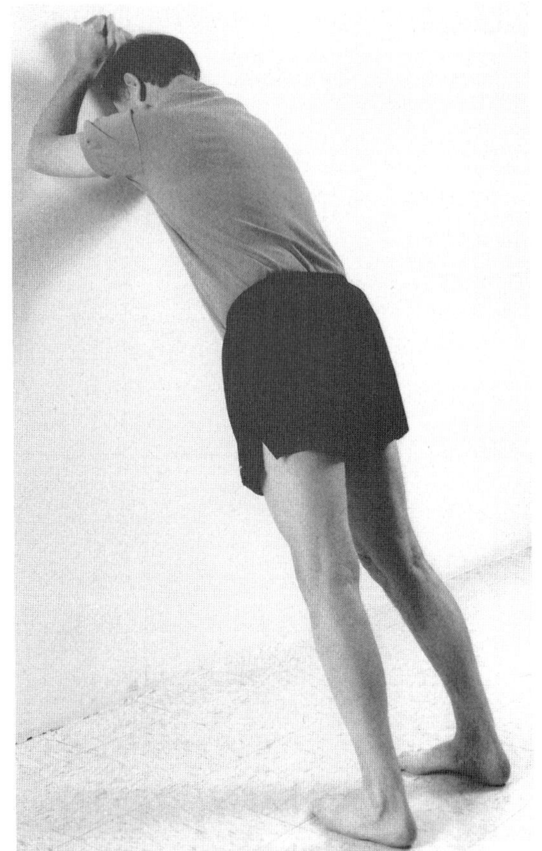

FIGURE 3-18 **Soleus muscle stretch.**

PURPOSE: Increase flexibility of the soleus muscle.

POSITION: Client standing with feet shoulder-width apart approximately 2 feet from wall with hips internally rotated (toes of feet pointed inward). Knees should be flexed to 20° to 30°.

PROCEDURE: While maintaining the flexed knees, client leans forward on the wall, providing support with forearms. While leaning forward, the pelvis should be held in, and not protruded. The heels should not come off the floor. A mild tension should be felt in the lower third of the posterior leg. If it is not felt, client should stand farther away from the wall before leaning forward. If discomfort or pain are felt, client should move closer to the wall before leaning forward.

NOTE: During the procedure, it is important to maintain the original internally rotated position of the hips and flexion of the knees.

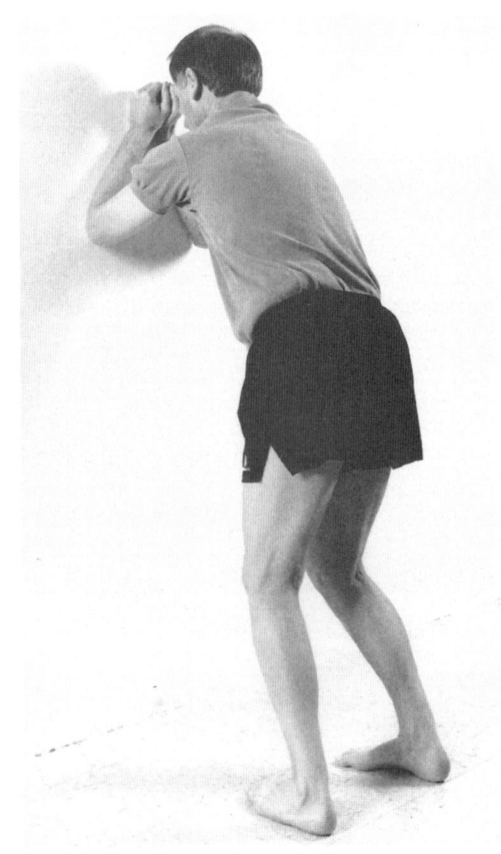

FIGURE 3-19 **Pectoral stretch (with assistance).**

PURPOSE: Increase flexibility of the pectoralis major muscle.

POSITION: Client lying supine, grasping hands behind the head.

PROCEDURE: While keeping the hands grasped behind the head, client relaxes the arms, allowing them to drop down to the support surface. A mild tension should be felt in the anterior shoulder bilaterally. To accentuate this stretch, the clinician applies a gentle force to the elbows bilaterally to push the elbows down toward the support surface. The force should be gentle, and the clinician must ensure that client feels mild tension in the anterior shoulder. The force should not cause pain or discomfort.

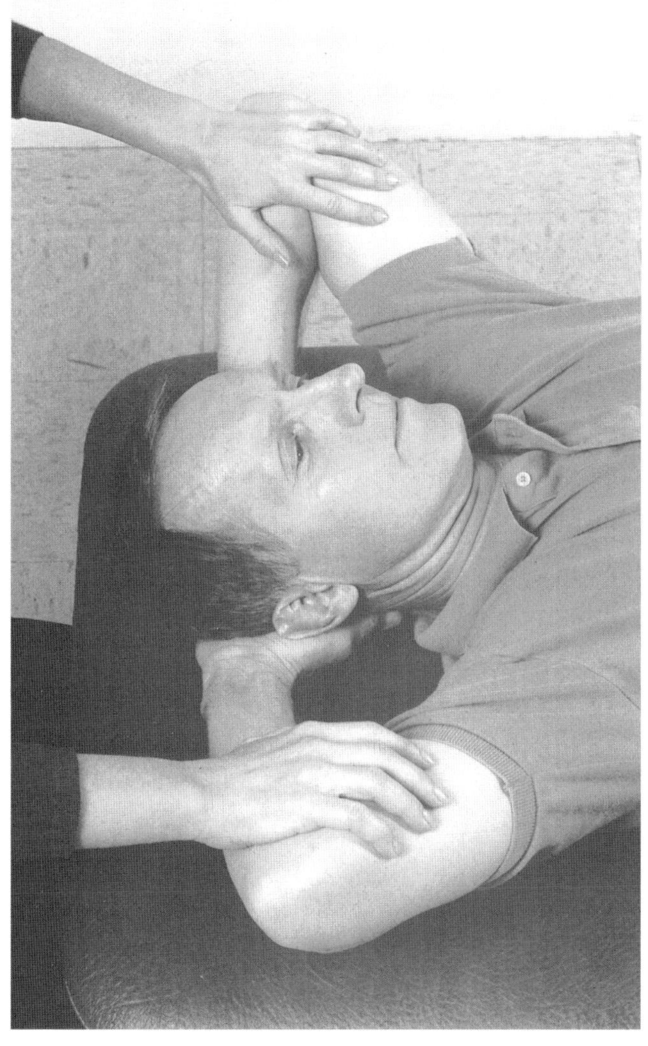

FIGURE 3-20 **Horizontal adduction stretch.**

PURPOSE: Increase flexibility of muscles of the posterior rotator cuff.

POSITION: Client sitting or standing. Client horizontally adducts the shoulder across the chest, with the elbow kept relatively extended. Client grasps the horizontally adducted shoulder proximal to the elbow.

PROCEDURE: With the grasping hand, client pulls the shoulder across the chest into more horizontal adduction until a mild tension is felt in the posterior aspect of the shoulder.

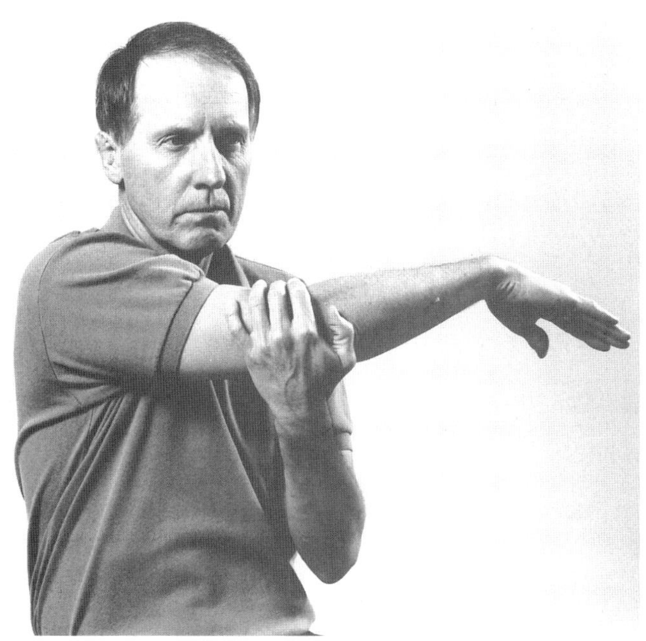

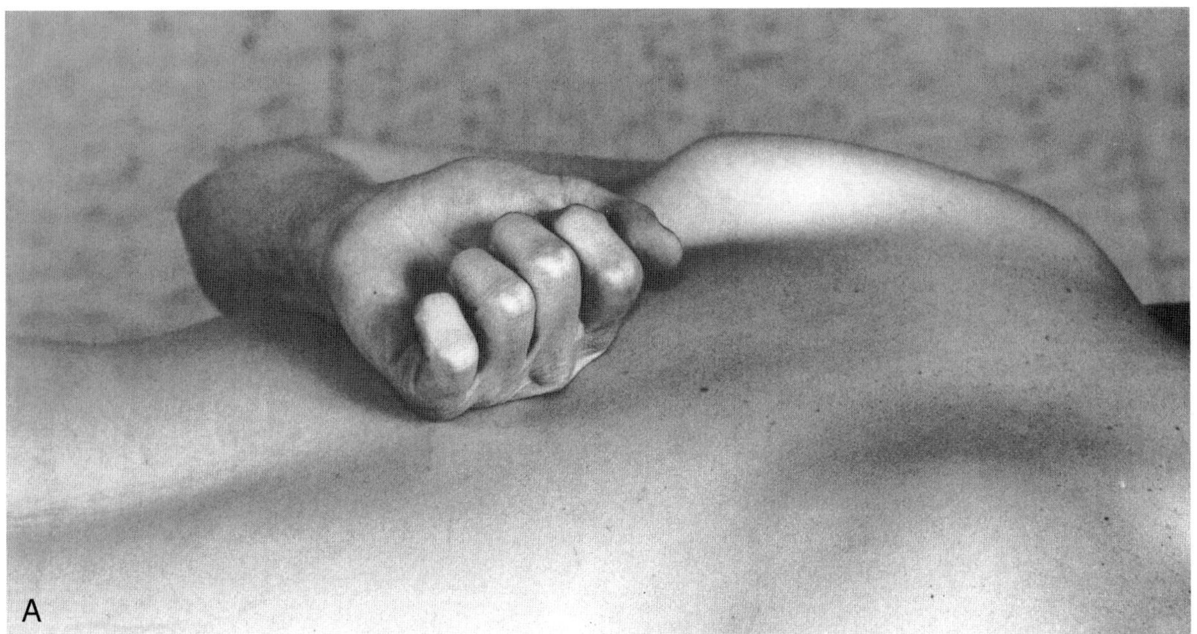

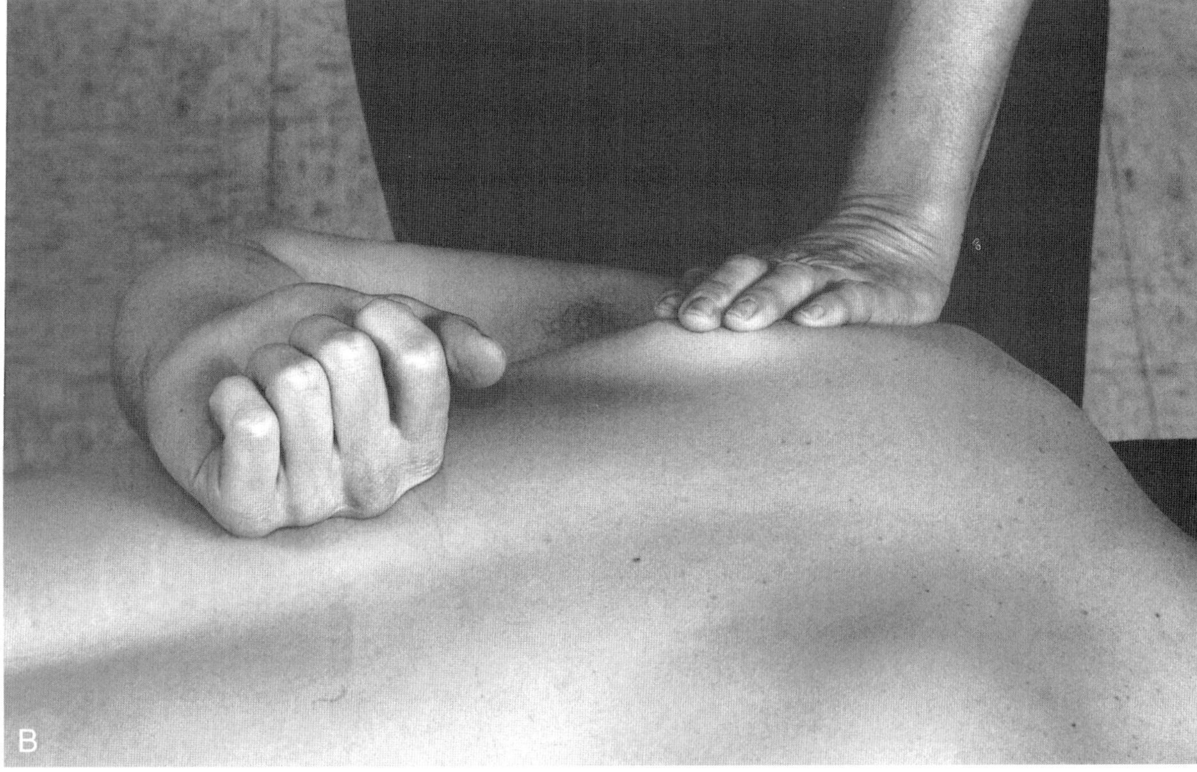

FIGURE 3-21 **Internal rotation stretch (with assistance).**

PURPOSE: Increase internal rotation flexibility.

POSITION: Client lying prone with shoulders internally rotated by placing the hand of the shoulder to be stretched behind the back. In most cases, this position will cause winging of the scapula (panel A).

PROCEDURE: Clinician places one hand on the client's winging scapula and applies gentle pressure, pushing it anteriorly against the rib cage until a mild tension is felt by client in the posterior shoulder (panel B).

NOTE: The amount of stretch felt by client can be increased or decreased by moving client's hand farther up or down the spine, respectively.

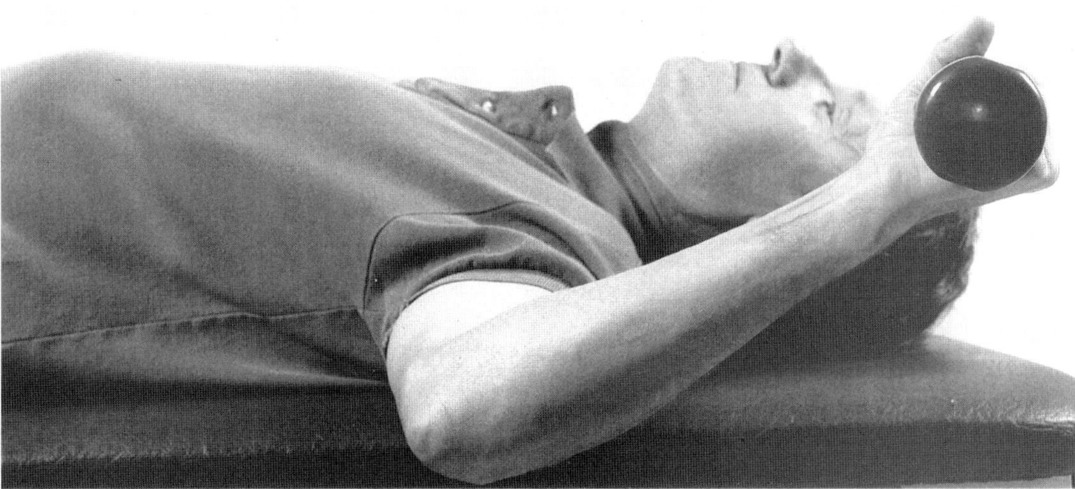

FIGURE 3-22 **External rotation stretch.**

PURPOSE: Increase external rotation flexibility.

POSITION: Client lying supine with shoulder abducted 90°, holding just the elbow over the edge of the support surface. Client externally rotates the shoulder.

PROCEDURE: Client is given a weight to hold, while maintaining the initial position. Client should be encouraged to relax the shoulder muscles completely while grasping the weight, allowing the hand to move toward the floor (external rotation). Clinician recommends the amount of weight that allows mild tension to be felt by client in the anterior shoulder.

NOTE: The amount of shoulder abduction used for this stretch can be varied to stretch the shoulder for different functional activities, especially for athletes involved in overhead activities. Commonly used ranges of abduction in which external rotation stretch is applied are 45°, 90°, and 135°.

FIGURE 3-23 **Towel stretch for rotation.**

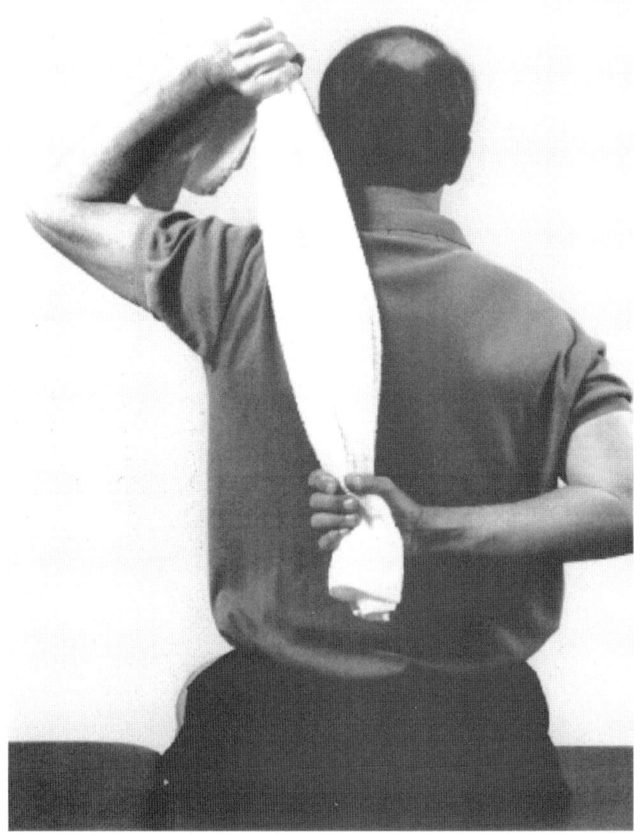

PURPOSE: Increase flexibility of internal and external rotation.

POSITION: Client sitting with feet shoulder-width apart. For external rotation of the left shoulder, client grasps a towel in the left hand and throws the towel over the left shoulder (placing the left shoulder into external rotation) allowing the towel to hang down to the lumbar spine. Client places the right arm behind the back and reaches up the spine to grasp the towel.

PROCEDURE: By gently pulling inferiorly on the towel with the right hand, client increases the amount of external rotation in the left arm (which continues to grasp the towel at the shoulder). Client pulls down with the right hand until a mild tension is felt in the anterior aspect of the left shoulder.

NOTE: The stretch can be reversed to an internal rotation stretch of the right shoulder by using the left arm to pull superiorly. The left hand grasping the towel from above (shoulder) pulls superiorly while the right hand maintains the grasp of the towel from below (lumbar spine), causing an increase in internal rotation of the right shoulder.

FIGURE 3-24 **Biceps brachii muscle stretch (with assistance).**

PURPOSE: Increase flexibility of the biceps brachii muscle.

POSITION: Client standing upright with arms behind body and elbows fully extended. Clinician standing behind client.

PROCEDURE: Ensuring that both elbows maintain full extension and the forearms are maintained in neutral position, clinician grasps client's hands with own hands and gently pulls client's upper extremity into shoulder extension. Client's upper extremities are pulled into shoulder hyperextension until a gentle tension is felt in the anterior aspect of the upper arm.

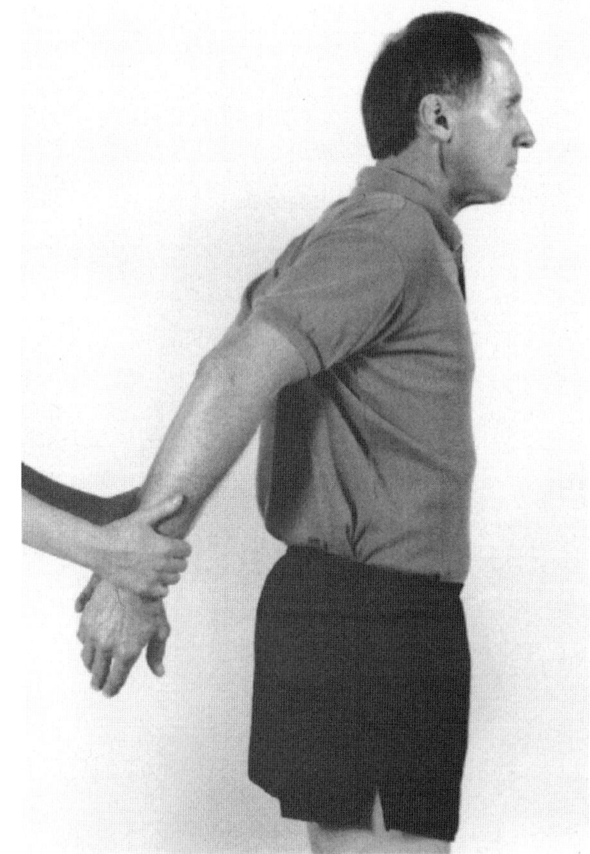

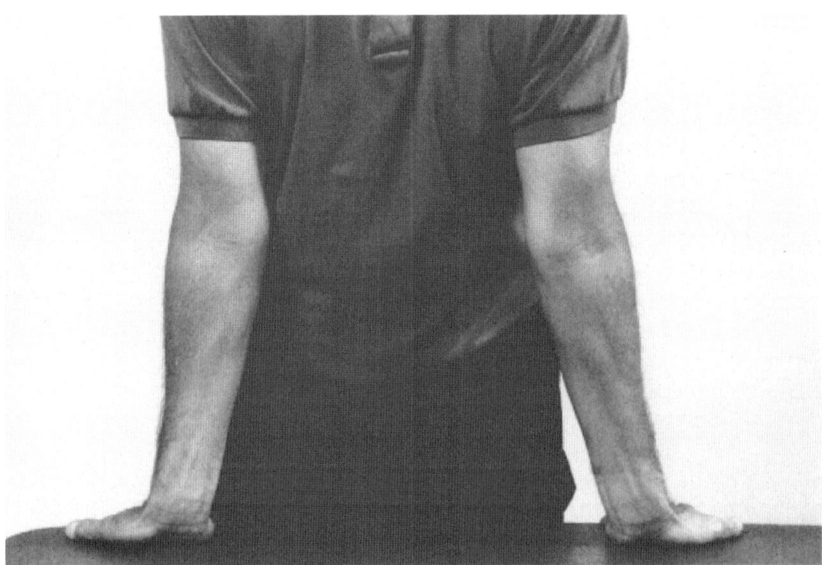

FIGURE 3-25 **Wrist extension stretch.**

PURPOSE: Increase wrist extension flexibility.

POSITION: Client standing, facing waist-high support surface.

PROCEDURE: Client leans forward on waist-high surface, placing hands with the palm down on surface, keeping the elbows fully extended. Client then leans the trunk forward over the hands, ensuring that the elbows are extended, causing hyperextension of the wrists. Client leans forward until a mild tension is felt on anterior aspect of forearms.

NOTE: This procedure can be modified to increase wrist flexion: (1) The dorsal surface of the hands are placed on the weight-bearing surface. (2) Client leans slightly backward until a mild tension is felt in the posterior aspect of the forearms.

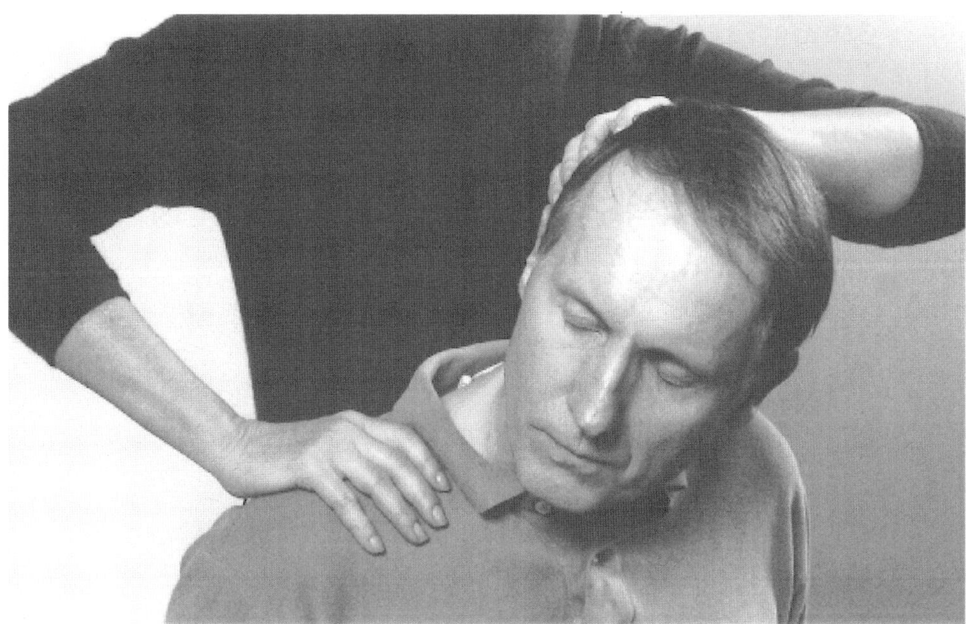

FIGURE 3-26 Trapezius muscle stretch (with assistance).

PURPOSE: Increase flexibility of trapezius muscle.

POSITION: Client sitting in chair. Clinician standing behind client and with one hand at the back of the client's head and the other on the shoulder of the side to be stretched.

PROCEDURE: To stretch the right trapezius muscle, clinician uses the hand on the back of the head to gently push client's head into flexion, left lateral flexion, and right rotation. The clinician's hand on the right shoulder gently depresses the shoulder to provide a counterforce to cervical movement. Gentle force should be applied by the clinician until a mild tension in the posterolateral aspect on the right side of the cervical spine is reported by client.

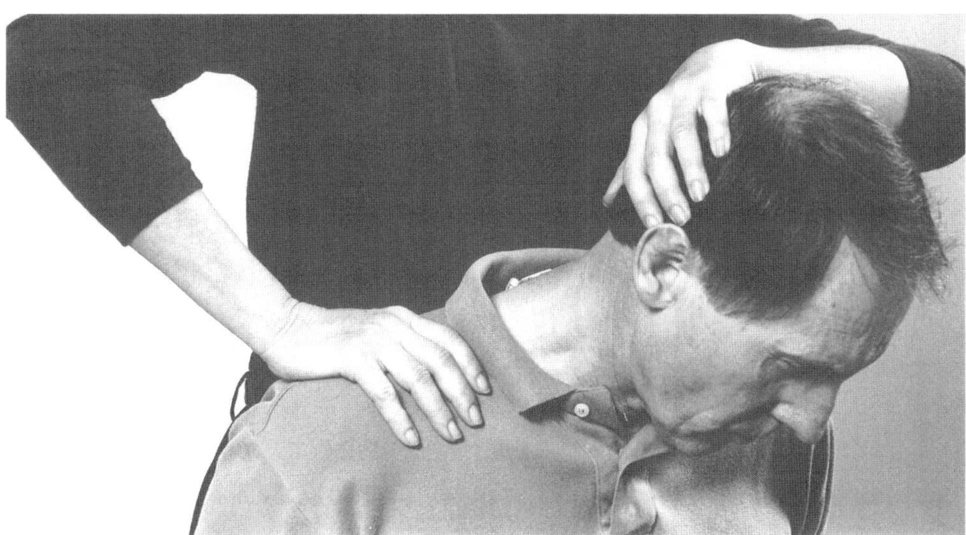

FIGURE 3-27 Levator scapulae muscle stretch (with assistance).

PURPOSE: Increase flexibility of the levator scapulae muscle.

POSITION: Client sitting in chair. Clinician standing behind client with one hand at the back of the head and the other on the shoulder of the side to be stretched.

PROCEDURE: To stretch the right levator scapulae muscle, clinician uses the hand on the back of the head to gently push the client's head into flexion, left lateral flexion, and left rotation. The clinician's hand on the right shoulder gently depresses the shoulder to provide a counterforce to cervical movement. Gentle force should be applied by the clinician until a mild tension in the posterolateral aspect on the right side of the cervical spine is reported by client.

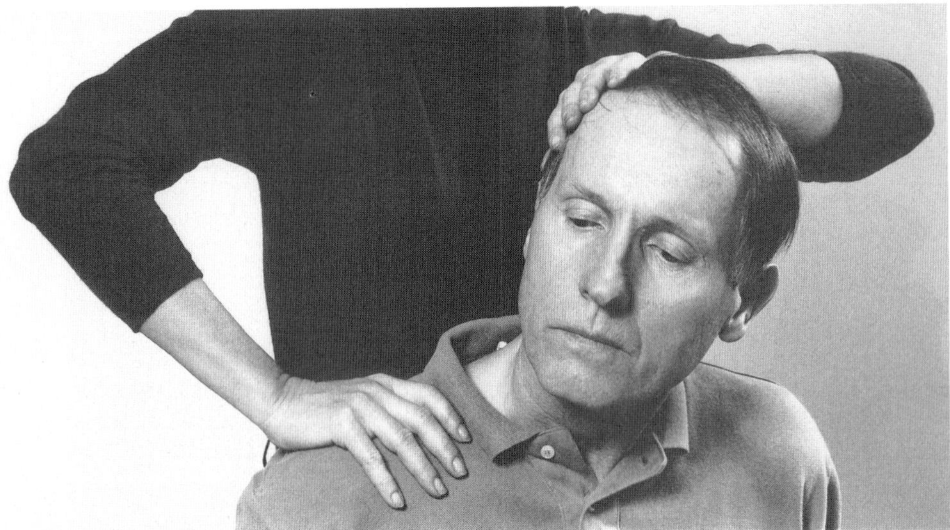

FIGURE 3-28 Scalenes muscle stretch (with assistance).

PURPOSE: Increase flexibility of the scalene muscles.

POSITION: Client sitting in chair. Clinician standing behind client with one hand on the back of the head and the other on the shoulders of the side to be stretched.

PROCEDURE: To stretch the right scalene muscle, clinician uses the hand on the back of the head to gently push the client's head into left lateral flexion and right rotation (no flexion). The clinician's hand on the right shoulder gently depresses the shoulder to provide a counterforce to cervical movement. Gentle force should be applied by the clinician until a mild tension in the anterolateral aspect on the right side of the cervical spine is reported by client.

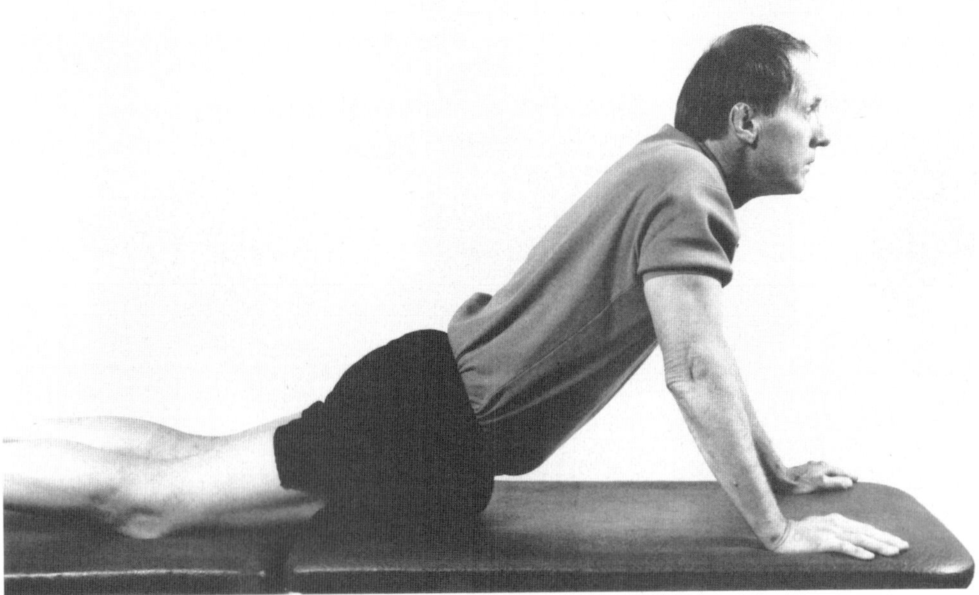

FIGURE 3-29 Prone press up.

PURPOSE: Increase extension flexibility of lumbar spine.

POSITION: Client lying prone with hands under shoulders.

PROCEDURE: Client pushes down with hands, lifting the upper trunk. During the procedure, it is vital that the client use muscles of the upper extremities and proximal stabilizers of the trunk. The lumbar spine must be relaxed. The pelvis should remain on the supporting surface as much as possible. Once full extension of the lumbar spine is reached, client pauses at that position for 1 to 2 sec. This hyperextended position should not be maintained for more than 5 sec. After the hold, client lowers himself or herself, with control, to the starting position. The lumbar spine must be relaxed during the entire activity.

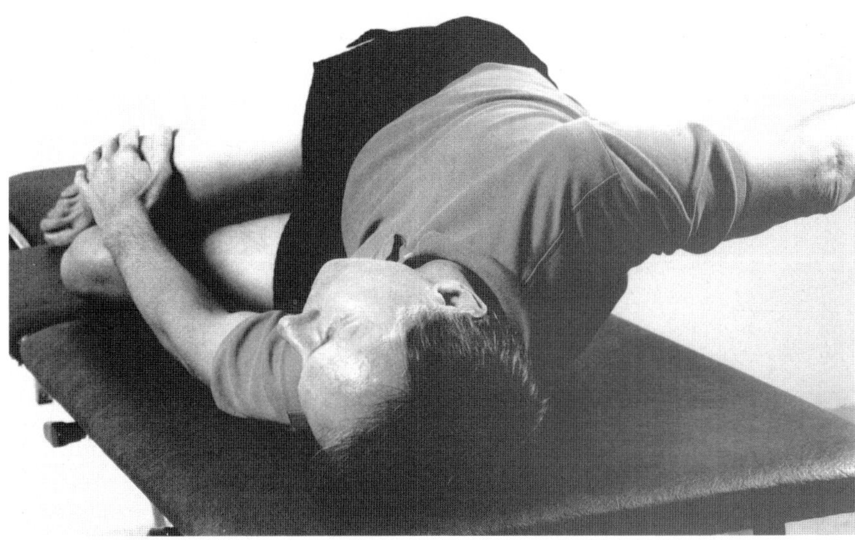

FIGURE 3-30 **Rotation in side lying.**

PURPOSE: Increase rotation flexibility of lumbar spine.

POSITION: Client side lying with hips and knees flexed. The amount of hip and knee flexion depends on the goal. To increase flexibility of the lower thoracic and upper lumbar spine, the hips and knees should be maximally flexed. To increase flexibility of the lower lumbar spine, the hips and knees should be minimally flexed. A good method is to monitor where client feels the stretch and adapt the flexion of the hips and knees accordingly.

PROCEDURE: To increase right rotation of the lumbar spine, client lies on the left side, keeping the left lower extremities on the support surface and rotating the shoulders to the right until a mild tension is felt in the lumbar spine. Client holds this position anywhere from 1 to 2 sec (cyclic movement) to 30 sec (prolonged hold) before returning to starting position.

FIGURE 3-31 **Rotation in sitting.**

PURPOSE: Increase rotation flexibility of the lumbar spine.

POSITION: Client sitting on support surface.

PROCEDURE: To increase left rotation of the lumbar spine, client rotates the shoulders to the left until mild tension is felt in the lumbar spine. To accentuate the stretch, client can place fingers of both hands on the support surface lateral to the left hip. Neutral position of the spine should be maintained.

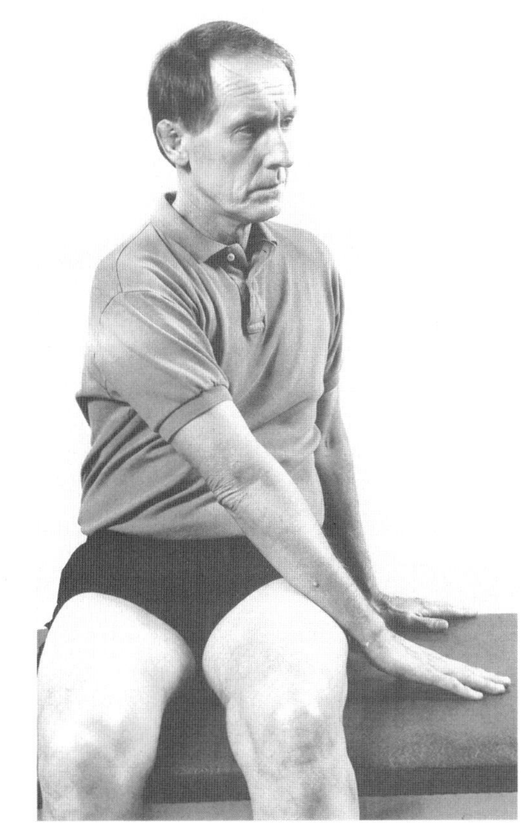

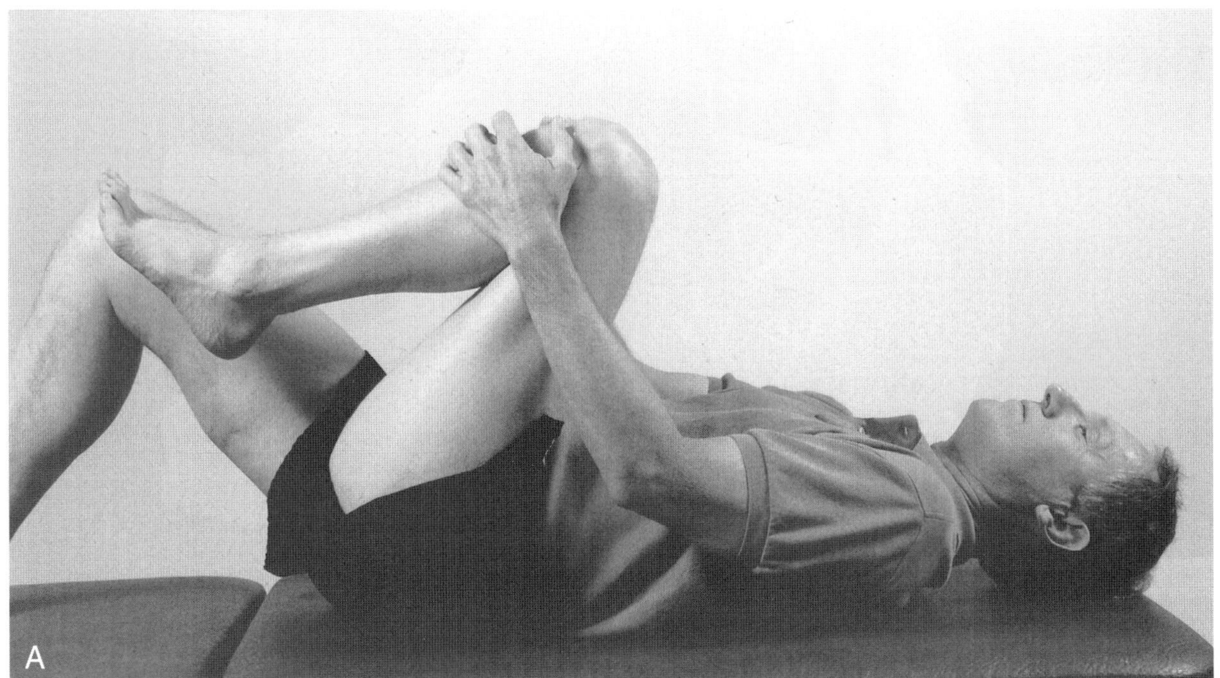

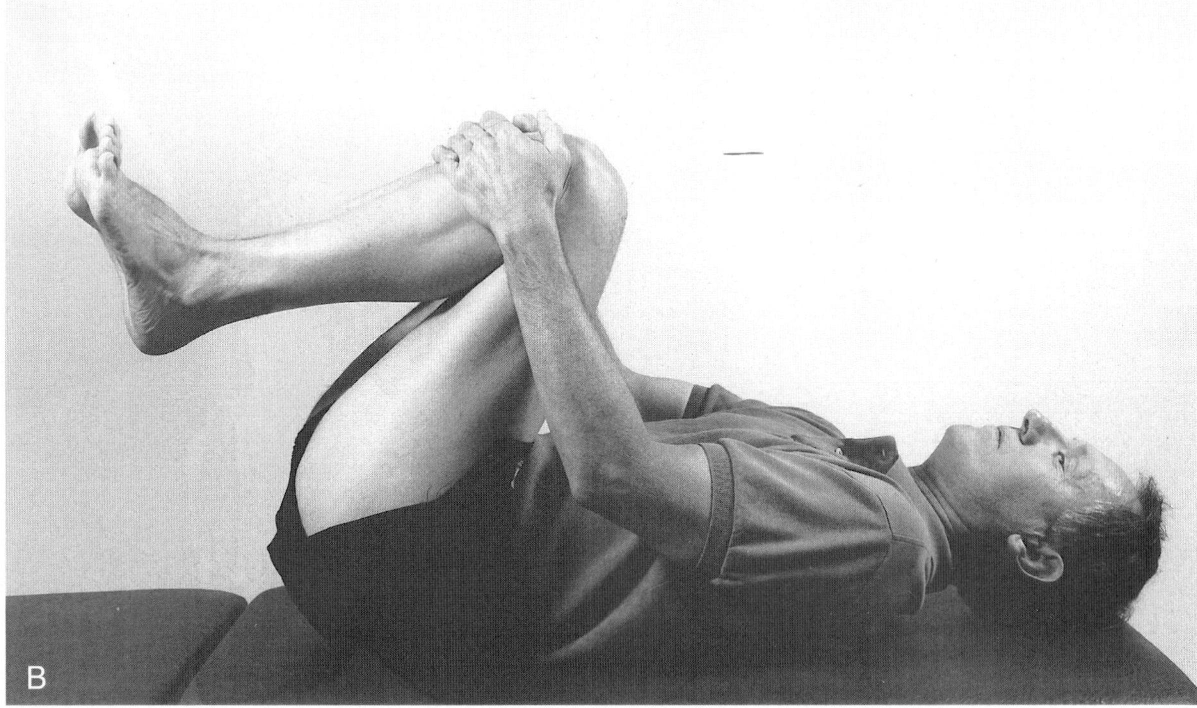

FIGURE 3-32 **Single and double knee to chest.**

PURPOSE: Increase flexion flexibility of the lumbar spine.

POSITION: Client lying supine with bilateral hips and knees flexed so the feet are positioned on the support surface.

PROCEDURE: Client flexes the hip of one leg, grasps the leg with both hands around the knee, and pulls the leg into more flexion until a mild tension is felt in the lumbar spine. The stretching activity is then repeated with the other leg (panel A).

NOTE: For a more aggressive stretch, client flexes both hips, grasps both legs with both hands around the knees, and pulls them into more flexion until a mild tension is felt in the lumbar spine (panel B).

CASE STUDY

PATIENT INFORMATION

The patient was a 45-year-old male who complained of pain in the legs below the knees bilaterally. The patient indicated that for the previous 3 weeks he had been running 2 miles, 4 days per week. He indicated that his lower legs hurt all the time and the pain became worse when he ran.

The examination indicated pain with palpation to the anterolateral aspect of the length of lower legs bilaterally. Passive plantarflexion range of motion was full in both legs, but the patient complained of pain with overpressure at the end of range. Examination of muscle flexibility indicated tightness in the gastrocnemius and soleus muscles. More specifically, left and right passive dorsiflexion with the knee extended (gastrocnemius muscle flexibility) was 0° degrees. Left and right passive dorsiflexion with the knee flexed to 20° (soleus muscle flexibility) was 7°. All resisted movement of the muscles around the ankle was strong and painless.

The patient was diagnosed with inflammation and possible tendinitis of the tibialis anterior muscle, commonly referred to as shin splints. Although shin splints have many origins, it was hypothesized that the pain and inflammation in the lower legs of this patient were caused by a weak tibialis anterior muscle having to dorsiflex against the tight calf muscle in a repetitive fashion.

LINKS TO

Guide to Physical Therapist Practice* and *Athletic Training Educational Competencies

Pattern 4E of the *Guide*[19] relates to the diagnosis of this patient. This pattern is described as "impaired joint mobility, motor function, muscle performance, and range of motion associated with localized inflammation." Included in the patient diagnostic group of this pattern is tendinitis. The anticipated goals are increasing the quality and quantity of movement between and across body segments through stretching.

The therapeutic exercise domain in the *Competencies*[20] refers to the treatment of athletes by using flexibility activities. Note that the teaching objectives under this domain list PNF stretching but not static stretching.

INTERVENTION

An initial goal of intervention was to decrease inflammation (pain). Because the patient was complaining of pain in the lower legs all the time and not just when running or immediately after running, he was instructed to stop all running and walking training activities. Owing to the severe nature of the inflammation that caused the constant pain, it was thought that stopping training was required. The patient reluctantly agreed.

The second goal was to begin to increase the flexibility of the calf muscles gradually in an attempt to decrease the amount of work being performed by the tibialis anterior muscle in pulling against the tight structures of the calf. While in the clinic, PNF contract–relax stretching was performed on the bilateral gastrocnemius muscles to attempt to increase length of the muscle.

Finally, the patient was instructed in a home program consisting of statically stretching the gastrocnemius muscle using a wall stretch (Fig. 3-17). He was told to perform the exercise two times per day (morning and night), holding the stretch for 30 sec.

PROGRESSION

One Week After Initial Examination

The patient stated that the pain in the lower leg was no longer constant and expressed a desire to begin to run again. Examination indicated that the patient still had slight pain on palpation to the anterolateral aspect of bilateral lower legs, but much less than the initial visit

Re-examination indicated that passive dorsiflexion range of motion measured with the knee extended (gastrocnemius flexibility) was 3° (3° gain since initial examination). Passive dorsiflexion range of motion measured with the knee flexed to 20° (soleus flexibility) was 7° (no change). Goals for intervention at this point were to continue to increase flexibility of the calf muscle and to strengthen the tibialis anterior muscle to assist the muscle in repetitive dorsiflexion during the swing phase and the deceleration of the foot after initial contact (heel strike), which occurs during running.

Again, while in the clinic, PNF contract–relax stretching was performed on the bilateral gastrocnemius muscles to attempt to increase length of the muscle. The home program was progressed as follows:

1. Continue static stretching to the gastrocnemius muscle: 30 sec two times per day.
2. Static stretching to the soleus muscle (Fig. 3-18): 30 sec two times per day.
3. Isotonic strengthening of the dorsiflexors (Fig. 6-19) using elastic tubing: three sets of 12 repetitions one time per day.
4. Initiate a walking program: limited to a maximum of 1 mile three times per week. Ice the lower legs immediately after the walking session.

Two Weeks After Initial Examination

Patient indicated that he had no pain during walking. Palpation of the legs bilaterally indicated no pain. Passive dorsiflexion range of motion measured with the knee extended (gastrocnemius flexibility) was 5° (5° gain since initial examination). Passive dorsiflexion range of motion measured with the knee flexed to 20° (soleus flexibility) was 10° (3° gain). Goals for the program were not changed (continue to increase flexibility of the calf muscle and strengthen the tibialis anterior muscle).

The patient was instructed to continue the home exercise program already established. He was given permission to begin running 1 mile two times per week with at least 2 days separating each running session. If no problems occurred after 1 week of running, the patient was instructed to increase to 2 miles two times per week. He was encouraged to ice after the running sessions and to return for re-examination and follow-up after 2 weeks.

Five Weeks After Initial Examination

The patient had been scheduled to return 4 weeks after initial examination, but he was unable to return until the 5th week. He complained of being out of shape during his initial runs but reported no discomfort to his lower legs during his weeks of running 2 miles two times per week. Re-examination indicated that gastrocnemius flexibility was 10° and soleus flexibility was 15°. Palpation indicated that the lower legs remained pain free.

No treatment was provided. The patient was instructed to gradually increase his training frequency by adding two 1-mile runs that week to the two 2-mile runs, for a total of 6 miles per week. If no problems occurred with the increase in training, the patient was given permission to return to his previous level of running (2 miles four times per week). In addition, he was instructed to continue stretching the gastrocnemius and soleus muscles one time per day for 30 sec. The patient was discharged and instructed to return if any problems developed.

OUTCOME

Patient sought treatment for bilateral shin splints and presented with tight gastrocnemius and soleus muscles. After a 5-week intervention in which stretching the tight muscles was emphasized along with some strengthening activities, the patient returned to his running pain-free.

SUMMARY

- The ultimate goal of any stretching programs is to increase the ability of the muscle to efficiently elongate through the necessary ROM. This chapter reviewed the three types of stretching activities most frequently referred to in the literature: ballistic stretching, PNF, and static stretching. Although extensive research has been performed on the effectiveness of these three stretching activities, no absolute recommendation can be made for the most appropriate method for increasing flexibility. All three stretching techniques will improve muscle flexibility.
- Ballistic stretching involves quick bobbing and jerking motions imposed on the muscle. Although some clinicians believe that ballistic stretching may have a role in an advanced stretching program of an athlete, this type of stretching poses the greatest potential for microtrauma to the muscle.
- Using a variety of types of muscle contractions to facilitate the sensory receptors to inhibit and relax the muscle being stretched, PNF has been documented to be an effective stretching technique. However, because PNF requires one-on-one intervention with a clinician, the time and expertise required to perform PNF appropriately make the stretching techniques somewhat cumbersome.
- Static stretching is a technique in which a stationary position is held for a period of time while the muscle is in its elongated position. Static stretching may be the most desirable stretching technique for an individual in terms of results, time, and comfort, because once the individual is properly trained, he or she can perform the technique independently.

GERIATRIC *Perspectives*

- The age-related effect of connective tissue stiffening is of particular importance for the older adult. A decrease in tissue water content, an increase in collagen bundling, and an increase in elastin cross-links result in a decrease in the distensibility and tensile strength of muscles, fascia, tendons, skin, and bones. Consequently, ballistic stretching is particularly problematic. Static stretching may potentially be more effective for older adults if applied slowly and held for a slightly longer duration (30 to 60 sec).[1]
- Modified dynamic flexibility, or functional flexibility, refers to an active type of stretching exercise involving movement of varying degrees and speeds to meet or enhance the ROM typically used during specific activities. It is an important consideration in initiating a stretching program for older adults.[2] Functional flexibility and ROM related to a minimum level of safe performance in activities of daily living have been defined through biomechanics research.[3]
- Stretch weakness is a theoretic phenomenon associated with muscle aging combined with disuse. Stretch weakness is thought to be the result of prolonged stretch applied beyond the physiologic resting length.[4] The phenomenon may be evidenced by altered muscle synergies (e.g., agonist–antagonist imbalances or agonist–antagonist co-contraction). Stretch weakness may also be related to pathologic age-related changes (e.g., postural malalignment and gait changes resulting from the disease process of degenerative joint disease and scoliosis). Stretch weakness should be addressed via a thorough examination of ROM and evaluation of muscle length before initiation of a flexibility or stretching program.
- Static stretching techniques are most effective if used in conjunction with active contraction. Hold–relax and contract–relax further enhance the therapeutic benefits of static stretching by allowing the agonist to relax. However, the stretch weakness phenomenon may preclude effective use of these PNF techniques. In the presence of agonist stretch weakness, passive stretching of the antagonist is recommended.
- Cognitively impaired patients are not usually candidates for a stretching program because of problems relaxing the muscle to be lengthened.
- A warmup and mild stretching program may be useful in the management of chronic pain and loss of joint range associated with some musculoskeletal and neuromuscular diseases (e.g., arthritis and Parkinson disease).
- The most effective stretching program should be based on the individual functional needs of the older individual. The primary outcome should be restoration or maintenance of physical independence.

1. Bandy WD, Irion JM, Briggler M. The effect of time and frequency of static stretching on flexibility of the hamstring muscles. Phys Ther 1997;77:1090–1096.
2. Stevens K. A theoretical overview of stretching and flexibility. Am Fitness 1998;16:30–37.
3. Young A. Exercise physiology in geriatric practice. Acta Med Scand 1986;711(suppl):227–232.
4. Kauffman TL. Geriatric rehabilitation manual. New York: Churchill Livingstone, 1999.

PEDIATRIC *Perspectives*

- The developing individual exhibits much greater mobility and flexibility than the mature individual.[1] Muscle inflexibility, when present, aggravates and predisposes children and adolescents to a variety of overuse injuries, including traction apophysitis.[2] Flexibility deficits that may occur in children and adolescents can be effectively treated using common stretching techniques (as described in this chapter).
- Ballistic stretching may be the least appropriate stretching technique for children for the same reasons that it is not recommended for sedentary and geriatric individuals. In addition, ballistic stretching may put excessive strain on the apophyses and epiphyses of developing bone.
- Muscle stretching is imperative for treatment of juvenile rheumatoid arthritis (JRA). The shortening of muscle and tendon and the resulting joint contractures (see chapter 4), may become a major cause of disability. The greater soft tissue flexibility and hypermobility in disease-free children under 8 years of age suggest the need for early intensive therapy for children with JRA in preventing long-term disability.[3] No evidence exists as to which stretching methods are the most efficacious for children with JRA. Low-load prolonged stretching using splinting methods may be appropriate.[3]

1. Kendall HO, Kendall FP, Boynton DA. Posture and pain. Melbourne, FL: Krieger, 1971.
2. Krivickus LS. Anatomical factors associated with overuse sports injuries. Sports Med 1997;24:132–146.
3. Wright FV, Smith E. Physical therapy management of the child and adolescent with juvenile rheumatoid arthritis. In: JM Walker, A Helewa, eds. Physical therapy in arthritis. Philadelphia: Saunders, 1996:211–244.

REFERENCES

1. Zachazewski J. Flexibility for sports. In: B Sanders, ed. Sports physical therapy. Norwalk, CT: Appleton & Lange, 1990:201–238.
2. Anderson B, Burke ER. Scientific, medical, and practical aspects of stretching. Clin Sports Med 1991;10:63–86.
3. Jonagen S, Nemeth G, Griksson F. Hamstring injuries in sprinters: the role of concentric and eccentric hamstring muscle strength and flexibility. Am J Sports Med 1994;22:262–266.
4. Worrell TW, Perrin DH, Gansneder B, Gieck J. Comparison of isokinetic strength and flexibility measures between hamstring injured and non-injured athletes. J Orthop Sports Phys Ther 1991;13:118–125.
5. Gordon J, Ghez C. Muscle receptors and spinal reflexes: the stretch reflex. In: ER Kandel, JH Schwartz JH, eds. Principles of neural science. 3rd ed. New York: Elsevier, 1991:564–580.
6. Lundy-Ekman L. Neuroscience: fundamentals for rehabilitation. Philadelphia: Saunders, 1998:85–106.
7. Waxman SG, deGroot J. Correlative neuroanatomy. Norwalk, CT: Appleton & Lange, 1995.
8. Sady SP, Wortman M, Blanke D. Flexibility training: ballistic, static or proprioceptive neuromuscular facilitation? Arch Phys Med Rehabil 1982;63:261–263.
9. Knott M, Voss DE. Proprioceptive neuromuscular facilitation: patterns and techniques. New York: Harper & Row, 1968.
10. Etnyre BR, Lee EJ. Chronic and acute flexibility of men and women using three different stretching techniques. Res Q 1988; 59:222–228.
11. American Academy of Orthopaedic Surgeons. Athletic training and sports medicine. 2nd ed. Rosemont, IL: AAOS, 1991.
12. Allerheiligen WB. Exercise techniques: stretching and warm-up. In: TR Baechle, ed. Essentials of strength training and conditioning. Champaign, IL: Human Kinetics, 1994:289–313.
13. Cornelius WL, Ebrahim K, Watson J, Hill DW. The effects of cold application and modified PNF stretching techniques on hip flexibility in college males. Res Q Exer Sport 1992;63: 311–314.
14. Osternig LR, Robertson R, Troxel R, Hanson P. Differential response to proprioceptive neuromuscular facilitation (PNF) stretch technique. Med Sci Sports Exerc 1990;22:106–111.
15. Gajdosik RL. Effects of static stretching on the maximal length and resistance to passive stretch of the hamstring muscles. J Orthop Sports Phys Ther 1991;14:250–255.
16. Madding SW, Wong JG, Hallum A, Medeiros JM. Effects of duration on passive stretching on hip abduction range of motion. J Orthop Sports Phys Ther 1987;8:409–416.
17. Bandy WD, Irion J. The effect of time of static stretch on the flexibility of the hamstring muscles. Phys Ther 1994;74:845–850.
18. Bandy WD, Irion JM, Briggler M. The effect of time and frequency of static stretching on flexibility of the hamstring muscles. Phys Ther 1997;77:1090–1096.
19. American Physical Therapy Association. Guide to physical therapist practice, second edition. Phys Ther 2001;81:1–768.
20. National Athletic Trainers' Association. Athletic training educational competencies. 3rd ed. Dallas: NATA, 1999.

CHAPTER 4

Joint Mobilization

Clayton F. Holmes, EdD, PT, ATC

Ginny Keely, MS, PT (Case Study)

Many synovial joints in the body are characterized with what Mennell[1] referred to as a capsular excess: a loose folding in the capsule that is necessary for the joint to achieve full range of motion (ROM). For example, the capsular excess can be easily observed at the shoulder in the inferior folds of the capsule (Fig. 4-1). This excess is important in the shoulder, because the loose folds of the inferior capsule allow for full, normal active flexion and abduction. In fact, capsular excess allows a joint to have some give, commonly called joint play.[1] Joint play movement in humans is a prerequisite for normal active ROM; and in turn, normal active ROM is a prerequisite for effective therapeutic exercise. Perhaps the most direct way for the clinician to improve joint play (and thus range of motion) is by a manual therapy procedure in which the clinician introduces a passive force, usually in a transverse direction, through a joint.[1]

The appropriate term for the manual therapy procedure in which a passive force is used to take advantage of the joint play to increase ROM has been a matter of debate. Currently, disagreement exists in regard to whether *mobilization* or *manipulation* is the appropriate term. The terms are often used interchangeably, which causes both confusion and disagreement in the health-care arena.[2,3] In Europe, the term *manipulation* is reserved almost exclusively for procedures involving high-velocity thrust movements.[2] In the United States, the term *manipulation* is often used to include all passive forms of joint motion.

For clarity, this chapter operationally defines mobilization and manipulation according to the *Guide to Physical Therapist Practice.*[4] Mobilization, a more general term than manipulation, is "a skilled passive hand movement that can be performed with variable amplitudes at variable speeds." Manipulation is defined as one type of mobilization. More specifically, manipulation is the "skilled passive hand movement that usually is performed with a small amplitude at a high velocity." In other words, the term *mobilization* refers to a passive movement technique performed at any velocity, including the high-velocity manipulation that some clinicians classify as a grade 5 mobilization (described later in this chapter).[5]

THEORETICAL MODELS IN MANUAL THERAPY

Manual therapy, once known as manual medicine, has been in existence since the time of Hippocrates. From ancient Greece through the Middle Ages, knowledge about the human body increased and intervention techniques changed and developed. By the 1700s, those who performed manual intervention in England were called "bone setters."[5] Within the last two centuries, several approaches (schools of thought) to manual therapy have developed.

Osteopathic Model

The osteopathic model is perhaps the root of manual therapy in the United States. This model can be traced to an American doctor named Still (1828–1917).[2] From anecdotal evidence, Still developed a theory he called the Law of the Artery. Initially, his claim was that all disease processes were a direct result of interference with arterial blood that carried vital nutrients to a body part. He believed that by performing joint manipulation he could maintain and improve blood flow. In 1892, Still opened the first school of osteopathy, and the ideas he fostered became the basis of the osteopathic model.[6] Over time, this school of thought has gained more acceptance in the United States; in Europe, however, osteopathic ideas are less accepted.[3]

Through the years, osteopathic physicians migrated from manual therapy into other areas of traditional medicine; and, today, these physicians no longer subscribe wholly to the Law of the Artery. A number of the manual techniques developed by osteopathic physicians, including muscle energy techniques and articulatory techniques, have demonstrated therapeutic value and are widely used

FIGURE 4-1

Capsular excess in the axillary recess of the inferior folds of the capsule of the glenohumeral joint.

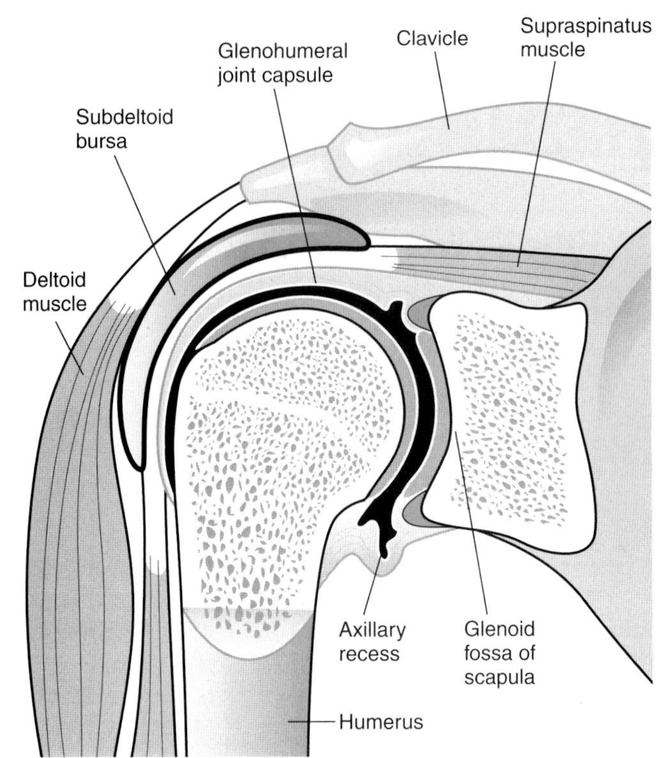

by practitioners who subscribe to many different schools of thought.

Chiropractic Model

The chiropractic model was founded by a grocer named Palmer (1845–1913) who founded the Palmer College of Chiropractics in 1895. Palmer based his theory on what he called the Law of the Nerve. He believed that vital life forces were cut off from any body part by small vertebral subluxations. By performing manual intervention, Palmer believed that the vital life forces could be maintained or improved.[6]

Today, some chiropractors, referred to as "straights," continue to embrace Palmer's philosophy. Another group of chiropractors, called "mixers," combine manual interventions with other more traditional interventions, such as passive agents and therapeutic exercise. Because of these differing opinions within the profession, the chiropractic model is currently in a state of flux.[3]

Current Orthopedic Approaches to Manual Therapy

In the 1900s, many innovative health professionals from around the world influenced the course of manual therapy in the United States. For example, practitioners at St. Thomas Hospital in London pioneered the development of current manual intervention. Two physicians who worked at St. Thomas—James Mennell[1] and, later, Cyriax[7]—each published works that proposed manual intervention as an effective mode of treatment for joint pathology.

More recently, Kaltenborn,[8] Maitland,[9] and John Mennell[1] contributed to the body of knowledge regarding manual therapy. Kaltenborn developed what has been called the Scandinavian approach to manual intervention. As a chiropractor, osteopath, and physiotherapist, he blended the different perspectives into a systematic process of examination and intervention. One manual intervention emphasized by Kaltenborn is joint mobilization. In fact, he is one of two professionals who have described grades (or levels) of mobilization.[10]

Maitland, a physical therapist from Australia, also worked out a specific description of mobilization grades. His categorization includes five grades of mobilizations, whereas Kaltenborn's has only three grades. In addition, Maitland has been a proponent of oscillatory mobilization, an intervention that has been widely accepted by physical therapists.[9,11]

Mennell, who practiced medicine in the United States, contributed, among other things, terms used to illustrate concepts relative to manual intervention: joint play, accessory motion, and joint dysfunction. Today, these terms have been widely accepted by manual therapists. For example, his idea that joint play is essential for normal motion is an almost inherent assumption held by many manual therapists.

These professionals are only a few of the many clinicians who have contributed to the body of knowledge relative to manual therapy. Each school of thought described in this section contains unique elements. Note, however, that many consistencies exist among the models as well. As Rothstein[12] stated in 1992: "We do a disservice to the pioneers of manual therapy when we worship their words and fail to advance the scientific basis of what they developed."

JOINT RESPONSE TO EXTERNAL FORCE: AUDIBLE POP

Traditional theories in health care suggest that it is quite common for normal joints to produce an audible pop.[13] Bourdillon and Day[3] refer to this audible pop as a "crackling noise" and suggest that it occurs as a result of "cavitation." As the synovial joint is pulled apart and the opposing surfaces move farther and farther apart, a negative pressure develops in the synovial fluid driving out carbon dioxide and releasing nitrogen from solution in a gaseous form. This gaseous bubble occupies the increased space. Once the surfaces are separated, the "pressure within the joint exceeds that in the bubble, and the bubble collapses causing a crackling noise."[13]

In addition, pathologic joints routinely create a popping or crackling sound, which is caused by (1) an unstable joint that subluxes during certain movements; (2) a roughness in the edges of the joint surfaces, possibly owing to articular surface degeneration; or (3) a thickening of any scar tissue surrounding the joint. If a joint subluxes frequently or the joint surfaces have become roughened, hypermobility may result. On the other hand, scarring around a joint will most likely cause hypomobility. In all cases, movement at the affected joints could cause a crackling or popping sound.[5]

Thus, because it is possible for normal, hypermobile, and hypomobile joints to create a popping sound, the therapeutic goal of a manual intervention should not be an audible pop. An audible pop may indicate that the joint surfaces have moved. However, when the pop does not occur, it does not indicate that the joint has not been moved. Rather, to determine if the joint has moved the clinician must develop what Maitland[11] refers to as "feel." Once this feel is developed, a clinician can confidently evaluate whether a joint is normal, hypermobile, or hypomobile. If a joint is hypomobile and mobilization is used as an intervention, feel can again be used to assess if mobility has been improved, regardless of whether a pop was heard during the mobilization procedure. An increase in function, or restoration of normal motion, of the hypomobile joint is the ultimate therapeutic goal of mobilization.

The osteopathic and chiropractic models do not agree with more traditional theories in medicine and physical therapy in regard to the cause of the audible pop at the joint. These models define three barriers to movement: anatomic, elastic, and physiologic. The anatomic barrier is the total ROM from one extreme to the other (Fig. 4-2). Movement beyond the anatomic barrier can occur only with fracture, dislocation, or rupture of ligaments. The elastic barrier is the range of motion within the total ROM in which the examiner can passively move the joint. The normal end feel felt by the examiner at the end of passive range of motion is this elastic barrier. The physiologic barrier is the ROM actively available to the individual and is generally smaller than the passive range.[14]

According to the osteopathic and chiropractic models, a space called the "paraphysiologic space" is found between the elastic and anatomic barriers. The primary goal of manipulation for the osteopath and chiropractor is to achieve movement into the paraphysiologic space, and thus to produce an audible pop. The popping sound that results from a high-velocity, low-amplitude thrust indicates that the clinician has reached this space. According to these models, if the pop occurs, the practitioner knows with certainty that the end of the ROM has been reached.[14]

Little research exists to support the concept of the paraphysiologic space, and little information is available on

FIGURE 4-2

Range of motion and barriers to movement according to the osteopathic and chiropractic models.

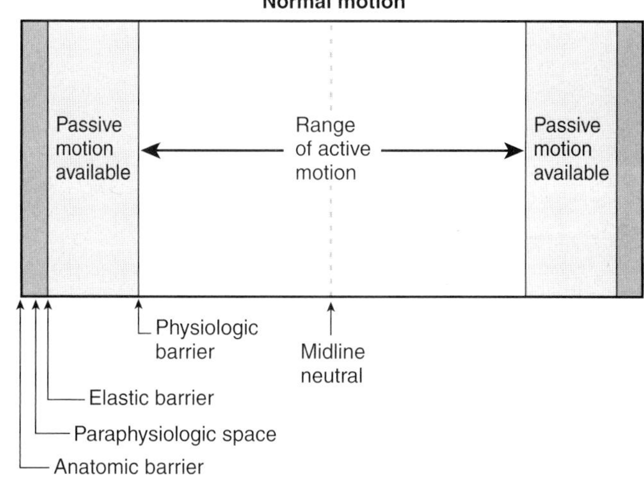

cavitation or gas release. Thus this chapter will not address the function of mobilization within the paraphysiologic space. This does not mean that the clinician should not embrace other components of specific approaches that subscribe to the idea of this space. Although an audible pop often occurs with manual therapy and may provide evidence that increased motion has occurred, this chapter assumes that an audible pop is not required for effective application of manual therapy for improving joint ROM and function.

■ *Scientific Basis*

BIOMECHANICAL BASIS FOR MOBILIZATION

Several biomechanical terms that derive from the field of engineering have been adopted by manual therapists, including arthrokinematics and osteokinematics.

Arthrokinematics

Arthrokinematics refers to movements of joint surfaces in relation to one another.[15] When two bones move, the articulating ends of the bones move along with the two long levers of the bones. For example, when the tibia moves on the femur (the long lever of the bones) during knee flexion and extension, the condyles of the tibia move on the condyles of the femur (the articulating ends of the bones). Two types of arthrokinematic motions that have been described in the literature are roll and slide (or glide) (Fig. 4-3). Roll occurs when new points on one joint surface meet new points on another surface. Slide has been called "pure translatory motion"[15] and occurs when one joint surface moves across a second surface so that the same point on one surface is continually in contact with new points on the second surface. The sliding that occurs during normal motion is caused by joint play and is a critical function of each joint. Slide is the movement most affected during mobilization.

Most synovial joints have articular surfaces that are either concave or convex in shape, with the convex end of a bone fitting into the concave end of the adjacent bone. Not only does this congruent arrangement allow for enhanced intrinsic stability of the joint but the convex–concave relationship dictates arthrokinematic motion. Specifically, "when a convex surface is moving on a fixed, concave surface, the convex articulating surface moves (slides) in a direction opposite to the direction traveled by the shaft of the bony lever."[15] The glenohumeral joint is an example of a convex surface (humeral head) moving on a fixed concave surface (glenoid fossa). In this example, the humeral head is the moving articulating surface, which must slide inferior as the humerus (the shaft of the bony lever) moves superior into abduction, in the opposite direction (Fig. 4-4A). Therefore, if the goal of the mobilization intervention is to increase shoulder abduction in light of capsular restriction, the appropriate manual intervention is mobilization in the inferior direction (inferior glide).

When a concave surface is moving on a stable convex surface, sliding occurs in the same direction as the bony lever.[15] The tibiofemoral joint is an example of a concave surface, tibia and meniscus, moving on a fixed convex surface, the femoral condyles. For example, in flexion, the tibia is the moving articulating surface, sliding posterior as the femur moves posterior into flexion (Fig. 4-4B). Therefore, if the goal of the mobilization intervention is to increase knee flexion in light of capsular restriction, mobilization of the tibial anterior surface is in the posterior direction.

Osteokinematics

Osteokinematic motion includes the quality and degree of the motion actually observed in the bony lever and is determined by the underlying, unseen arthrokinematic motion. The amount of slide (or glide) and roll occurring at the articular surfaces of a joint ultimately determines how much visible, functional movement occurs at that same joint. For example, during the osteokinematic movement of shoulder abduction, the arthrokinematic motion of the humerus sliding inferiorly occurs. When a capsular restriction exists, preventing the downward slide of the humeral head, the concomitant osteokinematic motion of humeral elevation cannot occur normally. Thus the

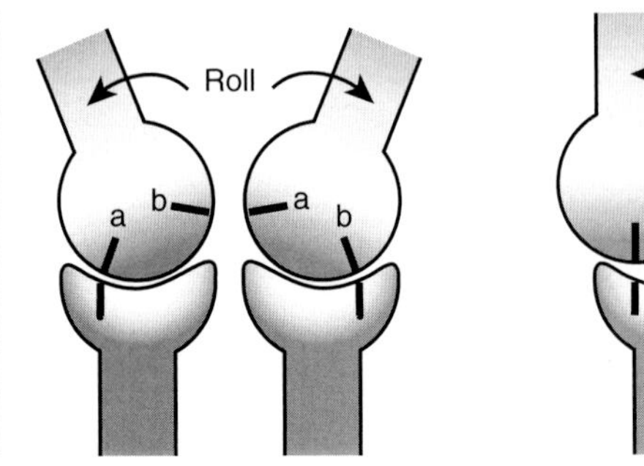

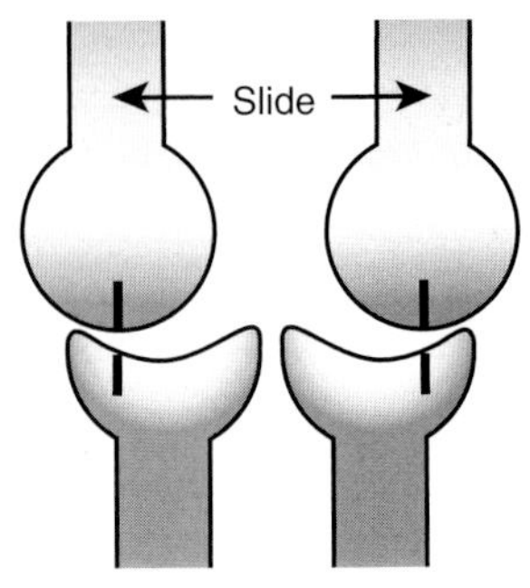

FIGURE 4-3 Arthrokinematic motions of roll and glide.

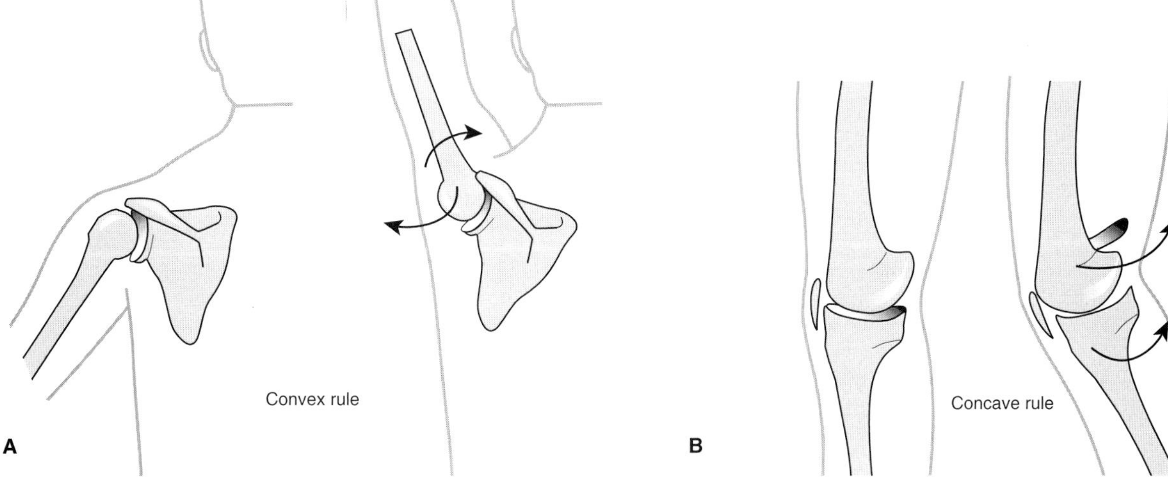

FIGURE 4-4 **The convex and concave rules at the shoulder and knee.**

(Panel A) When moving the convex surface, the head of humerus (convex surface) moves on the glenoid fossa (fixed concave surface), the head of the humerus must slide inferior as the shaft of the humerus moves superior into abduction, or in the opposite direction (convex rule). (Panel B) When the tibial plateau (moving concave surface) moves on the femur (fixed convex surface), the tibial plateau must slide posterior as shaft of the tibia moves into flexion, or in the same direction (concave rule).

most important reason to perform joint mobilization is to improve and maintain osteokinematic motion through restoration or maintenance of arthrokinematic motion.

EFFECTS OF JOINT MOBILIZATION

Tissue Response

Surrounding each joint is the joint capsule, with its outside layer made of dense, irregular collagen connective tissue. If the joint becomes inflamed as a result of injury or is immobilized for a period of time, the capsule may become thickened because of increased collagen production or by the binding together of individual collagen fibers. Mobilization to increase the restricted ROM will stress the capsule, causing plastic deformation of the collagen.[16,17] With effective mobilization, the collagen fibers are loosened and rearranged, and adhesions in the joint capsule may be broken. These changes in the collagen of the capsule will restore joint mobility.[5]

Neurophysiologic Basis

Low-grade mobilization can be effective in alleviating pain. The decrease in pain is thought to occur via two mechanisms. First, mobilization assists in improving the overall nutrition of the joint through movement of the synovial fluid. Second, mobilization activates type I and II mechanoreceptors in the joint capsule. Stimulation of these mechanoreceptors reduces pain. Through either or both of these mechanisms, low-grade mobilization has been effectively used for pain control.[18]

Clinical Guidelines

INDICATIONS FOR MOBILIZATION

The most important indication for mobilization is a limitation in active ROM, which is often concurrent with a limitation in passive ROM. Motion limitation most often results from joint hypomobility, which many clinicians categorize according to the following mobility scale:[8]

1. Ankylosed.
2. Considerable restriction.
3. Slight restriction.
4. Normal.
5. Slight increase.
6. Considerable increase.
7. Unstable.

A second indication for mobilization is a capsular end feel. The end feel of a joint motion is examined by applying gentle overpressure at the end of the ROM to determine the quality of the joint at that point. Several types of end feel exist in the body, including muscle, bone to bone, springy block, empty, and capsular.[5] If the end point feels thick—described by Cyriax[7] as leathery—and lacks the resiliency of normal tissue, a capsular end feel is present. In general, limitation of motion with a capsular end feel indicates a capsular lesion. In such cases, mobilization of the limited joint is one of the most effective means of restoring normal motion.

Pain is another indication for mobilization of the affected joint. Lower-grade mobilization may be used to stimulate joint receptors and decrease pain perception by the central nervous system. In addition, small distraction forces may be useful in reducing abnormal, pain-producing compression of joint surfaces.[18]

GRADES OF MOBILIZATION

As noted, Kaltenborn and Maitland have both described graded mobilizations. Kaltenborn[8] defined three grades:

Grade I: loosening—a low-level distraction force.
Grade II: tightening—a force that takes up available joint play.
Grade III: stretching—a force that stretches the tissue around the joint after grade II has been applied.[8]

For clinical application, the Maitland[11] grades—with the addition of grade 5 as defined by Saunders and Saunders[5]—are embraced in this chapter. In essence, the system is as follows (Fig. 4-5):

Grade 1: a tiny amplitude movement near the beginning of the range.
Grade 2: a large amplitude movement that carries well into the range but does not reach the limit of the range (this motion can occupy any part of the range).
Grade 3: a large amplitude that reaches to the limit of the range.
Grade 4: a tiny amplitude movement at the limit of the available range (the end range).
Grade 5: thrusting movements performed beyond the limit of the available range (the end range).

As Maitland[11] indicates, the "most important factor in achieving effective mobilization is learning to sense or feel movement." In addition, he states that no set rate exists at which to perform oscillations; however, a general guide would be two to three oscillations per second. He also suggested that oscillatory movements be applied for 20 sec or more at a time. This is consistent with other clinicians who have indicated that most of the desired effects have occurred after 30 sec of mobilization.[19] Maitland further points out that "learning to control the gentleness of Grade 1 is as important as learning to control the smoothness and rhythm of Grades 2 and 3, and all of these 'lower grades' should be used more often than Grade 4, for all joint dysfunction, both chronic and acute." In other words, the use of grades 1, 2, and 3 is as essential for increasing ROM as the use of grades 4 and 5.

PRINCIPLES FOR MOBILIZATION

A variety of principles and guidelines should be kept in mind when performing any mobilization technique.

- The patient should be relaxed and not exhibit muscle guarding.
- The clinician should be in the appropriate position, ideally one that allows him or her to maximize energy output for the entire length of the treatment.
- The clinician's grasp should be firm yet painless.[18]
- One bone should be stabilized with clinician's hand, belt, wedge, or treatment table and the other bone should be acted on with the clinician's hand or belt.
- When mobilizing the extremities, a grade 1 traction force should be applied at all times.
- Both the stabilization force and the mobilization force should be as close to the joint line as possible.
- Because discomfort may cause muscle guarding, pain should be monitored and minimized during the treatment.
- Only one joint should be mobilized at a time.
- As advocated by the osteopathic model, the clinician

FIGURE 4-5 **Maitland's five grades of mobilization.**

(Reprinted with permission from Saunders HD, Saunders R. Evaluation, treatment, and prevention of mobilization disorders. Vol 1. Spine. Bloomington, MN: Educational Opportunities, 1993.)

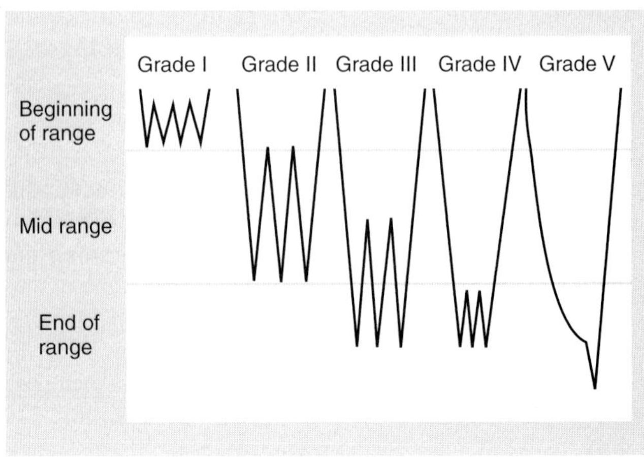

should re-examination joint play after each treatment to determine the effectiveness of the treatment.[5,18]

■ Techniques

SPINE

Figures 4-6 to 4-10 describe basic mobilization techniques for the spine. Included in these procedures are mobilization of the cervical and lumbar areas and mobilization of the sacroiliac joint.

EXTREMITIES

Figures 4-11 to 4-30 present mobilization techniques of the upper and lower extremities. Note that the techniques presented here are only a sampling of the available mobilization techniques.

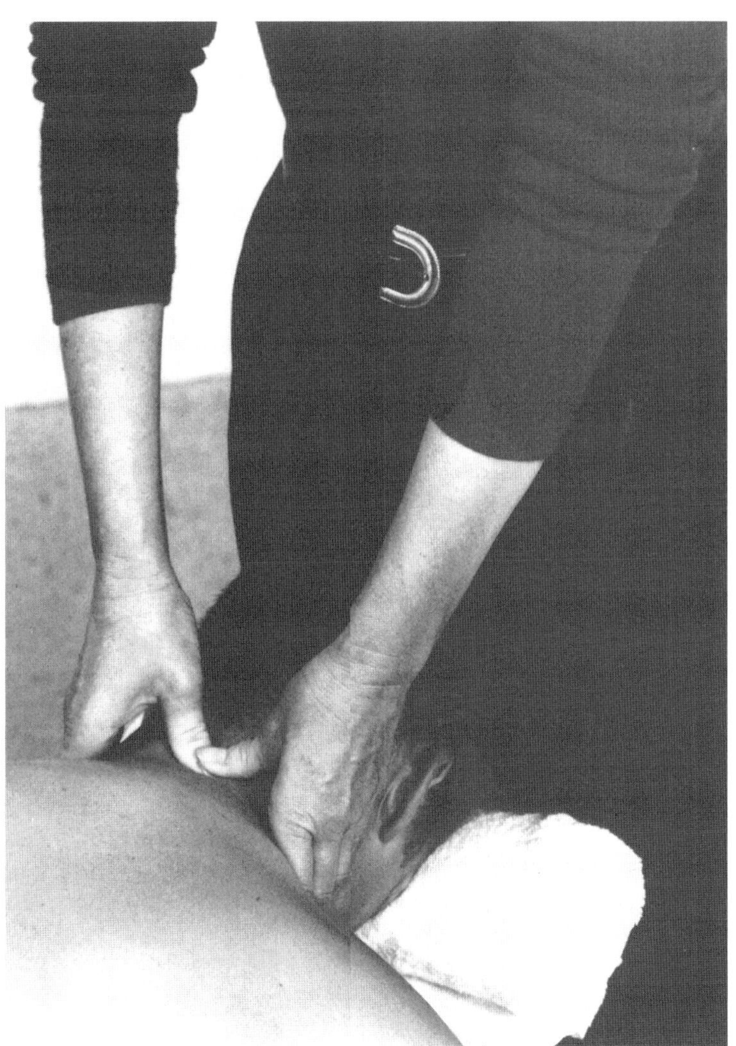

FIGURE 4-6 Cervical posterior to anterior glide.

PURPOSE: Increase segmental mobility.

POSITION: Client lying prone with a towel under forehead; cervical spine in neutral position. Clinician standing at end of table at client's head with hands placed at side of client's neck. Clinician's fingers take up slack in skin; one thumb placed directly over spinous process of selected vertebrae. Other thumb placed over thumb already positioned and is the mobilizing thumb that applies force.

PROCEDURE: Mobilizing thumb presses in a posterior to anterior direction on the spinous process.

FIGURE 4-7 Cervical transverse glide.

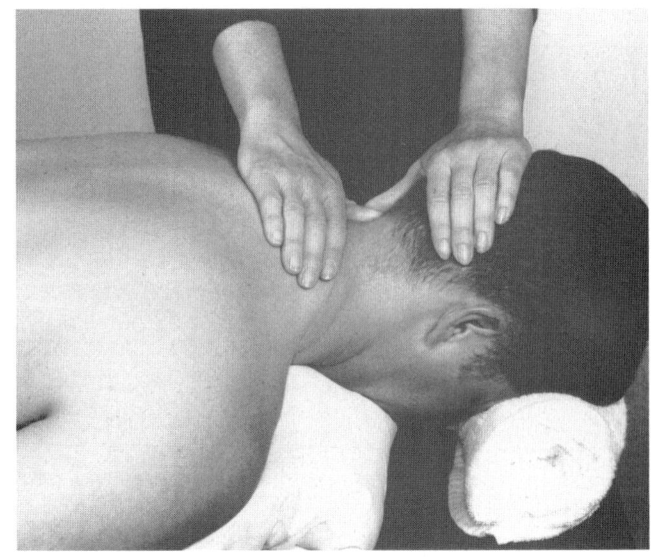

PURPOSE: Increase segmental mobility.

POSITION: Client lying prone with a towel under forehead; cervical spine in neutral position. Clinician standing on side opposite the direction the spinous process will be moved. One thumb placed on side of spinous process. Other thumb placed over thumb already positioned and is the mobilizing thumb that applies the force.

PROCEDURE: Mobilizing thumb presses away from clinician's body, pressing spinous process laterally away from clinician.

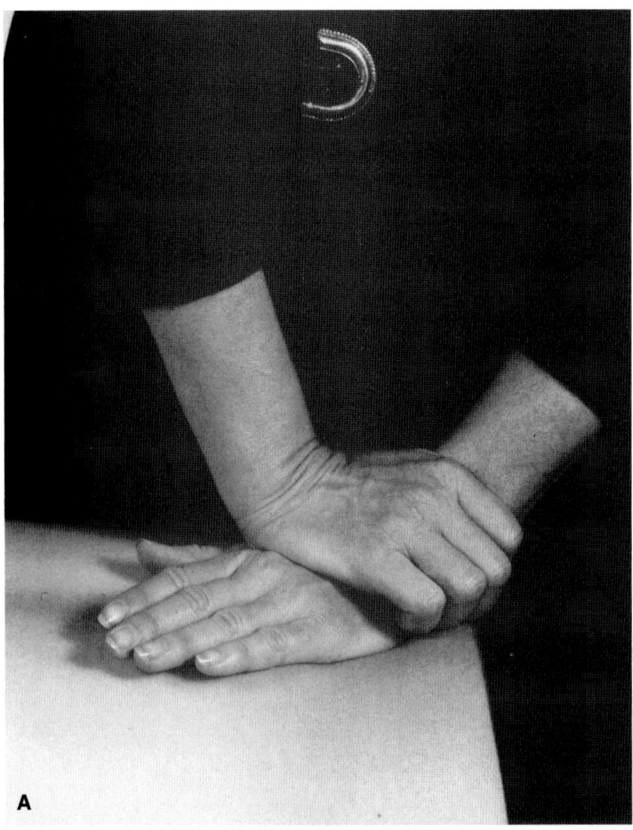

A

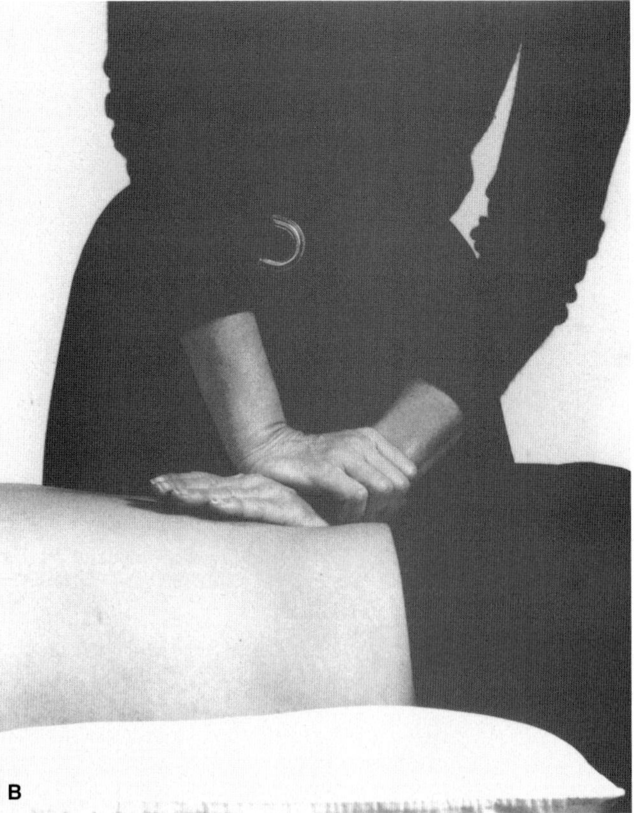

B

FIGURE 4-8 Lumbar posterior to anterior glide.

PURPOSE: Increase segmental mobility.

POSITION: Client lying prone with pillow under waist. Clinician standing next to table. Pisiform of mobilizing hand placed over client's spinous process. Other hand overlaps mobilizing hand (panel A). Clinician's arms fully extended, as much as possible, over client's spinous process (panel B).

PROCEDURE: Clinician pushes through arms in a posterior to anterior direction on spinous process; elbows are kept straight.

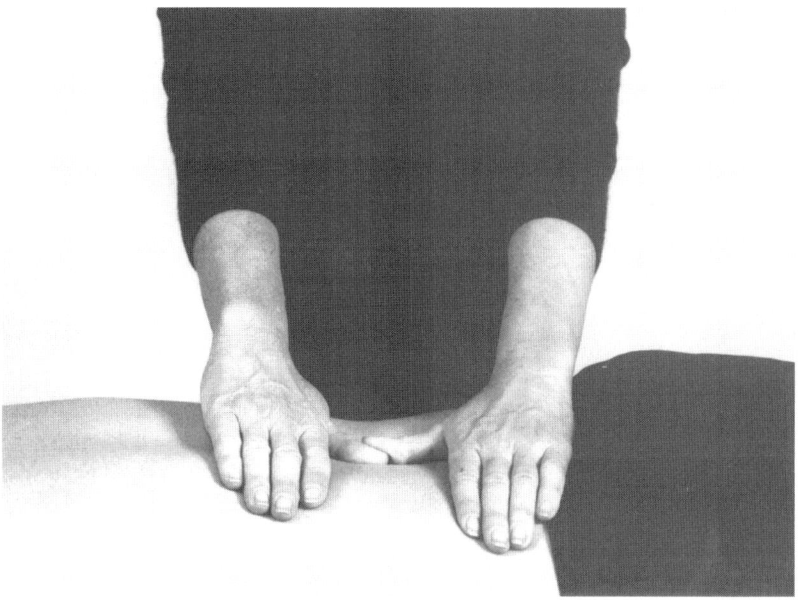

FIGURE 4-9 **Lumbar transverse glide.**

PURPOSE: Increase segmental mobility.

POSITION: Client lying prone with pillow under waist. Clinician standing on side opposite the direction the spinous process will be moved. One thumb placed on side of spinous process. Other thumb placed over thumb already positioned and is the mobilizing thumb that applies the force.

PROCEDURE: Mobilizing thumb presses away from clinician's body, pressing spinous process laterally away from clinician.

FIGURE 4-10 **Counternutation mobilization.**

PURPOSE: Move a nutated sacrum into counternutation.

POSITION: Client lying prone with pillow under waist. Clinician places palms of overlapping hands over inferior aspect (apex) of client's sacrum; fingers point toward head. Clinician's arms fully extended, as much as possible.

PROCEDURE: As client inhales, palm of mobilizing hand presses on apex of sacrum in an anterior direction; elbows are kept straight.

NOTE: A counternutated sacrum can be mobilized by pressing palm of mobilizing hand over superior aspect (base) of client's sacrum as client exhales.

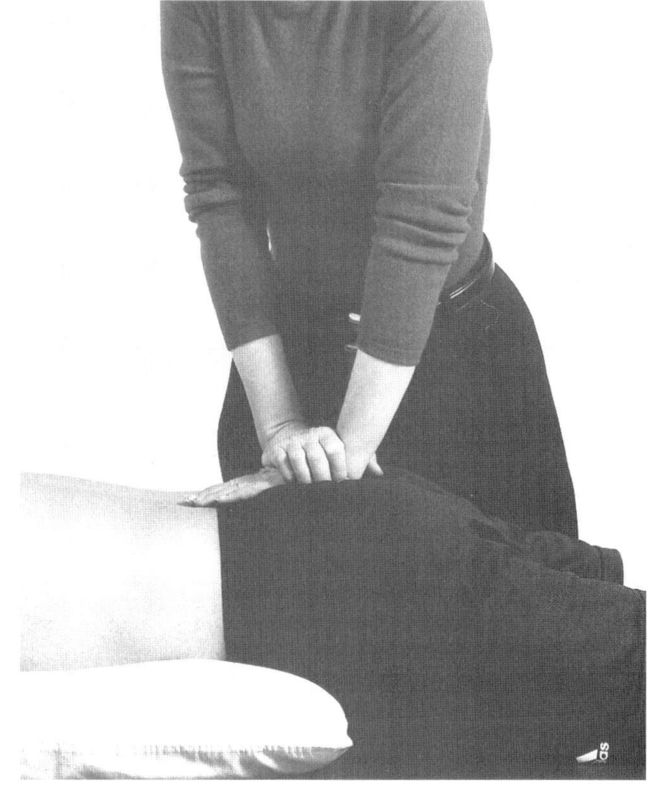

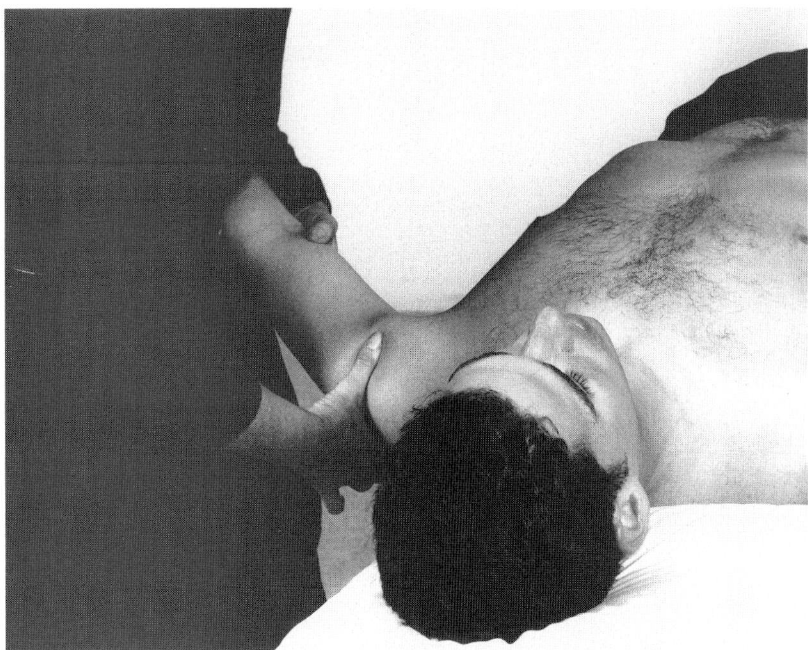

FIGURE 4-11 **Shoulder inferior glide.**

PURPOSE: Increase shoulder abduction and flexion.

POSITION: Client lying supine, shoulder abducted to 45°. Clinician standing on involved side. Stabilizing hand placed under arm, holding at elbow; mobilizing hand placed at joint line distal to acromion.

PROCEDURE: Mobilizing hand presses humerus toward client's feet.

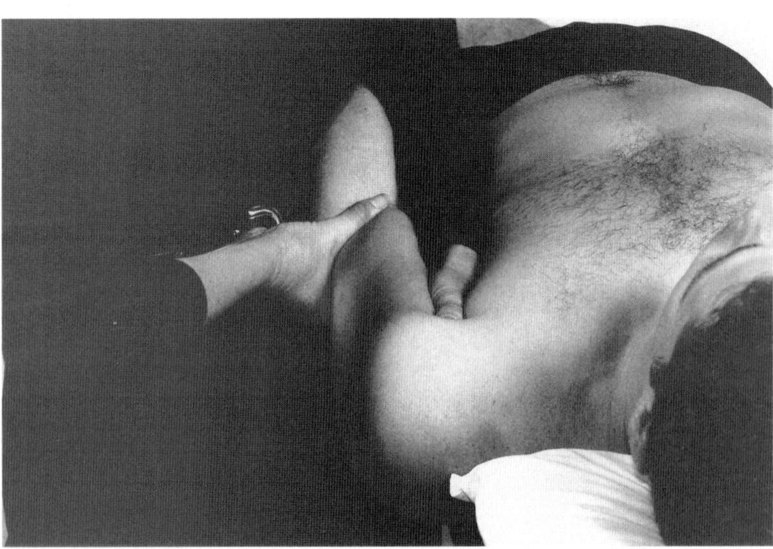

FIGURE 4-12 **Shoulder inferior glide (long-axis distraction).**

PURPOSE: Increase shoulder abduction and flexion.

POSITION: Client lying supine with arm at side. Clinician standing on involved side. Stabilizing hand placed in axilla area of client, pressing into ribs and superior in an attempt to block at inferior surface of glenoid neck. Mobilizing hand grasps elbow.

PROCEDURE: Mobilizing hand slowly pulls arm in inferior direction with stabilizing hand in axilla.

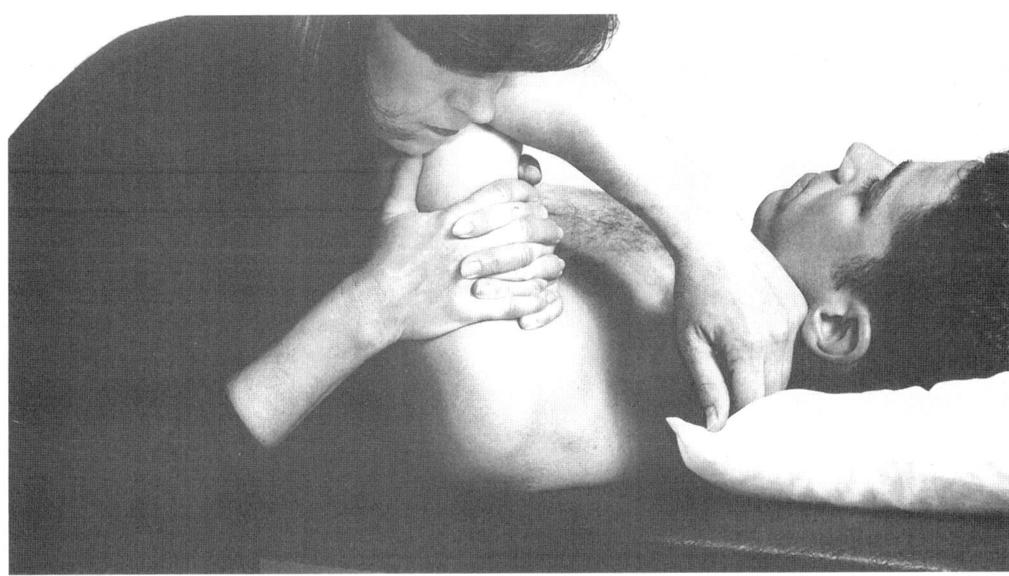

FIGURE 4-13 **Shoulder inferior glide.**

PURPOSE: Increase shoulder flexion and abduction.

POSITION: Client lying supine with shoulder near edge of table and flexed to 90°. Clinician, bending at hips, places client's elbow on top of clinician's shoulder. Clinician's interlocked fingers cupping over biceps, near joint line of shoulder.

PROCEDURE: Keeping clinician's trunk stable and using clinician's shoulder as fulcrum, clinician pulls humerus inferior.

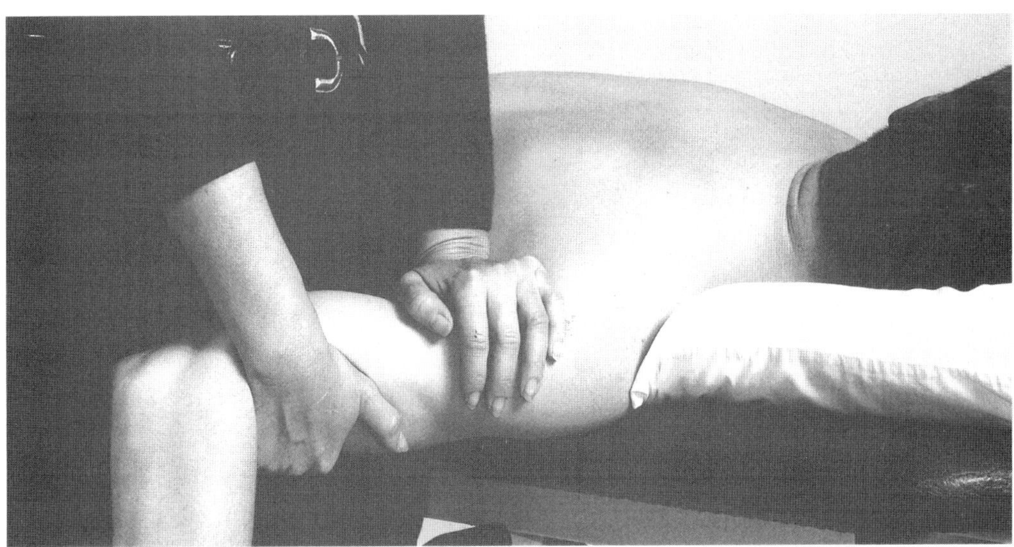

FIGURE 4-14 **Shoulder anterior glide.**

PURPOSE: Increase shoulder external rotation and extension.

POSITION: Client lying prone with shoulder at edge of table and abducted to 90°; elbow flexed to 90°. Clinician standing on involved side. Mobilizing hand placed over posterior shoulder, distal to joint line, with elbow fully extended. Stabilizing hand cradles biceps, holding the extremity.

PROCEDURE: Mobilizing hand presses anterior toward the floor; elbow is extended.

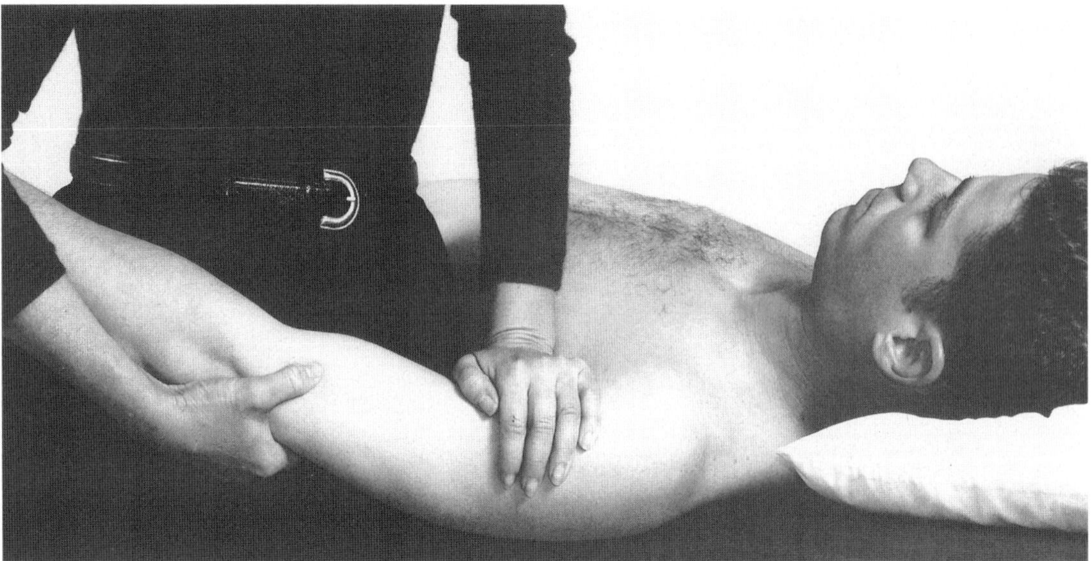

FIGURE 4-15 **Shoulder posterior glide.**

PURPOSE: Increase shoulder internal rotation and flexion.

POSITION: Client lying supine with shoulder at edge of table and abducted to 45°. Clinician standing on involved side. Mobilizing hand placed over anterior shoulder, distal to joint line, with elbow fully extended. Stabilizing hand cradles triceps, holding the extremity.

PROCEDURE: Mobilizing hand presses posterior toward the floor; elbow is extended.

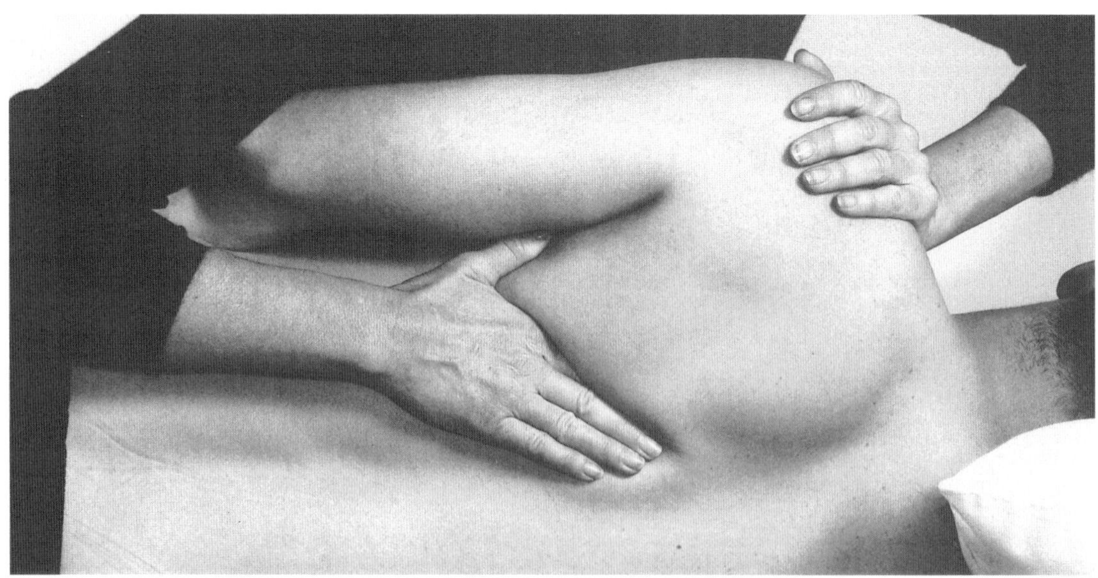

FIGURE 4-16 **Scapular mobilization.**

PURPOSE: Increase scapular mobility (general).

POSITION: Client side lying with involved side up. Clinician standing at the side of table in front of client. Stabilizing hand placed over anterior shoulder; mobilizing hand placed under inferior angle of scapula with index finger along inferior medial aspect of scapula.

PROCEDURE: As stabilizing hand pushes shoulder posteriorly, mobilizing hand moves under scapula (between scapula and ribs). Once this position is achieved, mobilizing hand performs protraction, retraction, upward rotation, and downward rotation of scapula.

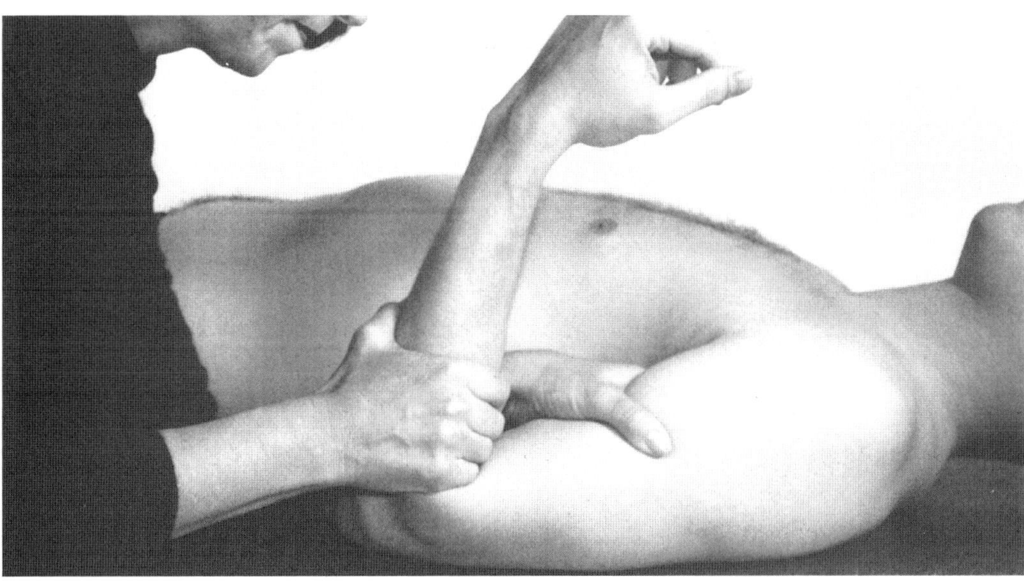

FIGURE 4-17 **Elbow (proximal radioulnar joint) distraction.**

PURPOSE: Increase elbow flexion or extension at the humeral-ulnar joint.

POSITION: Client lying supine with elbow flexed. Clinician standing on involved side. Stabilizing hand grips biceps to hold humerus; mobilizing hand grips ulna just distal to joint.

PROCEDURE: Mobilizing hand pulls the ulna distally (traction) and then attempts to flex (to increase flexion) or extend (to increase extension) the elbow.

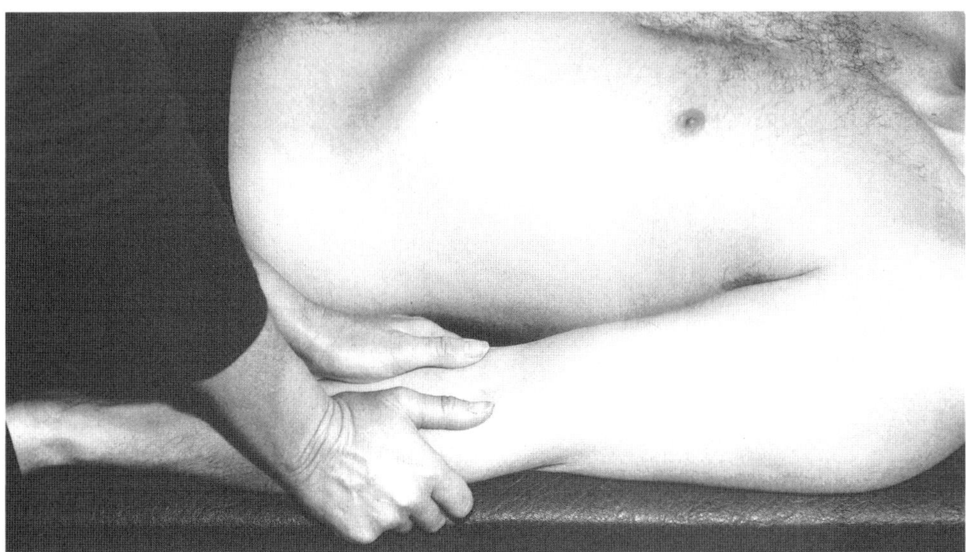

FIGURE 4-18 **Elbow (proximal radioulnar joint) anterior/posterior glide.**

PURPOSE: Increase elbow supination (anterior glide) and pronation (posterior glide).

POSITION: Client lying supine or sitting with limb supinated on table. Clinician standing on involved side. Stabilizing hand grasps proximal end of ulna between thumb and index finger. Mobilizing hand grasps proximal end of radius in same manner.

PROCEDURE: Mobilizing hand presses radius toward the table, causing a posterior glide and increasing pronation.

NOTE: Posterior glide shown. For anterior glide, same position is used, except client's arm is pronated. Mobilizing hand presses radius toward the table, causing an anterior glide and increasing supination.

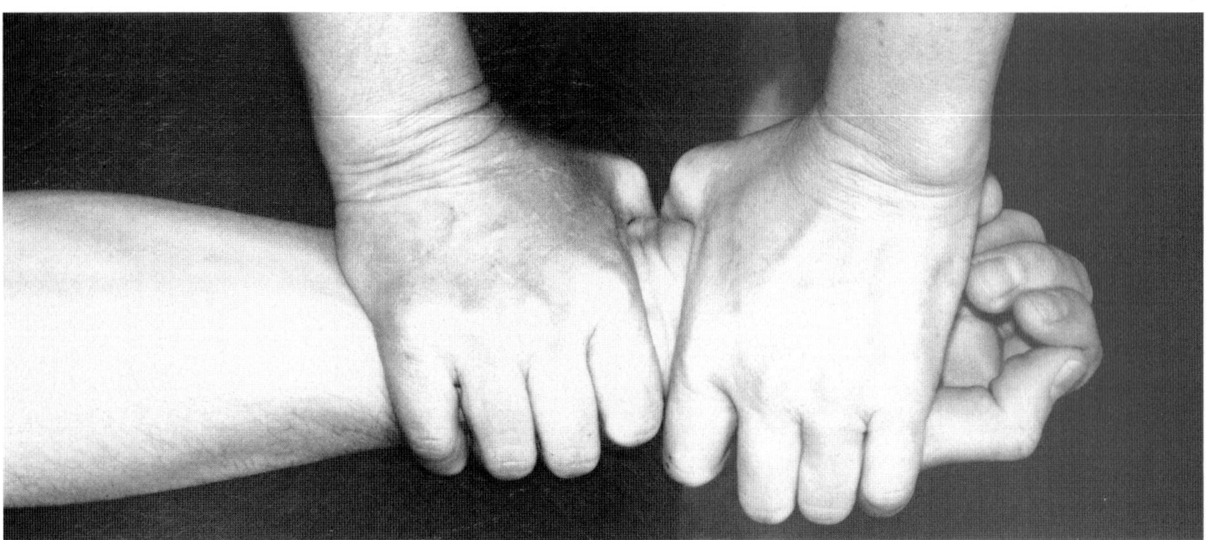

FIGURE 4-19 **Wrist anterior/posterior glide.**

PURPOSE: Increase wrist flexion (posterior glide of carpel bones as a group) and extension (anterior glide of carpel bones as a group).

POSITION: Client sitting in chair with supinated limb resting at edge of table. Clinician standing on involved side. Stabilizing hand grasps radius and ulna between thumb and index finger. Mobilizing hand grasps proximal row of carpel bones (as a group) in same manner.

PROCEDURE: Mobilizing hand presses proximal row of carpel bones (as a group) toward the floor.

NOTE: Posterior glide shown. For anterior glide, same position is used, except client's arm is pronated. Mobilizing hand presses proximal row of carpel bones (as a group) toward the floor, causing an increase in extension.

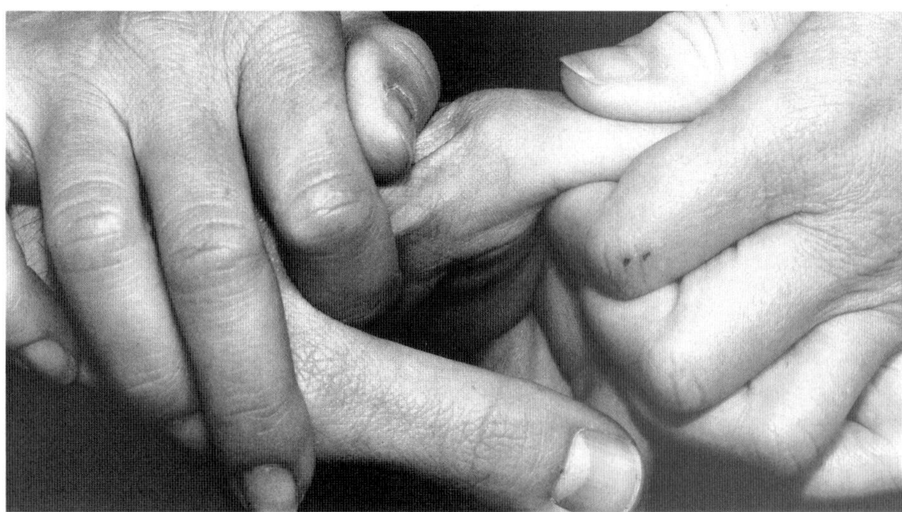

FIGURE 4-20 **Finger anterior/posterior glide.**

PURPOSE: Improves finger flexion (anterior glide) and extension (posterior glide).

POSITION: Client sitting with involved arm resting on table. Clinician standing on involved side. Stabilizing hand grasps distal segment of metacarpal (above joint line) with thumb and index finger. Mobilizing hand grasps proximal end of proximal phalange in same manner.

PROCEDURE: Mobilizing hand pushes proximal phalange in anterior direction to increase flexion or pulls in posterior direction to increase extension.

NOTE: May be performed by stabilizing proximal phalange and mobilizing middle phalange in an anterior/posterior direction. May be performed by stabilizing middle phalange and moving distal phalange in an anterior/posterior direction.

FIGURE 4-21 Hip inferior glide using belt.

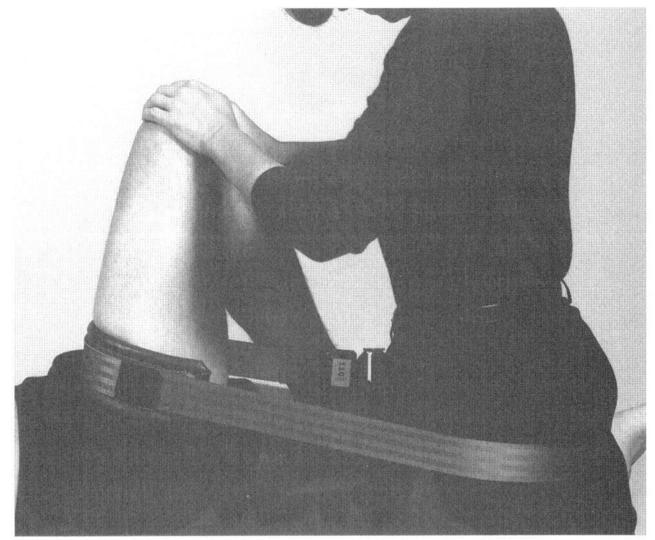

PURPOSE: Increase hip abduction and flexion.

POSITION: Client lying supine with hip flexed at 90° and knee fully flexed. Clinician standing at foot of client on involved side, facing client's head. Mobilization belt placed at client's proximal hip and around clinician's pelvis. Clinician places both hands on client's knee and acts as a fulcrum (stabilization).

PROCEDURE: Maintaining fulcrum/stabilization with hands, clinician mobilizes client's hip in an inferior direction (along the line of the client's lower extremity) using pelvic movements and causing an inferior glide.

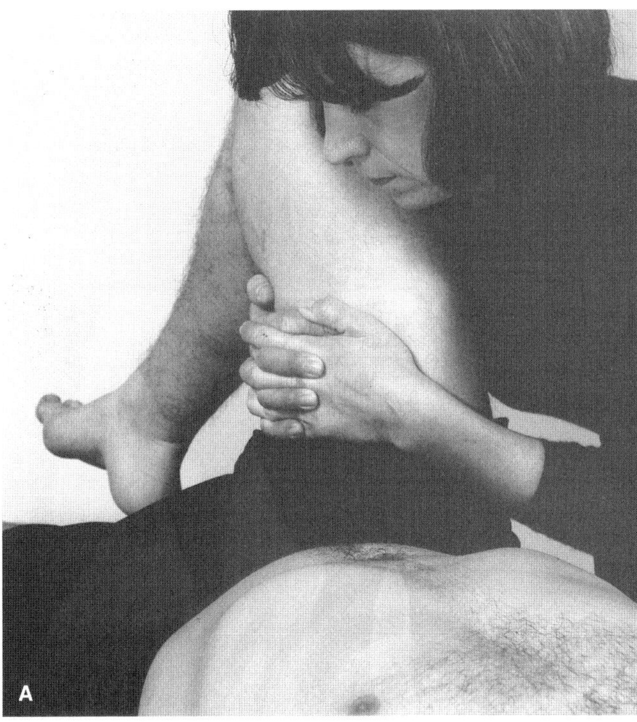

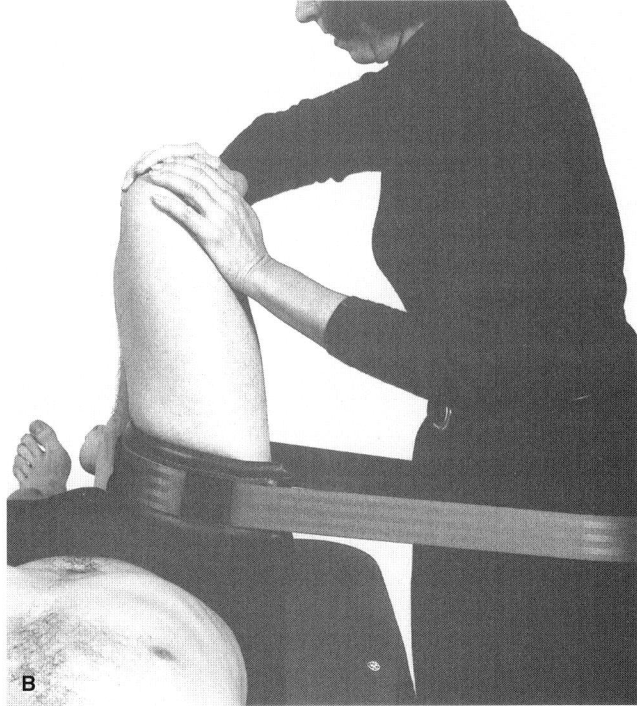

FIGURE 4-22 Hip lateral glide.

PURPOSE: Increase hip adduction; may be used as a general glide for all hip motions.

POSITION: Client lying supine with hip flexed at 90° and knee fully flexed. Clinician standing on involved side. Clinician's shoulder against lateral femur to act as a fulcrum. Clinician's interlocked fingers around the client's proximal femur.

PROCEDURE: Clinician stabilizes client's thigh against shoulder and pulls femur in a lateral distraction force. Clinician must not move his or her trunk when pulling on the femur with the arms (panel A).

NOTE: May be done with the use of a mobilization belt (panel B). Client in same position. Clinician standing at foot of client on involved side. Mobilization belt placed at client's proximal hip and around clinician's pelvis. Clinician places both hands on client's knee and act as a fulcrum (stabilization). Maintaining fulcrum/stabilization with hands, clinician mobilizes client's hip laterally using pelvic movements and causing a lateral glide.

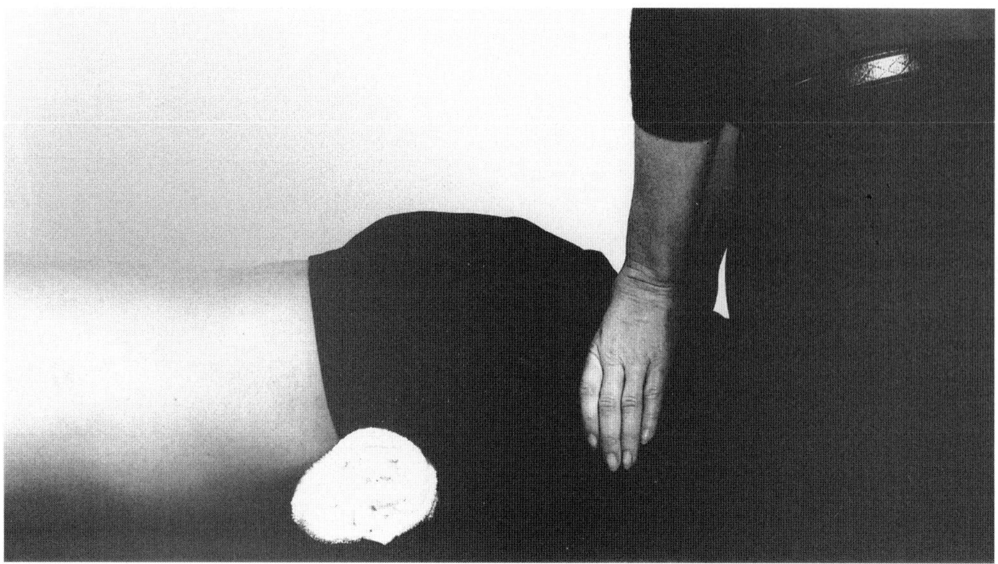

FIGURE 4-23 Hip anterior glide.

PURPOSE: Increase hip external rotation and extension.

POSITION: Client lying prone with the knee flexed to 90°; towel roll placed just proximal to the hip joint. Clinician standing on involved side. Both mobilizing hands placed at gluteal fold (just distal to joint line).

PROCEDURE: Mobilizing hands press anterior toward the table.

FIGURE 4-24 Hip posterior glide.

PURPOSE: Increase hip internal rotation and flexion.

POSITION: Client lying supine with the hip flexed to 90°; towel roll placed just proximal to hip joint. Clinician standing on involved side, holding leg in 90° degrees of hip flexion with both hands.

PROCEDURE: Using body weight, clinician applies a downward force, pushing through the femur.

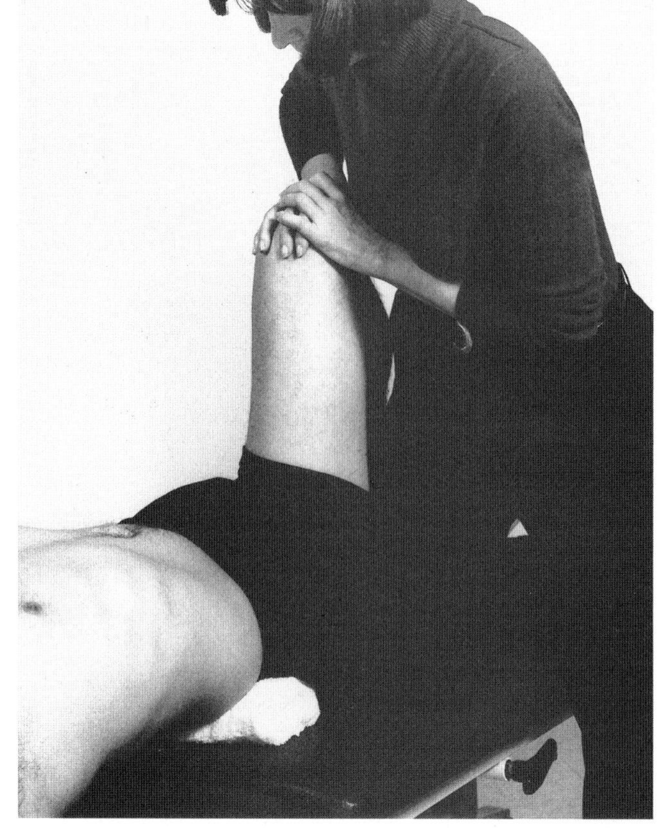

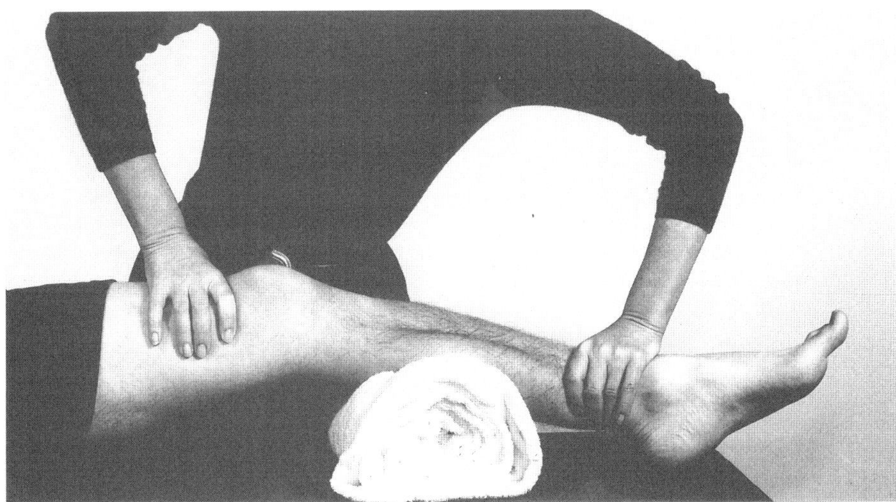

FIGURE 4-25 Knee anterior glide (of tibia).

PURPOSE: Increase knee extension.

POSITION: Client lying supine with towel roll under lower leg (towel roll must be placed distal to popliteal fossa). Clinician standing on same side as involved extremity with stabilizing hand across medial and lateral malleoli of the ankle. Mobilizing hand placed at distal end of femur, just proximal to knee joint.

PROCEDURE: While stabilizing hand firmly fixes foot against table by pushing down on distal tibia across medial and lateral malleoli of ankle (causing the tibia to be stabilized in flexion, given the towel roll under the lower leg), mobilizing hand pushes the femur posteriorly.

NOTE: Pushing down on femur with the tibia stabilized causes a posterior glide of the femur, which, in effect, results in an anterior glide of the tibia.

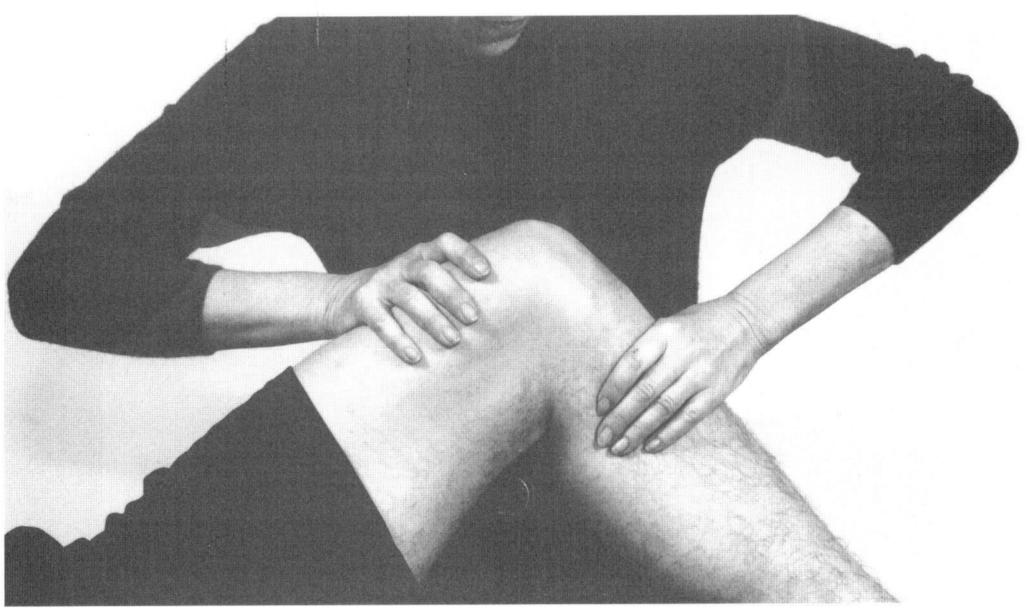

FIGURE 4-26 Knee posterior glide.

PURPOSE: Increase knee flexion.

POSITION: Client lying supine with involved knee flexed to 90°. Clinician standing on involved side. Stabilizing hand placed over distal end of femur; mobilizing hand grasping tibia just below joint line.

PROCEDURE: With stabilizing hand limiting abduction/adduction of the femur, mobilizing hand provides a posteriorly directed force to tibia.

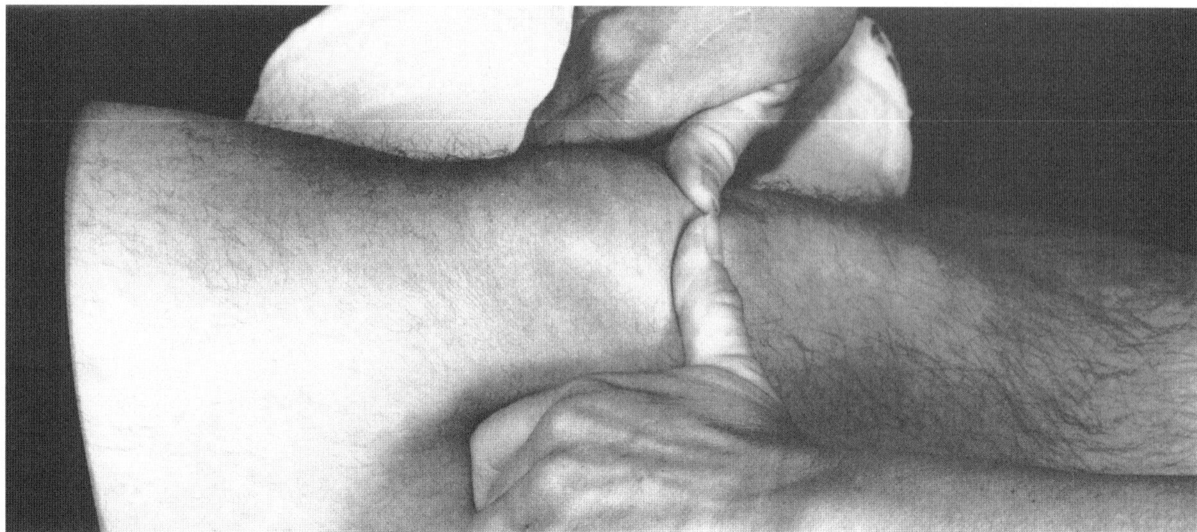

FIGURE 4-27 **Patella superior/inferior glide.**

PURPOSE: Increases knee extension (superior glide) and flexion (inferior glide).

POSITION: Client lying supine with small towel roll under knee, placing knee in slight flexion. Clinician sitting or standing on involved side. Mobilizing thumbs placed side by side on inferior pole of the patella. Index fingers placed on medial and lateral sides of patella.

PROCEDURE: Thumbs press patella in superior direction.

NOTE: Superior glide shown. For inferior glide, same position is used, except clinician places thumbs side by side on superior pole of knee. Thumbs press patella in inferior direction, causing an increase in flexion.

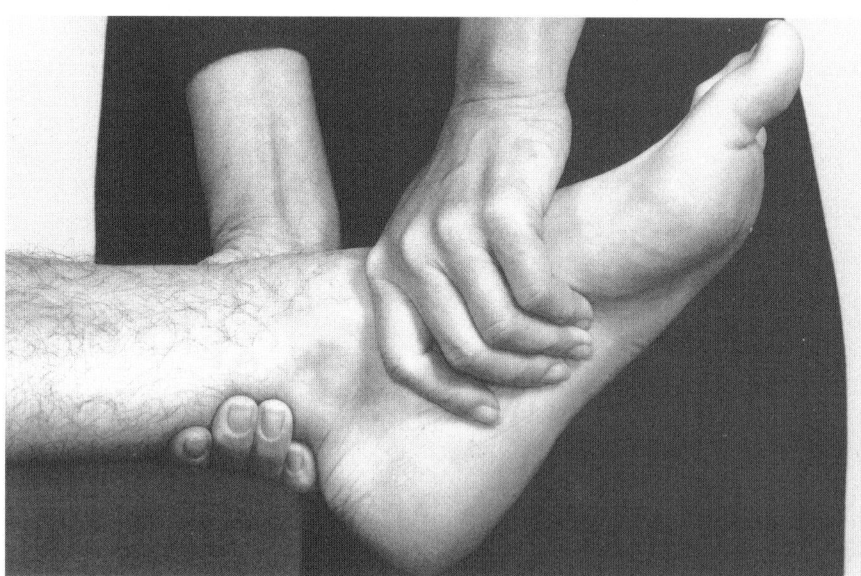

FIGURE 4-28 **Ankle posterior glide.**

PURPOSE: Increase dorsiflexion.

POSITION: Client lying supine with involved foot hanging off table. Clinician standing at end of table. Stabilizing hand grasps tibia and fibula at medial and lateral malleoli; mobilizing hand grasps anterior surface of foot, just distal to joint line.

PROCEDURE: With stabilizing hand limiting movement of tibia and fibula, mobilizing hand presses the foot in posterior direction, relative to the malleolus.

FIGURE 4-29 **Ankle anterior glide.**

PURPOSE: Increase plantarflexion.

POSITION: Client lying prone with involved foot hanging off table. Clinician standing at end of table. Stabilizing hand grasps tibia and fibula at medial and lateral malleoli; mobilizing hand grasps calcaneous, just distal to joint line.

PROCEDURE: With stabilizing hand limiting movement of the tibia and fibula, mobilizing hand presses foot in anterior direction, relative to the malleolus.

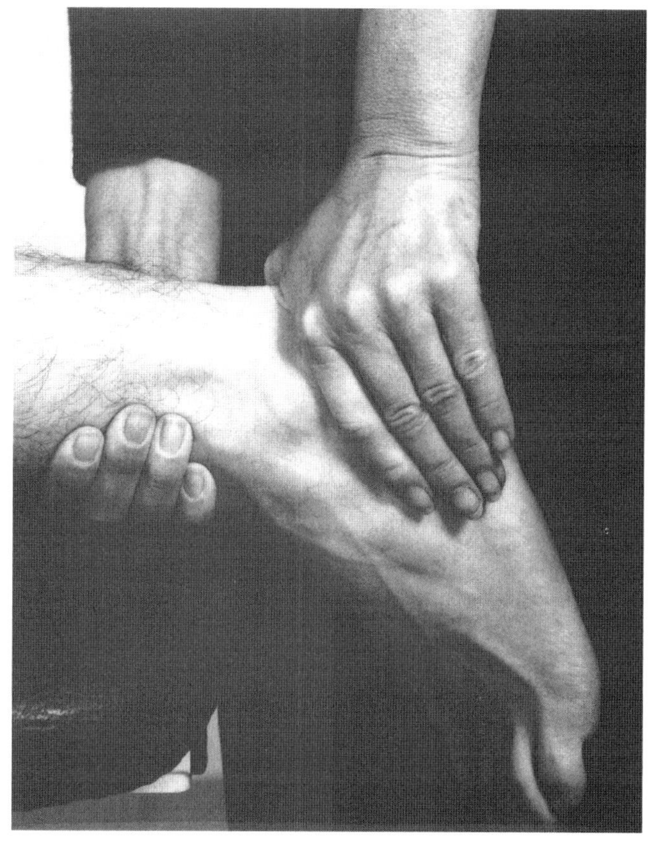

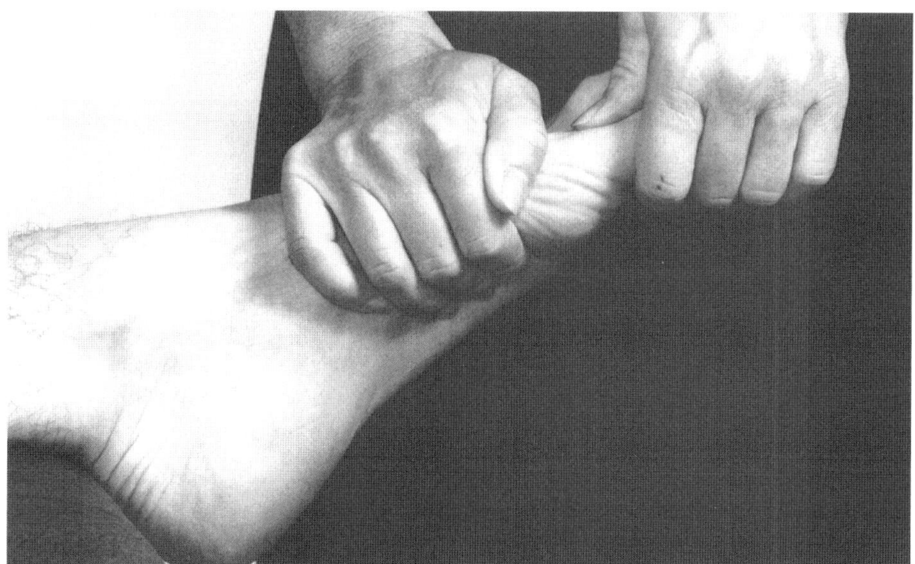

FIGURE 4-30 **Metatarsal/phalange mobilization.**

PURPOSE: Increase flexion and extension of toes.

POSITION: Client lying supine with involved foot hanging off table. Clinician standing at end of table. Stabilizing hand grasps the head of the metatarsal between thumb and index finger; mobilizing hand grasps proximal phalange in same manner.

PROCEDURE: Mobilizing hand provides a distraction force while pressing the toe into flexion and extension.

GERIATRIC *Perspectives*

- Older adults can benefit from appropriately applied mobilization to decrease pain and restore limited joint motion. Specific joint hypomobility in older adults may be related to decreased use and maintained joint position. Joint mobilization is appropriate if mobility is limited by capsular or ligamentous tightness during specific motions.
- Arthrokinematic and osteokinematic joint changes occur with aging and may limit the level of mobilization to grade 1, 2, or 3. For example, a decrease in water content in articular cartilage results in a decrease in tensile strength of the joint capsule, making use of grade 4 or 5 questionable. In addition, changes in joints and soft tissue make the whole musculoskeletal system more susceptible to microtrauma.
- An increase in the diameter of type II collagen fibers and an increase in cross-linking affect plastic deformation, resulting in potentiation of hypomobility.[1] Furthermore, age-related capsular thickening may affect the capsular end feel and limit the indicators associated with a capsular lesion.
- Application of mobilization requires the use of a firm, yet painless grasp. The clinician should be aware that water content and elasticity of the skin occur with aging, making the skin more susceptible to tears and bruising. Client positioning (especially prone positioning) may cause discomfort and muscle guarding in older adults.

1. Tallis RC, Fillit HM, Brocklehurst JC. Brocklehurst's textbook of geriatric medicine and gerontology. 5th ed. New York: Churchill Livingstone, 1998.

CASE STUDY

PATIENT INFORMATION

A 46-year-old male media technician presented to the clinic with the diagnosis of rotator cuff strain. He reported burning, nagging, clawing pain in the right posterior upper back, radiating to the shoulder, and sharp pain in the shoulder when removing his shirt overhead. The onset of pain was insidious and of approximately 2 years' duration, and the symptoms seemed to be worsening. He rated the pain as varying between 0/10 and 7/10. Working at the computer, writing, reaching across the body, and weightlifting increased the pain. The symptoms decreased when he was not at work. The patient's goals were to learn the origin of the pain, abolish the pain, and resume lifting weights.

Postural examination revealed downward rotation of the right scapula, forward head position, and excessive thoracic kyphosis. Range of motion was slightly limited in right internal rotation and extension. Muscle testing demonstrated 4/5 strength of the right shoulder external rotators and biceps, 4−/5 strength of the lower trapezius, and 4+/5 strength of the middle trapezius. Neurologic testing was normal and symmetrical. Mobility tests revealed slight anterior laxity on the right; posterior and inferior capsular mobility were moderately restricted on the left. Spring testing of the thoracic spine demonstrated mild limitations at T4-T7. Palpation revealed moderate soft tissue restrictions of the pectorals and upper trapezius and a trigger point located in the right infraspinatus muscle belly.

LINKS TO

Guide to Physical Therapist Practice and *Athletic Training Educational Competencies*

This patient's diagnosis is related to pattern 4D of the *Guide*.[4] This pattern is described as "impaired joint mobility, motor function, muscle performance, and range of motion associated with connective tissue dysfunction." Included in the diagnostic group of this pattern are rotator cuff syndrome of the shoulder and allied disorders. Anticipated goals include improved "joint integrity and mobility" and an increase in the "tolerance to positions and activities." Specific direct interventions include "joint mobilization."

In the *Competencies*,[20] the use of joint mobilization is listed as a tool for the treatment of athletes. Specifically, the *Competencies* notes that an individual should "demonstrate appropriate application of contemporary therapeutic exercises including joint mobilization."

INTERVENTION

Initial goals of intervention were to improve the client's tolerance to work activities and to assist him in returning to a weightlifting routine without exacerbation of symptoms. The patient was seen two times a week for the following intervention:

1. Soft tissue mobilization to the right upper trapezius, pectorals, and trigger point area of the infraspinatus muscle.
2. Mobilization: grade 4 posterior to anterior glides at T4-T7 (Fig. 4-8), grade 3 to 4 shoulder inferior glides (Fig. 4-11), grade 3 to 4 shoulder posterior glides (Fig. 4-15).
3. Postural education (Chapter 12) and discussion of proper workstation setup.

PROGRESSION

One Week After Initial Examination

One week later, the client described his pain as occasional and at a 5/10 level, but he was able to abolish the symptoms with postural correction, which he was doing approximately 10 times per hour. In addition, the patient had modified his workstation as recommended and reported less incidence of pain while at work.

Examination revealed improvement in glenohumeral and thoracic mobility. Thus the goals of intervention were revised to further address strength limitations:

1. Continue mobilization to thoracic spine and shoulder; twice a week.
2. Strengthening: proprioceptive neuromuscular facilitation (D2 flexion) while maintaining scapular stabilization (see Fig. 8-7); twice a week.
3. Daily home program of proprioceptive neuromuscular facilitation with elastic tubing (Fig. 8-20).

Two Weeks After Initial Examination

After two weeks of intervention, the patient presented with improved thoracic alignment and improved strength: 4+/5 middle trapezius, external rotator, and biceps strength and 4/5 lower trapezius strength. Although anterior capsular laxity remained, glenohumeral alignment was improved as posterior/inferior capsular mobility approached normal. The goals of intervention were to continue to improve strength. Intervention consisted of following:

1. Continue mobilization to shoulder and thoracic spine; twice a week.
2. Strengthening: multiple-position external rotation exercises using elastic tubing (at side and at 45° and ~80° abduction; see Fig. 6-13) and manually resisted scapular/glenohumeral stabilization (rhythmic stabilization; see Fig. 8-23); twice a week.
3. Continue daily home exercise program.

Three Weeks After Initial Examination

After 3 weeks of intervention, the patient presented with 5/5 strength throughout the shoulder complex. Posterior glenohumeral mobility was normal, but inferior mobility remained slightly restricted. The patient continued to exercise during the workday to control symptoms and expressed a desire to return to weightlifting. Intervention at this point was as follows:

1. Continue home exercise program.
2. Instruction in an appropriate weightlifting program (Chapter 5), emphasizing the posterior upper back, shoulder biceps, and functional patterns.

OUTCOME

After 3 weeks of intervention, the patient was able to control his shoulder and upper back symptoms and had resumed prior activities. He had met all goals and was discharged to a home exercise program to be completed three times per week and a weightlifting program to be completed two to three times per week (two to three sets per exercise).

SUMMARY

- A variety of schools of thought regarding manual therapy were introduced. The terms mobilization and manipulation were used as defined in the *Guide,* and the graded oscillations described by Maitland were adopted.
- The causes of the audible pop heard during the performance of mobilization procedures were discussed. The pop, however, was not assumed to be the therapeutic goal of mobilization as discussed in this chapter.
- The scientific basis for mobilization was introduced. The biomechanical basis of mobilization maintains that for normal osteokinematic motion to occur, normal arthrokinematic motion must occur. The neurophysiologic basis recognizes that lower grades of mobilization can alleviate pain. Clinical indications for mobilization were provided along with specific mobilization techniques for some of the major articulations in the body.

PEDIATRIC *Perspectives*

- The developing individual exhibits much greater mobility and flexibility than the adult.[1] The degree of joint mobility varies widely among normal children.[2] Hypermobile joints (not caused by injury) throughout the body result from ligamentous laxity and are common in infancy, less common in childhood, and relatively uncommon in adulthood.[2]
- Active ROM and functional/play activities may suffice for return of normal joint mobility in the child. Be sure to make the activities fun.
- Epiphyseal plates in the preadolescent are vulnerable to shear and torsion stresses.[3] These plates are weaker than their associated joint capsules and ligaments.[2] Although epiphyseal injuries usually are a result of trauma,[2] the possibility of injury to immature growth plates, particularly during growth spurts, implies the need to be cautious when using joint mobilization in children and preadolescents.[4]
- For children with central nervous system disorders such as cerebral palsy, joint contractures occur secondary to the immobilization that results from spasticity.[4] Proceed with caution when mobilizing in the presence of spasticity.
- Down syndrome is characterized by hypermobile joints secondary to ligament laxity. Joint mobilization is contraindicated for children with Down syndrome and those with neurodevelopmental disabilities or delays that exhibit hypotonia and ligament laxity.
- Children with juvenile rheumatoid arthritis often develop joint contractures. These contractures should be treated early and aggressively to minimize secondary contractures in adjacent joints and subsequent functional deficits.[5]

1. Kendall HO, Kendall FP, Boynton DA. Posture and pain. Rpt. ed. Melbourne, FL: Krieger, 1971.
2. Salter RB. Textbook or disorders and injuries of the musculoskeletal system. 3rd ed. Baltimore: Williams & Wilkins, 1999.
3. Speer DP, Braun JK. The biomechanical basis of growth plate injuries. Phys Sportsmed 1985;13:72–78.
4. Harris SR, Lundgren BD. Joint mobilization for children with central nervous system disorders: indications and precautions. Phys Ther 1991;71:890–895.
5. Wright FV, Smith E, Physical therapy management of the child and adolescent with juvenile rheumatoid arthritis. In: JM Walker, A Helewa, eds. Physical therapy in arthritis. Philadelphia: Saunders, 1996:211–244.

REFERENCES

1. Mennell JM. The musculoskeletal system: differential diagnosis from symptoms and physical signs. Gaithersburg, MD: Aspen Publishers, 1992.
2. Basmajian JV, Nyberg R. Rational manual therapies. Baltimore: Williams & Wilkins, 1993.
3. Bourdillon JF, Day EA. Spinal manipulation. London: Heinemann Medical, 1987.
4. American Physical Therapy Association. Guide to physical therapist practice, second edition. Phys Ther 2001;81:1–768.
5. Saunders HD, Saunders R. Evaluation, treatment and prevention of musculoskeletal disorders. Vol. 1 Spine. Bloomington, Minnesota: Educational Opportunities, 1993.
6. Hertling D, Kessler RM. Management of common musculoskeletal disorders. Philadelphia: Lippincott-Raven, 1996.
7. Cyriax JH, Cyriax J. Textbook of orthopaedic medicine, 8th ed. London: Bailliere Tindall, 1982.
8. Kaltenborn FM. The spine: basic evaluation and mobilization techniques. Minneapolis: Orthopedic Physical Therapy Products, 1993.
9. Maitland GD. Vertebral manipulation. Boston: Butterworth, 1977.
10. Lehmkuhl LD, Smith LK. Brunnstrom's clinical kinesiology. 4th ed. Philadelphia: Davis, 1983.
11. Maitland GD. Peripheral manipulation. Boston: Butterworth, 1977.
12. Rothstein, JM. Manual therapy: a special issue and a special topic [Editor's note]. Phys Ther 1992;72:839–841.
13. Tortora GJ. Principles of human anatomy. 5th ed. New York: Harper & Row, 1989.
14. Greenman PE. Principles of manual medicine. Baltimore: Williams & Wilkins, 1989.
15. Norkin CC, Levangie PK. Joint structure and function: a comprehensive analysis. 2nd ed. Philadelphia: Davis, 1992.
16. Soderberg GL. Kinesiology: application to pathological motion. 2nd ed. Baltimore: Williams & Wilkins, 1997.
17. Bogduk N, Twomey LT. Clinical anatomy of the lumbar spine. London: Churchhill Livingstone, 1991.
18. Edmond SL. Manipulation and mobilization: extremity and spinal techniques. St. Louis: Mosby, 1993.
19. Lee R, Evans J. Towards a better understanding of spinal posteroanterior mobilization. Physiotherapy 1994;80:68–73.
20. National Athletic Trainer's Association. Athletic training educational competencies. 3rd ed. Dallas: NATA, 1999.

SECTION

Strength, Power, and Endurance

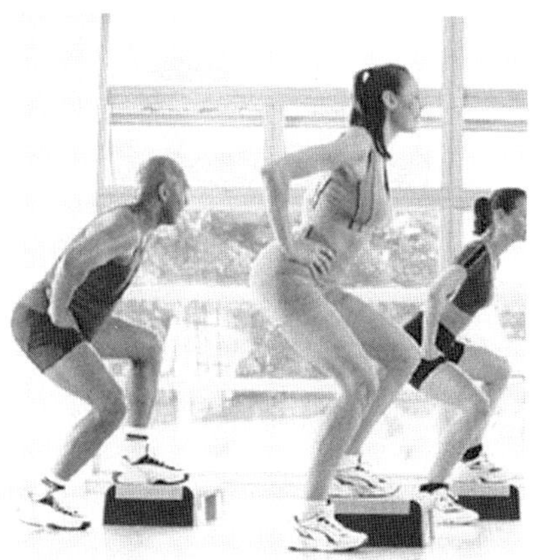

CHAPTER

Principles of Resistance Training

Michael Sanders, EdD
Barbara Sanders, PhD, PT, SCS

Background

The clinician frequently addresses the concepts of strength and resistance training, characteristics of muscular performance. Strength is defined as the maximal voluntary force that can be produced by the neuromuscular system, usually demonstrated by the ability to lift a maximal load one time, called the one repetition maximum (1 RM). Increase in strength occurs as a result of resistance training (defined as lifting heavy loads for a relatively low number of repetitions for all types of contractions) and involves a complex set of interactions: neurologic, muscular, biomechanical.[1] The importance of a strong theoretical background in strength and resistive training allows not only a common language and standardization of terminology but also practical applications of muscle training theory. Research has demonstrated that many health and fitness benefits result from engaging in muscle training. Several authors[2,3] have provided copious data on the positive physiologic responses to training programs. The concepts discussed in following sections provide an important background to the physiological parameters and practical adaptations of muscle training.

MUSCLE LOSS

Adults who do not strength train lose between 5 and 7 lb of muscle every decade.[2] Although endurance exercise improves cardiovascular fitness, it does not prevent the loss of muscle tissue. Only muscle training maintains muscle mass and strength throughout the mid-life years.

METABOLIC RATE

Because muscle is active tissue, muscle loss is accompanied by a reduction in resting metabolism rate. Information from Keyes et al.[4] and Evans and Rosenberg[2] indicates that the average adult experiences a 2 to 5% reduction in metabolic rate every decade of life. Regular muscle training prevents muscle loss and the accompanying decrease in resting metabolic rate.

In fact, research reveals that adding 3 lb of muscle mass increases resting metabolic rate by 7% and daily calorie requirements by 15%.[5] At rest, 1 lb of muscle requires about 35 calories per day for tissue maintenance; and during exercise, muscle energy use increases dramatically. Adults who replace muscle through sensible strength training use more calories all day long, thereby, reducing the likelihood of fat accumulation.

MUSCLE MASS

Because most adults do not perform resistance training, they need first to replace the muscle tissue that has been lost through inactivity. Fleg and Lakaha[6] reported that a standard strength-training program can increase total muscle area by 11.4%. This response is typical for men who train at 80% of 1 RM, three days per week.

BODY COMPOSITION

Misner and co-workers[5] reported that after 8 weeks of training, adults who were given a constant diet were able to lower their percent body fat. Weight training with low repetition, progressive load activity increased fat-free weight through increased muscular development.

BONE MINERAL DENSITY

The effects of progressive resistance exercise are similar for muscle tissue and bone tissue. The same muscle training stimulates increases in the bone mineral density of the upper femur after 4 months of exercise.[5] Appropriate application of progressive resistance exercise is the key to increasing bone mineral density and connective tissue strength. Support for this premise comes from several studies that compared bone mineral densities of athletes with those of nonathletes.[7–9] These studies suggest that exercise programs specifically designed to stimulate bone growth should consider specificity of loading, progressive overload, and variation. Exercises should involve many muscle groups, direct the force vectors through the axial skeleton, and allow larger loads to be used. For example, running may be a good stimulus for the femur but would not be effective for the wrist.

GLUCOSE METABOLISM

Hurley[3] reported a 23% increase in glucose uptake after 4 months of resistance training. Because poor glucose metabolism is associated with adult-onset diabetes, improved glucose metabolism is an important benefit of regular strength exercise. The rates of muscle glycogen use, muscle glucose uptake, and liver glucose output are directly related to the intensity and duration of exercise in combination with diet. Exercise programs alter skeletal muscle carbohydrate metabolism, enhancing insulin action and perhaps accounting for the benefits of exercise in insulin-resistant states.

GASTROINTESTINAL TRANSIT TIME

A study by Koffler et al.[10] showed a 56% increase in gastrointestinal transit time after 3 months of resistance training. This increase is a significant finding, because delayed gastrointestinal transit time is related to a higher risk of colon cancer.

RESTING BLOOD PRESSURE

Resistance training alone has been shown to significantly reduce resting blood pressure.[11] One study revealed that strength plus aerobic exercise is effective for improving blood pressure readings.[5] After 2 months of combined exercise, participants' systolic blood pressures dropped by 5 mm Hg and their diastolic blood pressure by 3 mm Hg.

BLOOD LIPID LEVELS

Although the effects of resistance training on blood lipid levels need further research, at least two studies revealed improved profiles after several weeks of strength exercise. Note that improvements in blood lipid levels are similar for both endurance and strength exercise.[12,13]

■ *Scientific Basis*

ANATOMIC CONSIDERATIONS OF MUSCLE

Muscle Structure

A muscle is composed of many thousands of cells, called muscle fibers. Each muscle fiber has a thin sheath-like covering of connective tissue, called the endomysium. Individual muscle fibers are collected into bundles (fasciculi), which are covered with a thicker layer of loose connective tissue (perimysium). The perimysium sends connective tissue partitions (trabeculae) into the bundles to partially subdivide them. A number of fasciculi bundles make up the total belly of the muscle. The muscle belly is covered externally by a loose connective tissue (epimysium or deep fascia), which is continuous with the perimysium of the bundles. At the end of the muscle, the epimysium merges with the connective tissue material of the tendon[14,15] (Fig. 5-1).

Each single muscle fiber does not run through the entire length of the muscle or even through a fasciculus. A muscle fiber can begin in the periosteum and end in the muscle, begin in the tendon and end in the muscle, or begin in the muscle and end in the muscle. Because muscle fiber does not run the length of the whole muscle, the connective tissue sheaths—endomysium around the single fiber, perimysium around the fasciculus, and epimysium around the whole muscle—are necessary to transmit the force of muscle contraction from fiber to fiber to fasciculus and from fasciculus to fasciculus to the tendons, which act on the bones.[14,15]

Muscle Fiber Structure

Each individual muscle fiber is made up of threads of protein molecules called myofibrils, which are enclosed in a special membrane called the sarcolemma. Each myofibril contains fine threads of protein molecules called actin (thin filaments) and myosin (thick filaments). The actin and myosin make up the contractile element of the muscle.[14,15] Detailed descriptions of skeletal muscle and muscle fiber, including the sliding filament theory, are available elsewhere.[15,16]

REGULATION OF MUSCLE CONTRACTION

Motor Unit

The final pathway by which the nervous system can exert control over motor activity is the motor unit. The motor unit is the functional unit of skeletal muscle and consists of a single motor cell (with the body contained in the anterior horn of the spinal cord), its axon and terminal branches, and all the individual muscle fibers supplied by the axon. The actual number of muscle fibers in a particular motor unit varies. Muscles involved in delicate movements of the eye have an innervation ratio (the total number of motor axons divided by the total number of muscle fibers in a muscle) of 1:4. Large postural muscles that do not require a fine degree of control have an innervation ratio as large as 1:150. It is important to note that the motor unit functions on an "all or none" principle, thus all of the fibers within the unit contract and develop force at the same time.[15,17,18]

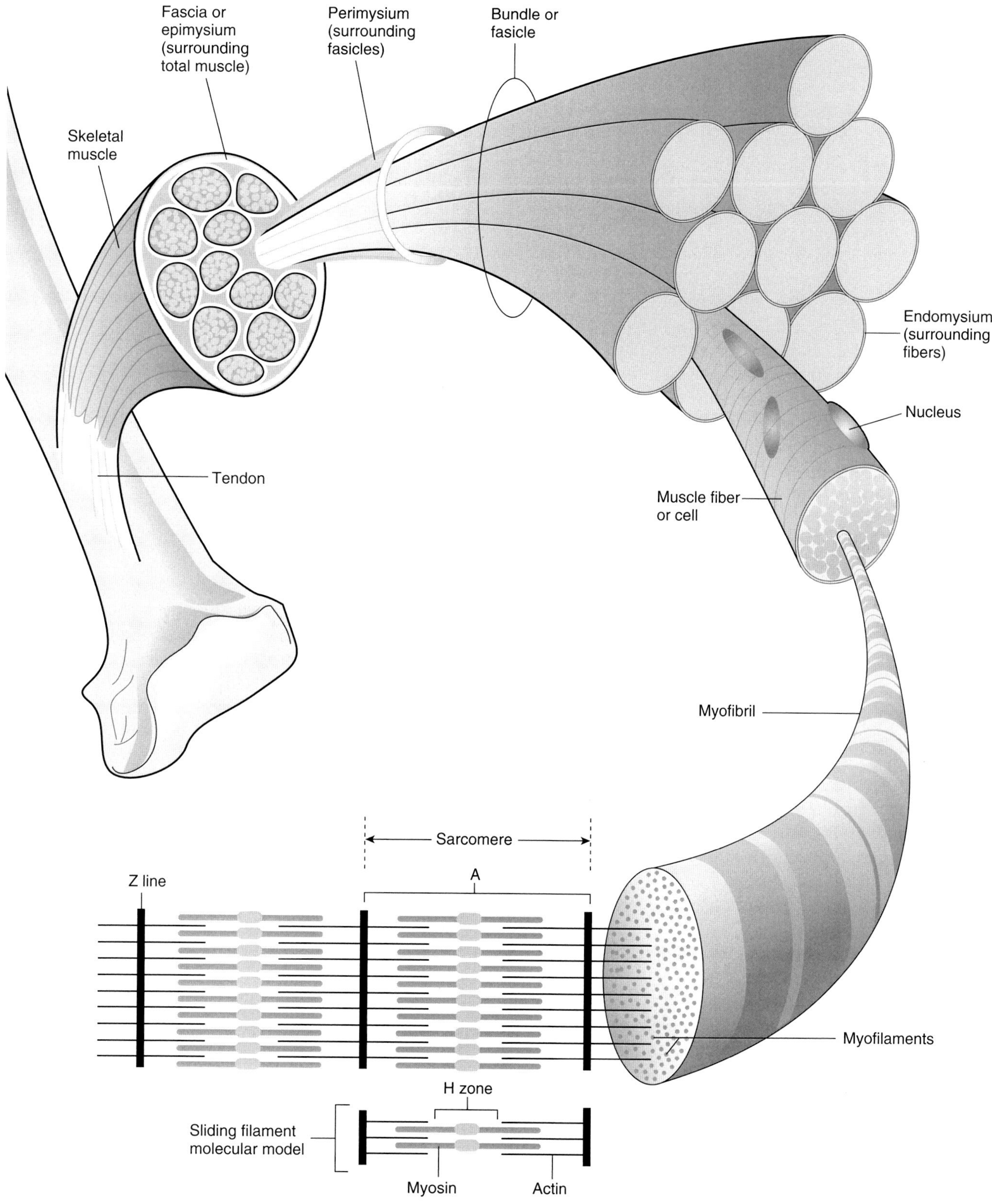

FIGURE 5-1 The structure of muscle.

Motor Unit Recruitment

Motor units can cause an increase in muscle tension through two primary mechanisms. First, the strength of a muscle contraction is affected by the number of motor units recruited. Increased strength of contraction is primarily accomplished by summing the contractions of different numbers of muscle fibers at once. Because all the fibers making up a motor unit contract in unison and to their maximum (if they contract at all), variations in the strength of contractions partly depend on the number of motor units employed. This type of summation, in which different numbers of motor units are brought into play to produce gradations of strength, is called multiple motor unit summation. During this type of summation, only a few motor units are contracted simultaneously when a weak contraction is desired and a great number of motor units are contracted at the same time when a strong contraction is desired. Should all the motor units contract at the same time, the contraction would be maximal. Therefore, the strength of a muscle contraction can be varied by changing the number of motor units contracting at the same time.[15,19]

Second, the strength of a muscle contraction is affected by the frequency of stimulation. When a muscle fiber is stimulated many times in succession with contractions that occur close enough together so that a new contraction starts before the previous one ends, each succeeding contraction adds to the force of the preceding one, increasing the overall strength of the contraction. This type of summation, in which gradations in strength are produced by variations in the frequency of stimulation of the fibers, is called wave summation. Wave summation is characterized by the production of a weak contraction when the fiber is stimulated only a few times per second and a strong contraction when the fiber is stimulated many times per second. A maximum contraction occurs when all the individual muscle twitches become fused into a smooth, continuous contraction called a tetanized contraction.[15,20]

During submaximal efforts, the force of a muscle contraction is obtained by using a combination of multiple motor unit summation and wave summation. The force of a submaximal muscle contraction is obtained by contracting the different motor units of a muscle a few at a time but in rapid succession so that the muscle tension is always of a tetanic nature rather than a twitching one. In a weak contraction, only one or two motor units contract at only two or three times per second, but the contractions are spread one after another among different motor units to achieve a tetanized state. Relatively smooth performances are achieved by low discharge rates of motor units firing asynchronously or out of phase, so that when one group of muscles is contracting another group is resting. When a stronger contraction is desired, a greater number of motor units is recruited simultaneously and fire more frequently. If the majority of the motor units are discharging together at maximal frequency, the force of the muscle will be greater, and the motor units are said to be synchronous, or in phase.[15,20]

Cross-Sectional Area

Research performed on muscle has shown that the larger the physiologic cross-section of a muscle, the more tension produced during a maximal contraction.[15,21] This relationship between the strength of a muscle contraction and the cross-sectional area is also influenced by anatomic factors, such as fiber orientation of the muscle. The fibers of most pennate muscles are arranged obliquely to the angle of pull, in contrast to fusiform muscles in which the fibers are typically arranged parallel to a central tendon. Although fusiform muscle contracts through a greater range of motion than pennate muscle, the cross-sectional area of pennate muscle is usually much greater. As a result, pennate muscle fibers have a greater potential for generating more tension during muscle contraction than the fusiform muscle fibers (Fig. 5-2).[15]

Force Velocity

The velocity at which a muscle contracts affects the amount of force a muscle can develop. For concentric contractions, muscular tension tends to decrease as the velocity of the shortening contraction increases; and as the velocity of the contraction decreases, muscular tension increases. Conversely, during eccentric exercise, the maximal contractile force tends to increase with increasing velocity. It has been theorized that the high stretching force that takes place during lengthening contractions produces an optimal overlap between the actin and myosin filaments, allowing optimal cross-bridge formation and increased muscle tension.[15]

MUSCLE FIBER TYPE

Human skeletal muscle is composed of different percentages of fiber types. The percentage of composition of these fiber types varies widely between muscles and among individuals.[22] Many classifications have been used to differentiate fiber types based on physiologic, histochemical, and biochemical properties.[23,24]

For many years, researchers used physiologic techniques to examine the contractile properties of muscle and the speed at which a fiber could produce peak tension. Two fiber types were identified: fast twitch (FT) and slow twitch (ST). Fast twitch fibers develop high tension quickly but maintain that tension for only a short period of time. Slow twitch fibers develop less tension more slowly and are resistant to fatigue. While FT fibers are primarily recruited during short-term, high-intensity work (resistance training), ST fibers are primarily used for long-term, low-intensity work (endurance training).[23,24]

FIGURE 5-2 **Fiber orientation of muscle: pennate and fusiform.**

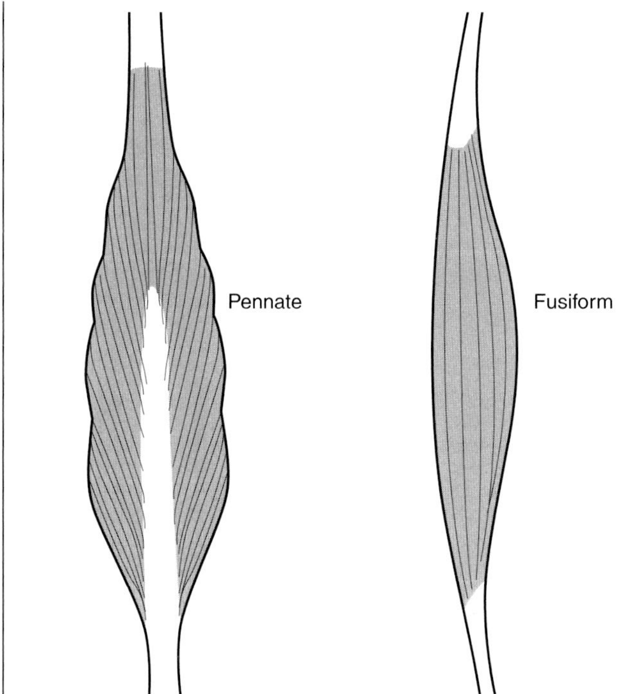

Recent research involving new staining techniques and electron microscopy have led to a classification system that defines three fiber types:[23,24] slow oxidative (or ST), fast oxidative glycolytic (or FT-fatigue resistant), and fast glycolytic (or FT-fast fatigable). Table 5-1 presents the structural and functional characteristics of these fibers.

ADAPTATION OF MUSCLE IN RESPONSE TO RESISTANCE TRAINING

The increased ability of a muscle to generate increased force after resistance training is the result of two important changes: the adaptation of the muscle and the extent to which the motor unit can activate the muscle. Muscle adaptations include an increase in cross-sectional area, primarily caused by increase in size (hypertrophy) of the muscle fiber. This hypertrophy of the muscle fiber is caused by the increased synthesis of the myofibrillar proteins actin and myosin.[25–27]

Improvement in the ability of the motor unit to activate the muscle after resistance training has been inferred on the basis of reports of increases in strength without changes in the cross-section of the muscle. The literature has referred to these "learned" changes in the nervous system as a result of strength training as "neural adaptation."[25,27] One common method for evaluating neural adaptation of muscle is to record the motor unit activity (via electromyography) during a maximal voluntary contraction before and after resistance training. Motor unit activation (via increases in multiple motor unit summation and wave summation) during maximal contraction has been shown to increase after muscle training.[25]

EXERCISE TRAINING PRINCIPLES

Overload

Within the human body, all cells possess the ability to adapt to external stimuli, and general adaptations occur continually. In addition to everyday adjustments, adaptation also occurs more specifically as a result of training. When an increased training load challenges an individual's current level of fitness, a response by the body occurs as an adaptation (such as an increase in muscle strength) to the stimulus of the training load. This increase in training load that leads to an adaptation in muscle is called overload. The initial response is fatigue and adaptation to the training load. Overload causes fatigue, and recovery and adaptation allow the body to overcompensate and reach higher level of fitness.[26]

Intensity and Volume

The stress placed on the body in training, both physiologic and psychological, is called the training load or stimulus. The training load is quantified as the intensity and volume of training, which are integrally related and cannot be separated. One depends on the other at all times.[28] Intensity and volume are defined in this section, and their use in a training model (periodization) is presented later in this chapter.

TABLE 5-1 Structural and Functional Characteristics of Muscle Fibers

Characteristic	Slow Oxidative	Fast Oxidative Glycolytic	Fast Glycolytic
Diameter	Small	Intermediate	Large
Muscle color	Red	Red	White
Capillary bed	Dense	Dense	Sparse
Myoglobin content	High	Intermediate	Low
Speed of contraction	Slow	Fast	Fast
Rate of fatigue	Slow	Intermediate	Fast
Motor unit size	Small	Intermediate to large	Large
Conduction velocity	Slow	Fast	Fast
Mitochondria	Numerous	Numerous	Few

Intensity is the strength of the stimulus or concentration of work per unit of time; often thought of as the quality of effort. Examples of the quantification of intensity include endurance or speed expressed as a percent of maximum oxygen consumption ($\dot{V}O_2max$), maximum heart rate (HR) (Chapter 11), speed (in meters per second), frequency of movement (stride rate per activity), strength (kilograms or pounds per lift), or jumping and throwing (height or distance per effort).

Also referred to as the extent of training, volume is the amount (quantity) of training performed or the sum of all repetitions or their duration. Examples of the quantification of volume include kilograms lifted, meters run (sprint training), kilometers or miles run (distance training), number of throws or jumps taken, number of sets and repetitions performed, or minute or hours of training time.[28]

The beginner or the deconditioned individual should use small loads to avoid too much overload and possible injury. Care must be taken not to recommend too great a volume increase per training session, which can lead to excess fatigue, low efficiency of training, and increased risk of injury. Therefore, if the client requires more training, but the volume of training per session is already adequate, the best alternative is to increase the number of training sessions per week, rather than increase the volume per training session. This concept relates to the idea of density of training, which is the number of units of work distributed per time period of training.[28] More information on intensity and volume will be presented later in this chapter.

Specificity

The concept of specificity is that the nature of the training load determines the training effect. To train most effectively, the method must be aimed specifically at developing the type of abilities that are dominant in a given sport. In other words, each type of exercise has its own specific training effect, which results in the specific adaptations to imposed demands (SAID) principle. The load must be specific to the individual and to the activity for which he or she is training. As a corollary to the law of specificity, general training must always precede specific training.[28,29]

Cross-Training

The principle of cross-training suggests that despite the idea of specificity of training, athletes may improve performance in one mode of exercise by training in another mode. Although cross-training occasionally provides some transfer effects, the effects are not as great as those that could be obtained by increasing the specific training by a similar amount.

For example, a distance runner may want to participate in an alternative training session that would continue to help increase her aerobic endurance, and she would like to pursue something different from running to put variety in her exercise program. This runner may decide to use swimming as a cross-training technique to meet her goals. Although the athlete may benefit from swimming, the cross-training activity will not increase her performance in running as much as if she had spent the same training time actually running. In other words, the cross-training (swimming) of this athlete may have increased her performance to a certain level; but if she had spent the same amount of time and intensity running (specific training), she would have realized even more gains.

Although cross-training benefits are sometimes observed, they are usually noted in physiologic measures and rarely in performance. Therefore, cross-training is an inefficient method for increasing performance capacity.[28]

Overtraining

A progressive increase in training stimulus is necessary for improvements in fitness levels. However, in attempts to achieve this increased level of fitness, an individual may not take sufficient time to fully recuperate after chronic bouts of training. Overtraining is thought to be caused by training loads that are too demanding of the individual's ability to adapt, resulting in fatigue, possible substitution patterns, and injury. Overtraining occurs when the body's adaptive mechanisms repetitively fail to cope with chronic training stress, resulting in performance deterioration instead of performance improvement.[30]

Overtraining may lead to physiologic and psychomotor depression, chronic fatigue, depressed appetite, weight loss, insomnia, decreased libido, increased blood pressure, and muscle soreness. In addition, other metabolic, hormonal, muscular, hypothalamic, and cardiovascular changes often accompany the overtrained state. Overtraining can be characterized by negative affective states such as anxiety, depression, anger, lack of self-confidence, and decreased vigor.[30]

Studies have used a variety of terminology to describe overtraining and its affiliated states. For example, Mackinnon and Hooper[31] describe the following progressive stages: staleness, overtraining, and burnout. Mackinnon et al.[32] later suggested that overtraining can lead to staleness; but overtraining reflects a process and staleness represents an outcome or product. Despite the continuing debate of semantics, try to keep the terminology simple when speaking to an individual unfamiliar with the subject.

Not surprisingly, rest has been suggested to alleviate many of the symptoms caused by overtraining. After an intense training session, an individual typically recuperates within 24 hr. Other methods to help avoid staleness (which can be caused by overtraining) include mini break periods and occasional changes in routine; furthermore, the client may benefit if the pressure to perform is eased. Severe overtraining and staleness may require a long recovery period and should be expected to be slow.[31]

Modifications to the workout may help prevent overtraining. Training should include stresses to the metabolic pathways and motor skills needed for the athlete's particular activity. All cross-training should be secondary and occur during off-season training; it may even be eliminated during seasonal training. For example, an activity primarily requiring power or speed may compromise performance training for cardiovascular endurance, particularly during the sports season.

Overtraining should not be considered as an absolute state. In actuality, overtraining and any of its related states should be viewed as a continuum: from optimally recuperated to extremely overtrained. It is conceivable that a person may be slightly overtrained yet still achieve modest gains in performance. Obviously, the more desirable situation would be optimal recuperation and, consequently, greater gains.[31]

Precautions

The clinician should consider several precautions when developing a muscle training program. For cardiovascular reasons, the client should not hold his breath during exertion (Valsalva maneuver). This maneuver can be avoided during muscle training by encouraging the client to breathe properly during exercise. Encourage him to count, talk, or breathe rhythmically during exercise. The individual can also be instructed to exhale during the lift and inhale during recovery.

Muscle soreness may develop as a result of exercise and should be of relatively short duration. Delayed onset muscle soreness (DOMS) develops 24 to 48 hr after exercise and resolves within 1 week. Eccentric exercise causes more DOMS than concentric exercise. It can be reduced by having the client perform both warm-up and cool-down stretching exercises. In addition, the client should be cautioned about the potential soreness owing to exercise.

Fatigue and overtraining, described earlier, are important considerations in the design of any exercise program. Adequate recovery should be built into the program.

■ *Clinical Guidelines*

TRAINING PROGRAMS

Training programs address all types of muscle action, including static and dynamic activities. Static muscle action is called isometric, in which force is developed without motion. In other words, a muscle that contracts isometrically is one in which tension is developed, but no change occurs in the joint angle. All other muscle actions are dynamic. Isotonic exercise is one in which muscles contract while lifting a constant resistance. The actual muscle tension generated by the muscle varies over the full range of motion (ROM) owing to the change in muscle length and the angle of pull as the bony lever is moved. Isotonic exercise can be divided into concentric actions, which are muscle-shortening contractions, and eccentric actions, which are muscle-lengthening movements. Isokinetic exercise involves muscle contractions in which the speed of movement is controlled at a constant rate, stimulating maximal contraction of the muscle throughout the complete ROM. Isokinetic exercise can be both eccentric and concentric. More detailed information on isometric, isotonic, and isokinetic exercise (including suggestions for clinical use) is presented in Chapter 6.

The concept of open- and closed-kinetic-chain exercises has received considerable attention in the scientific literature, particularly in terms of rehabilitation.[33,34] A closed-kinetic-chain (CKC) exercise is one in which the distal segment is fixed and a force is transmitted directly through the foot or the hand in an action, such as a squat or a pushup. An open-kinetic-chain (OKC) exercise is one in which the distal segment is not fixed and the segment can move freely, such as leg extensions. Open- and closed-kinetic-chain exercises produce markedly different muscle recruitment and joint motions. Most human movements, such as walking and running, contain a combination of open- and closed-chain aspects.[34] The clinician should address both CKC and OKC activities for the rehabilitation of an individual (Chapters 6 through 9).

EXERCISE GUIDELINES

The first step in beginning an exercise program for most individuals is consultation with a health-care professional. To be successful, the exercise program must be effective, safe, and motivating to the participant. To be effective and achieve physiologic benefits, an exercise routine must have the appropriate mode, duration, frequency, and intensity.

In addition to the training period, individuals should be instructed to include 5 to 10 min of warm-up and cool-down exercises in their routine. Programs should be individually tailored to the needs and interests of participants. Any exercise routine that includes adequate warm-up and cool-down periods, incorporates proper stretching exercises, and is designed to progress slowly in intensity is unlikely to result in injuries.

An exercise routine must have some motivational appeal if individuals are to adhere to program long enough to achieve the desired results. A program with incremental, achievable goals and a mechanism to measure progress is likely to encourage participation. Perhaps of even greater importance is the ongoing examination of the participant's response to exercise, including monitoring for changes in balance, strength, and flexibility.

The American College of Sports Medicine[35] (ACSM) recommendations for resistance training exercise are presented in Table 5-2. Further recommendations for the warm-up period are presented in Table 5-3.

TABLE 5-2 ACSM Recommendations for Resistance Training Exercise

Perform a minimum of 8 to 10 exercises that train the major muscle groups.
Workouts should not be too long; programs longer than 1 hr are associated with high dropout rates.
Perform one set of 8 to 12 repetitions to the point of volitional fatigue.
More sets may elicit slightly greater strength gains, but additional improvement is relatively small.
Perform exercises at least 2 days per week.
More frequent training may elicit slightly greater strength gains, but additional improvement is relatively small.
Adhere closely to the specific exercise techniques.
Perform exercises through the full ROM.
Elderly trainees should perform the exercises in the maximum ROM that does not elicit pain or discomfort.
Perform exercises in a controlled manner.
Maintain a normal breathing pattern.
Exercise with a training partner when possible.
A partner can provide feedback, assistance, and motivation.

PERIODIZATION

Periodization is the gradual cycling of specificity, intensity, and volume of training to achieve optimal development of performance capacities; it consists of periodic changes of the objectives, tasks, and content of training. Periodization can be further explained as the division of the training year to meet specific objectives. The objectives make up a year-long program for optimal improvement in performance and preparation for a definitive climax to a competitive season. The goals are met through systematic planning of all segments of the training year or season. Periodization prevents a plateau response from occurring during a prolonged training regimen by providing manipulation of the different variables and continual stimulation to the client in phases or cycles.[36,37]

The trend has been to increase both the intensity and volume of training at all levels of development, making the proper manipulation of these two variables extremely important when avoiding overtraining and breakdown. Increases in both intensity and volume do not necessarily yield improved performances. To realize meaningful results while observing the law of specificity, exercises should be performed near the absolute intensity limit only 55 to 60% of the total training time during a preparation period. The intensity is increased to 80 to 90% during a competitive period.

The level of development of the client determines the proportion and distribution of intensity and volume. For the beginner, progress is illustrated by a linear increase in intensity and volume; however, volume should take precedence. At the elite level, a linear increase will not yield desired results. At this level, sudden jumps in volume and intensity (load leaping) may be required to simulate further improvement. It is important to understand the relationship of volume and intensity to the major demands of the

TABLE 5-3 ACSM Recommendations for Warm-Up Exercises

- Perform 12 to 15 repetitions with no weight before the workout set, with 30 sec to 4 min of rest before the workout set.
- A specific warm-up is more effective for weight training than a general warm-up. Example of a general warm-up: jumping jacks.
- No warm-up set is required for high-repetition exercises, which are not as intense and serve as a warm-up in themselves. Example: 20–50 repetitions for abdominal training.
- Perform a second warm-up if the muscles and joints involved may be more susceptible to injury. Example: squats and bench press may require second warm-up.

event. When speed and strength are the main demands, intensity must be emphasized to facilitate improvement; this is especially true during the competitive period of the season. When endurance is the main demand, volume represents the principal stimulus for progress.

Periodized training, in essence, is a training plan that changes the workout sessions at regular time intervals. Figure 5-3 presents the classic interaction of intensity and volume and how these variables can be manipulated to emphasize the different aspects of training by "phasing," or cycling the workouts. The following sections explain Figure 5-3 and present a suggested training program that uses periodization for high-performance athletes.[36,37]

Preparation Phase (Preseason)

Hypertrophy

The goal of hypertrophy subphase is a major gain in strength to provide the foundation for obtaining power, muscular endurance, speed, and skill in later phases of the periodization cycle. This subphase encourages neuromuscular adaptation by using high repetitions of many exercises (large volume) and, therefore, demanding maximal neuromuscular recruitment. The training should be performed three times per week. By applying the correct stress level to the muscles being trained and allowing adequate recuperation/regeneration time (2 to 3 min), maximum muscular hypertrophy can be achieved. Training parameters used in this phase are outlined in Table 5-4.

Strength/Power

During the strength/power subphase, muscle strength and power are the main training goals. The role of this subphase is to make the difficult transition from the emphasis on volume to an emphasis on intensity and skill. Power refers to the ability of the neuromuscular system to pro-

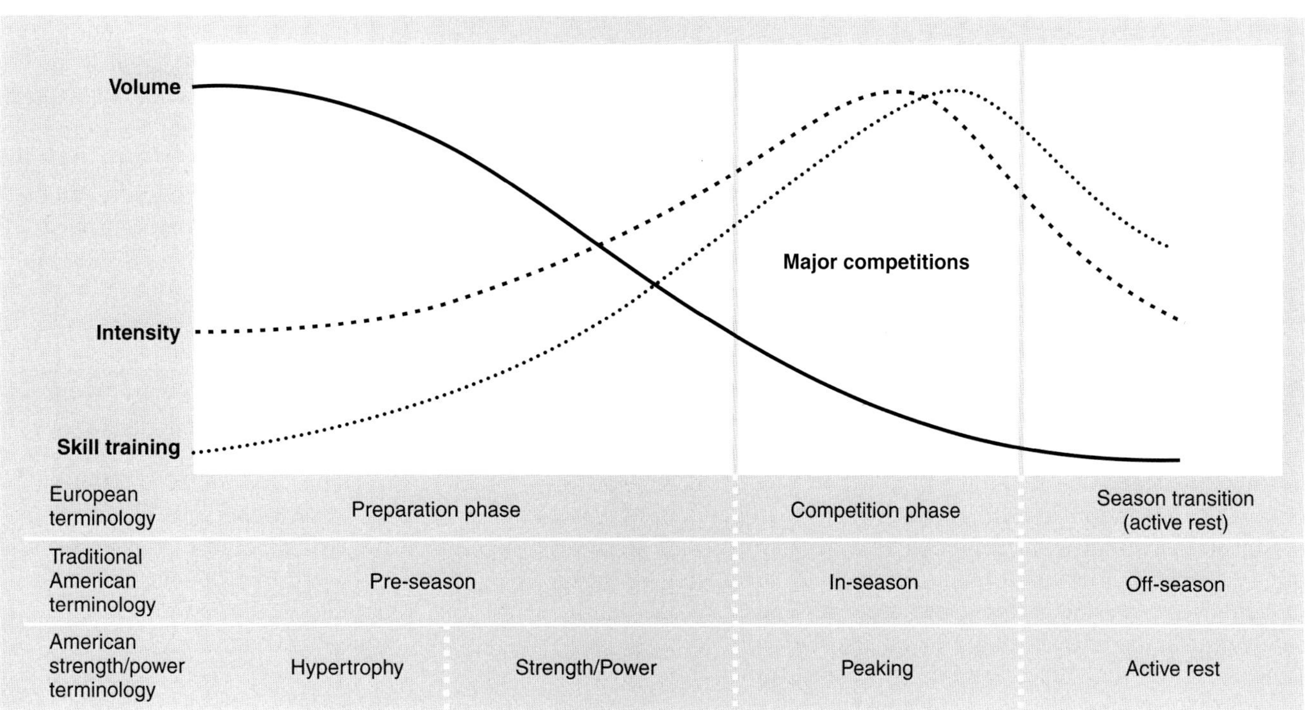

FIGURE 5-3 Periodization training phases.

TABLE 5-4 Principles of Periodization Training for High-Performance Athletes

Preparation phase

Hypertrophy

Occurs during the early stages of off-season preparation

Goals are to develop a strength/endurance base for future, more intense training

Training begins with low-intensity skills at high volume

Repetitions are gradually decreased and resistance levels are gradually increased

Strength/power

Intensity level is gradually increased to > 70% of the athlete's 1 RM for five to eight repetitions

Volume of training is decreased and intensity is slowly increased; training for intensity and skill are increased and speed work intensifies to near competition pace

Competition phase

Early maintenance (early in season)

Goal is to maintain strength, while gradually reducing total volume

Program becomes sport specific

Peaking (late in season)

Greater reduction of volume as maximum performance date or season nears

Reduction of load to ≤ 70%

May totally stop resistance training 3 to 5 days before peak competition

Transition phase

Goal is to allow body to recover from rigors of competitive season

Resistance training is stopped to allow muscles, tendons, and ligaments to heal

Performing other activities (outside of lifting) is preferred over total rest; cross-training

duce the greatest amount of force in the shortest amount of time. Specific power training needs to be incorporated to convert maximum strength gains into explosive, dynamic athletic skill. Careful planning can help enhance power output while maintaining maximum strength.

Several methods exist that can be used to improve power (e.g., free weights, plyometrics). These loads must be performed dynamically to create maximal acceleration. The number of repetitions depends on the training stimulus; the range is from 6 to 20. The clinician must be extremely selective when choosing the appropriate exercises for power training. The program should consist of no more than two to four exercises. The rest interval should be 3 to 5 sec. Training parameters used in this subphase of the preparation phase are outlined in Table 5-2.

Competition Phase (In Season, Peaking)

To avoid deleterious de-training effects during the competitive season, the athlete must continue to follow a sport-specific resistance-training program. The resistance-training aspect of the program, however, progresses to a minimum maintenance phase, while the training for specific skills needed to participate in the sport takes priority, increasing in intensity and progressing to a maximum phase. The specific program is based on the dominant physiologic demands of the sport (power or muscular endurance).

The sports-specific maintenance program is performed in conjunction with other tactical and technical skills. Therefore, the number of exercises must be kept low (two to three) and only two strength-training sessions should be performed each week. The length of the training sessions should be 20 to 30 min. The total number of sets performed is kept low, usually one to four, depending on whether power or muscular endurance is being trained. For power and maximum strength, two to four sets should be used. For muscle endurance one to two sets of higher repetitions (10 to 15) should be performed and the rest intervals should be longer than normally suggested (Table 5-4).

Transition Phase (Off-Season, Active Rest)

After a long competitive season, athletes are physiologically and psychologically fatigued. They need to engage in an active rest period for least 4 weeks. The transition phase bridges the gap between two annual training periodization cycles. During this phase, athletes continue to train so they do not lose their overall fitness level. Training should occur two to three times per week and a low intensity (40 to 50%). Stress is undesirable during this phase (Table 5-4).

Techniques

Specific techniques for improving muscular strength are extensive and no one universal approach has been established as being the best. The components of a resistive-training program include the amount of resistance, the number of repetitions, the number of sets, and the frequency of training. Regardless of the techniques used, the level of the participant must be examined and a satisfactory overload component planned. The amount of resistance and the number of repetitions must be sufficient to challenge the muscle to work at a higher intensity than normal.

GERIATRIC *Perspectives*

- The ability to generate an appropriate force of contraction appears to decline by 0.75 to 1.0% per year between the ages of 30 to 50 years, followed by a more accelerated decline in later years (15% per decade between 50 and 70 years; 30% loss between 70 and 80 years).[1,2] Maximum isometric force, contraction time, relaxation time, and fatigability demonstrate different degrees of age-related change.[3–5] The loss of muscle strength with aging is largely associated with the decrease in total muscle mass that is known to occur after age 30 (age of peak performance). This loss of total muscle mass is the result of a combination of physiologic phenomena, including specific decreases in the size and number of muscle fibers, changes in biochemical capacity and sensitivity, changes in soft tissue and fat, and a general loss of water content in connective tissue.[6]
- Age-related loss of muscle strength is not uniform across muscle groups and types. In general, muscle strength of the lower extremities declines faster than muscle strength of the upper extremities. Isometric strength (force generated against an unyielding resistance) is better maintained than dynamic strength (1 RM contraction). The disproportionate decline in muscle strength may be more related to disuse than to aging.[7]
- Functionally, the age-related loss of muscle strength results in a general slowing down of muscle contraction and fatigability, which affects the type and duration of muscle training. Training programs that use slow-velocity contractions, repeated low-level resistance, and contractions over a range (from small to large) improve the strength outcome. To avoid an increase in intrathoracic pressure, breath holding should be avoided when lifting the weight.
- Males are more able to maintain muscle strength than females. However, when the ratio of lean muscle to fat, weight, and height differences are considered, the sex differences are less obvious.
- Based on a review of existing literature, Welle[8] recommended that the intensity of muscle training be kept at about 80% of maximum capacity, performing two to three sets of 8 to 12 repetitions for each exercise at this level of intensity, with rest periods between sets. This regime should be repeated two to three times a week. As maximum capacity increases, the amount of resistance should be increased accordingly.
- Increased muscle oxidative capacity, increased use of circulating nutrients, and strength gains from 30 to 100% have been documented in older and frail adults after strength training.[8,9] Risk of late-onset muscle soreness may be increased in older adults secondary to the slowed reabsorption of lactates. In addition, certain medications may affect blood flow to the exercising muscle; therefore, a good history and screen are strongly advised before initiating a muscle training program for older individuals. Unfortunately, no standardized screening protocol exists to identify which individuals should avoid muscle training. In the current medical system, routine screening using exercise testing equipment is not cost-effective. One option is to more closely screen individuals with specific conditions, such as hypertension, using electrocardiogram and blood pressure monitoring during a weight-lifting stress test.[10]
- Endurance or fatigability of the aged muscle is much greater than in young muscles. Using an animal model, Brooks and Faulkner[11] reported a maximum sustained power of old muscles to 45% of the muscles in young mice. However, if muscle fatigue and endurance are examined relative to strength, older individuals were found to be comparable to younger individuals.[12]
- Resistance training does result in strength gains in older adults; however, the relationships of increased strength to improvement in physical performance and to the remediation of disabilities have not been clearly defined.[13]
- Resistive training has been tolerated well by older adults.[14] Judge[15] recommended a strengthening program using moderate velocities of movements with graded resistance, placing emphasis on the following muscle groups: gluteals, hamstrings, quadriceps, ankle dorsiflexors, finger flexors, biceps, triceps, and combined shoulder and elbow musculature.

1. Era P, Lyyra AL, Viitasalo J, Heikkinen E. Determinants of isometric muscle strength in men of different ages. Eur J Appl Physiol 1992;64:84–91.
2. LaForest S, St-Pierre DMM, Cyr J, Gayton D. Effects of age and regular exercise on muscle strength and endurance. Eur J Appl Physiol 1990;60:104–111.
3. Brooks SV, Faulkner JA. Contractile properties of skeletal muscles from young, adult and aged mice. J Physiol 1988;404:71–82.
4. Frontera WR, Hughes VA, Lutz KJ, Evans WJ. A cross-sectional study of muscle strength and mass in 45- to 78-yr-old men and women. J Appl Physiol 1991;71:644–650.
5. Overend TJ, Cunningham DA, Kramer JF, et al. Knee extensor and knee flexor strength: cross-sectional area ratios in young and elderly men. J Gerontol Med Sci 1992;47:M204–M210.

6. Gabbard C. Motor behavior across the lifespan. Dubuque, IA: Brown, 1992.
7. Spirduso WW. Physical dimensions of aging. Champaign, IL: Human Kinetics, 1995.
8. Welle S. Resistance training in older persons. Clin Geriatr 1998; 6:1–9.
9. Fiatarone MA, O'Neill EF, Ryan ND, et al. Exercise training and nutritional supplementation for physical frailty in very frail elderly people. N Engl J Med 1994;330:1769–1775.
10. Evans WJ. Reversing sarcopenia: how weight training can build strength and vitality. Geriatrics 1996;51:46–53.
11. Brooks SV, Faulkner JA. Skeletal muscle weakness in old age: underlying mechanisms. Med Sci Sports Exerc 1994;26:432–439.
12. Lindström B, Lexell J, Gerdle B, Downham D. Skeletal muscle fatigue and endurance in young and old men and women. J Gerontol Bio Sci 1997;52A:B59–B66.
13. McClure J. Understanding the relationship between strength and mobility in frail older persons: a review of the literature. Top Geriatr Rehabil 1996;11:20–37.
14. Porter MM, Vandervoort AA. High intensity strength training for the older adult: a review. Top Geriatr Rehabil 1995;10:61–74.
15. Judge JO. Resistance training. Top Geriatr Rehabil 1993;8:38–50.

Later chapters in this book build on the background presented here. There, the reader will find details, specific techniques and protocols, and case studies that pull all this information together, allowing for a more complete understanding of the effective and efficient management and intervention for the client.

SUMMARY

- Individuals gain many health and fitness benefits from participation in a resistance training program.
- Connective tissue, called the endomysium, serves as a cover for the single muscle fiber. Muscle fibers are bundled together into fascicles, which are covered by perimysium. A number of fascicle bundles make up the belly of the muscle, which is covered by the epimysium.
- The performance of muscle is affected by motor unit activation, cross-sectional area of the muscle, and the force–velocity relationship. Muscle is composed of different fiber types, including slow oxidative, fast glycolytic, and fast oxidative glycolytic. Training allows the muscle to generate more force, which is the result of increased muscle size and neural adaptation.
- Training principles that affect performance include the concepts of overload, intensity and volume, specificity, cross-training, overtraining, and precautions. A wide variety of training programs lead to increased muscle strength. Such programs use, for example, isometric, isotonic, and isokinetic contractions; open- and closed-chain activities; and periodization. A more complete understanding of the structures and function of muscle combined with a base knowledge of resistance training principles allows the clinician to guide a client in an effective and efficient muscle training exercise program.

PEDIATRIC *Perspectives*

- Absolute muscular strength increases linearly with chronologic age from early childhood in both sexes until age 13 or 14 years. Total muscle mass increases more than 5 times in males and 3.5 times in females from childhood to adulthood. Increases in strength relate closely to increases in mass during growth throughout childhood.[1]
- During adolescence, a significant acceleration occurs in the development of strength, most notably in boys. In boys, peak growth in muscle mass occurs both during and after peak weight gain, followed by gains in strength. In girls, peak strength development generally occurs before peak weight gain.[1,2]
- Weight training in children has been controversial because of concerns regarding potential injury and questionable efficacy in actual strength improvements, owing to low circulating androgens.[3] In particular, experts have noted the potential for injuries (epiphyseal fractures, disk injuries, bony injuries to the low back) from heavy muscle overload in children. Therefore, moderate strength training is recommended; maximal resistance training should be avoided because of the sensitivity of joint structures, especially the epiphyses. In fact, most researchers agree that maximal lifts of any kind should be avoided in the prepubescent.[4,5]
- Recommendations from various sources regarding strength training of children are relatively consistent and include the following requirements:[1,2,4–7]
  - Close, trained supervision during training.
  - Employment of concentric muscle actions with high repetitions (8 to 12 repetitions; no less than 6 to 8) and relatively low resistance.
  - Adequate warm-up before training.
  - Emphasis on proper form throughout exercise performance.
  - Inclusion of stretching
- Furthermore, children should not be allowed to exercise to exhaustion. To avoid injury, it is essential that any strength training equipment or machinery used during training be adjustable or adaptable to the proper size for children.[1]
- Available evidence indicates that with proper strength training children can improve muscular strength without adverse effects on bone, muscle, or connective tissues.[4,6,7] Children of both sexes may realize increases in muscle strength as great as 40% as a result of resistance training.[4]
- Resistive training in prepubescents has been shown to increase strength without hypertrophy, because hormone levels are not high enough to support hypertrophy.[8] Increases in strength that occur in these children as a result of strength training are hypothesized to be the result of neural adaptation or increased coordination of muscle groups during exercise.[5,8]
- There are many proposed benefits of strength training in children, including increased strength and power, improved local muscular endurance, improved balance and proprioception, prevention of injury, positive influence on sport performance, and enhancement of body image.[6,8] Additionally, training with weights can be fun, safe, and appropriate for a child.[2,6]

Basic Guidelines for Resistance Exercise Progression in Children.[a,b]

Age (years)	Considerations
≤ 7	Introduce child to basic exercises with little or no weight; develop the concept of a training session; teach exercise techniques; progress from body-weight calisthenics, partner exercises, and lightly resisted exercises; keep volume low
8–10	Gradually increase number of exercises; practice exercise technique in all lifts; start gradual progressive loading of exercises; keep exercises simple; gradually increase training volume; carefully monitor toleration to exercise stress
11–13	Teach all basic exercise techniques; continue progressive loading of each exercise; emphasize exercise techniques; introduce more advanced exercises with little or no resistance
14–15	Progress to more advanced youth programs in resistance exercise; add sport-specific components; emphasize exercise techniques; increase volume
≥ 16	Move child to entry-level adult programs after all background knowledge has been mastered and a basic level of training experience has been gained

[a]If a child of any age has no previous experience, start the program at previous age level and move the child to more advanced levels as exercise toleration, skills, amount of training time, and understanding permit.

[b]Reprinted with permission from Thein L. The child and adolescent athlete. In: JE Zachezewski, DJ Magee, WS Quillen. Athletic injuries and rehabilitation. Philadelphia: Saunders, 1996:933–956.

1. American College of Sports Medicine. ACSM's guidelines for exercise testing and prescription. 3rd ed. Baltimore: Williams & Wilkins, 1998.
2. American Academy of Pediatrics, Committee on Sports Medicine. Strength, training, weight and power lifting, and body building by children and adolescents. Pediatrics 1990;86:801.

3. Campbell SK. Physical therapy for children. Philadelphia: Saunders, 1995.
4. Sewall L, Michelli LJ. Strength training for children. J Pediatr Orthop 1986;6:143–146.
5. Thein L. The child and adolescent athlete. In: JE Zachezewski, DJ Magee, WS Quillen. Athletic injuries and rehabilitation. Philadelphia: Saunders, 1996:933–956.
6. Kraemer WJ, Fleck SJ. Strength training for young athletes. Champaign, IL: Human Kinetics, 1993.
7. Rians CB, Weltman A, Janney C, et al. Strength training for pre-pubescent males: Is it safe? Am J Sports Med 1987;15: 483–488.
8. Falkel JE, Cipriani DJ. Physiological principles of resistance training and rehabilitation. In: JE Zachezewski, DJ Magee, WS Quillen. Athletic injuries and rehabilitation. Philadelphia: Saunders, 1996:206–226.

REFERENCES

1. Vogel JA. Introduction to the symposium: physiological responses and adaptations to resistance exercise. Med Sci Sports Exerc 1988;20:S131–S134.
2. Evans W, Rosenberg I. Biomakers. New York: Simon & Schuster, 1992.
3. Hurley B. Does strength training improve health status? Strength Condition J 1994;16:7–13.
4. Keyes A, Taylor HL, Grande F. Basal metabolism and age of adult man. Metabolism 1973;22:579–587.
5. Misner JE, Boileau RA, Massey BH, Mayhew JL. Alterations in the body composition of adult men during selected physical training programs. J Am Geriatr Soc 1974:22:33–37.
6. Fleg HL, Lakaha EG. Role of muscle loss in the age-associated reduction in VO_2 max. J Appl Physiol 1988;60:1147–1151.
7. Dudley DA, Dyamil R. Incompatibility of endurance and strength modes of exercises [Abstract]. Med Sci Sports Exer 1985:17:184.
8. Fiore CF, Corttini E, Fargetta C, et al. The effects of muscle-building exercise on forearm bone mineral content and osteoblast activity in drug free and anabolic steroids self administering young men. Bone Miner 1991;13:77–83.
9. Granhead H, Johnson R, Hansson T. The loads on the lumbar spine during extreme weight lifting. Spine 1987;12:146–149.
10. Koffler K, Menkes A, Redmond A, et al. Strength training accelerates gastrointestinal transit in middle-aged and older men. Medi Sci Sports Exerc 1992;24:415–419.
11. Harris K, Holly R. Physiological response to circuit weight training in borderline hypertensive subjects. Med Sci Sports Exerc 1987;19:246–252.
12. Stone M, Blessing D, Byrd R, et al. Physiological effects of a short term resistive training program on middle aged untrained men. Natl Strength Condition Assoc J 1982;4:16–20.
13. Hurley B, Hagberg J, Goldberg A, et al. Resistance training can reduce coronary risk factors without altering VO_2 max or percent body fat. Med Sci Sports Exerc 1988;10:150–154.
14. Lehmkuhl D. Local factors in muscle performance. Phys Ther 1966;46:473–484.
15. Irion G. Physiology: the basis of clinical practice. Thorofare, NJ: Slack, 2000.
16. American College of Sports Medicine. ACSM's guidelines for exercise testing and prescription. 3rd ed. Baltimore: Williams & Wilkins, 1998.
17. Freund HJ. Motor unit and muscle activity in voluntary motor control. Physiol Rev 1983;63:387–436.
18. English A, Wolf SL. The motor unit. Anatomy and physiology. Phys Ther 1982;62:1763–1772.
19. Milner-Brown HS, Stein RB, Yemm R. The orderly recruitment of human motor units during voluntary isometric contractions. J Physiol 1973;230:359–370.
20. Kukula CG, Clamann HP. Comparison of the recruitment and discharge properties of motor units inhuman brachial biceps and adductor pollicis during isometric contractions. Brain Res 1981;219:45–55.
21. Young A, Stokes M, Round JM. The effect of high resistance training of the strength and cross-sectional area of the human quadriceps. Eur J Clin Invest 1983;13:411–417.
22. Gollnick PD, Matoba H. The muscle fiber compositions of skeletal muscle as a predictor of athletic success. Am J Sports Med 1984;12:212–217.
23. Peter JB, Barnard RJ, Edgerton VR, et al. Metabolic profiles of three fiber types of skeletal muscle. Biochemistry 1972;11: 2627–2633.
24. Burke RE, Levine DN, Tsairis P, et al. Physiological types and histochemical profiles in motor units of the cat gastrocnemius. J Physiol 1973;234:723–748.
25. Sale DG. Neural adaptation to resistance training. Med Sci Sports Exerc 1988;20:S135–S145.
26. Fleck SJ, Kraemer WJ. Resistance training: physiological responses and adaptations [Part 2 of 4]. Phys Sportmed 1988;16: 75–107.
27. Fleck SJ, Kraemer WJ. Resistance training: physiological response and adaptations [Part 3 of 4]. Phys Sportmed 1988;16: 108–124.
28. Baechle TR. Essentials of strength training and conditioning. Champaign, IL: Human Kinetics, 1994.
29. Kegerreis S. The construction and implementation of functional progression as a component of athletic rehabilitation. J Orthop Sport Phys Ther 1983;5:14–19.
30. Fleck SJ, Kraemer WJ. Designing resistance training programs. Champaign, IL: Human Kinetics, 1997.
31. Mackinnon LT, Hooper SL. Plasma glutamine and upper respiratory tract infection during intensified training in swimmers. Med Sci Sports Exerc 1996;28:285–290.
32. Mackinnon LT, Hooper SL, Jones S, et al. Hormonal, immunological and hematological responses to intensified training in swimmers. Med Sci Sports Exerc 1997;29:1637–1645.
33. Beynnon D, Johnson RJ. Anterior cruciate ligament injury rehabilitation in athletics. Sports Med 1996;22:54–64.
34. Palmitier RA, Kai-Nan A, Scott SG, Chao EYS. Kinetic chain exercise in knee rehabilitation. Sports Med 1991;11:402–413.
35. American College of Sports Medicine. Principles of exercise prescription. Baltimore: Williams & Wilkins, 1995.
36. Bompa TO. Periodization of strength: the new wave in strength training. Toronto: Varitas, 1993.
37. Bompa TO. Theory and of training: the key to athletic performance. 3rd ed. Dubuque, IA: Kendall/Hunt, 1994.

CHAPTER

Open-Chain Resistance Training

William D. Bandy, PhD, PT, SCS, ATC

Recent literature on the rehabilitation of selected pathologies has been documented in the areas of plyometrics, closed-kinetic-chain activities, and functional rehabilitation.[1] Although quite valuable for selected pathologies, these activities put tremendous stress on the joint structures and the surrounding muscles. If incorporated into the rehabilitation program too soon, tissue damage and delayed healing can occur. Proper progression to these more aggressive activities is of considerable importance. It has been recommended that "the neuromuscular system . . . be adequately trained to tolerate the imposed stress during functional tasks."[1] Adequate training includes the proper use of a comprehensive, progressive, open-chain resistance training program.

An integral part of a progressive rehabilitation protocol is the proper implementation of an open-chain resistance training program. The clinician is frequently responsible for designing, monitoring, and supervising a resistance training program with the goal of increasing muscular strength. Appropriate use of open-chain resistance training allows a safe progression to a more aggressive rehabilitation program.

Despite recent excitement about aggressive rehabilitation programs used in the advanced stages of healing, it is imperative that the clinician remember the basic principles of open-chain resistance training, including the three primary types of exercise: isometric, isotonic, and isokinetic (Table 6-1). This chapter presents a brief review of the adaptation of muscle to resistance training and emphasizes the appropriate use of each type of exercise in the clinical setting.

■ Scientific Basis

ISOMETRIC EXERCISE

The term *isometric* means "same or constant" (*iso*) "length" (*metric*). In other words, a muscle that contracts isometrically is one in which tension is developed but no change occurs in the joint angle, and the change in muscle length is minimal. The joint angle does not change because the external resistance against which the muscle is working is equal to or greater than the tension developed by the muscle. In this case, no external movement occurs, but considerable tension develops in the muscle[2,3] (Fig. 6-1).

Gains in Strength

The rate of increase in strength after isometric training was first assessed as 5% per week by Hettinger and Muller[4] in 1953. Later, Muller[5] suggested that strength gains produced during isometric contractions depend on the state of training of the subjects involved in the research; weekly gains varied from 12% per week for individuals in a poor state of training to 2% per week for those in a high state of training. Strength gains after participating in a variety of other isometric training programs have been reported at 2% to 19% per week.[6,7]

Magnitude

The ideal magnitude of isometric contraction, measured in terms of percent maximal contraction, was first reported to be 67% (two thirds), because loads above that had no additional effect.[4] Cotton[7] studied daily isometric exercise of the forearm flexors and found a significant increase in strength for groups exercising at 50%, 75%, and 100% maximal contraction but found no increase in strength in groups training at 25% of maximal. In addition, he reported that the strength gains were similar in the groups using 50%, 75%, and 100% maximal contraction, supporting Hettinger and Muller.[4] In contrast, Walters et al.[6] noted that isometric training was most effective when each contraction was performed maximally. They found that one 15-sec maximal isometric contraction daily produced significantly greater strength gains than the same exercise protocol at two thirds maximal contraction.

TABLE 6-1 Types of Muscle Contractions for Open-Chain Resistance Training

Type of Contraction	Action Possible	Example
Isometric	Tension developed; no movement	Pushing against a fixed object (e.g., another person, another body part, a wall)
Isotonic	Concentric, eccentric	Using resistance (e.g., free weights, dumbbells, elastic tubing, cuff weights, pulleys)
Isokinetic	Concentric, eccentric	Using a dynamometer (e.g., Biodex, Cybex)

Duration

The optimal duration of an isometric contraction necessary to produce strength gains has not been documented. The duration used in research on isometric training has varied from 3 to 100 sec.[8,9] The majority of studies reviewed that report strength gains after isometric training used 6-sec contractions; however, no investigation has compared this to any other duration.

Frequency

Liberson and Asa[10] compared one 6-sec isometric contraction daily to twenty 6-sec contractions daily. The exercise program incorporating twenty repetitions produced greater strength gains than the exercise program using just one repetition per session.

Specificity of Isometric Training

Although support exists for the use of isometric training, the literature regarding its correct use in rehabilitation is controversial. Some research indicates that isometric training performed at one angle results in strength gains only at the angle trained (angular specificity),[8] but other reports indicate that it also increases strength at adjacent angles.[11]

Bandy and Hanten[11] compared three experimental groups that isometrically trained the knee extensor muscles, each at a different angle of knee flexion (shortened, medium, lengthened) to a control group. They reported at least a 30° transfer of strength regardless of the length of the muscle and at least a 75° transfer of strength after exercise in the lengthened position. Results of this study have some interesting clinical implications concerning isometric exercise. If the goal is to provide general strength increases for rehabilitation from pathology or disuse but pain, effusion, or surgical constraints dictate the use of isometric exercise, an efficient way to increase strength throughout the entire range of motion (ROM) is to exercise the muscles in the lengthened position.

FIGURE 6-1 Isometric contraction.

Muscle tension occurs in the biceps (*arrows*), but the forearm does not move.

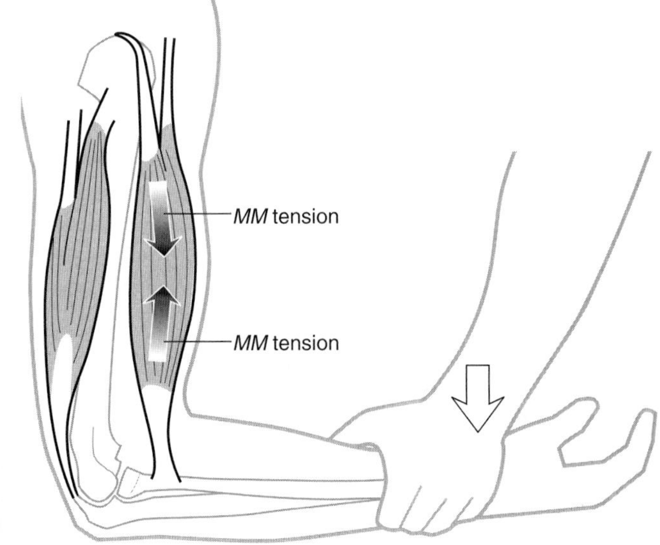

ISOTONIC EXERCISE

The term *isotonic* means "same or constant" (*iso*) "tension" (*tonic*). In other words, an isotonic exercise is ideally one that produces the same amount of tension while shortening to overcome a given resistance. In reality, an isotonic contraction is one in which the muscles contract while lifting a constant resistance, and the muscle tension varies somewhat over the full ROM owing to changes in muscle length, the angle of pull as the bony lever is moved, and the horizontal distance from the resistance to the joint axis of movement (Fig. 6-2).[2,3]

The definition of isotonic exercise is further differentiated into concentric (shortening) and eccentric (lengthening) contractions, depending on the magnitude of the muscle force and the resistance applied. Concentric refers to a muscle contraction in which the internal force produced by the muscle exceeds the external force of the resistance, allowing the muscle to shorten and produce movement (Fig. 6-3). Eccentric refers to a muscle contraction in an already shortened muscle to which an external resistance greater than the internal muscle force is added, allowing the muscle to lengthen while continuing to maintain tension (Fig. 6-4).[2,3]

Length and Tension

Measurements of the tension created by stimulated muscle fiber show that isometric tension is maximal when the initial length of the muscle at the time of stimulation is stretched to about 20% beyond the normal resting length (defined as muscle fiber that is not stimulated and has no external forces acting on it). The strength of the active contractile component decreases as the muscle is shortened or lengthened from the optimal muscle length.

The sliding filament theory was proposed to explain changes in tension as muscle length changes from the resting length. It suggests that the force developed by the active contractile component of the muscle is governed by the relative position of the actin and myosin filaments of each sarcomere. The most efficient length of muscle fiber is the slightly elongated position, when the cross-bridges of the actin and myosin seem to couple most effectively and produce the greatest tension. During both lengthening and shortening of the muscle, effective coupling of the cross-bridges cannot take place; thus the tension of the muscle contraction decreases.[12,13]

Biomechanical Advantage

The amount of force a muscle is able to generate during a contraction is influenced by the length of the moment arm.

FIGURE 6-2 Variance of muscle tension during isotonic contraction.

Although the resistance (*R*) is constant, the actual muscle tension varies owing to the changing distance (*D*) from the resistance to the elbow axis of motion. Specifically, the distance (D_1) from the resistance (R_1) to the axis of motion at 90° of elbow flexion is greater than the distance (D_2) from the resistance (R_2) to the axis of motion in which the elbow is more flexed and D_1 is greater than the distance (D_3) from the resistance (R_3) to the axis of motion in which the elbow is more extended.

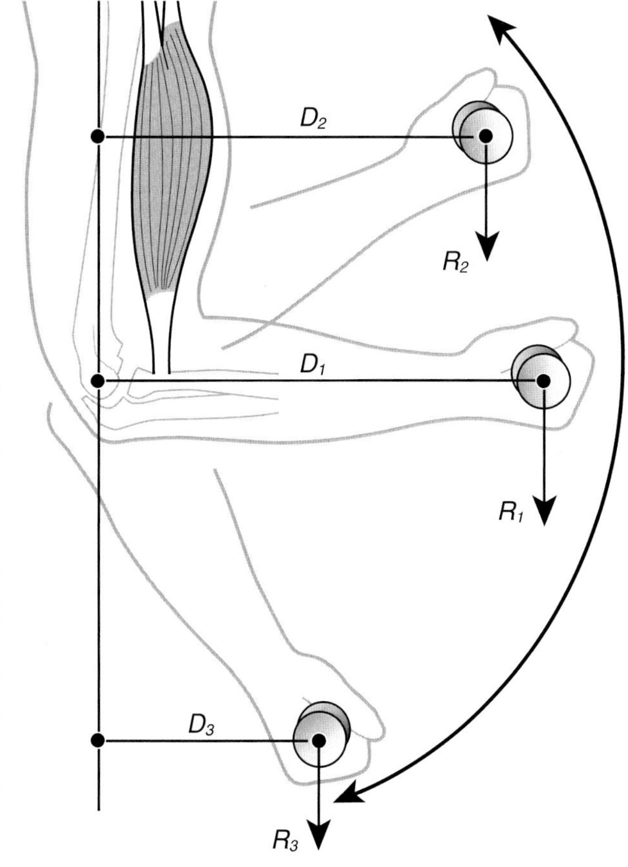

FIGURE 6-3 Concentric contraction, or shortening of muscle against resistance.

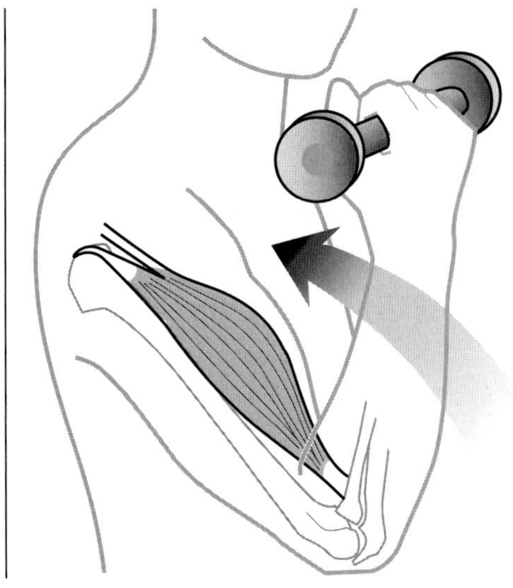

The moment arm of the muscle is defined as the perpendicular distance from the axis of motion to the line of action of the muscle. The amount of torque produced by the muscle is determined by multiplying the magnitude of the force of the muscle by the moment arm. The farther away from the joint axis the muscle inserts into the bone, the greater the moment arm and, therefore, the greater the force produced by the muscle contraction[12,13] (Fig 6-5).

The amount of force produced by a muscle contraction is also determined by the angle at which the muscle inserts into the bone. A 90° angle of attachment is optimal for producing a purely rotational force. At angles of attachment greater or less than this optimum angle, the muscle will produce the same amount of force, but some of the rotational force will be lost to distraction or compression forces at the joint. Therefore, the muscle contraction will not be able to exert the same amount of torque.[13] Because of the influence of changing muscle length (length and tension) and the changing leverage of the muscle on the bone (biomechanical advantage), muscle tension during isotonic exercise is less than maximal through the full ROM. Therefore, the ability of the mus-

FIGURE 6-4 Eccentric contraction, or lengthening of muscle against resistance.

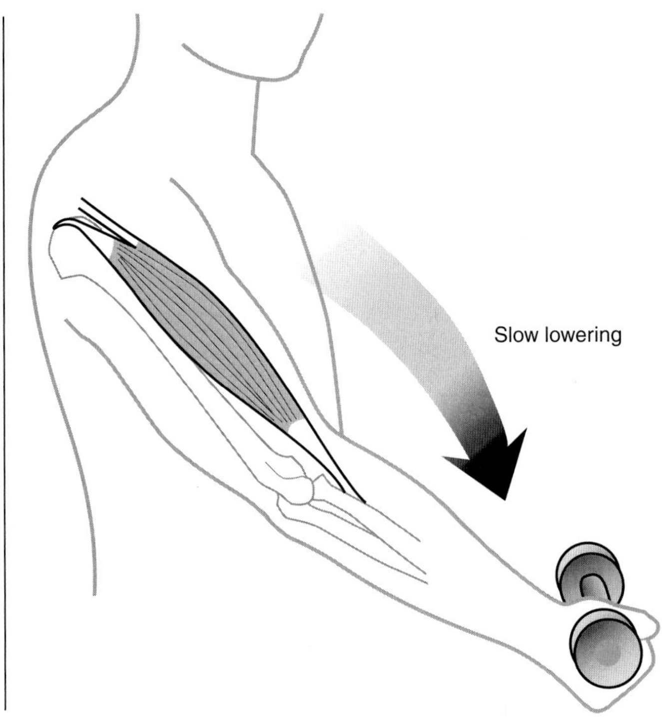

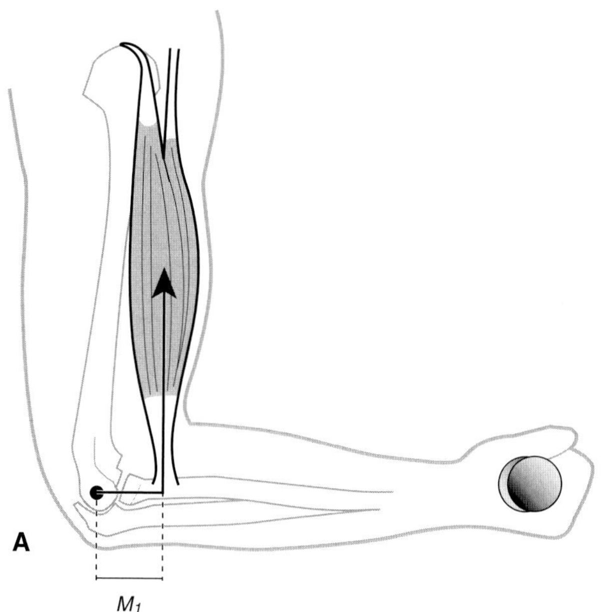

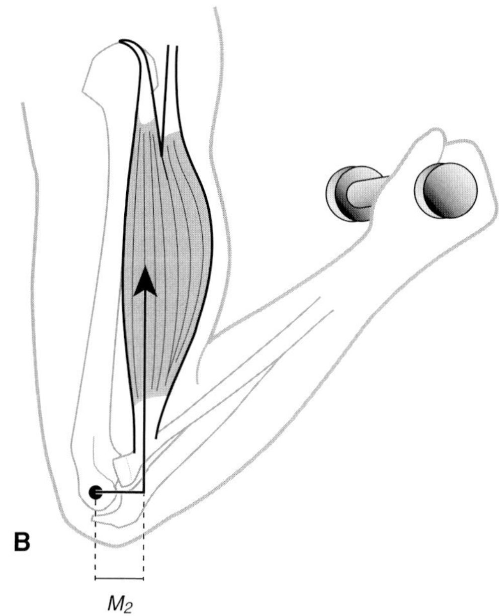

FIGURE 6-5 Biomechanical advantage.

During elbow flexion, the perpendicular distance from the axis of motion to the angle of muscle insertion (moment arm, M) is greater in panel A (M_1) than in panel B (M_2), resulting in a larger biomechanical advantage and a greater potential to produce force in the 90° angle of insertion.

cle to move a load throughout the ROM is limited by the weakest point in the range.

Eccentric Muscle Contractions

A muscle acting eccentrically responds to the application of an external force with increased tension during physical lengthening of the musculotendinous unit. Instead of the muscle performing work on the resistance, the resistance is said to perform work on the muscle during eccentric loading, a phenomenon referred to as negative work. Examples of the integral nature of eccentric muscle actions in the performance of functional activities are the tibialis anterior controlling foot descent from initial contact to foot-flat during gait, the posterior deltoid slowing the forward movement of the arm during the deceleration phase of throwing, the hamstrings acting as eccentric decelerators of the lower leg during the terminal portion of the swing phase of gait during running, and the eccentric control of forward bending of the trunk into gravity by the spinal extensors. These examples emphasize the importance of including eccentric exercise in resistance training.[14]

Delayed Onset Muscle Soreness

Delayed onset muscle soreness (DOMS) is a common occurrence after exercise. Postexercise soreness is more pronounced after eccentric than after concentric exercise. Symptoms associated with DOMS include dull, diffuse pain, stiffness, and tenderness to direct pressure. These symptoms may last up to 1 week, although most cases resolve in 72 hr. Symptom intensity generally peaks at 48 hr. Signs associated with eccentrically mediated DOMS include edema formation in muscle, loss of active range of motion, and a decreased ability to produce force by the muscle for up to 1 week after intense exercise.[15,16]

Eccentric muscular contractions result in mechanical microtrauma to participating tissues, including direct myofibril and connective tissue damage. This finding has significant implications in the clinical use of resistance training. One important clinical consideration is DOMS because it poses a potential threat to unimpeded progression through a therapeutic exercise continuum. Inappropriate implementation of eccentric training may result in an inflammatory microtraumatic response, potentially compromising the patient's function and ability to participate maximally in therapeutic exercise until the inflammatory response subsides.

The deleterious effects of DOMS can be minimized by controlling the frequency of significant eccentric work performed by the patient. Given the recovery period of 3 to 7 days after eccentric exercise, it is proposed that individuals should perform maximal eccentric exercise no more than two times per week. Studies that incorporated four eccentric training sessions per week demonstrated either minimal strength gains (2.9%) or an actual decrease in force production. Allowing 3 days of recovery between sessions may allow tissue healing and repair to occur.[17,18]

ISOKINETIC EXERCISE

Isokinetic exercise involves muscle contractions in which the speed of movement is controlled mechanically so that the limb moves at a predetermined, constant velocity. Electromechanical machinery maintains the preselected speed of movement during activity; and once the limb is accelerated to that velocity, a sufficient amount of resistance is applied to prohibit the limb from accelerating beyond the target speed. This accommodating resistance varies as the muscle force varies as a result of changing muscle length and angle of pull, allowing for maximal dynamic loading of the muscles throughout the full ROM. Therefore, isokinetic exercise devices stimulate maximal contraction of the muscle throughout the complete range of motion.[19] The use of isokinetic exercise in rehabilitation has received great attention because of its accommodating resistance and its ability to exercise at higher speeds of contraction, more closely mimicking functional speed. Isokinetic exercise can involve a dynamic shortening contraction of the muscle with the velocity of movement held constant (concentric isokinetic loading) or involve lengthening contractions at controlled angular velocities (eccentric isokinetic loading).

Although an interesting and exciting adjunct to the area of open-chain resistance training, isokinetic exercise is not a panacea. No research to date has indicated that one type of exercise (isometric, isotonic, isokinetic) is better than another; instead, all forms of muscular activity are needed to provide the patient with an integrated and progressive resistance training program.

Quantification

Modern isokinetic equipment contains computer-assisted dynamometers designed to provide the clinician or researcher with a plethora of quantitative information regarding muscle function. Before the design of isokinetic technology, such objective information was not easily obtainable. Among the most commonly used isokinetic parameters are peak torque, work, and power.[20]

Limitations

Isokinetic exercise is, of course, not without its limitations. Human muscle function is not characterized by a constant speed of movement but, rather, by a continuous interplay of acceleration and deceleration. Also, work is most often performed against a fixed (rather than accommodating) resistance. Functionally, muscle groups work together synergistically with particular activation patterns, which vary from task to task and are not simulated by isokinetic exercise. Therefore, isokinetic training does not simulate normal muscle function. An additional and considerable limitation in the clinical use of isokinetic exercise is the cost of the equipment, which, relative to other types of therapeutic exercise, may be prohibitive.

■ *Clinical Guidelines*

ISOMETRIC EXERCISE

Generally, isometric exercises are used in the early stages of a rehabilitation program for an acute injury or immediately after surgery when open-chain resistance exercises through full ROM are contraindicated because of pain, effusion, crepitus, or insufficient healing. An isometric program may be best until the condition has healed. The exercise program can then be progressed to the point at which the resistance training can occur through the full ROM.[2,3]

Some studies report that isometric contractions do not necessarily need to be maximally performed to achieve strength gains.[7] The use of submaximal isometric training to increase strength may be important for a patient early in the rehabilitation program, when maximal contractions may be painful. Submaximal isometric contractions can be used to increase strength until the patient can be progressed to maximal contractions, as the condition and tolerance to pain allows.

As noted, no research defines the optimal duration for performing an isometric contraction, although some reports suggest that strength gains are achieved after isometric contractions of 6 to 10 sec in duration, which is the current suggested duration. In addition, the literature[20] suggests multiple repetitions of the 6- to 10-sec contractions with the muscle in the lengthened position. If no increase in symptoms occurs after the exercise sessions, the isometric program can probably be performed by the patient every day. If an increase in symptoms occurs or new problems arise, the isometric program should be performed on alternate days.

ISOTONIC EXERCISE

Isotonic exercise is probably the most common type of resistance training because of its ease of performance and low cost. A number of isotonic programs have been proposed for incorporating the optimal amount of resistance and repetitions to produce maximal gains in muscular strength. These programs vary from the classic progressive resistance exercise (PRE) protocol using three sets of 10 repetitions (proposed by Delorme[21] in 1945) to an extremely aggressive program for advanced stages of rehabilitation using more weight and 4 to 6 repetitions (proposed by Stone and Kroll[22] in 1982). Tables 6-2 through

TABLE 6-2 Delorme's Progressive Resistance Exercise

Set	Weight[a]	Repetitions
1	50% of 10 RM	10
2	75% of 10 RM	10
3	100% of 10 RM	10

[a]10 RM, repetition maximum means maximum amount of weight that can be lifted 10 times. For example, if the maximum amount of weight that can lifted 10 times is 50 lb, the first set is 25 lb for 10 repetitions, the second set is 37.5 lb for 10 repetitions, and the final set is 50 lb for 10 repetitions.

TABLE 6-4 Guidelines for Determining Adjusted Working Weight for the DAPRE Technique

Number of Repetitions Performed for Set 3	Adjusted Working Weight for Set 4
0–2	Decrease 5–10 lb
3–4	Decrease 0–5 lb
5–6	No change
7–10	Increase 5–10 lb
≥ 11	Increase 10–15 lb

6-6 present suggested training protocols reported in the literature.[21–23]

Although each program in the tables has documentation showing that strength gains occur when overloading the muscle using that method, no literature exists indicating that any one of these programs is better than the others. In other words, no single combination of sets and repetitions has been documented to be the optimal resistance program for increasing strength for everyone. If the basic principles of overloading the muscle to a higher level than it is accustomed are understood (chapter 5) and if continued adjustments are made to ensure that the overload principle is progressed as the individual accommodates to the given load, then a wide range of isotonic resistance programs can be incorporated into the treatment of patients.

Caution should be used when progressing a patient through an isotonic resistance program. Frequent examination of the patient is necessary to ensure that the exercise program does not lead to an increase in pain, crepitus, and swelling. Although many resistance training programs have been shown to increase strength in normal individuals, using a relatively low number of repetitions with high resistance may cause problems in the patient with a musculoskeletal pathology. The critical factor in the success of an exercise program is to avoid causing swelling and discomfort, while having the patient work to his or her maximum of exercise tolerance. To this end, high repetitions and relatively low resistance should be used early in the isotonic phase of intervention. Two to three sets of 10 to 12 repetitions is recommended for the initial stages when using an isotonic protocol.

In addition, when using isotonic exercise programs, the clinician must be aware of the healing constraints of the pathology and progress the patient along open-chain resistance training programs in a way that is consistent with fibrous healing. To ensure safety, the patient should not be introduced to maximal stress immediately but be guided in a sequence of resistance exercises involving submaximal work. The proper progression should incorporate limited ROM exercise first, progressing to full ROM while still using a submaximum workload, finally culminating in unrestricted ROM with maximum effort.

TABLE 6-3 The Daily Adjustable Progressive Resistance Exercise (DAPRE) Technique

Set	Weight	Repetitions
1	50% of working weight	10
2	75% of working weight	6
3	Full working weight	Maximum[a]
4	Adjusted working weight[a]	Maximum[b]

[a]Used to determine the weight for the fourth set (see Table 6-4).
[b]Used to determine the weight for the third set of the next session (see Table 6-5).

TABLE 6-5 Guidelines for Determining Full Working Weight for the DAPRE Technique

Number of Repetitions Performed for Set 4	Full Working Weight for Set 3 of Next Session
0–2	Decrease 5–10 lb
3–4	No change
5–6	Increase 5–10 lb
7–10	Increase 5–15 lb
≥ 11	Increase 10–20 lb

TABLE 6-6 Aggressive Resistance-Training Program

Set	Weight[a]	Repetitions
1	50% of 4 RM	8
2	80% of 4 RM	8
3	90% of 4 RM	6
4	95% of 4 RM	4
5	100% of 4 RM	4

[a]4 RM, repetition maximum means maximum amount of weight that can be lifted four times. For example, if the maximum amount of weight that can lifted four times is 100 lb, the first set is 50 lb for eight repetitions, the second set is 80 lb for eight repetitions, the third set is 90 lb for six repetitions, the fourth set is 95 lb for four repetitions, and the fifth set is 100 lb for 4 repetitions.

ISOKINETIC EXERCISE

The clinician must be aware of the unique advantages and limitations when considering the implementation of isokinetic exercise for optimizing outcomes of intervention. The clinical advantages of isokinetic exercise include the ability to control the velocity of movement of the exercising limb segment, the accommodating resistance that allows for maximal muscle loading throughout the ROM, and the quantitative nature of performance assessment afforded by computer interfacing. However, isokinetic training differs significantly from normal function in a number of ways, a deficiency that underscores the importance of integrating all means of open-chain resistance training in rehabilitation.

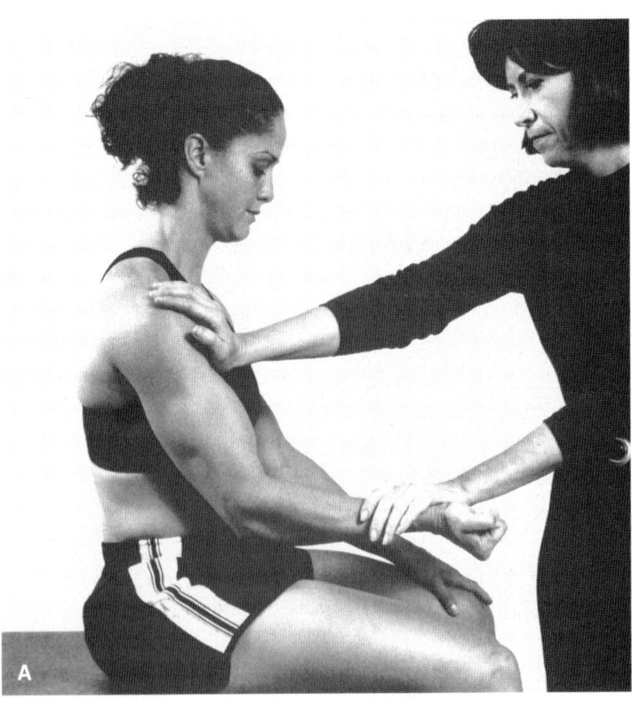

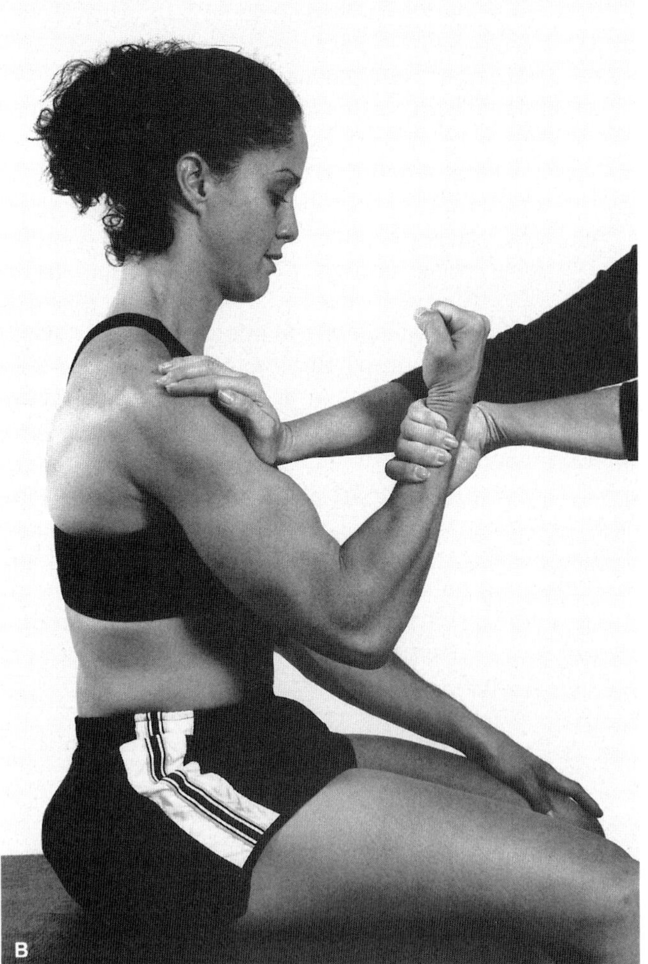

FIGURE 6-6 Isometric elbow flexion with clinician assistance.

PURPOSE: Strengthening biceps muscle of the elbow in two parts of the ROM.

POSITION: Patient sitting with hips and knees flexed to 90°. Clinician places distal hand on client's wrist and proximal hand on client's shoulder. Panel A, exercise at 45° of elbow flexion; panel B, exercise at 90° of elbow flexion.

PROCEDURE: Client flexes arm as clinician provides isometric resistance to the movement with distal hand. Resistance should be held for 6 to 10 sec per repetition.

When implementing isokinetic exercise, certain clinical considerations must be addressed. The clinician must select the speed at which the patient will be exercising the involved muscle, keeping in mind that the best approach is to have the individuals train at speeds as close as possible to those encountered functionally. One suggested protocol is to have the patient exercise across a variety of speeds (sometimes referred to as a velocity spectrum) such as 8 repetitions at a relatively slow speed (e.g., 60°/sec), 10 repetitions at a moderate speed (e.g., 180°/sec), and 12 repetitions at a fast speed (e.g., 300°/sec).

The most appropriate ROM should be selected, factoring in soft tissue healing constraints and the range in which pain occurs. If preferential recruitment of fast-twitch muscle fibers is desired, maximal isokinetic exercise should be considered, because the allowance for optimal recruitment of fast-twitch fibers through the full ROM. Isokinetic training should incorporate both concentric and eccentric exercise, if possible.

■ *Techniques*

ISOMETRIC EXERCISES

Early in the resistance-training program, the patient may exercise by doing simple isometric exercises called muscle sets, especially in the lower extremity. The most common of these muscle sets are gluteal sets, quadriceps sets, and hamstring sets. The gluteal set is performed by having the patient tighten the gluteal muscles by pinching the muscles of the buttocks together and holding in an isometric contraction for 6 to 10 sec. The quadriceps set, most easily performed in supine, is performed by tightening the quadriceps muscle by straightening the knee and holding the contraction isometrically. The hamstring set is also most easily performed in supine by pushing the heel of the foot into the surface under the heel, thereby, causing an isometric hip extension activity.

The patient can be assisted by a clinician or, with

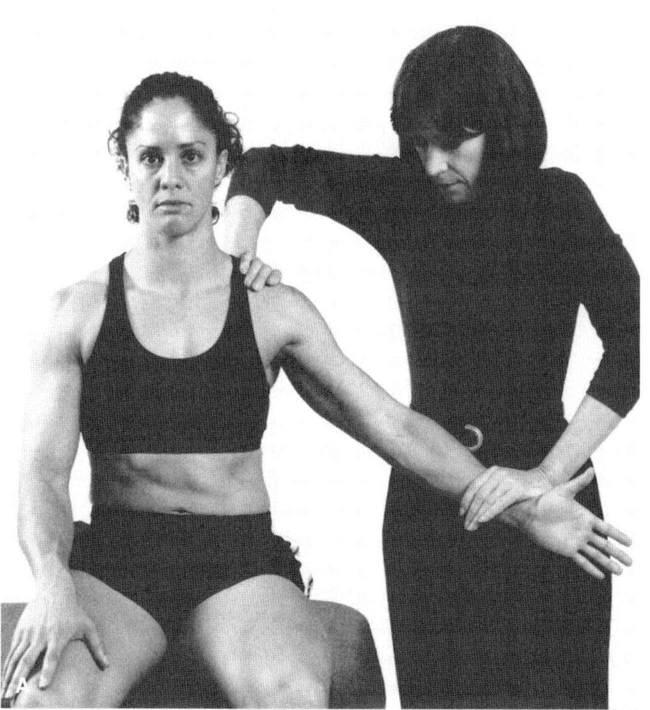

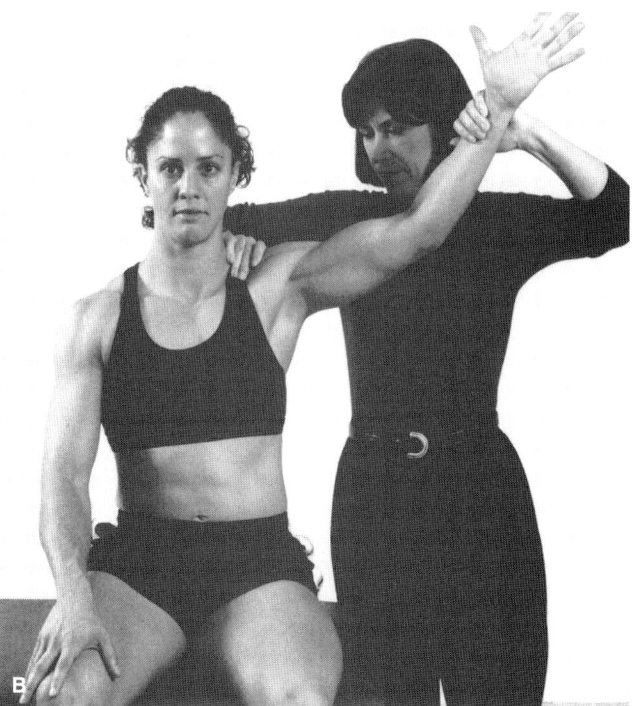

FIGURE 6-7 Isometric shoulder abduction in the plane of the scapula with clinician assistance.

PURPOSE: Strengthening abductor muscles of the shoulder in the plane of the scapula in two parts of the ROM.

POSITION: Patient sitting with hips and knees flexed to 90°. Clinician places distal hand on client's wrist and proximal hand on client's shoulder. Panel A, exercise at 45° of shoulder abduction; panel B, exercise at 100° of shoulder abduction. Shoulder is held in abduction in the plane of the scapula (30° horizontally adducted from the frontal plane).

PROCEDCURE: Client abducts arm as clinician provides isometric resistance to the movement with distal hand. Resistance should be held for 6 to 10 sec per repetition.

imagination, can use his or her own body for resistance. Figures 6-6 through 6-10 depict a few isometric exercises that can be performed early in the intervention phase for a patient requiring initial strengthening activities.

ISOTONIC EXERCISES

Isotonic exercise can be performed by using cuff weights, elastic tubing, dumbbells, and a variety of machines. In addition, the creative clinician will be able to work with the patient to develop resistive devices that do not cost as much as high-tech exercise equipment. Creative devices include purses or backpacks filled with soup cans or books (weighed on a home scale to check that the correct total weight is used). This chapter emphasizes economic and efficient techniques that can be used by the patient at home or in the office. Figures 6-11 through 6-19 present a wide range of isotonic exercises that can be effectively used for rehabilitation of upper- and lower-extremity dysfunction.

ISOKINETIC EXERCISE

Since the 1970s, no other mode of resistance training has received more attention among researchers and clinicians than has isokinetic exercise. To determine if isokinetic exercise is appropriate for a patient, the clinician must have a proper understanding of the scientific rationale underlying the method and the clinical rationale for its use. Figure 6-20 shows a common isokinetic dynamometer used in the treatment of patients today. The isokinetic dynamometer shown has the ability to exercise upper and lower extremities.

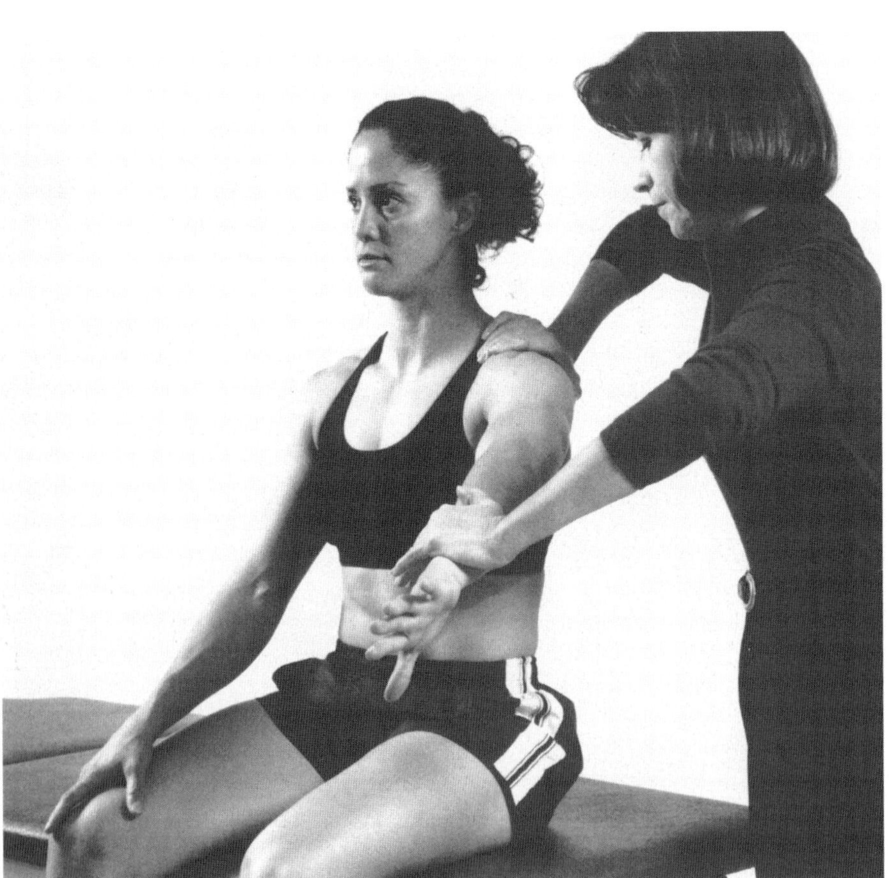

FIGURE 6-8 **Isometric exercise applied in the empty can position with clinician assistance.**

PURPOSE: Strengthening supraspinatus muscle of the shoulder.

POSITION: Patient sitting with hips and knees flexed to 90°. Clinician places distal hand on client's wrist and proximal hand on client's shoulder. Client holds arm in empty can position of abduction, internal rotation, and slight forward horizontal adduction.

PROCEDURE: Client abducts arm as clinician provides isometric resistance to the movement with distal hand. Resistance should be held for 6 to 10 sec per repetition.

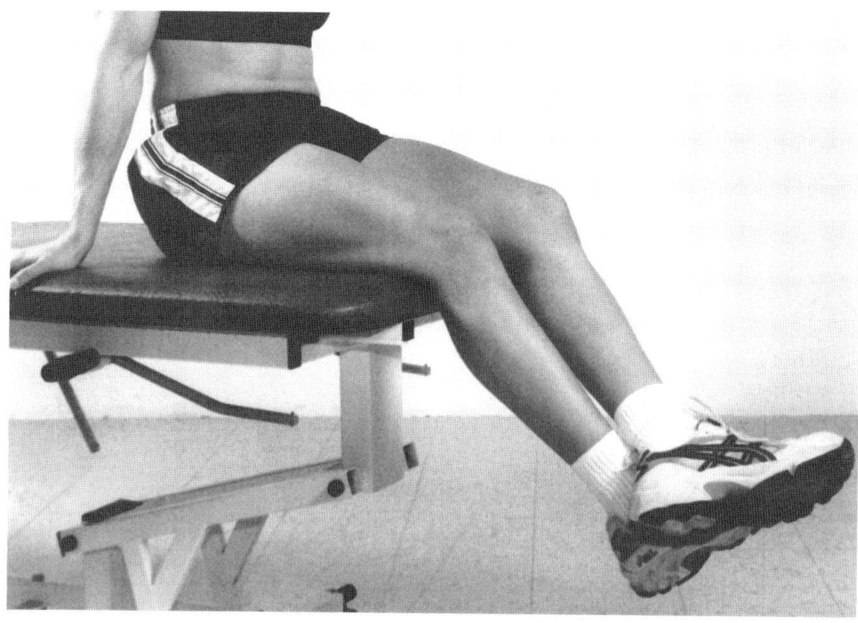

FIGURE 6-9 Isometric knee extension exercise for independent home program.

PURPOSE: Strengthening quadriceps muscles.

POSITION: Client sitting with both legs flexed to 45°. The left leg placed on the anterior surface of the right leg.

PROCEDURE: The client uses left leg to flex and provides isometric resistance against anterior surface of right leg. Right leg attempts to extend against resistance of left leg. Resistance should be held for 6 to 10 sec per repetition.

FIGURE 6-10 Isometric ankle dorsiflexion exercise for independent home program.

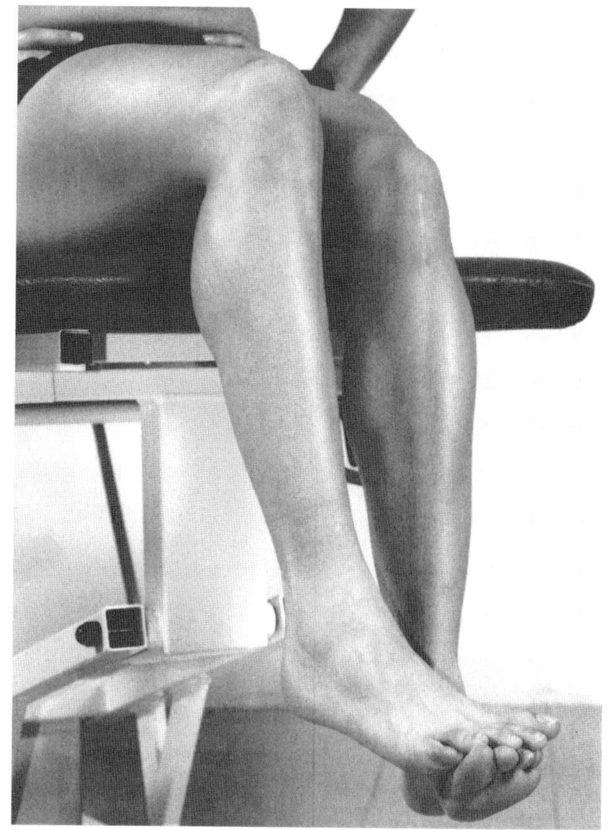

PURPOSE: Strengthening tibialis anterior muscle of the ankle.

POSITION: Patient sitting with hip and knee flexed at 90°. Client places right foot on anterior surface of left foot.

PROCEDURE: The client uses right foot to plantarflex and provide resistance against anterior surface of left foot. Left foot attempts to dorsiflex against resistance of right foot. Resistance should be held for 6 to 10 sec per repetition

FIGURE 6-11 Isotonic exercise applied in the "empty can" position with dumbbell.

PURPOSE: Strengthening supraspinatus muscle of the shoulder.

POSITION: Client standing with arm at side, internally rotated, and in the plane of the scapula (30° horizontally adducted from the frontal plane) holding dumbbell.

PROCEDURE: Client abducts arm (concentric), to less than 90° in the plane of the scapula while maintaining upper extremity in internal rotation and elbow extended. It is important that arm stay below the horizontal and not be elevated above 90°, to avoid impingement of the shoulder. Following a brief pause at 90°, shoulder is slowly lowered to original position (eccentric).

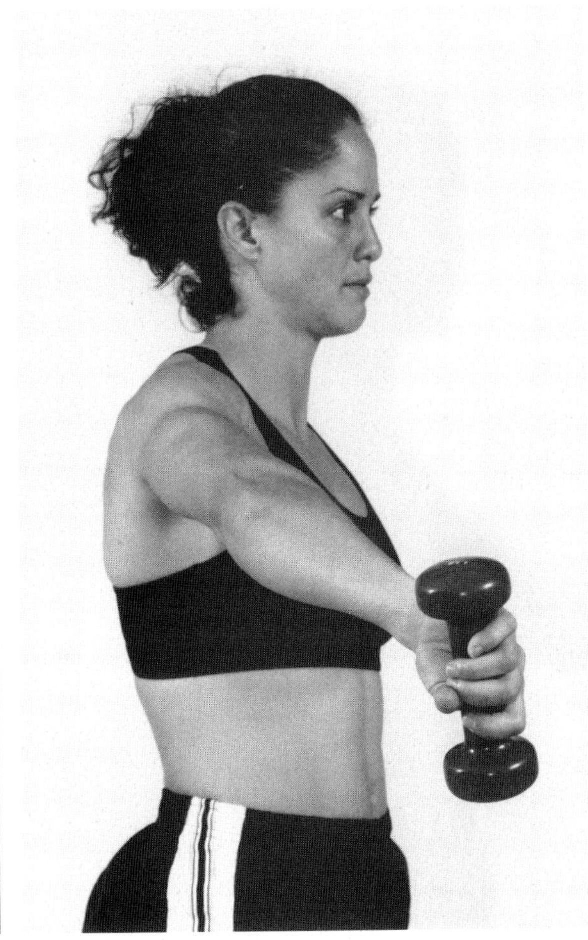

FIGURE 6-12 Isotonic exercise for shoulder external rotation with dumbbell.

PURPOSE: Strengthening external rotator muscles of the rotator cuff of the shoulder (infraspinatus, teres minor).

POSITION: Client lying prone with upper arm (shoulder to elbow) stabilized on the table and the forearm (elbow to hand) hanging off the table holding dumbbell. Hand is allowed to hang from the table.

PROCEDURE: Client externally rotates shoulder (concentric), pauses at end range of external rotation, and then slowly lowers arm back to original position (eccentric).

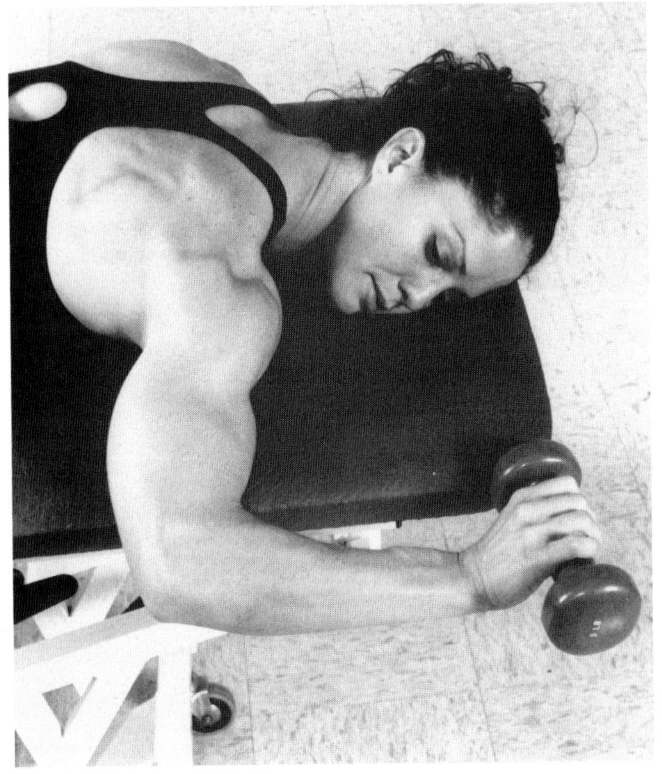

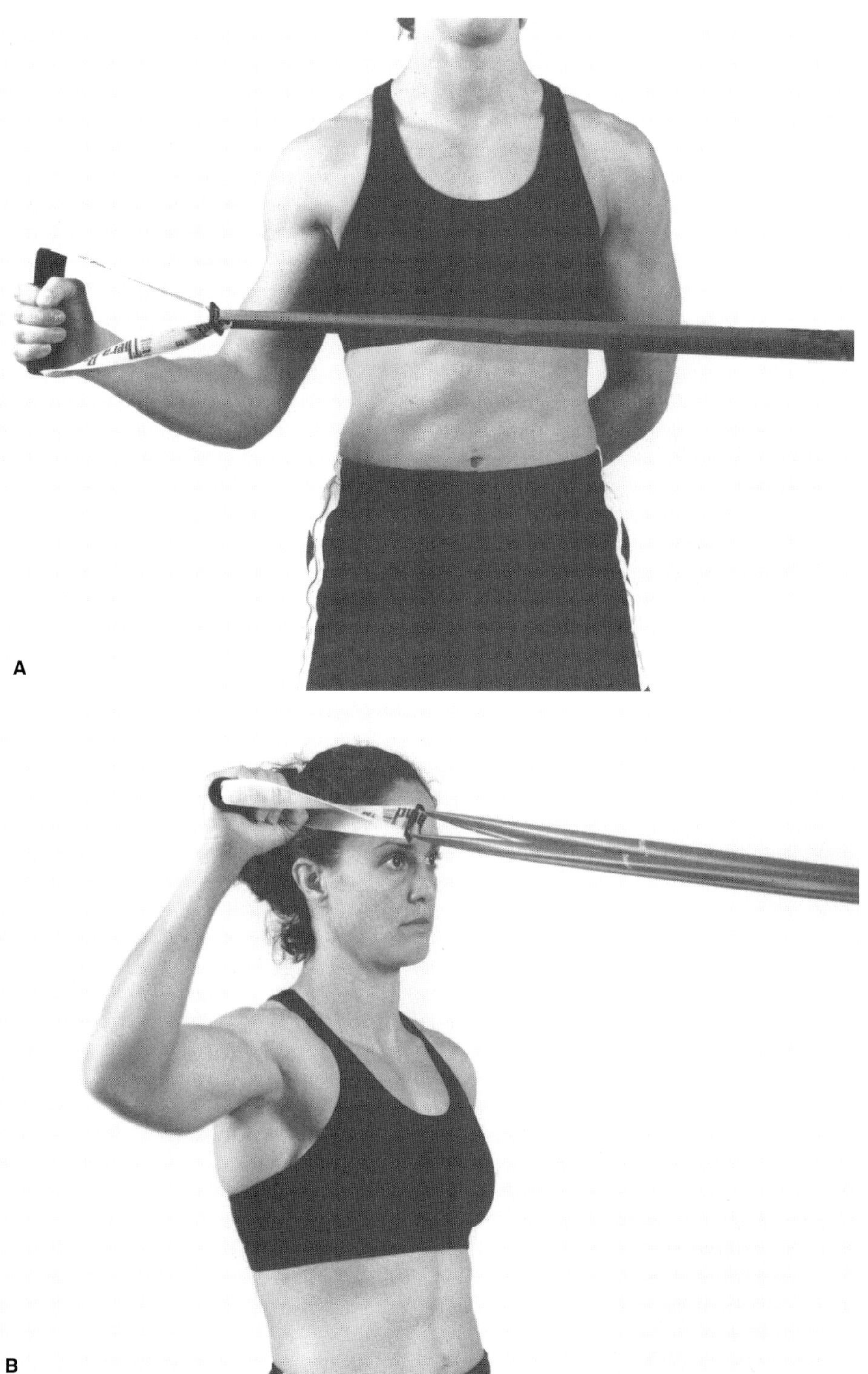

FIGURE 6-13 **Isotonic exercise of shoulder external rotation with elastic tubing.**

PURPOSE: Strengthening external rotator muscles of the rotator cuff of the shoulder (infraspinatus, teres minor) in two different positions of shoulder abduction.

POSITION: Client positions shoulder in a conservative position of adduction next to the body (panel A) or a more aggressive position of the shoulder in external rotation at 90° of abduction (panel B). Client grasps elastic tubing.

PROCEDURE: From an internally rotated position, client externally rotates shoulder against resistance of the elastic tubing (concentric), pauses at end range of external rotation. Then, slowly and with control, the client allows the arm to return to the starting position (eccentric).

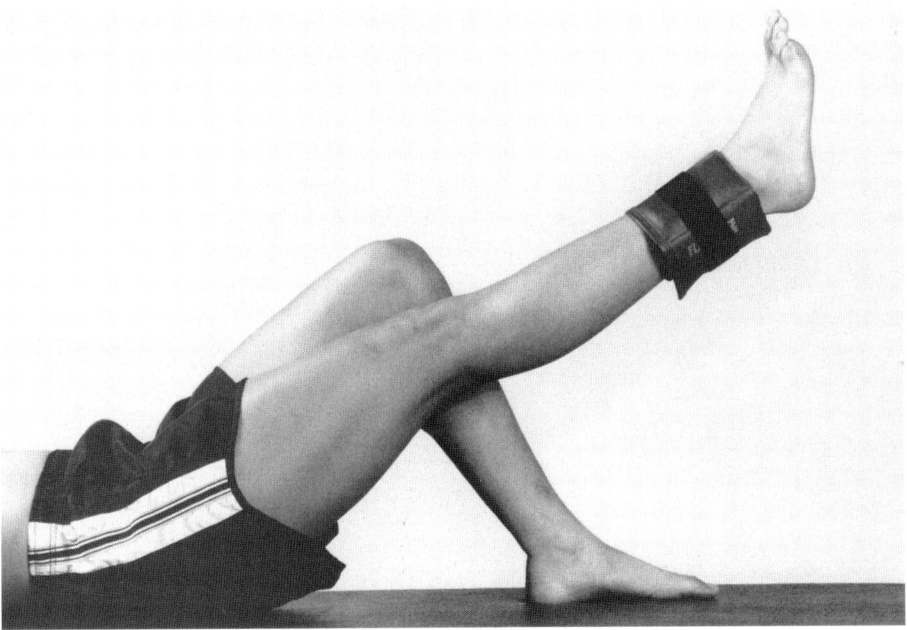

FIGURE 6-14 Isotonic straight leg raise with cuff weight.

PURPOSE: Strengthening hip flexors using straight leg raise.

POSITION: Client lying supine with cuff weight strapped around ankle. Opposite leg may be flexed for comfort of client.

PROCEDURE: Client raises leg (concentric), holds briefly in flexed position, and slowly lowers (eccentric) leg to starting position.

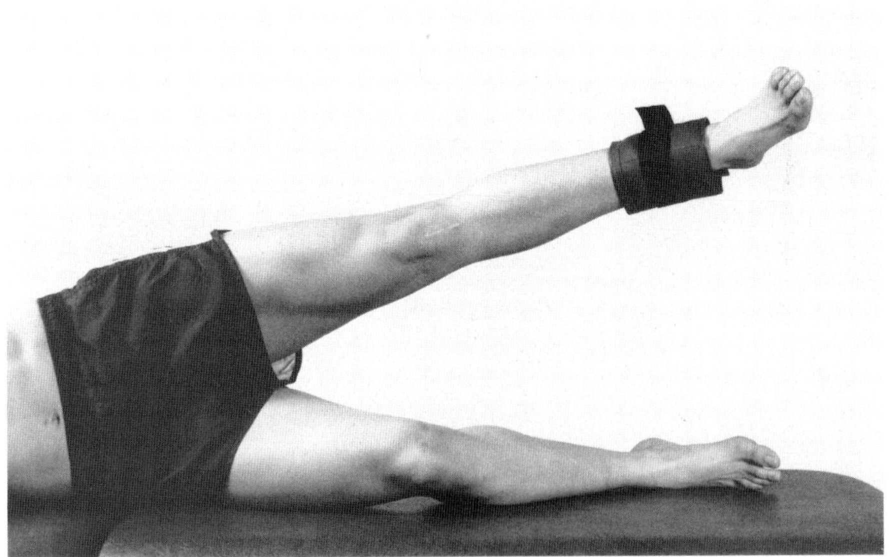

FIGURE 6-15 Isotonic exercise of hip abduction with cuff weight.

PURPOSE: Strengthening hip abductor muscles.

POSITION: Client lying on side with cuff weight strapped around ankle of leg closest to ceiling. Opposite leg may be flexed for comfort of client.

PROCEDURE: Client raises leg (concentric), holds briefly in abducted position, and slowly lowers (eccentric) the leg to starting position.

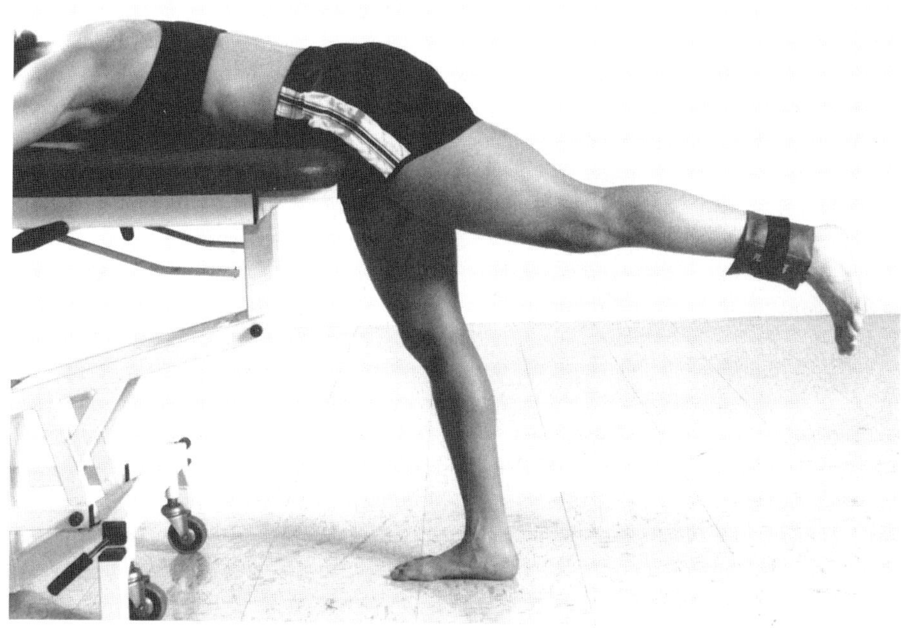

FIGURE 6-16 **Isotonic exercise for hip extension with cuff weight.**

PURPOSE: Strengthening hamstring muscles of the knee.

POSITION: Client lying prone with leg held over edge of plinth. Cuff weight strapped around ankle.

PROCEDURE: Client slowly lowers leg to the floor (eccentric). After a brief pause, client lifts leg into hip extension (concentric).

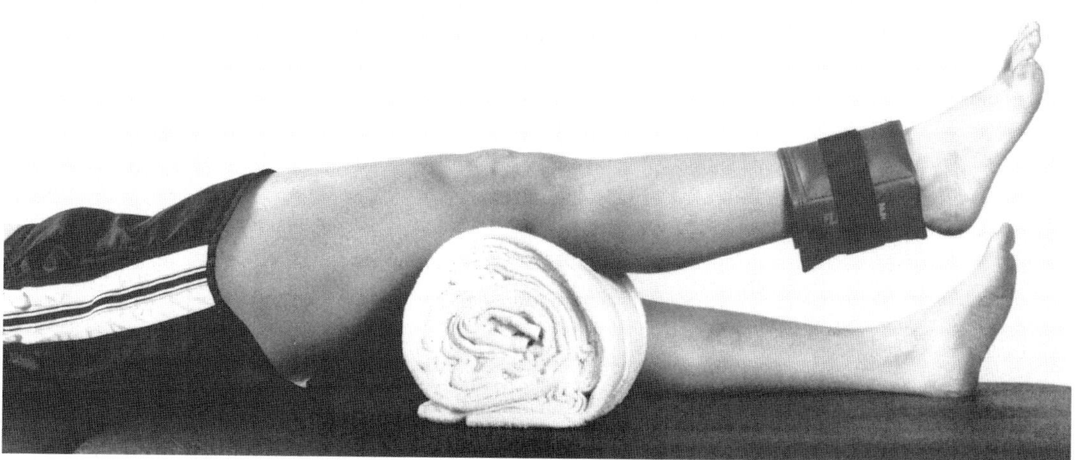

FIGURE 6-17 **Isotonic knee extension exercise through limited ROM with cuff weight.**

PURPOSE: Strengthening quadriceps muscles of the knee in a limited or protected ROM.

POSITION: Client lying supine with cuff weight strapped around ankle. A bolster or towel roll is placed under client's knee allowing a limited ROM (shown, 30° of full extension).

PROCEDURE: Client extends knee (concentric) through partial ROM (shown, 30° to full extension). Once fully extended, client pauses briefly, holding knee in extended position, and then slowly lowers leg with control from full extension (eccentric).

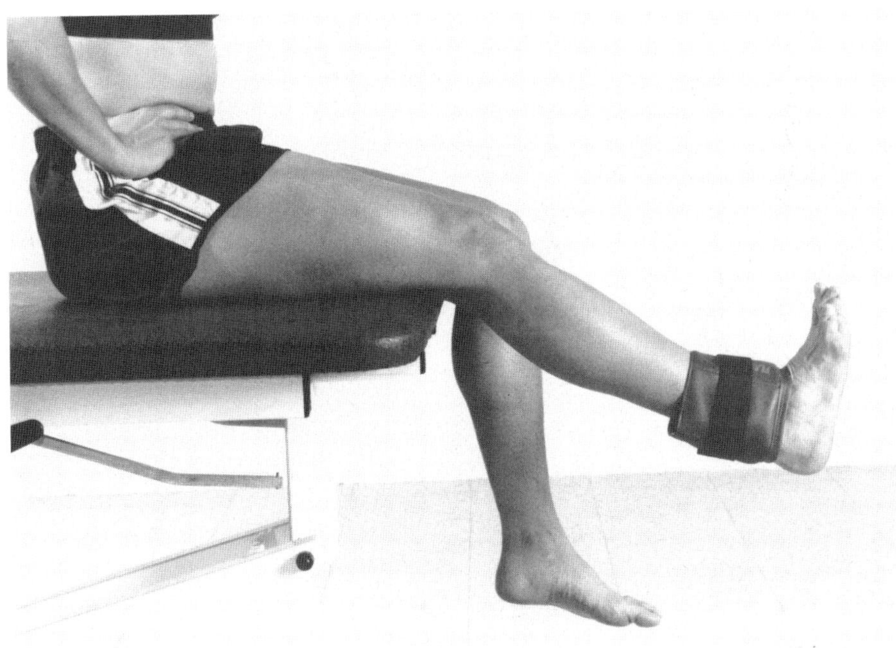

FIGURE 6-18 **Isotonic knee extension exercise through full ROM with cuff weight.**

PURPOSE: Strengthening quadriceps muscles of the knee in full ROM.

POSITION: Client sitting with cuff weight strapped around ankle.

PROCEDURE: Client extends knee through the full ROM (concentric). Once fully extended, client pauses briefly holding knee in extended position, and then slowly lowers leg with control from full extension (eccentric).

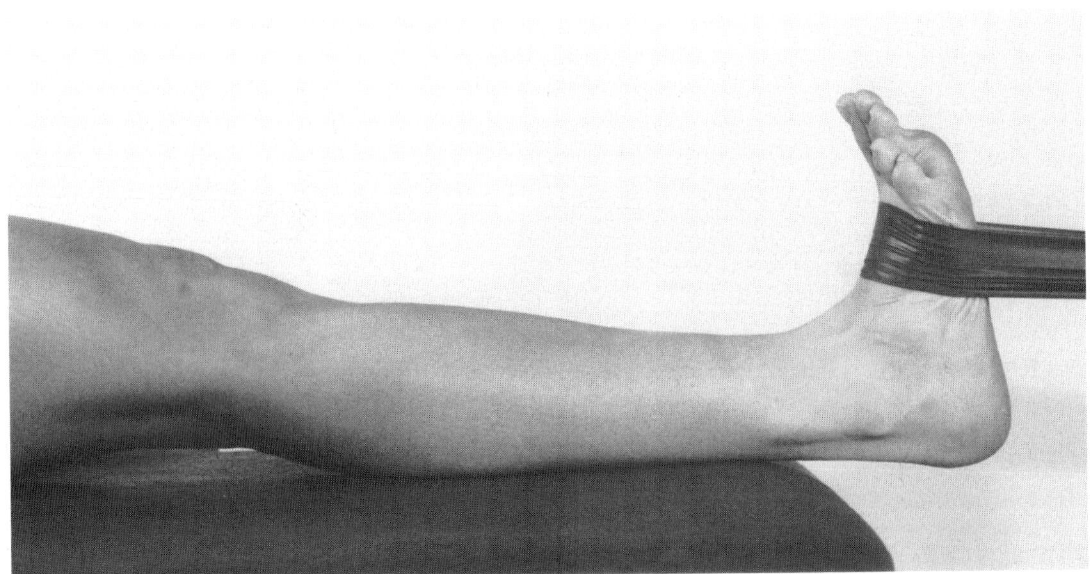

FIGURE 6-19 **Isotonic exercise of ankle dorsiflexion with clinician assistance and elastic tubing.**

PURPOSE: Strengthening tibialis anterior muscle.

POSITION: Client long sitting with one end of elastic across the dorsum of foot. Clinician holds other end of elastic tubing.

PROCEDURE: From the plantarflexed position, client dorsiflexes ankle (concentric), pauses at end range of dorsiflexion, and then slowly allows foot to return to starting position (eccentric).

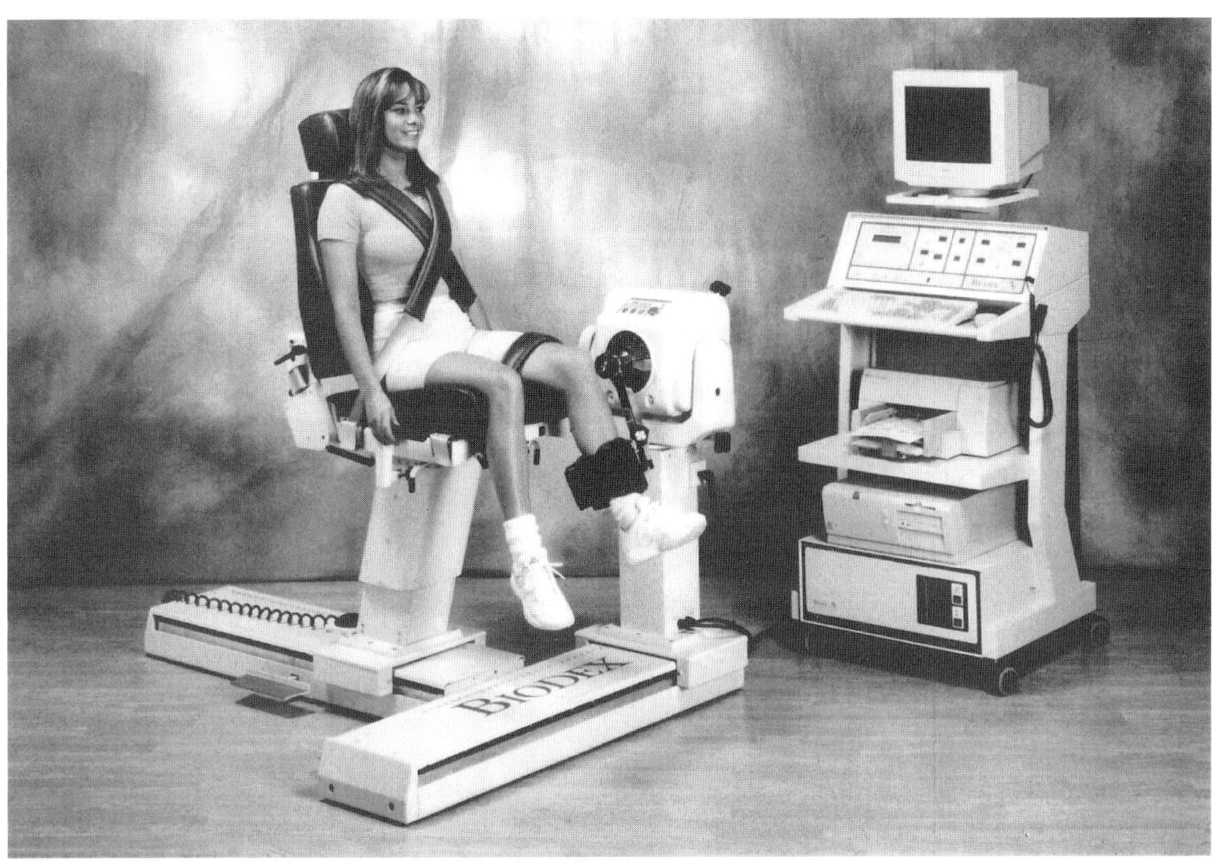

FIGURE 6-20 **Isokinetic exercise for the lower extremity with Biodex dynamometer.**

PURPOSE: Isokinetic strengthening of knee extensors.

POSITION: Client sitting on chair of dynamometer with stabilization straps placed around chest, pelvis, and thigh. Lower part of leg (near ankle) is also stabilized to the isokinetic device.

PROCEDURE: Client extends knee as fast and as hard as possible against accommodating resistance provided by device (concentric). At end of full knee extension, client immediately flexes knee as fast and as hard as possible against accommodating resistance (concentric contraction of reciprocal muscle). Or client immediately resists lever arm as it pushes leg into flexion (eccentric contraction of the ipsilateral muscle).

NOTE: The exact nature of the type of contraction depends on how the isokinetic dynamometer is programmed. The example given here is but one of many options available with a computer-generated isokinetic dynamometer.

(Courtesy Biodex Medical Systems, Shirley, NY.)

CASE STUDY

PATIENT INFORMATION

A 21-year-old college football player (linebacker) presented to the clinic complaining of pain and weakness in the right arm near the cubital fossa. He described the injury as occurring in the third quarter of a football game two days earlier when he made an arm tackle of an opposing ball carrier. During the tackle, his right arm was forcibly horizontally abducted behind his back while he pulled the ball carrier to the ground by flexing his elbow. Immediately, he felt severe pain in his upper arm, which subsided to a dull pain after 5 min. The patient indicated that he was able to complete the game with minimal pain. The following day (1 day before coming into the clinic), he complained of upper arm pain and an inability to extend the elbow without pain.

(continued)

GERIATRIC *Perspectives*

- Open-chain resistance activities are appropriate for all age groups, even the oldest-old, with few modifications. These activities for senior adults may be exemplified by functional tasks, such as carrying a plate of food or a bag of groceries.
- Open-chain activities are associated with shearing forces across the joint. Of particular importance are the shearing forces that occur parallel to the tibiofemoral joint during open-chain activities. The use of such exercises with added resistance may be problematic after some surgeries, such as total knee replacement.
- Although open-chain resistance training is not particularly functional, the training provides a means of isolating muscle groups. For example, quadriceps strength is known to decrease with aging. The strength loss has been associated with increased chair rise time and difficulty climbing stairs.
- With aging, the peak force generated during a single maximal contraction against a constant force (isometric strength) and the peak force generated as the muscle is shortening (concentric strength) decrease and the muscle fatigues more quickly.[1–3] Furthermore, the speed of the response to stimuli (reaction time and contraction response) slows progressively with aging.[3]
- In designing a training program that uses open-chain activities for older individuals, a taxonomy of exercise is the recommended choice. The progression should begin with holding muscle contractions (isometric), proceed to control during muscle lengthening (eccentric), and finally progress to a shortening contraction (concentric). Within each level of training, the amount of resistance, duration, and frequency may be progressed.
- Submaximal isometric training (up to 75% of the maximum amount of weight that can be lifted once) for 3 months has been shown to significantly increase strength and cross-sectional area of muscle in older individuals.[4] Use of techniques such as PNF and task-specific strengthening (Chapter 8) may improve functional carryover to open-chain resistance training and thus may increase the effect performance.

1. Spirduso WW. Physical dimensions of aging. Champaign, IL: Human Kinetics, 1995.
2. Overend TJ, Cunningham DA, Kramer JF, et al. Knee extensor and knee flexor strength: cross-sectional area ratios in young and elderly men. J Gerontol Med Sci 1992;47:M204–M210.
3. Shephard RJ. Aging, physical activity, and health. Champaign, IL: Human Kinetics, 1997.
4. Pyka G, Lindenberger E, Charette S, Marcus R. Muscle strength and fiber adaptations to a year-long resistance training program in elderly men and women. J Gerontol Med Sci 1994;49:B22–B27.

Examination indicated acute inflammation, including pain and palpable heat at the anterior surface of the upper arm. In addition, swelling was present at the anterior aspect of the elbow joint. Passive ROM was full but painful at full elbow extension. Resisted elbow flexion was painful and weak (manual muscle testing grade 3/5); resisted shoulder flexion was strong (5/5) but with slight pain. All other examination procedures were pain free. Based on the examination, the patient was diagnosed with a strain to the biceps brachii muscle.

LINKS TO

Guide to Physical Therapist Practice and *Athletic Training Educational Competencies*

Pattern 4D of the *Guide*[24] relates to the diagnosis of this patient. The pattern is described as "impaired joint mobility, motor function, muscle performance, and range of motion associated with connective tissue dysfunction." Included in this diagnostic group is muscle strain, and anticipated goals include increasing strength using resistive exercises (including concentric, dynamic/isotonic, eccentric, isokinetic, isometric).

The *Competencies*[25] refers to the treatment of athletes using isometric, isotonic, and isokinetic exercise techniques. The teaching objectives listed under the competencies of this domain indicate that "the student will demonstrate the ability to instruct the following exercises using isometric and progressive resistance techniques: . . . elbow flexion [and] elbow extension."

INTERVENTION

Initial goals of intervention were to decrease inflammation (swelling, pain), maintain full ROM, and diminish loss of

PEDIATRIC *Perspectives*

- Open-chain exercises are appropriate and often a first option for strengthening in children. Open-chain activities provide isolation of muscle groups and are simple to teach. These activities are common in many upper- and lower-extremity movements used by children, such as reaching, throwing, and kicking.
- It is common to use both open- and closed-kinetic-chain modes of exercise in a therapeutic exercise program designed for children. Both are used for improvement of overall strength and function. Open-chain training may be the superior activity in young children for some upper-extremity tasks because children may lack the proximal strength (scapular stabilizers) and alignment to safely support closed-kinetic chain exercises. An example of this is the scapular prominence that diminishes with age.[1]
- The same concern applies to some lower-extremity and trunk movements, for which open-chain training may be superior to closed chain. Very young children may lack the trunk strength needed to correctly perform some lower-extremity closed-kinetic-chain activities. An example of this is the sway back posture of toddlers and youth.[1]

1. Kendall FP, McCreary EK. Muscles: testing and function. 4th ed. Baltimore, MD: Williams & Wilkins, 1994.

strength during healing. The patient was instructed in a home program consisting of

1. Ice before treatment.
2. Active flexion and extension ROM exercises to the elbow; 15 repetitions in the morning and in the evening (Fig. 2-26).
3. Isometric exercises to elbow flexors in two parts of the range (45° and 90°) using submaximal (pain-free) contractions: 20 repetitions in the morning and in the evening (Fig. 6-6).
4. Ice after treatment.
5. Return to clinic in 1 week.

PROGRESSION

One Week After Initial Examination

The patient had no pain with passive ROM of the elbow, decreased pain with resisted elbow flexion, no swelling at the elbow, and no pain with resisted shoulder flexion. Given that inflammation was decreased, the goals of intervention were to promote healing (influence proper collagen deposition, increase blood flow) and to increase strength of the biceps brachii. The home program was progressed as follows:

1. Isotonic elbow flexion exercises using a 2-lb cuff weight: three sets of 12 repetitions twice a day.
2. Isotonic shoulder flexion exercise using a 5-lb weight: two sets of 12 repetitions twice a day.
3. Ice after treatment.

Two Weeks After Initial Examination

The examination indicated no pain with any resisted movements but a slight loss of strength with elbow flexion (4+/5). The goals of intervention at this point were to aggressively strengthen the biceps brachii.

In the clinic, the patient exercised isokinetically by performing 8 repetitions of concentric elbow flexion and elbow extension at 60°/sec, 10 repetitions at 180°/sec, and 12 repetitions at 300°/sec. The program was repeated three times (three sets at each speed). The patient was able to perform these exercises without any pain or complaints of any kind. He was iced after the exercise session. After the intervention session, the patient was instructed to perform a daily home exercise program of three sets of 15 repetitions of isotonic elbow flexion using elastic tubing.

OUTCOME

Three weeks after the initial examination, the patient was pain free for all movements and the strength of elbow flexion on the right was equal to the left, as indicated by manual muscle testing (5/5). The patient was discharged from care with instructions to call or return if problems developed.

SUMMARY

- The three common modes of exercise (isometric, isotonic, isokinetic) were defined, and research was presented as a review of the exercise types and to enhance the understanding of their use in clinical intervention.

- Isometric exercises are used most commonly early in the rehabilitation program to avoid open-chain resistance exercises through the full ROM, which may cause increased pain, effusion, or crepitus. Isometric exercises can also be used at various points in the ROM to enhance more effective strengthening at that part of the range and, therefore, can be used throughout the entire rehabilitation program, rather than only during the acute or inflammatory phase.
- Isotonic resistance programs are common, and their effectiveness in increasing strength is well documented. Isotonic exercise should be performed both concentrically and eccentrically for the most functional result. A potential disadvantage to isotonic exercise is that the actual tension developed varies as the muscle changes length and maximal resistance is not achieved throughout the full ROM.
- Isokinetic exercise is performed at a fixed speed against accommodating resistance. Electromechanical mechanisms vary the resistance to accommodate the fluctuations in muscle force owing to changing muscle length and angle of pull. Therefore, isokinetic exercise devices stimulate maximal contraction of the muscle throughout the complete ROM.
- The clinician must be aware of potential adverse responses of the patient to the open-chain resistance-training program (pain, crepitus, swelling) and of healing constraints that may affect the program. The specific program must be individualized to each patient.

REFERENCES

1. Bandy WD. Functional rehabilitation of the athlete. Orthop Phys Ther Clin North Am 1992;1:1–13.
2. Falkel J, Cipriani D. Physiological principles of resistance training and rehabilitation. In: J Zachazewski, D Magee, W Quillen, eds. Athletic injuries and rehabilitation. Philadelphia: Saunders, 1996:206–228.
3. Arnheim D, Prentice W. Principles of athletic training. 8th ed. Baltimore: Mosby Year Book, 1993:32–73.
4. Hettinger T, Muller EA. Muskelleisting and muskeltraining. Arbeitphysiologic 1953;15:111–126 [Cited in Hislop HJ. Quantitative changes in human muscular strength during isometric exercise. Phys Ther 1963;43:21–38.]
5. Muller EA. Influence of training and of inactivity on muscle strength. Arch Phys Med Rehabil 1970;51:449–462.
6. Walters L, Steward CC, LeClaire JF. Effort of short bouts of isometric and isotonic contractions on muscular strength and endurance. Am J Phys Med 1960;39:131–141.
7. Cotton D. Relationship of duration of sustained voluntary isometric contraction to changes in endurance and strength. Res Q 1967;38:366–374.
8. Belka D. Comparison of dynamic, static, and combination training on dominant wrist flexor muscles. Res Q 1966;49:245–250.
9. Knapik JA, Mawdsley RH, Ramos MU. Angular specificity and test mode specificity of isometric and isokinetic strength training. J Orthop Sports Phys Ther 1983;5:58–65.
10. Liberson WT, Asa MM. Further studies on brief isometric exercises. Arch Phys Med Rehabil 1959;40:330–333.
11. Bandy WD, Hanten WP. Changes in torque and electromyographic activity of the quadriceps femoris muscles following isometric training. Phys Ther 1993;73:455–467.
12. Norkin C, Levangie, P. Joint structure and function: a comprehensive analysis. 2nd ed. Philadelphia: Davis, 1992:92–124.
13. Soderberg G. Kinesiology. Application to pathological motion. 2nd ed. Baltimore: Williams & Wilkins, 1997:29–57.
14. Albert M. Eccentric muscle training in sports and orthopaedics. New York: Churchill Livingstone, 1991.
15. Smith LL. Acute inflammation: the underlying mechanism in delayed-onset muscle soreness? Med Sci Sports Exerc 1991;23: 542–551.
16. Stauber WT, Clarkson PM, Fritz VK, Evans WJ. Extracellular matrix disruption and pain after eccentric muscle action. J Appl Physiol 1990;69:868–874.
17. Howell JN, Chelboun G, Conaster R. Muscle stiffness, strength loss, swelling and soreness following exercise-induced injury in humans. J Physiol 1993;464:183–196.
18. Ebbling CB, Clarkson PM. Muscle adaptation prior to recovery following eccentric exercises. Eur J Appl Physiol 1990;60:26–31.
19. American Academy of Orthopaedic Surgeons. Athletic training and sports medicine. 2nd ed. Park Ridge, IL: AAOS, 1991.
20. Bandy WD, Lovelace-Chandler V. Relationship of peak torque to peak work and peak power of the quadriceps and hamstrings muscles in a normal sample using an accommodating resistance measurement device. Isok Exerc Sci 1991;1:87–91.
21. Delorme TL. Restoration of muscle power by heavy resistance exercise. J Bone Joint Surg [Am] 1945;27:645–667.
22. Stone WJ, Kroll WA. Sports conditioning and weight training: programs for athletic conditioning. Boston: Allyn & Bacon, 1982.
23. Knight K. Knee rehabilitation by the daily adjustable progressive resistance exercise technique. Am J Sports Med 1979;7: 336–337.
24. American Physical Therapy Association. Guide to physical therapist practice, second edition. Phys Ther 2001;81:1–768.
25. National Athletic Trainers' Association. Athletic training educational competencies. 3rd ed. Dallas: NATA, 1999.

CHAPTER 7

Medical Exercise Training

J. Allen Hardin, MS, PT, SCS, ATC

Introduction

Medical exercise training (MET), also referred to as medical exercise therapy and training therapy, is a system of progressively graded exercise directed toward the maintenance and improvement of one's health. Using a functional approach to examine and treat patients with musculoskeletal dysfunction, the principles of strength, speed, endurance, power, coordination, work capacity, and aerobic training are applied to achieve highly specific results. The progressive exercise system is designed to restore normal function through principles of mobilization and stabilization. This system focuses on various aspects of prevention, rehabilitation, education, and training. Medical exercise training has gained in international popularity among clinicians, becoming recognized as an essential treatment tool because of the emphasis on pain-free rehabilitation and the ability to both examine and treat a patient in the same functional position.

DESCRIPTION

According to Torstensen,[1] MET was developed during the early 1960s by the Norwegian physiotherapist Holten and was sanctioned in 1967 by the Norwegian Health Authorities as a treatment method with its own defined criteria. Medical exercise training uses specific exercises for mobilizing hypomobile areas and stabilizing exercises for hypermobile areas, thereby normalizing function. The theory focuses on applying graded exercises for treating and preventing dysfunction in the musculoskeletal system. The prescribed exercises are graded in such a way that the patients work in trunk flexion, extension, and rotation; exercising the abdominal and back musculature as well as the upper and lower extremities.[2]

Medical exercise training is considered to be a component of both manual and exercise therapy. It is classified as a special form of treatment based on specific criteria.[3] The patient performs exercises with minimal manual assistance but with constant monitoring by the clinician. The exercises are designed to optimally stimulate neuromuscular, arthrogenic, circulatory, and respiratory components while allowing the patient to exercise pain free, because they are based on the concept of unloading (reducing the effects of gravity).[4] It is essential that the clinician closely monitor the patient to ensure proper exercise grading in relation to the pathologic reactions of the tissues and the patient's tolerance for pain and to obtain high-quality performance by the patient through continuous dialogue. Medical exercise training is based on a minimum of 1 hr of work for effective treatment within a group of no more than five patients.[4]

The exercises are typically performed with the use of specially designed exercise equipment, such as wall pulley, lateral pulley, angle bench, multipurpose bench, incline board, wall bar, unloading frame, dumbbells, and barbells.[2] This chapter illustrates specific exercises for clinical application and recognizes that the need for specific, often costly, equipment (not available to all clinicians in every setting) is a limitation.

Medical exercise training is a treatment modality that has found useful application in various disciplines, including the field of manual therapy. Although few, if any, manual contacts are made during treatment, manual therapists often use the MET approach to satisfy the patient's functional needs through exercise therapy. Medical exercise training allows manual therapy clinicians to look beyond the joint itself to the periarticular structures, achieving optimal neurogenic control through either mobility or stability. In recent years, these exercises have become extremely valuable for manual therapists in obtaining increased range of motion (ROM), decreased pain and guarding, and normalized somaticovisceral reflexes.[5–8]

ROLE OF THE EXAMINATION

The design of MET, like any individualized exercise program, depends completely on the initial examination. The initial examination is the basis for choosing the appropriate exercises and their grading.[2] The examination should consist of past and present medical history, active and passive tests, muscle tests, specific joint tests, and functional tests.[9,10] From the examination, a diagnosis is established and an individually designed exercise program is created, which is related to symptoms, specific tissues involved, the nature and stage of the lesion, clinical diagnosis, patient needs, and the anticipated level of functional recovery (expectations).[2] The program also consists of re-examination and adjustment when appropriate.

The purpose of the examination is to identify structures that can influence general or localized joint mobility and should be based on a thorough understanding of joint anatomy and physiology, including the anatomic joint with its surrounding and related soft tissues. Only with the knowledge gained through examination can the clinician prescribe an exercise program that is specific for each patient's needs in terms of resistance, repetitions, sets, rest between sets, speed, and ROM with reference to functional qualities.

FUNCTIONAL TESTING

The examination is incomplete without some assessment of functional activities. The purpose of the functional testing as it relates to MET is to identify structures that can influence general or localized mobility. It should be based on a thorough knowledge of joint anatomy and physiology, including the bony articulation, cartilage, ligaments, and intra-articular tissues as well as the surrounding and related soft tissues (including the vascularity and innervation). Changes noted through functional testing involve degeneration or regeneration of damaged articular structures, muscular dysfunction, neurologic deficits, coordination disturbances, somatic dysfunction, and tissue texture abnormalities.[11] The functional test, as a component of the examination, incorporates movements that simulate activities of daily living (ADLs) or athletic activities and is objectively quantified through a standardized tool or test. The examination may involve task analysis or simply observation of specific activities. It should be performed in conjunction with the overall examination so a complete picture of the patient and the patient's dysfunction can be developed.

JOINT MOBILITY

The term *hypomobility* denotes a decrease in the ROM in an extremity joint or a spinal segment. Active or passive joint motion restriction may be caused by structural or function problems in articular structures or the periarticular soft tissues. The goal of treatment for hypomobility is to move the restricted joint or spinal segments via soft tissue or joint techniques, including massage, stretching, and mobilization. The goals of such treatment are pain reduction and improvement of ROM.

The term *hypermobility* refers to an increase in the ROM in an extremity joint or spinal segment. Neither generalized hypermobility nor segmental or localized hypermobility is necessarily accompanied by pain but should be considered pathologic in the presence of pain. Pain may be caused by postural imbalance or motor performance abnormalities and may be relieved by active compensatory movement. Treatment of hypermobility emphasizes stability and is made up of exercises that decrease joint mobility and improve muscle strength, endurance, and coordination along with education regarding physiologically correct movement patterns.

■ *Scientific Basis*

THEORETICAL CONSIDERATIONS

The concept of MET is wholly based on an individually adapted approach that integrates the concepts of examination, exercise, and manual therapy. The method encompasses the principle that the prescribed treatment is individual to the pathology and tissue tolerance of each patient and specifically designed to comply to his or her optimal progression.[8] The emphasis of the individual treatment regimen focuses on reducing acute inflammatory symptoms and improving functional tissue tolerance through what Grimsby[8] refers to as the "specificity approach." This approach emphasizes three components of modified therapeutic exercises: "specific motion of specific joints in specific directions, specific input of specific dosage to obtain specific functional qualities, [and] specific facilitation for specific tissue regeneration."

CLINICAL EVIDENCE

The application of MET into a standard rehabilitation program enhances functional outcomes through not only symptom reduction, improved tissue tolerance, and tissue regeneration but also facilitated muscle fiber recruitment, improved neuromuscular control and coordination, muscular hypertrophy, and muscular endurance. The literature supports the use of MET in the treatment of various pathologies, including lower lumbar instability, chronic low back pain and dysfunction, habitual shoulder dislocation, supraspinatus rupture, and chronic supraspinatus tendinitis.[2,4,12] Findings support the theoretical framework of using MET for tissue regeneration and tendon repair from the biomechanical stresses of exercise, for objective improvements in strength and work capacity, and for subjective improvements in pain.[9,12] In addition, patient satisfaction and return-to-work rates are significantly improved.[2]

DESIGNING A PROGRAM

Designing an individualized exercise program, within the guidelines of MET, requires that the emphasis be placed on specificity of training. Exercise specificity implies that the muscle groups targeted in an exercise program must be the same muscles that are responsible for carrying out functional activities. Specificity of training is not unique to MET but is tantamount to its success. The variables in MET must match the demands and requirements placed on the patient during performance of functional activities.

Purpose of Exercise

There are many reasons to engage in exercise, most notably to improve or maintain physical well-being. For MET, the primary reason to exercise is to improve function, which can be achieved by increasing strength, flexibility, endurance, coordination, agility, balance, timing, and speed. It is difficult to compare the effectiveness of different exercise programs because of the great number of variables. Therefore, testing as a basis for exercise programs becomes essential. The first step is to establish a baseline by which improvement can be measured.

Measurement of Progress

Measurement of progress specifically related to functional status is an essential component of any prescribed exercise program. Results of testing can serve as a motivational tool when progress is noted. Clinicians routinely use standardized testing procedures (e.g., manual muscle testing) and technical information (e.g., tensiometer readings, isokinetic data, and goniometric measurements) in an attempt to document progress objectively. Other testing methods, however, have been advocated as perhaps more accurate reflections of functional status. These tests provide functionally relevant measures of strength, flexibility, and endurance and include such activities as sit-ups, push-ups, jumping activities (single and double leg), and throwing activities. Baseline data are recorded at the initiation of treatment and are collected at regular intervals. Clinicians are limited only by their imaginations. The key to successful monitoring is establishing a baseline by which improvement can be measured; outcomes must be quantifiable and functional.

■ *Clinical Guidelines*

CRITERIA FOR INTERVENTION

An individualized, specific treatment approach is incorporated in MET to improve functional status. Each stimulus is specific and is followed by a specific response. The stimulus must be appropriately created so that a specific functional improvement occurs. The following criteria must be considered when using a MET program as a treatment intervention:[11]

- MET is a form of treatment in which the prescribed exercises are exclusively active exercises; no manual intervention is required. It is individualized training with optimal stimulation.
- Exercises are prescribed with consideration of such factors as ROM, maximal resistance, and number of repetitions, thereby ensuring specific treatment aimed at improving muscle strength, muscle endurance, coordination, and function.
- The exercise program is customized to the individual patient's daily demands. The original design of the treatment plan is based on examination, and subsequent changes are based on re-examination.

PRECAUTIONS

Like other therapeutic procedures or modalities, MET has precautions. The relatively few precautions include the following[11]:

- A hypomobile or painful joint must be treated first when a shortened muscle traverses the segment. The shortened muscle should not be stretched over the joint until active joint gliding is established.
- Active joint gliding must be established before training a weakened muscle when the weakened muscle traverses a hypomobile joint.
- A shortened antagonist muscle must be stretched before strengthening a weakened muscle.
- Single specific motion patterns should be exercised before complex motor activities are prescribed.
- The patient should not initiate an exercise program without prior examination or when not feeling well.
- Although generalized and localized muscle soreness is acceptable, no joint pain should be experienced during the course of the exercise program.

TRAINING PRINCIPLES

Principles important to effective implementation of MET ensure an individually adapted exercise prescription aimed at reducing symptoms and improving function. Adhering to these principles helps the clinician achieve the desired functional outcomes:

- Avoid incorrect motor patterns.
- Stop the exercise if the patient becomes physically or psychologically too tired to perform the motor patterns correctly.
- Prescribe a training program that is consistent with the patient's goals.

- Remember that treatment success depends on the patient's intrinsic ability to perform functional tasks.

The patient must follow the MET program to obtain optimal motor pattern correction. Furthermore, the training sessions should be spaced out. A single, concentrated training period has less effect on motor learning and functional improvement than do shorter daily (or at least tri-weekly) exercise sessions, which enhance learning through repetition.[11]

EFFECTS OF TRAINING

The patient may be affected in numerous ways by MET: systemic and localized, subtle and obvious. Consistent performance of exercise based on the principles of MET may lead to improved muscle strength, muscle endurance, coordination, circulation, oxygen uptake and consumption, cardiovascular and respiratory function, and physiologic movement patterns.[11] The degree of improvement of systemic function depends on muscle mass and work performed. Patients and untrained athletes should begin a MET program at lower intensity than trained athletes. However, the same physiologic and scientific principles apply to all: the program intensity should be increased gradually.

Medical exercise training has specific localized effects on body structures. Intermittent pressure loading may stimulate the regeneration of bone and hyaline cartilage. Muscle strength can be improved through recruitment of motor units that were not previously used. Adipose tissue may be reduced.[11]

Increased strength and the rate at which it is obtained depend on individual's level of conditioning before initiation of the exercise program. Deconditioned clients will see greater gains in strength than will conditioned athletes. However, the first 1 to 2 months of training by deconditioned individuals are usually not accompanied by hypertrophy; changes in muscle cross-sectional area are not seen until after 6 weeks. For example, if an untrained individual improves her maximum bench press from 100 to 120 lb during the first 2 weeks of a training program, her improvement is 20%. A conditioned power lifter, however, could not make the same percentage gain (e.g., 350 to 420 lb) in the same period of time. Furthermore genetic endowment, sex, and age may effect strength gains and the rate of strength gains.

PHASES OF MET

Training for rehabilitation is typically divided into two phases (1) obtaining pain-free, coordinated mobility and stability around the physiologic axes through the ROM and (2) increasing tissue tolerance to the demands of activities of daily living. Initially, the primary goals are to reduce symptoms and increase blood circulation to improve protein synthesis of involved tissues. During this time, the patient is usually still functionally limited as a result of the impairment.[8] If joint mobility is limited and causes movement around a nonphysiologic axis, joint mobilization may be indicated (Chapter 4). When the symptoms have begun to resolve and the range of motion has increased, MET should be initiated. At this point, dosage must be minimal in regard to resistance, range, speed, and repetitions. As noted, the goal of phase 1 is to alleviate symptoms by applying graded exercise only. During this time, the use of unloaded positions may be most advantageous. Torstensen et al.[9] refer to this phase as "circulatory exercising." Once exercise is initiated, the primary goals are to increase circulation to the tonic system to prevent atrophy, increase protein synthesis, and reduce the level of metabolites, which can be achieved only through exercise and influencing muscular endurance.[8]

When the patient becomes asymptotic, phase 2 may be initiated. The primary goal of this phase is to increase the tissue tolerance for loading, thus preventing the return of symptoms. This often involves a reduced number of repetitions at an increased weight resistance.

EXERCISE GRADING

The goal of graded exercise is to allow pain-free performance of the prescribed exercise in accordance with the patient's pain level and the pathologic reactions of the tissues. Exercise grading is a unique component of MET and makes it possible for the patient to start exercising immediately without applying any passive treatment modalities.[9] The cornerstones of graded exercise are to promote exercise performance in the pain-free ROM and to reduce the effects of gravity through unloading. Application of these concepts allows dysfunctional tissues to receive optimal stimuli for regeneration through the biomechanical stresses created from the intermittent tension–tension release mechanism of exercise. Therefore, appropriate dosage of properly graded exercise is an essential component of MET, allowing sufficient stimulus to normalize pathology and increase tolerance for loading.

EXERCISE DOSAGE

The tolerance to exercise should mirror the patient's current level of physical activity and determines the grading of the load used for treatment. In practical terms, a resistance is chosen from experience, with an optimal load being the goal. However, the following questions remain: How does one decide the dosage with specific reference to each particular patient's exercise tolerance? How does one decide the number of repetitions, the amount of resistance, and the speed at which the patient can perform in a pain-free synergy? All factors are based on the patient's needs, or the amount of stress the tissue structures are put under during ADLs. In other words, it is important to understand the optimal regeneration stimulus of different tissues. The optimal regeneration stimulus is the external stimulus necessary to stress the involved tissues adequately enough to cause adaptation. Dysfunction is not necessarily solved by minimizing the resistance but optimizing it.[4] The fundamental principles of MET require giving the pathologic degenerated tissues their optimal regeneration stimulus.

Factors to consider in exercise dosage include starting position, resistance, ROM, repetitions, training rate, relaxation (rest period), and training interval. Positions used for training consist of prone, supine, side lying, standing, and sitting. These positions are selected based on situational positional unloading in an attempt to reduce the effects of gravity. For example, for a patient with chronic low back pain, exercise positions that apply minimal pressure to the intervertebral disks may be advantageous. Specific mobilization techniques may require positions that stabilize, eliminating concurrent motion in other vertebral areas. For hypermobility, the starting positions are selected so that the hypermobile segment becomes indirectly stabilized. Conversely, if the goal of treatment is mobilization of a hypomobile segment, the positions would be adjusted accordingly.

The results of the physical examination determine the starting position for each exercise. The principles of MET emphasize the functional aspects of exercise; therefore, the starting position, like the exercise itself, must be functional. The starting position must be adapted to the patient's condition and must allow exercise completion in a coordinated fashion.

Resistance should be based on a determination of the patient's optimal loading. The patient's tolerance should be examined through several ranges of motion: segmental, normal, and full.[11] These ranges use isotonic muscle contractions to approximate the origin and insertion from maximally contracted to maximally stretched positions. The goal of treatment is to establish motion throughout the entire range. When tissues with reduced elasticity and mobility are being targeted (hypomobility), the goal is to increase coordination, vascularity, and ROM. However, if functional hypermobility exists, too much ROM in articular structures can be detrimental. Thus the antagonistic muscles to the hypermobile range must increase their sensitivity to stretch during eccentric work. Providing resistance by working against gravity can be used to grade exercise as well. Therefore, all movements are performed against resistance, even though it may be only inertia that has to be overcome.

The number of prescribed repetitions for a daily workout session can be close to 500. Performance of such a large number of repetitions may possibly influence mechanisms such as endurance, circulation, and coordination.[2] The total number prescribed is, of course, patient dependent. Resistance should be chosen so that the patient can perform a minimum of three sets of 30 repetitions of one exercise. However, the prescribed number of repetitions depends on the resistance and the intent or goals of training. Fewer repetitions at high resistance tend to emphasize muscular strength, whereas more repetitions at low resistance targets muscular endurance.

The Holten diagram (Fig. 7-1) depicts the relationship between the maximum number of repetitions that can be performed and the percentage of maximal resistance in regard to muscular strength and endurance. The dia-

FIGURE 7-1 Holten diagram showing suggestions for number of repetitions and amount of resistance.

(Reprinted with permission from Tom Arild Torstensen, Medical exercise therapy for thoracic and low back pain—sciatica (course material). Published by Holten Institute, Oslo, Norway.

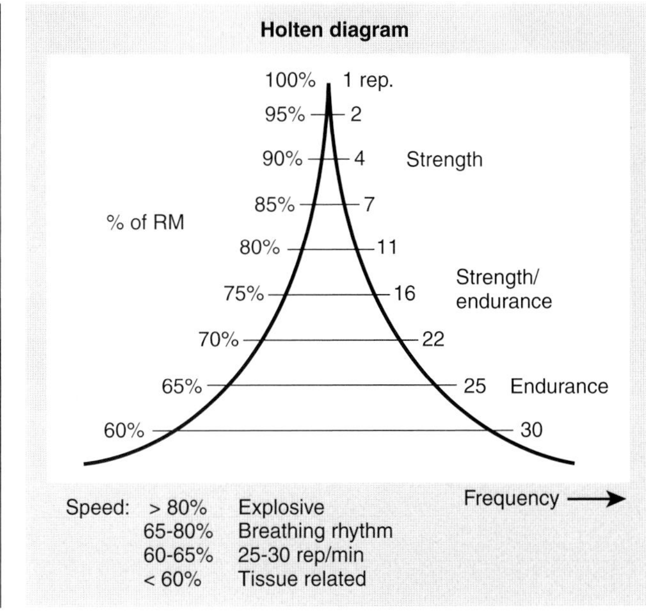

gram helps determine the muscular effect (alterations in muscular strength, endurance, or both). According to the diagram, exercise influences endurance when 30 or more repetitions are performed at 60% of one repetition maximum (RM) or less resistance. The prescribed training rate should be low for patients experiencing symptoms and when treating a specific joint. Overall, resistance increases as the training rate increases. The Holten diagram is an excellent resource for determining exercise dosage.

The relaxation phase, or rest period, is determined by the amount of time the patient needs to return to his or her starting respiratory rate. The break between sets may be as short as 30 sec or as long as 2 min, depending on the patient. The training interval should consist of a minimum of three exercise sessions per week, but can be increased to daily exercise if tolerated by the patient.

Clinical practice has demonstrated that a rather large exercise stimulus is necessary for normalizing function.[13] However, when designing the intensity of the prescribed exercise, clinicians must take into consideration such factors as the patient's general health status, pain, motion restrictions, and neurologic deficits as well as cardiovascular and respiratory status.

■ *Techniques*

MOBILIZATION

Mobilization is performed for the treatment of hypomobility. Chapter 4 presents the basis for treatment and a variety of techniques used for passive mobilization. Medical exercise training incorporates active mobilization, which is defined as self-mobilization of an extremity joint or spinal segment performed independently by the patient. Figures 7-2 to 7-5 show examples of active mobilization.

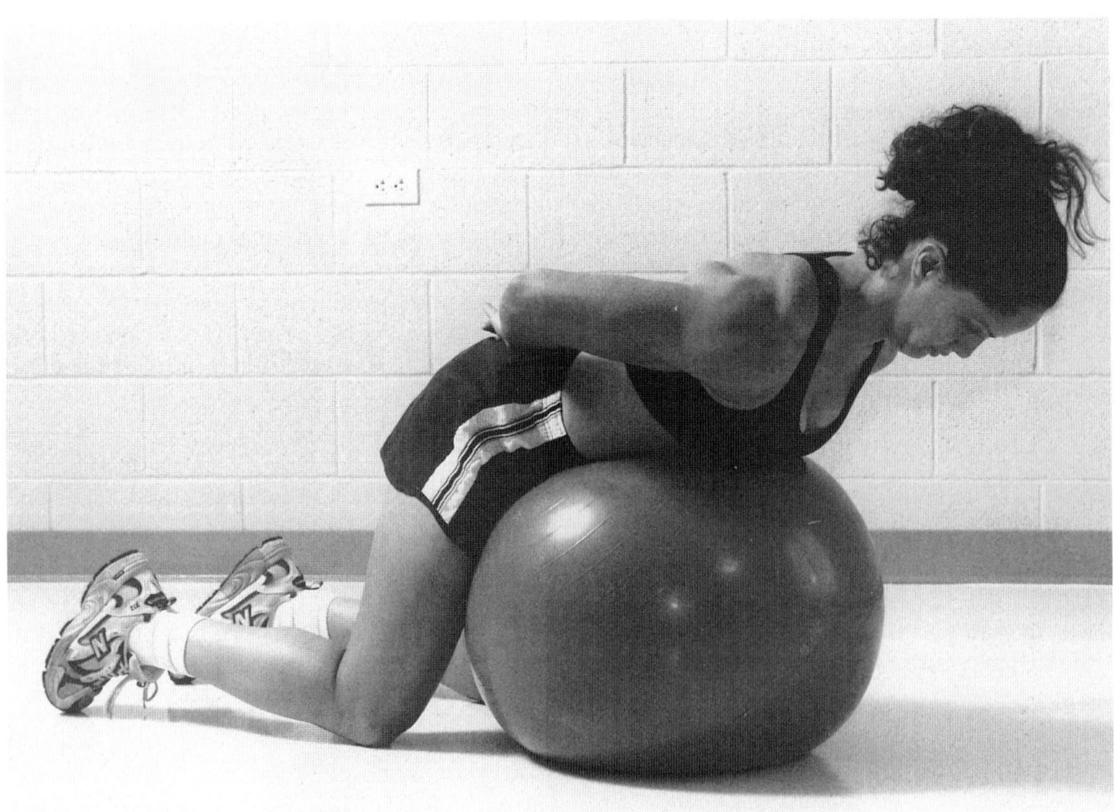

FIGURE 7-2 **Active mobilization to increase extension of spine.**

PURPOSE: Actively increase extension of spine.

POSITION: Client lying prone over therapeutic ball or stationary roll so apex of ball determines location of the axis of rotation. Spine flexed; hips and knees flexed; ankles dorsiflexed.

PROCEDURE: Client actively extends spine while simultaneously extending the cervical spine and retracting the scapulae.

FIGURE 7-3 **Active mobilization to increase extension and rotation of spine.**

PURPOSE: Actively increase extension, side bending, and rotation of spine while strengthening the spinal extensor and rotator musculature.

POSITION: Client sitting with hips and knees flexed to 90°, feet firmly on floor. Spine flexed, side bent left, and rotated left, allowing client to grasp pulley handle with both hands. Placement of roll determines the axis of rotation (panel A).

PROCEDURE: Client turns head and cervical spine to the right and extends the trunk while rotating to the right; arms raised overhead (panel B).

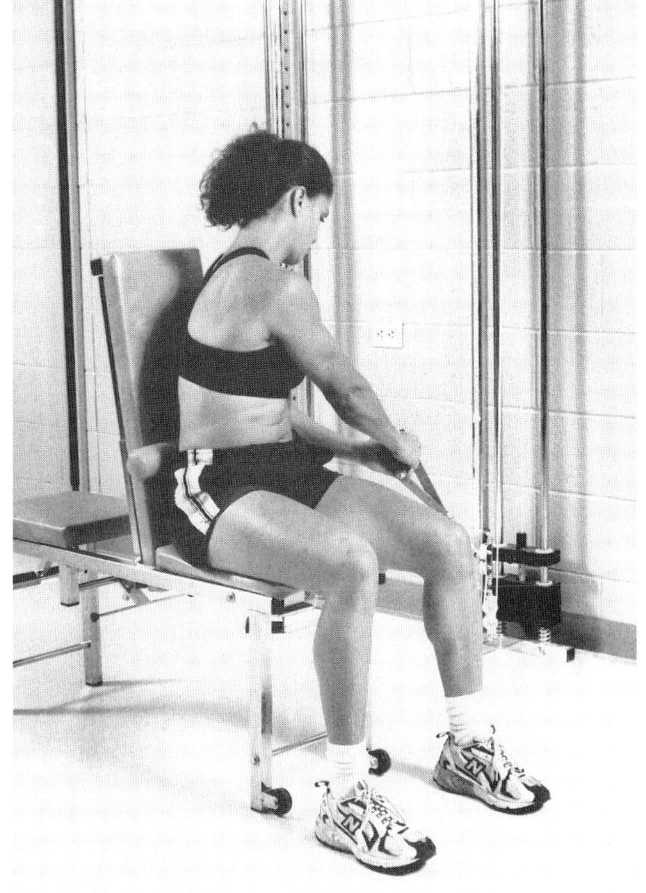

A

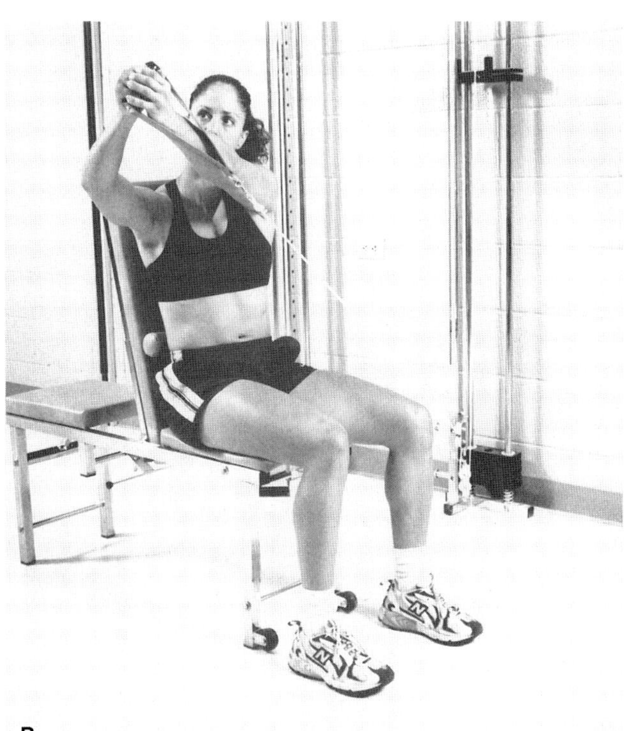

B

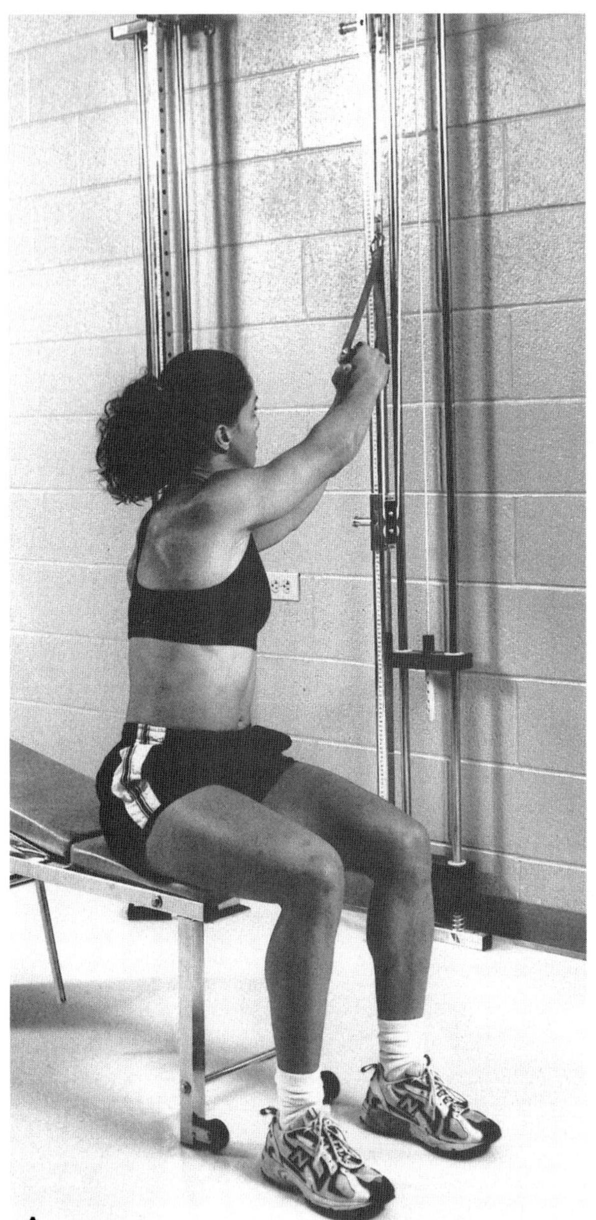
A

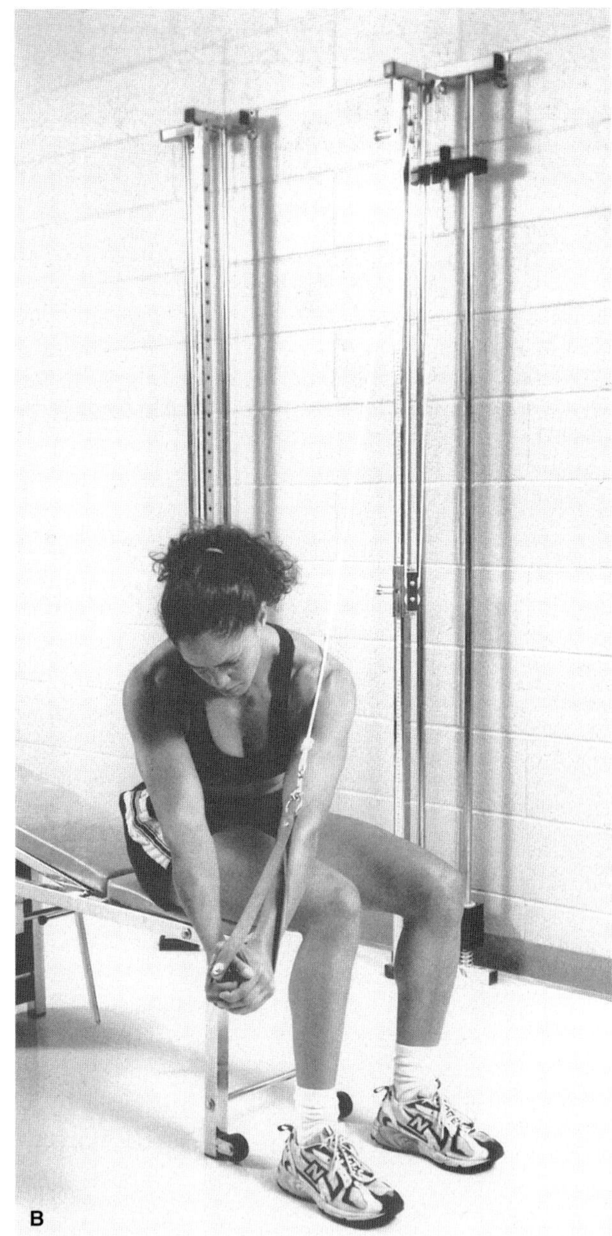
B

FIGURE 7-4 **Active mobilization to increase flexion, side bending, and rotation of spine.**

PURPOSE: Actively increase flexion, side bending, and rotation of spine while strengthening the abdominal musculature.

POSITION: Client sitting with hips and knees flexed to 90°, feet firmly on floor. Spine extended and rotated left, allowing client to grasp pulley handle with both hands (panel A).

PROCEDURE: Client actively turns head and cervical spine right; then flexes, side bends, and rotates spine right as pulley handle is pulled toward floor (panel B).

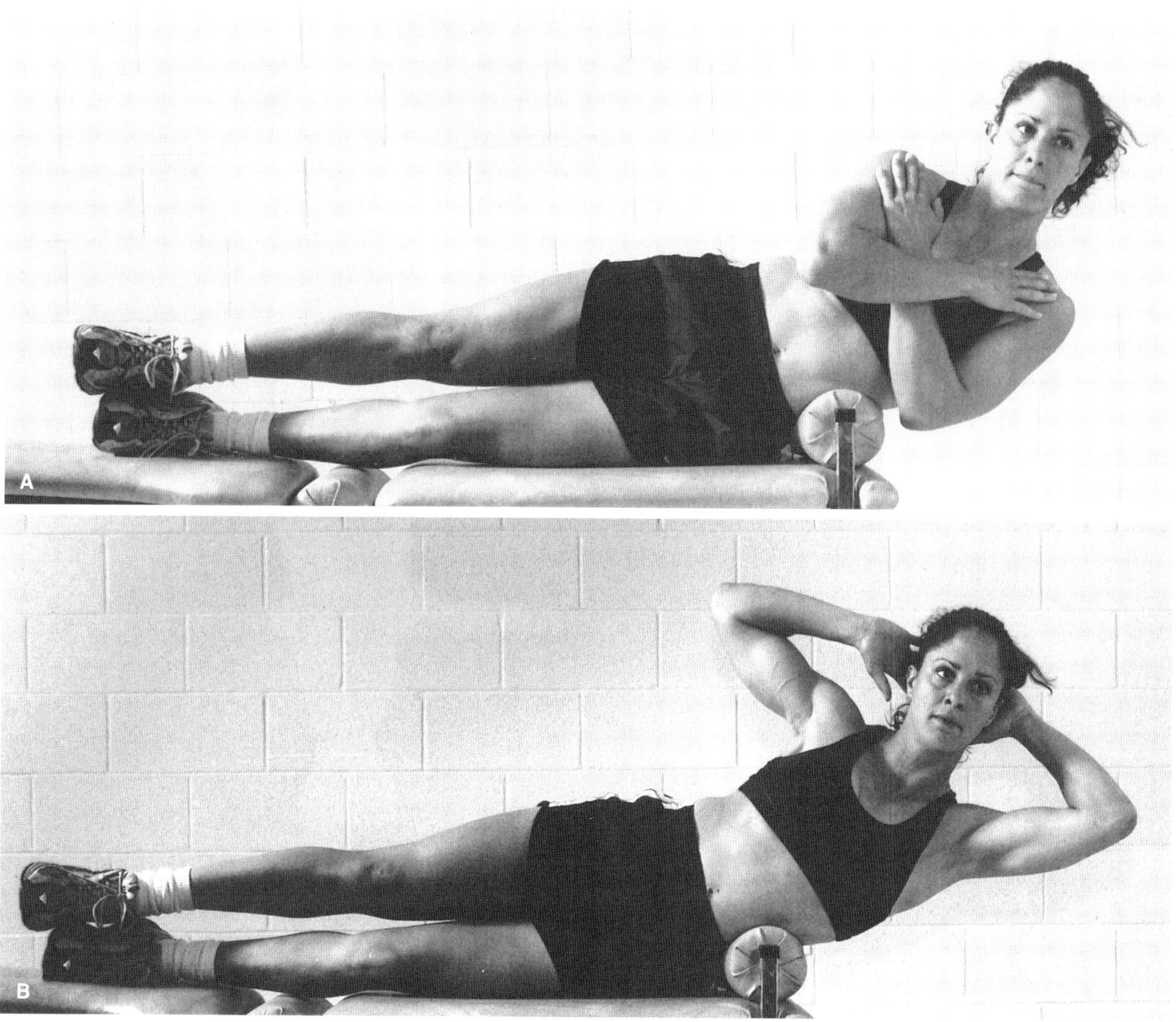

FIGURE 7-5 Active mobilization to increase side bending.

PURPOSE: Actively increase side bending of spine while strengthening the abdominal muscles, back muscles, and hip abductors.

POSITION: Client side lying on adjustable bench with trunk in 15° decline; hands can be placed on shoulders (panel A) or behind head (panel B; increases difficulty). To make exercise easier, lower extremities can be secured at ankles. Roll at trunk determines axis of movement. Spine is side bent to the left.

PROCEDURE: Client actively side bends to right.

STABILIZATION

Stabilization techniques are performed for hypermobility and often incorporate exercises and activities that facilitate stability through enhanced neuromuscular control. Figures 7-6 to 7-16 provide examples of stabilizing techniques that indirectly train the abdominal muscles along with the cervical, thoracic, and lumbar paraspinal muscles.

TRAINING

Training techniques are designed to improve muscle strength, endurance, and neuromuscular control. Figures 7-17 to 7-27 present common training techniques.

FIGURE 7-6 **Stabilization with reciprocal upper-extremity movement.**

PURPOSE: Stabilize spine; strengthen bilateral shoulder girdle.

POSITION: Client standing with trunk in neutral, stable position. Dumbbells may be used.

PROCEDURE: Client alternately raises one extremity while lowering the other.

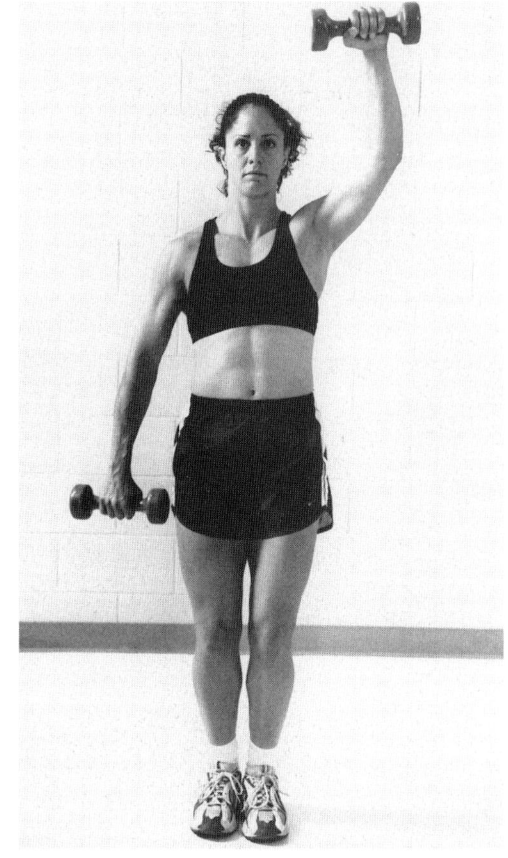

FIGURE 7-7 **Stabilization while strengthening upper trapezius muscles.**

PURPOSE: Stabilize spine; strengthen upper trapezius muscles.

POSITION: Client standing with trunk in neutral, stable position. Dumbbells may be used.

PROCEDURE: Client abducts both upper extremities simultaneously.

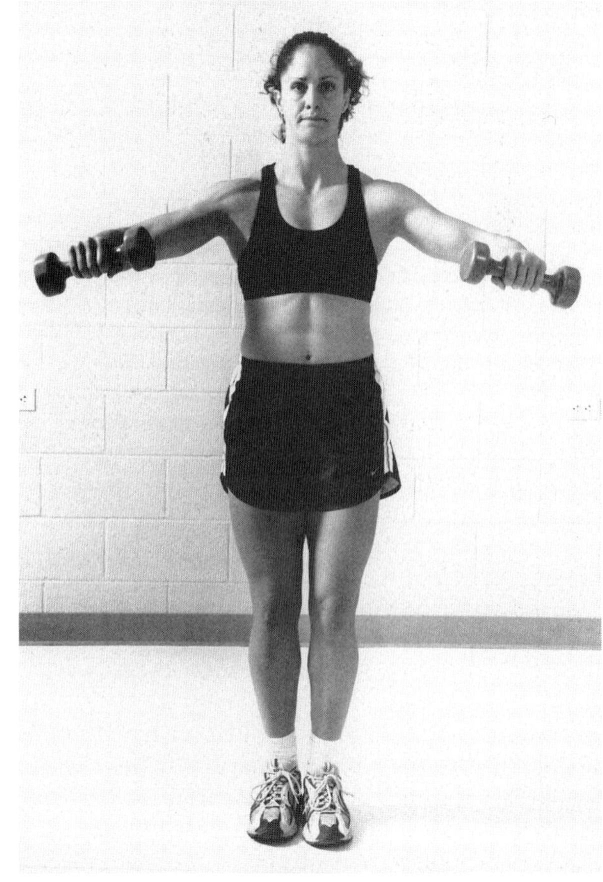

FIGURE 7-8 **Pull to chest.**

PURPOSE: Stabilize spine; strengthen posterior shoulder girdle and scapular stabilizing musculature.

POSITION: Client lying supine with hips and knees flexed. Shoulders flexed to allow for grasping of pulley bar.

PROCEDURE: Client pulls bar toward chest by flexing elbows, extending shoulders, and retracting scapulae.

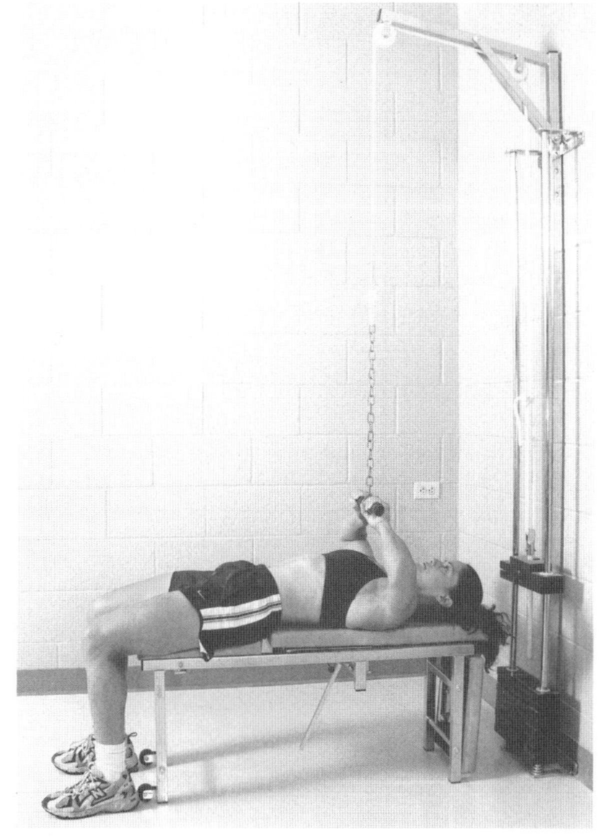

FIGURE 7-9 **Pull to chest.**

PURPOSE: Stabilize spine; strengthen biceps and scapular stabilizing musculature.

POSITION: Client sitting; hips and knees flexed to 90°; feet firmly on floor. Upper extremities in 90° of shoulder flexion to allow grasping of pulley bar.

PROCEDURE: Client pulls bar toward chest by flexing elbows, extending shoulders, and retracting scapula.

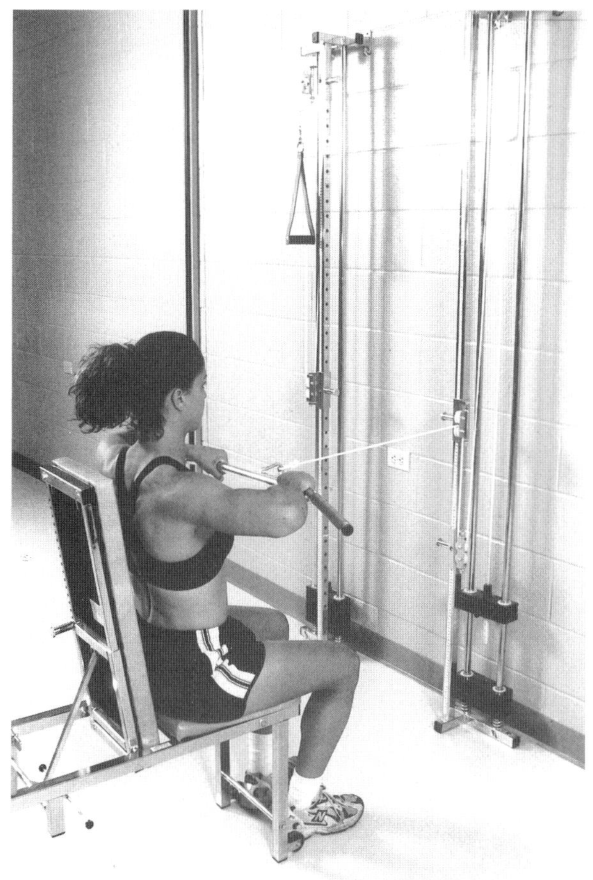

FIGURE 7-10 **Pull to chest from above.**

PURPOSE: Stabilize spine; strengthen teres major, latissimus dorsi, and scapular stabilizing musculature.

POSITION: Client sitting; hips and knees flexed; feet firmly on floor. Upper extremities in about 150° of shoulder flexion to allow grasping of pulley handle.

PROCEDURE: Client pulls pulley handle toward chest by flexing elbows, extending shoulders, and retracting scapulae.

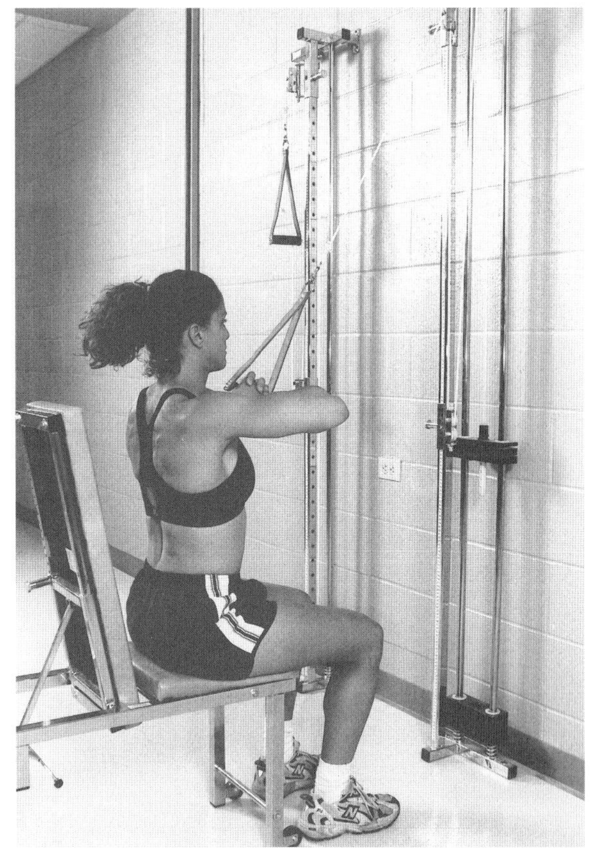

FIGURE 7-11 **Bar raise.**

PURPOSE: Stabilize spine; strengthen shoulder flexors, abductors, and external rotators.

POSITION: Client sitting; hips and knees flexed; feet firmly on floor. Arms at side with elbows flexed, grasping pulley bar.

PROCEDURE: Client lifts pulley bar overhead by flexing shoulders.

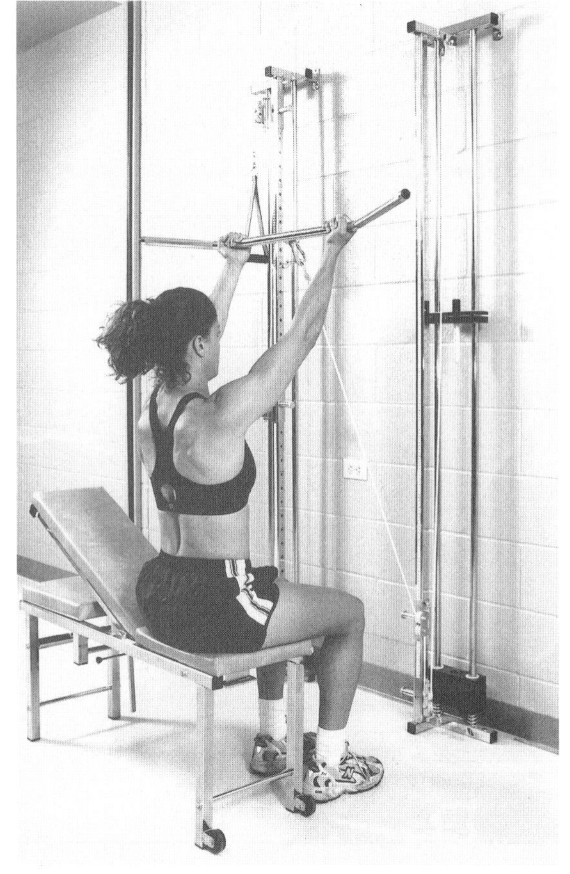

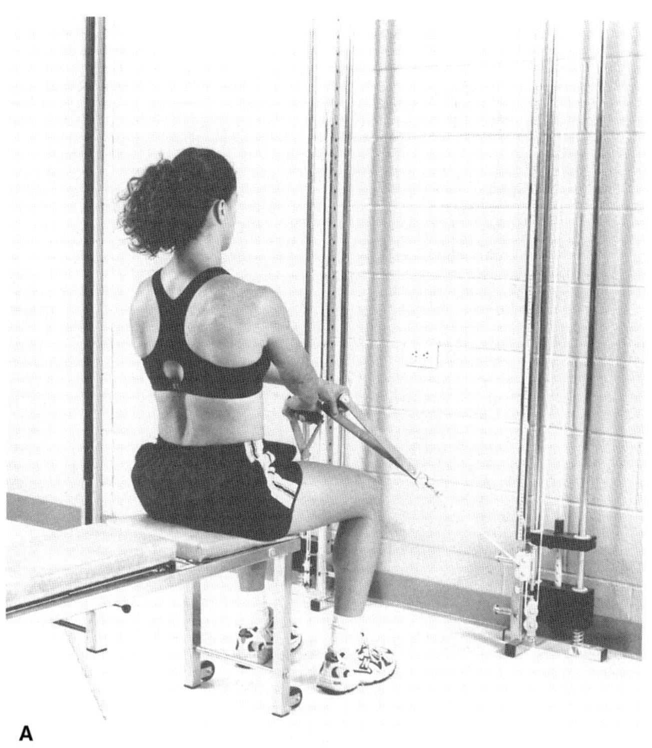

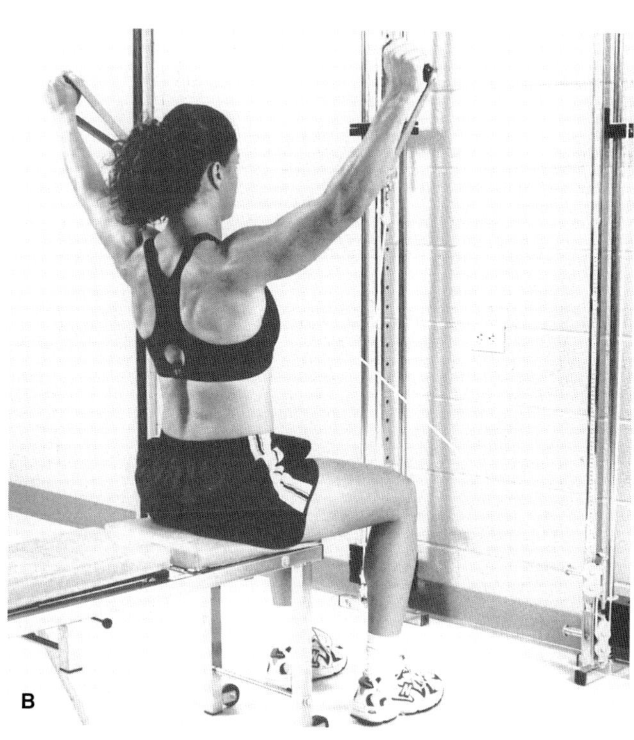

FIGURE 7-12 **Stabilization while strengthening upper extremity.**

PURPOSE: Stabilize spine; strengthen scapular retractors, shoulder flexors, abductors, and external rotators.

POSITION: Client sitting with hips and knees flexed; feet firmly on floor (panel A). Arms in position to allow for grasping of the contralateral pulley handles.

PROCEDURE: Client lifts pulley handles overhead by elevating arms (panel B).

FIGURE 7-13 **Shoulder abduction.**

PURPOSE: Stabilize spine; strengthen shoulder abductors.

POSITION: Client standing with arms at side, grasping pulley handle.

PROCEDURE: Client abducts arm to shoulder height in plane of the scapula.

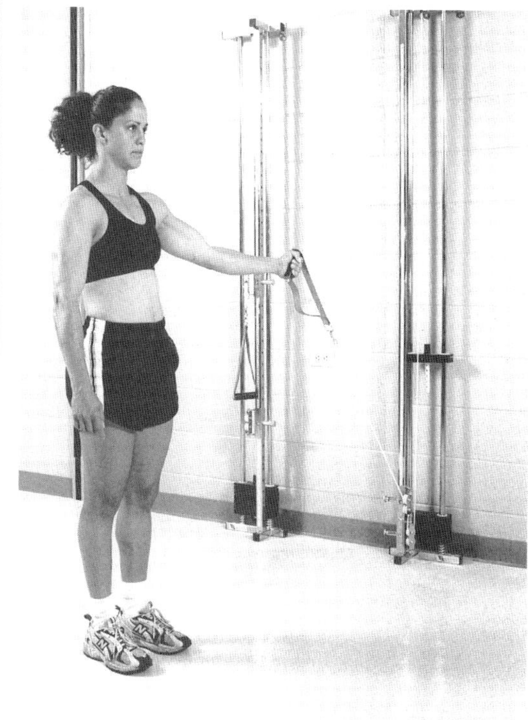

FIGURE 7-14 **Triceps exercise.**

PURPOSE: Stabilize spine; strengthen elbow extensors and scapular stabilizers.

POSITION: Client standing; arms at side with elbows flexed to grasp pulley bar.

PROCEDURE: Client extends elbows.

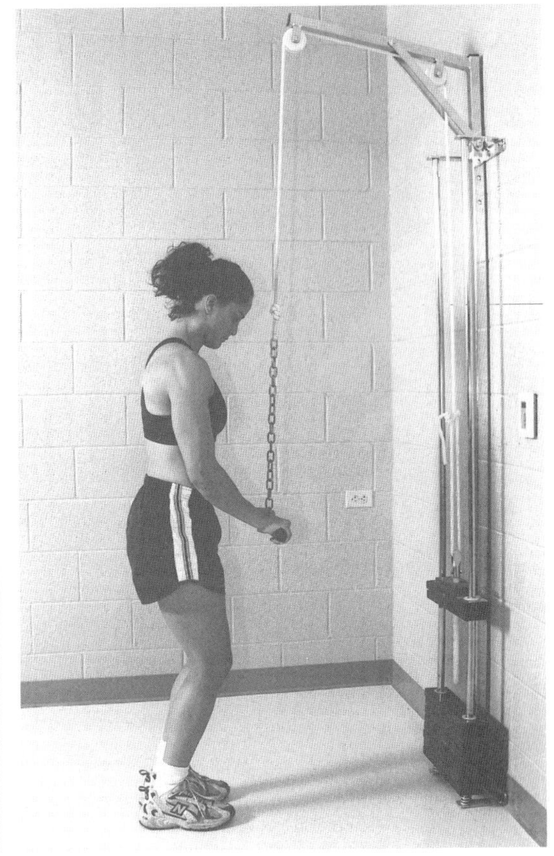

FIGURE 7-15 **Bar pull.**

PURPOSE: Stabilize spine; strengthen scapular retractors and shoulder abductors.

POSITION: Client standing; knees slightly bent; arms in front of body to allow grasping of pulley bar.

PROCEDURE: Client lifts pulley to chin by abducting shoulders and scapular retractors.

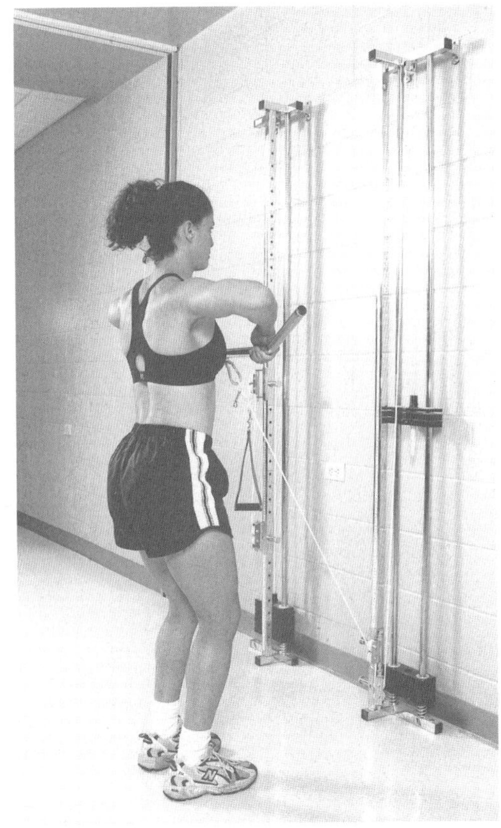

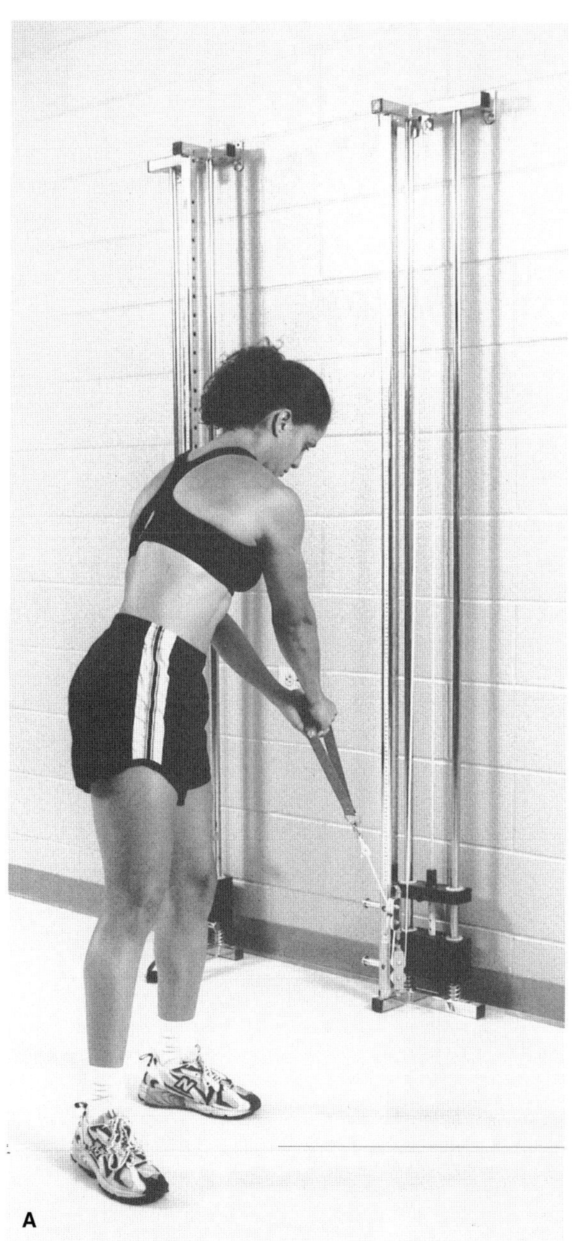

A

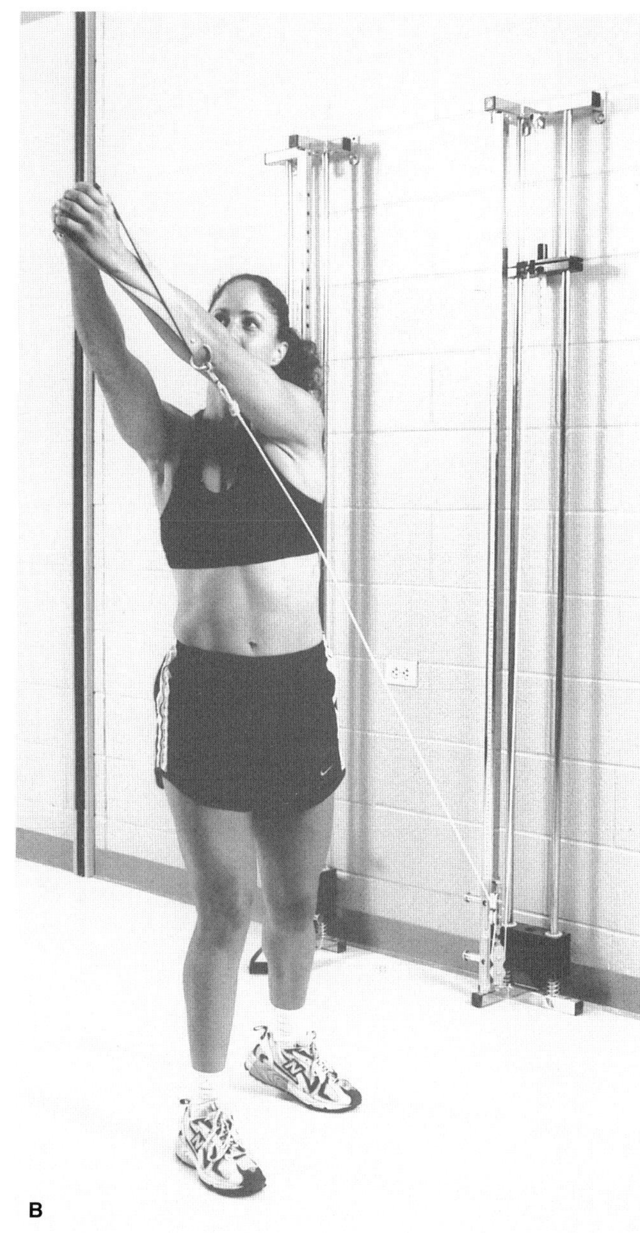

B

FIGURE 7-16 **Stabilization while performing diagonal movement patterns.**

PURPOSE: Stabilize spine; perform functional diagonal movement pattern.

POSITION: (Panel A) Client standing with feet staggered, weight on left leg, facing pulley. Client flexes, left side bends, and left rotates spine; allowing client to grasp pulley handle with both hands.

PROCEDURE: (Panel B) Weight is transferred to right leg. Client extends, side bends right, and rotates the spine right while lifting pulley handle in diagonal pattern.

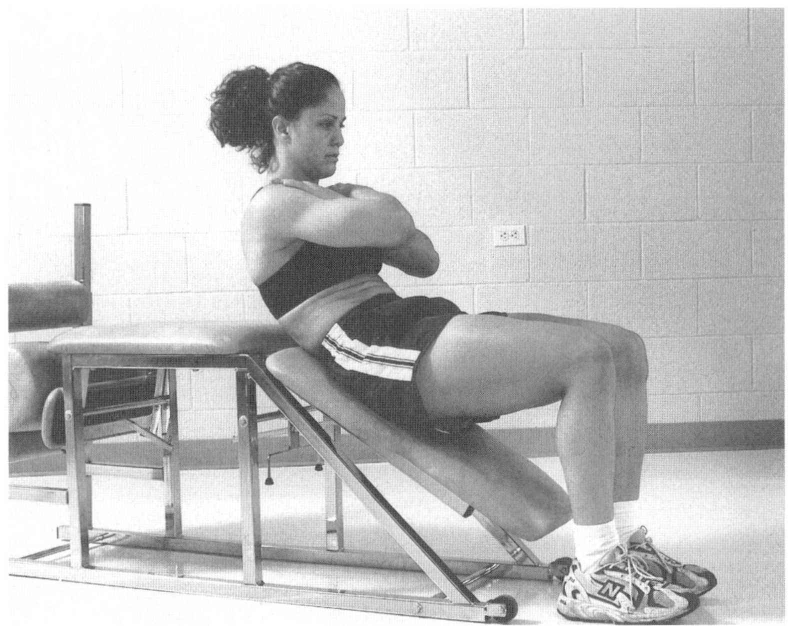

FIGURE 7-17 **Abdominal muscle strengthening.**

PURPOSE: Strengthen abdominal musculature.

POSITION: Client lying supine on incline bench with knees flexed and feet firmly on floor. Hands clasped in front of body.

PROCEDURE: Client gradually lifts head and trunk off bench until spine is flexed.

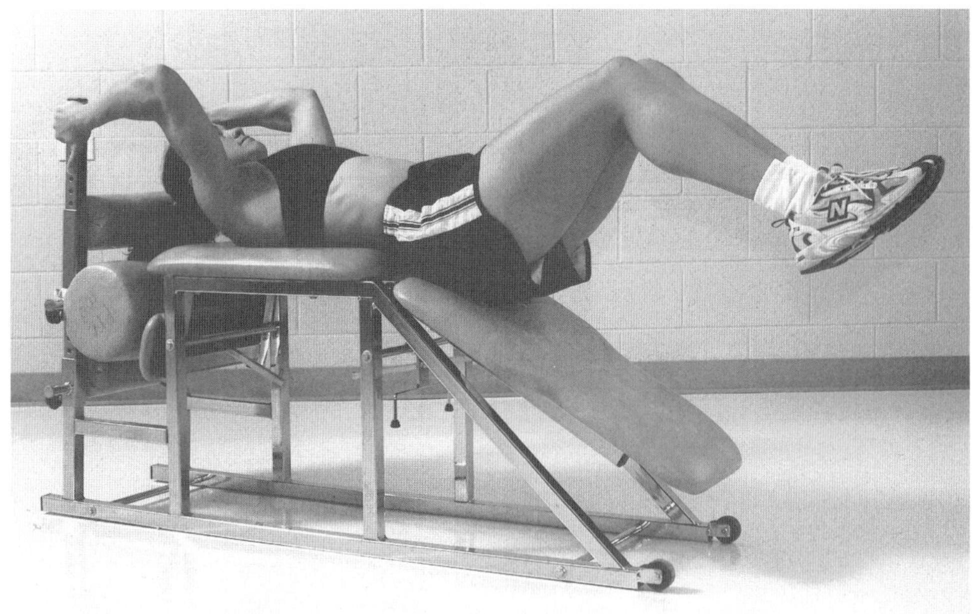

FIGURE 7-18 **Abdominal muscle strengthening.**

PURPOSE: Strengthen abdominal musculature.

POSITION: Client lying supine on incline bench with hips and knees held in extended position.

PROCEDURE: Client lifts pelvis and bilateral lower extremities off bench.

FIGURE 7-19 **Back muscle strengthening.**

PURPOSE: Strengthen back extensor musculature.

POSITION: Client kneeling on incline bench, toes on floor. Hips and spine in flexed position. Hands hold shoulders.

PROCEDURE: Client extends spine to neutral position, lifting body from bench.

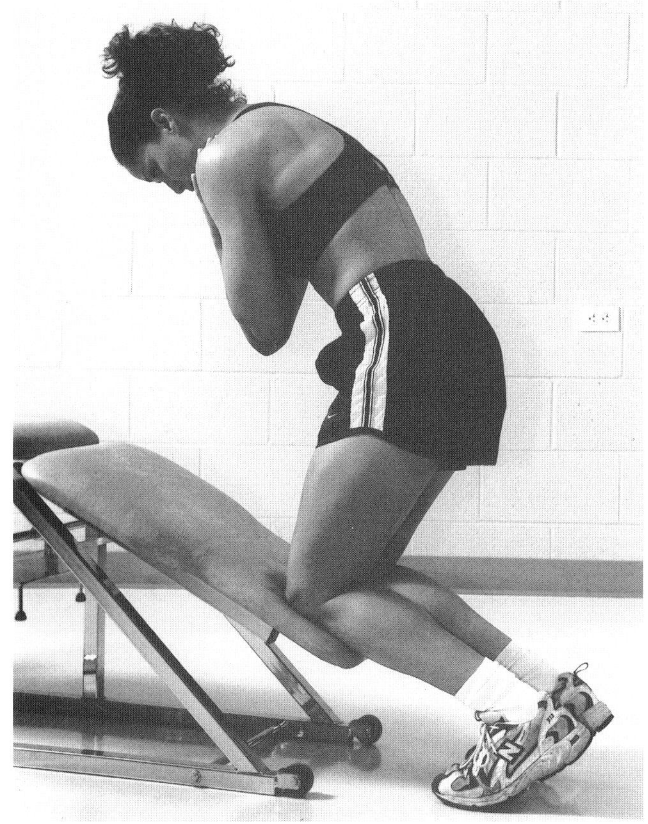

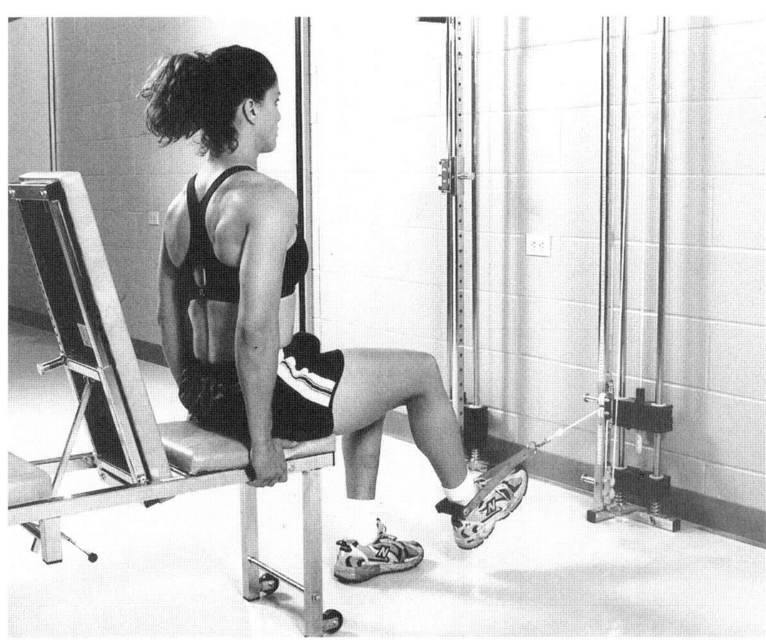

FIGURE 7-20 **Knee flexor muscle strengthening.**

PURPOSE: Strengthen knee flexor musculature.

POSITION: Client sitting on end of bench with ankle strapped to pulley.

PROCEDURE: Client flexes knee against resistance of pulley.

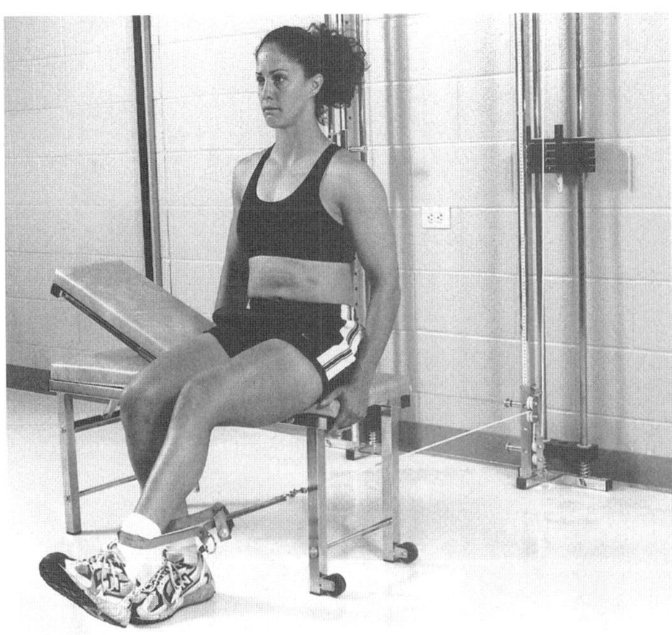

FIGURE 7-21 **Knee extensor muscle strengthening.**

PURPOSE: Strengthen knee extensor musculature.

POSITION: Client sitting with knee flexed at end of bench with ankle strapped to pulley.

PROCEDURE: Client extends knee against resistance of pulley.

FIGURE 7-22 **Unloaded mini-squats.**

PURPOSE: Lower-extremity strengthening and stabilization training with reduced weight bearing.

POSITION: Client standing; holding overhead pulley bar at mid-torso; elbows extended.

PROCEDURE: Keeping elbows extended, client performs mini-squat by flexing hips and knees and lowering body in direction of floor.

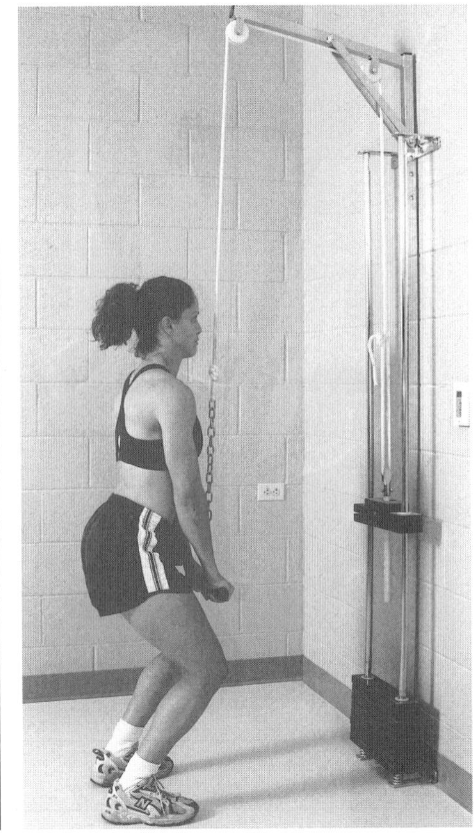

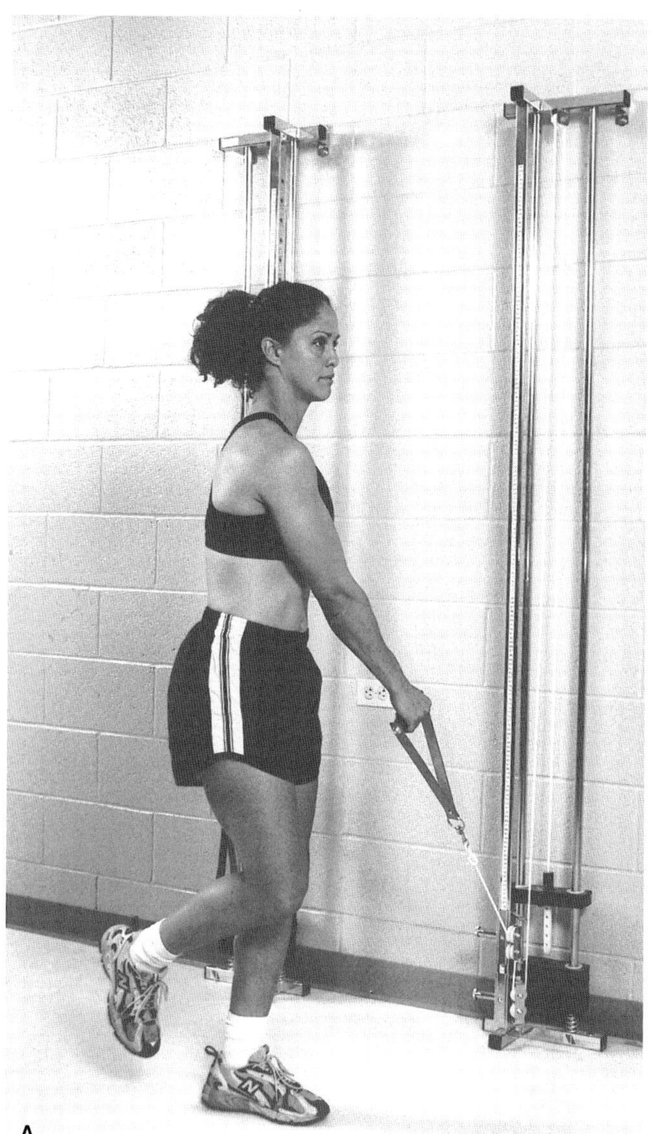

A

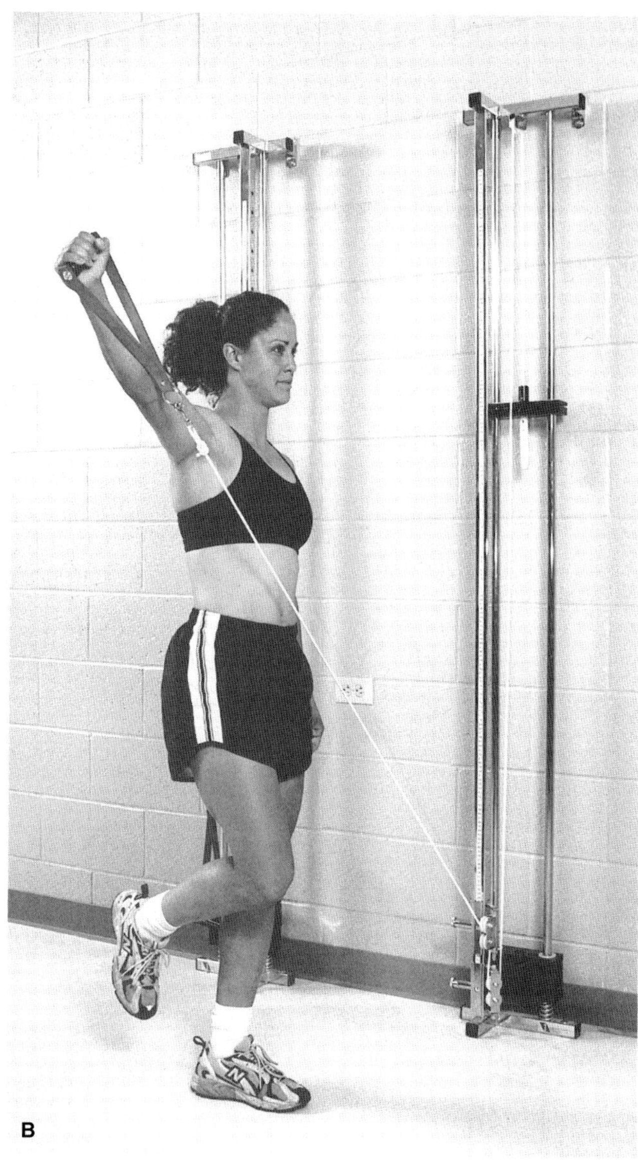

B

FIGURE 7-23 **Diagonal movement patterns with unilateral upper extremity.**

PURPOSE: Facilitate unilateral balance, coordination, and neuromuscular control using diagonal patterns.

POSITION: Client standing on left leg with unilateral support. Client left side bends and left rotates spine, allowing client to grasp pulley handle with right hand (panel A).

PROCEDURE: Client side bends and rotates the spine to the right while lifting pulley handle in diagonal pattern with right arm (panel B); client extends arms, resulting in perturbation while maintaining unilateral stance.

FIGURE 7-24 Lower-extremity stabilization.

PURPOSE: Facilitate unilateral balance, coordination, and neuromuscular control.

POSITION: Client standing on one leg with unilateral support. Upper extremities are flexed to grasp pulley handles.

PROCEDURE: Client gradually extends arms to neutral, resulting in perturbation while maintaining unilateral stance.

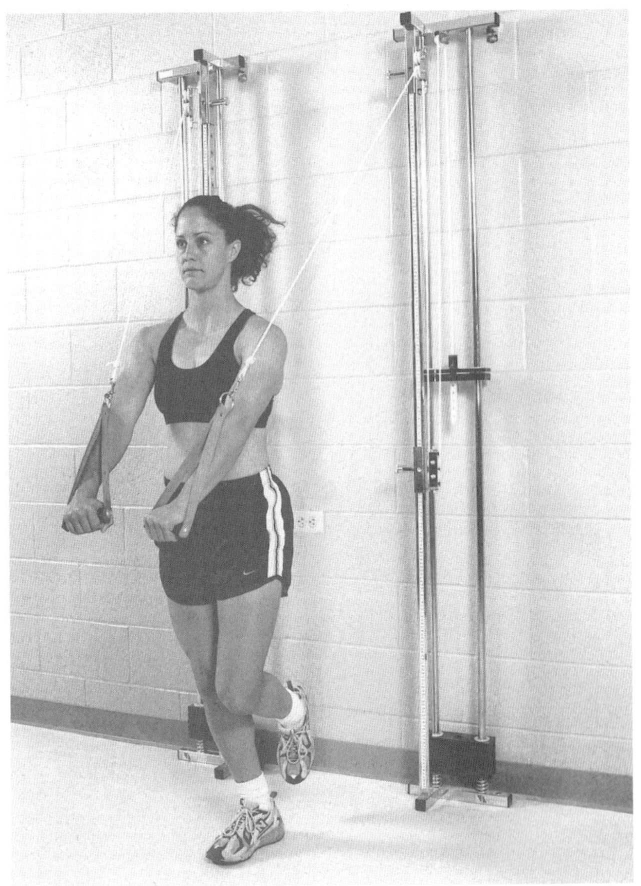

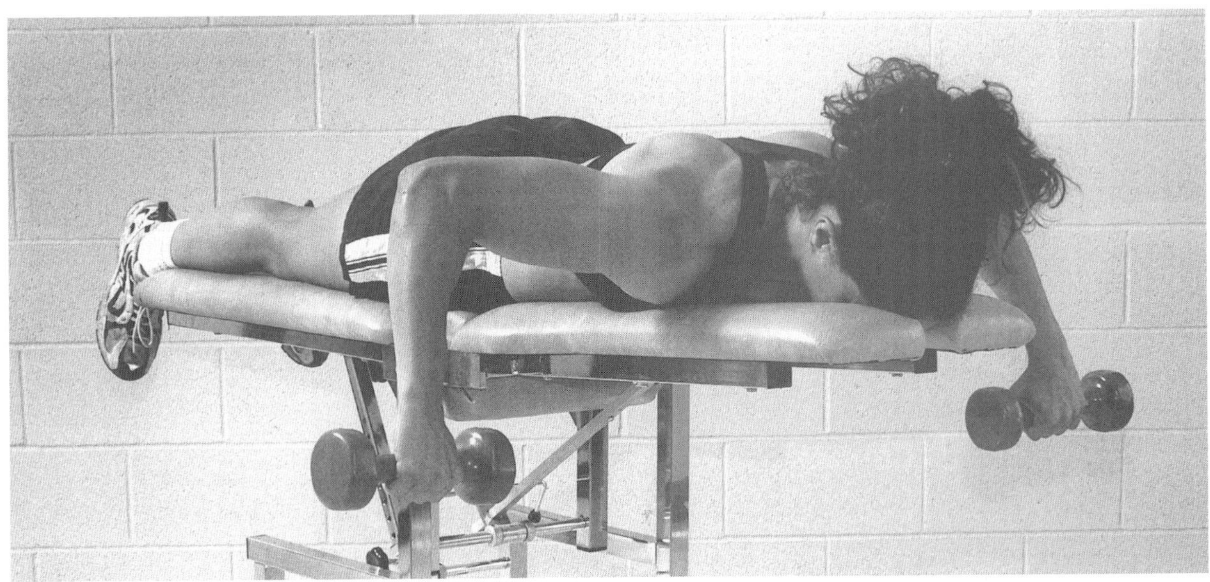

FIGURE 7-25 Horizontal adduction.

PURPOSE: Strengthen trapezius and scapular stabilizer musculature.

POSITION: Client lying prone on bench; arms hanging off edge of support surface. Dumbbells may be used.

PROCEDURE: Client horizontally abducts arms and retracts scapulae.

FIGURE 7-26 **Pull to chest.**

PURPOSE: Strengthen scapular stabilizer musculature.

POSITION: Client sitting on adjustable bench with support for anterior trunk. Arms in flexed position, allowing client to grasp pulley handles, one in each hand.

PROCEDURE: Client horizontally abducts arms and retracts scapulae.

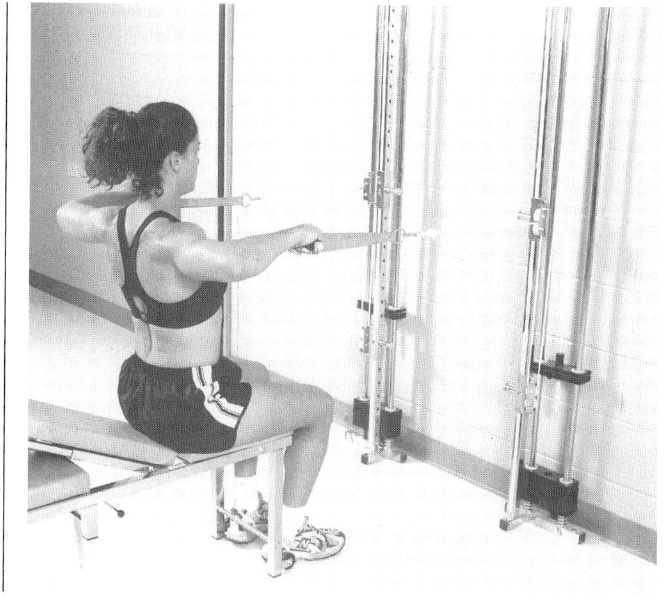

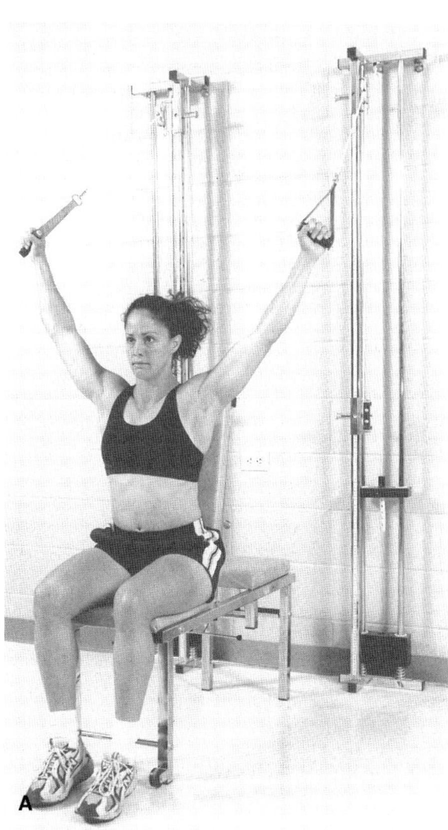

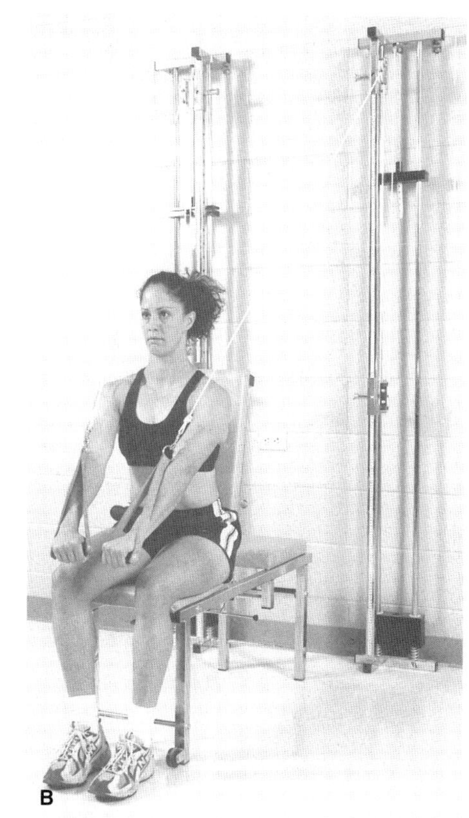

FIGURE 7-27 **Latissimus dorsi muscle strengthening.**

PURPOSE: Strengthen latissimus dorsi musculature.

POSITION: Client sitting on adjustable bench with support for posterior trunk. Hips and knees are flexed, feet firmly on floor. Arms are elevated overhead, allowing client to grasp pulley handles in each hands (panel A).

PROCEDURE: Client extends arms toward midline of body (panel B).

CASE STUDY

PATIENT INFORMATION

A 22-year-old intercollegiate baseball pitcher presented to the university sports medicine facility complaining of pain in his low back. He described the onset of symptoms as moderate low back pain noted while pitching nine innings during a game. The patient reported that the pain increased as the game progressed; however, he was able to complete the game. The following day he complained of low back pain with forward bending and noted mild soreness in his right (throwing) shoulder.

Physical examination revealed pain and palpable tenderness in the lumbar paraspinal musculature (bilateral) and increased skin temperature, indicating inflammation. Active forward bending was limited, as was left side bending and left rotation. Assessment of passive intervertebral movement indicated localized hypomobility in lumbar vertebral segments L3-4 and L4-5. Selected tissue tension testing and manual muscle testing of the trunk indicated strong and pain-free trunk flexor strength (4+/5) and strong and painful back extensor strength (4/5). In addition, testing of the right shoulder revealed strong and pain-free external rotation (4+/5) and pain-free but slightly weak scapular protraction and retraction (4/5). Left shoulder examination indicated strong external rotation (5/5) and strong scapular protraction and retraction (5/5). No upper- or lower-quarter neurologic signs were present. Gait was unaffected.

Based on the physical examination, the clinician diagnosed a lumbar paraspinal muscle strain. Right shoulder girdle (scapular stabilizer) weakness was also noted.

LINKS TO

Guide to Physical Therapist Practice and *Athletic Training Educational Competencies*

Pattern 4D of the *Guide*[14] relates to the diagnosis of this patient. This pattern is described as "impaired joint mobility, motor function, muscle performance, and range of motion associated with connective tissue dysfunction." Anticipated goals of therapeutic exercise in pattern 4D include decreasing pain; improving physical function; improving joint mobility; increasing strength, power, and endurance; and reducing risk of recurrence. Specific direct interventions related to this diagnosis include strengthening via active assistive, active, and resistive exercises.

The therapeutic exercise domain in the *Competencies*[15] refers to the treatment of athletes using "elastic, mechanical, and manual resistance." In addition, "exercises to improve dynamic joint stability, neuromuscular coordination, postural stability, and proprioception" are included.

INTERVENTION

Initial goals of intervention were to reduce symptoms, increase blood circulation, and decrease inflammation and muscle soreness while increasing active and passive lumbar movement. These goals were to be accomplished by performing pain-free, coordinated mobility and stability exercises around the physiologic axes through the available ROM. The patient was instructed to perform three sets of 30 repetitions and dosage was adjusted, as needed, each session. Tissue tolerance in the initial stage dictated that muscular endurance be emphasized; thus ensuring pain-free exercise performance. The following techniques were prescribed:

1. Active mobilization to improve lumbar spine flexion, left side bending, and left rotation (Fig. 7-4).
2. Abdominal muscle strengthening (Figs. 7-17 and 7-18).
3. Back extensor muscle strengthening (Fig. 7-19).
4. Trapezius and scapular stabilizer muscle strengthening (Fig. 7-25).
5. Ice the low back after exercise.

The patient performed these exercises daily under direct supervision in the clinic.

INTERVENTION

One Week After Initial Examination

During the first week of training, the patient's exercise program had advanced toward increasing the demands on the targeted tissues by decreasing repetitions (three sets of 22 repetitions) and increasing resistance, effectively emphasizing both muscular strength and endurance.

Examination indicated that the patient presented with full active movement (lumbar forward bending, side bending, and rotation) and improved strength in trunk flexion (5/5), trunk extension (4+/5), and scapular protraction and retraction (4+/5). Palpable tenderness and skin temperature changes were no longer present. Pain was not associated with any active movement or resisted testing. The initial goals of treatment were achieved. Therefore, the goal of continued treatment became to increase tissue tolerance to the demands of daily activity (pitching). The program was advanced to include the following techniques, which were initiated at three sets of 30 repetitions, adjusted as needed:

GERIATRIC *Perspectives*

- Little research is available to support or refute the use of MET in older adults. Because older adults demonstrate varied age-related changes in soft tissue, including decreased flexibility (hypomobility) and loss of muscle mass and endurance, MET should be beneficial for restoration of functional movement.
- Older adults have a decrease in type II fast-twitch muscle fibers; a phenomenon that may be related to disuse.[1] The fast-twitch fibers are recruited during high-intensity muscle demands.[2] Thus MET may offer unique training potential for older adults. Likewise, facilitated muscle fiber recruitment would maximize performance capabilities during functional activities.
- The length of sessions and repetitions may need to be altered to accommodate the limitations of the older adult. Similarly, positioning for exercise should consider age-related postural and bony changes. Careful monitoring of exercise response should be performed to decrease likelihood of injury and to ensure compliance with prescribed protocol.

1. Wilmore JH. The aging of bone and muscle. Clin Sports Med 1991;10: 231–244.
2. Fredericks CM. Skeletal muscle: the somatic effector. In: ???????, ed. Pathophysiology of the motor systems. Principles and clinical presentations. Philadelphia: Davis, 1995:???–???.

1. Back extensor muscle strengthening (Fig. 7-19).
2. Stabilization while strengthening the posterior shoulder girdle and scapular stabilizers (Figs. 7-6 to 7-15).

Two Weeks After Initial Examination

After 2 weeks of intervention, no pain, restricted movement, or weakness was reported. The patient's program had been advanced so that he was performing 3 sets of 12 to 16 repetitions of the previously prescribed exercises, using increased resistance. This progression was based on tissue tolerance, as the goal shifted toward increasing muscular strength.

The patient, however, had not attempted to return to pitching. Thus the goals of intervention became to return to pitching and prevent recurrence of symptoms. The individually prescribed program was progressed to include stabilization while performing diagonal movement patterns with bilateral upper extremities (Fig. 7-16). The patient was told to do three sets of 30 repetitions to meet the unique demands placed on the shoulder girdle by the overhead athlete (such as baseball pitcher, tennis player). In contrast to the other exercises, repetitions were increased as the patient progressed, rather than decreased, to continue to emphasize muscular endurance.

OUTCOME

The patient's program concluded with participation in a standardized interval throwing program to progress him toward returning to pitching. The interval throwing program was initiated at 3 weeks postinjury. He progressed from short toss to long toss to throwing from a pitching mound in 1 week's time. He pitched in his first game 4 weeks postinjury. He was then discharged to return to his previous level of function (pitching in the starting rotation) without complications or recurrence.

SUMMARY

- Medical exercise training is a system of progressively graded exercise that uses a functional approach to musculoskeletal disorders to assess and treat patients based on the principles of strength, speed, endurance, power, coordination, work capacity, and aerobic training. It is designed to restore function through the principles of active mobilization and stabilization. Active mobilization is performed for the treatment of hypomobility, and stabilization is performed for hypermobility.
- The MET program suggests that the clinician establish a baseline by which improvement can be measured. This requires implementation of functionally relevant measures of strength, flexibility, and endurance in conjunction with routinely used standardized testing procedures, such as manual muscle testing and goniometry. Accurate reflection of functional status requires testing that is both quantifiable and functional.
- Medical exercise training uses exclusively active exercise with optimal stimulation. The prescribed exercises consider factors such as ROM, maximal resistance, and

PEDIATRIC *Perspectives*

- There are no direct contraindications to the use of MET principles for children and adolescents.[1] However, clinicians should remember that children generally have some degree of normal hypermobility. Furthermore, children and adolescents may not have adequate hormonal support for the strength development that adults realize through MET's specificity approach.[1,2] Therefore, lower resistance and higher repetitions are indicated. Children and adolescents should not exceed 50 resistance repetitions.[1] Finally, to facilitate development of muscular coordination and strength, special attention must be paid to proper technique when using exercise training in children.[2]

1. Grimsby O. Personal communication, Oct 4, 1999.
2. Thein LA. The child and adolescent athlete. In: JE Zachezewski, DJ Magee, WS Quillen, eds. Athletic injuries and rehabilitation. Philadelphia: Saunders, 1996:933–958.

number of repetitions and are customized to the individual patient's daily demands. Proper exercise dosage is essential to the patient's functional return; exercise tolerance should mirror the patient's current level of physical activity. Exercise dosage is based on the patient's needs, including the amount of stress the tissue structures are put under during ADLs. Dysfunction is not corrected by minimizing the resistance, but optimizing it. Factors to consider when determining exercise dosage include starting position, resistance, ROM, repetitions, training rate, relaxation, and training interval.

- The goal of graded exercise is to allow pain-free performance of the prescribed exercise in accordance with pain and the pathologic reactions of the tissues. Exercise grading promotes exercise performance in the pain-free range of motion and reduces the effects of gravity through unloading.

REFERENCES

1. Torstensen TA. The physical therapy approach. In: JW Frymoyer, Ducker TB, Hadler NM, et al., eds. The adult spine: principles and practice. Philadelphia: Lippincott-Raven, 1997:1797–1805.
2. Torstensen TA, Ljunggren AE, Meen HD, et al. Efficiency and costs of medical exercise therapy, conventional physiotherapy, and self-exercise in patients with chronic low back pain. Spine 1998;23:2616–2624.
3. Holten O. Medical training therapy. Fysiterapeuten 1976;11: 9–14.
4. Holten O, Torstensen TA. Medical exercise therapy: the basic principles. Fysioterapeuten 1991;58:27–32.
5. Watson RR, Eisinger M. Exercise and disease. Boca Raton, FL: CRC Press, 1993.
6. Walker JM. Connective tissue plasticity: issues in histological and light microscopy studies of exercise and aging in articular cartilage. J Orthop Sports Phys Ther 1991;14:189–197.
7. Enwemeka CS. Connective tissue plasticity: ultrastructural, biomechanical, and morphometric effects of physical factors on intact and regenerating tendons. J Orthop Sports Phys Ther 1991; 14:198–212.
8. Grimsby O. Scientific therapeutic exercise progressions. J Man Manipulative Ther 1994;2:94–101.
9. Torstensen TA, Meen HD, Stiris M. The effect of medical exercise therapy on a patient with chronic supraspinatus tendinitis. Diagnostic ultrasound—tissue regeneration: a case study. J Orthop Sports Phys Ther 1994;20:319–327.
10. Magee DJ. Orthopedic physical assessment. Philadelphia: Saunders, 1992.
11. Gustavsen R, Streeck R. Training therapy: prophylaxis and rehabilitation. New York: Thieme Medical, 1993.
12. Torstensen TA. Medical exercise therapy. Paper presented at World Congress of Physical Therapy. London, 1991.
13. Tipton CM, Vailas CV, Matthes RD. Experimental studies on the influences of physical activity on ligaments, tendons, and joints. Acta Med Scand, Suppl. 1986;711:157–168.
14. American Physical Therapy Association. Guide to physical therapist practice, second edition. Phys Ther 2001;81:1–768.
15. National Athletic Trainers' Association. Athletic training educational competencies. 3rd ed. Dallas: NATA, 1999

CHAPTER

Proprioceptive Neuromuscular Facilitation

Marcia H. Stalvey, PT, MS, NCS

Proprioceptive neuromuscular facilitation (PNF) is a philosophy of treatment developed in the 1950s by Kabat[1,2] and expanded under the vision of physical therapists Knot and Voss.[3] The basic principles of PNF emphasize the need for maximal demands to achieve maximal potential. The strong segments are used to facilitate the weak; improvement in specific functional activities is always the goal. Traditionally used for individuals with neurologic diagnoses,[4,5] PNF has wide applications for the rehabilitation of individuals of musculoskeletal dysfunction. It is widely accepted that the central nervous system (CNS), through neural adaptation, plays a part in the strength gains beyond those attributable to increases in muscle hypertrophy.[6,7] Proprioceptive neuromuscular facilitation can be used effectively as part of an overall progressive rehabilitation program to hasten that neural adaptation through motor relearning, to improve strength and flexibility, and to promote a functional progression. The purposes of this chapter are to

- Review the philosophy, principles, and neurophysiologic basis of PNF.
- Review and illustrate the more commonly used PNF diagonal patterns.
- Describe and illustrate applications of selected PNF techniques.
- Provide specific examples of the clinical application of PNF.

Scientific Basis

Proprioceptive neuromuscular facilitation is one of the traditional neurophysiologic approaches to therapeutic exercise, based on the classic work of Sherrington[8] and a hierarchical concept of the nervous system.[1,2] We now know that motor control is far more complex than just a muscle spindle and "top-down" organization,[9,10] and the use of PNF for central nervous system deficits has been somewhat controversial in light of more contemporary models of motor control. However, the literature substantiates the basic principles of PNF and their application to a wide variety of diagnoses, including the injured athlete.[11–17] Proprioceptive neuromuscular facilitation is most commonly used to restore range of motion (ROM), decrease pain, increase strength and endurance, hasten motor learning, improve coordination, facilitate proximal stability, and begin functional progression.[11,12,15,18]

Kabat[1,2] based his concepts of facilitation on the neurophysiology of the muscle spindle, applying Sherrington's laws of reciprocal innervation and successive induction to a therapeutic exercise technique. Reciprocal innervation states that contraction of the agonist produces simultaneous relaxation (inhibition) of the antagonist.[10] Successive induction suggests that voluntary motion of one muscle can be facilitated by the action of another.[10] For example, contraction of the biceps (the agonist), followed by contraction of the triceps (antagonist) results in increased response of biceps (the agonist). Additional neurophysiologic rationale is provided when specific techniques and applications are described.

Clinical Guidelines

One of the most easily and widely modified approaches to therapeutic exercise, PNF is therefore readily applied to all stages of rehabilitation of the injured individual. In the acute stages of injury, isometric contractions, manual contacts, and an indirect approach are used to help guide and teach movements to the patient when swelling and pain interfere. Proprioceptive neuromuscular facilitation provides the clinician with a means of manually grading an activity, giving precise feedback tailored to the patient's needs, activities, and level of rehabilitation. Techniques and patterns can be modified to avoid pain and to protect the integrity of a surgical procedure and/or joint. Ultimately, PNF patterns and techniques can be used to provide isometric, concentric, and eccentric strengthening using high-tech devices (e.g., pulleys, elastic bands, and isokinetic devices) and low-tech procedures (manual contact).

BASIC PROCEDURES

Proprioceptive neuromuscular facilitation uses specific proprioceptive and other sensory inputs to facilitate motor responses and motor learning. These inputs (or procedures) include tactile stimulation through the clinician's manual contacts or grip, resistance, stretch, irradiation (overflow), traction, approximation, verbal commands, and visual cues.[3,19,20]

Manual Contact

The clinician should touch only the surface of the area being facilitated. This manual contact gives the clinician a means of controlling the direction of motion and eliminating, correcting, or minimizing substitution. The contact also applies a demand (referred to as the appropriate resistance) and gives specific cutaneous and pressure stimulation. Usually, one manual contact is placed distally and the other proximally to incorporate both distal movement and proximal stabilization of the musculature in the trunk, scapula, or pelvis. Precise placement depends on the relative strengths of the patient.

Resistance

One of the hallmarks of PNF and the cornerstone of many of its techniques is resistance. Resistance is a means of guiding movement, securing maximal effort, and aiding motor relearning. Optimal resistance is defined as resistance that is graded appropriately for the intention of the movement. Simply put, maximal resistance is the most resistance that can be applied by the clinician and still result in a smooth, coordinated motion for a particular activity performed by the client. Therefore, it is essential not to over-resist the movements being facilitated and to allow the motion to occur.

If the task requires concentric or eccentric muscle contractions, the intention is either a shortening or a lengthening movement. Optimal resistance can change constantly throughout the ROM, depending on strength, joint stability, pain, and ability of the patient. Examples include eccentric resistance for the glenohumeral rotators and scapular stabilizers for the throwing athlete and concentric control for the jumper or sprinter. The intention of isometric muscle work is not motion but rather postural stability. Resistance to isometric contractions is, therefore, built up gradually so that no motion occurs. Proprioceptive neuromuscular facilitation is especially suited for use with the injured athlete because of the emphasis on varying the type and speed of control needed, especially eccentric control.[15]

Manually resisted diagonal patterns and selected techniques allow the clinician to closely monitor the patient, finely grade the feedback, and change the challenge of the activity to meet the individual's needs. Patterns can be incorporated into independent and home programs using pulleys, weights, rubber tubing, and equipment, which are particularly necessary for muscle strength greater than 4/5 (as tested via manual muscle test).

Quick Stretch

Quick stretch is one of the most powerful neurophysiologic tools available.[2,3,9,10] When followed by resistance, quick stretch facilitates the muscle stretched. The stretch reflex is elicited by a gentle quick "nudge" or "tap" to the muscles under tension, either from a fully elongated starting position or superimposed on an active muscle contraction. Quick stretch is contraindicated with pain, fracture, or recent surgical procedure.[6,7]

Irradiation

Used together, quick stretch and resistance can result in irradiation (or overflow) from the stronger segments to the weaker. Overflow, as defined by Sherington,[9] occurs at the level of the anterior horn cell and is the "spread of facilitation with increased effort." Typically, overflow proceeds into muscles that are synergistic to the prime mover or to the muscles needed to stabilize that motion. This facilitation is directly proportional to the amount of strength in the resisted muscle groups and the amount of resistance applied. Irradiation is the key to using a strong motion to reinforce a weaker motion, such as facilitating ankle dorsiflexion through overflow from resistance applied to strong hip and knee flexion. Similarly, overflow may be used to promote proximal stabilization, such as strengthening trunk flexion through overflow from the resistance of strong bilateral lower extremity flexion. Irradiation can be especially helpful in re-establishing early active motion when pain is a factor. Because the patterns of irradiation are only partly predictable, closely monitoring the results and modifying the resistance are essential for best results.

Traction and Approximation

Manual traction and approximation are powerful facilitatory techniques that must be carefully modified in patients with pain or instability and after surgery.[11,12,20] Both procedures are contraindicated when joint instability, pain, or a recent surgical procedure is present. Use of traction and approximation can be gradually and cautiously reinstated as motor control and structural stability improve.

Traction is an elongating vector force applied along the long axis of the limb, slightly separating the joint surfaces. Traction is generally used to promote isotonic movement in phasic muscle groups, such as with pulling or antigravity motions (breast stroking in swimming).

Approximation is a compressive force applied through the long axis of the trunk or limb that facilitates stabilization, extension, and tonic muscle responses, especially in the lower extremities and trunk. For example, heel strike in gait provides a type of quick approximation that is followed by sustained approximation as the body weight progresses over the foot and extended hip. Closed-chain weight bearing on an aligned, extended arm facilitates scapular stabilization and control, in part, through the effects of approximation.

Verbal Commands

Verbal commands instruct the client what to do, when and how to perform a task, and how to correct a task.[19,20] These commands need to be simple, direct, and timed to coordinate the effort and motion. Softly spoken commands tend to be soothing and useful in the indirect approach with the patient with pain. Firm commands (louder) usually elicit stronger effort from the patient.

Visual Cues

Visual cues provide additional feedback for directional and postural control, assisting in the incorporation of appropriate head and trunk motions. Initially, vision can be substituted for proprioceptive loss, but care must be exercised to avoid visual dependence.

DIAGONAL PATTERNS

Proprioceptive neuromuscular facilitation is perhaps best known for the spiral and diagonal movement patterns identified by Kabat.[1,2] These patterns of synergistic muscle combinations offer a mechanical lever arm to therapeutic exercise, because they combine all planes of movement, cross midline, and are similar to normal functional movement. A narrow groove of motion exists, delineated by the shoulder in the upper extremity and the hip in the lower extremity, in which maximum power is achieved. Optimally, both the client and the clinician move in that groove. Each pattern has motion in flexion or extension, abduction or adduction, and external or internal rotation. The largest range of motion occurs in flexion and extension, the least in rotation. However, Kabat considers rotation to be the most important factor in eliciting strength and endurance changes.

Definition

The patterns of movement can be named two different ways: either by diagonal 1 (D1) or diagonal 2 (D2) or, more simply, for the motion occurring at the proximal joint. For example, shoulder flexion-abduction-external rotation (D2 flexion) or hip extension-adduction-external rotation (D2 extension). In this chapter, the motion of the proximal joint will be emphasized when describing patterns; reference to D1 and D2 will be secondary.

Tables 8-1 and 8-2 describe the components of the two upper- and lower extremity diagonals, each consisting of two antagonistic patterns. In the extremity patterns, certain combinations of motions occur together consistently. Rotation of the shoulder and forearm occur in the same direction: supination with external rotation and pronation with internal rotation. When the shoulder abducts, the hand and wrist extend; hand and wrist flexion occur with shoulder adduction. In the lower extremity, ankle dorsiflexion combines with hip flexion and plantar flexion with hip extension. Ankle eversion occurs with hip abduction; ankle inversion occurs with hip adduction. Internal hip rotation coincides with abduction motions; external rotation, with adduction motions. Therefore, memorizing every component of the pattern is not necessary.

The intermediate joint (elbow, knee) may remain straight, flexed, or extended, depending on the function required. Varying the elbow position changes the muscle activity at the shoulder, in part owing to the change in lever arm for the clinician.

Unilateral Versus Bilateral

Patterns may be performed unilaterally or bilaterally. Unilateral patterns focus on a specific motion of the joint. Bilateral patterns emphasize the proximal limb movement and the trunk by combining two extremities moving at the same time, either symmetrically (same diagonals, like the butterfly stroke), or asymmetrical (opposite diagonals, going toward the same side, as in throwing the hammer). Bilateral patterns permit the clinician to elicit overflow from a strong segment to facilitate weaker motions in the ipsilateral or contralateral extremity. Unilateral and bilateral patterns will be described in detail later in this chapter.

Normal Timing

The normal timing of the PNF patterns is distal to proximal, with the foot or hand leading the motion. For example, when performing a unilateral flexion adduction pattern (D1 flexion), the forearm and wrist supinate and flex first and then hold while the shoulder flexes and adducts. Shoulder external rotation initiates simultaneously with the distal wrist motion and completes as the shoulder approaches end range. Even when the ankle or hand has adequate strength, the recruitment pattern may be faulty, particularly in a normally functioning or highly trained individual. Correct sequencing or normal timing can be facilitated by manually restraining the proximal segments until the distal component is activated. This normal timing promotes motor learning.

TABLE 8-1 Upper Extremity Diagonal Patterns

Scapula	Anterior elevation	Posterior elevation
Shoulder	Flexion	Flexion
	Adduction	Abduction
	External rotation	External rotation
Elbow	Varies	Varies
Forearm	Supination	Supination
Wrist	Radial flexion	Radial extension
Fingers	Flexion	Extension
	D1 FLEXION	**D2 FLEXION**
	SHOULDER	
	D2 EXTENSION	**D1 EXTENSION**
Scapula	Anterior depression	Posterior depression
Shoulder	Extension	Extension
	Adduction	Abduction
	Internal rotation	Internal rotation
Elbow	Varies	Varies
Forearm	Pronation	Pronation
Wrist	Ulnar flexion	Ulnar extension
Fingers	Flexion	Extension

GENERAL TREATMENT DESIGN

In keeping with the PNF philosophy of using the strong to facilitate the weak, the clinician first identifies the individual's strength, which is usually an extremity or quadrant that is pain free, strong, and demonstrates controlled and coordinated motion. Impairments in ROM, strength, and control are noted next. Functional limitations, such as inability to jump without pain, are identified next; then specific goals are set.

The clinician must also understand the biomechanics of the specific functional movement pattern, the key muscle components, the types or range of muscle contractions, and the stage of motor control needed. Depending on the activity, upper extremity demands may be for closed-chain movements (as in parallel bar work in gymnastics) or open-chain movements (as in throwing a baseball). Most activities, however, require both open- and closed-chain activities. The clinician can then select appropriate PNF techniques and the corresponding PNF patterns to meet the functional goal.

Biomechanical considerations—such as the size of the base of support, the height of the center of gravity, the length of the lever arm, open- versus closed-chain activity, and the number of joints involved in the activity—can be varied to advance a therapeutic program. Proprioceptive neuromuscular facilitation can also be effectively combined with the use of therapeutic modalities, soft tissue techniques, and mobilization (Chapter 4). It is not necessary to do diagonal patterns to "do PNF," although the diagonal patterns are useful. Rather, the basic philosophy, principles, and techniques of PNF can be applied to functional activities to achieve a wide range of goals.

CLINICAL APPLICATION

Table 8-3 presents PNF diagonal pattern "helpers" that assist the clinician in applying PNF patterns effectively. These helpers emphasize the clinician's body position and preparation of the client and remind the clinician of key cues for PNF principles.

For clarity, most of the patterns in this chapter are shown in supine. However, all of the PNF patterns and techniques may be applied in any posture and should not be limited to supine. The hip flexion-abduction pattern in side lying emphasizes antigravity strengthening of the hip abductors. Lower extremity patterns should be progressed so the patient is able to perform them in an upright posi-

TABLE 8-2 Lower Extremity Diagonal Patterns

Pelvis	Anterior elevation	Posterior elevation
Hip	Flexion	Flexion
	Adduction	Abduction
	External rotation	Internal rotation
Knee	Varies	Varies
Ankle	Dorsiflexion	Dorsiflexion
Foot	Inversion	Eversion
Toes	Extension	Extension
	D1 FLEXION	**D2 FLEXION**
	HIP	
	D2 EXTENSION	**D1 EXTENSION**
Pelvis	Anterior depression	Posterior depression
Hip	Extension	Extension
	Adduction	Abduction
	External rotation	Internal rotation
Knee	Varies	Varies
Ankle	Plantarflexion	Plantarflexion
Foot	Inversion	Eversion
Toes	Flexion	Flexion

tion, often with narrowed base of postural support. upper extremity patterns combined with weight bearing in standing facilitate stability and controlled mobility essential to the development of skilled motion.[21] Bilateral-extremity patterns can be used in sitting to facilitate trunk control. Performance of these patterns in a functional posture can help achieve more complex movements.

The diagonal movement patterns are similar to the motions used in activities of daily living as well as in sports. For example, kicking a soccer ball is similar to the lower extremity flexion-adduction pattern (D1 flexion). The breaststroke is a widened version of upper extremity extension-abduction and internal rotation with the elbow flexing pattern (D1 extension). Cocking the arm for a throw corresponds to the flexion-abduction of the upper extremity pattern (D2 flexion); release, deceleration, and follow-through are similar to extension-adduction with internal rotation patterns (D2 extension).

Selected commonly used limb and trunk patterns are described in the following sections. It is beyond the scope of this chapter to detail all patterns and possible combinations. For further information on any other patterns or techniques, see the texts by Adler et al.[19] and Voss et al.[3]

UPPER EXTREMITY DIAGONAL PATTERNS

Scapular Patterns

Perhaps the most underused but most helpful of all the PNF patterns are the patterns for the scapula. Both stability and mobility of the scapulae are required if the upper extremity is to function normally and pain free. Most individuals presenting with shoulder dysfunction benefit from retraining of scapular stabilizers.[21] Scapular patterns can be initially performed in side lying and progressed to sitting or standing. Similarly, activities can begin in a closed-chain context and move to an open-chain context as control improves.

There are four scapular patterns, two in each of the corresponding upper extremity patterns. Scapular elevation patterns work with upper extremity flexion, and scapular depression patterns with upper extremity extension (Figs. 8-1 to 8-4).

Unilateral Upper Extremity Patterns

Unilateral upper extremity patterns offer the clinician a long lever arm from which to facilitate into the extremity and trunk (Table 8-1). When performing upper extremity patterns care must be exercised in those indi-

TABLE 8-3 PNF Diagonal Pattern Helpers

Clinician's position
Face the direction of motion
Shoulders and pelvis face the line of movement
Take up all the slack in all components of motion
Patient's position
Close to the clinician
Starting position is one of optimal elongation
Manual contacts
Combinations of proximal and distal
Quick stretch to initiate
Use body weight, not arm strength
Nudge
Move with the patient
Clinician's center of gravity *must* move
Distal component initiates motion
When performing reversals
Change distal manual contact first

viduals with anterior glenohumeral laxity or who have just had surgery. Motions should not exceed 90° flexion, abduction, or rotation in early treatment to avoid stressing unstable structures. Similarly, weight bearing on an extended arm, in quadruped or modified plantigrade, should be closely monitored in individuals with posterior instability. The key concept is to start with the pattern that is strongest, most stable, or least painful (Figs. 8-5 to 8-8).

Bilateral Symmetrical Upper Extremity Patterns

Any time two extremity patterns are combined, the emphasis shifts to the trunk and proximal extremity components. Symmetrical patterns eliminate the trunk rotation component of the movement and, as such, are ideal for the patient who cannot tolerate much trunk rotation. In general, full ROM in distal motions are sacrificed to facilitate proximal control. Although any combination of patterns is possible, the more commonly used patterns are shown in Figures 8-9 to 8-11. Bilateral symmetrical upper extremity patterns are particularly easy and effective when performed with pulleys.

Bilateral Asymmetrical Trunk Patterns

A strong trunk is essential for normal function and successful performance of many activities. Some sports, such as gymnastics, place a particularly high demand on trunk control. Trunk patterns for PNF, including upper extremity chops and lifts and bilateral symmetric lower extremity patterns (described later in this chapter), can be used to strengthen trunk musculature or to irradiate into the neck, scapula, and extremities. Chops and lifts are bilateral asymmetric patterns that can be done in supine, sitting, prone, or anywhere else in the biomechanical progression that challenges the individual. Because they are asymmetric patterns, significant trunk rotation and crossing of midline occurs, which may need to be moderated for some individuals.

Chops are combination of extension-abduction (D1 extension) in the lead arm and extension-adduction (D2 extension) in the grasping arm. Chops can also facilitate functional activities such as rolling or coming to sit (Fig. 8-12).

Lifts are a bilateral asymmetric pattern combining flexion-abduction (D2 flexion) in one arm with flexion-adduction (D1 flexion) in the other. Lifts are an effective tool for facilitating upper trunk extension and scapular stabilization at the end range (Fig. 8-13).

LOWER EXTREMITY DIAGONAL PATTERNS

Unilateral Lower Extremity Patterns

The two lower extremity diagonals are shown in Table 8-2. As in the upper extremity, the intermediate joint (knee) may flex, extend, or stay straight. Again, the starting position for each pattern is at the end of the antagonistic pattern. Common patterns are presented in Figures 8-14 to 8-17.

Bilateral Symmetrical Lower Extremity Patterns

Bilateral symmetrical lower extremity patterns involve the combination of both extremities working together. Holding the feet bilaterally while performing the bilateral pattern places the emphasis on the lower trunk moving on the upper trunk. These patterns emphasize irradiation from stronger to weaker segments or limb. The patterns are usually initiated in sitting (Fig 8-18), but can be performed in prone to facilitate knee flexion activities.

Bilateral lower extremity patterns are not used as frequently for musculoskeletal dysfunction as are bilateral upper extremity patterns and thus are not emphasized. For more information on bilateral patterns, the reader see the texts by Adler et al.[19] and Voss et al.[3]

PROGRESSION AND INTEGRATION WITH EQUIPMENT

All of the patterns described previously can be performed as part of an equipment-based program, most easily with a pulley program. The patterns can be adapted to more elaborate isokinetic equipment, with the rotational components

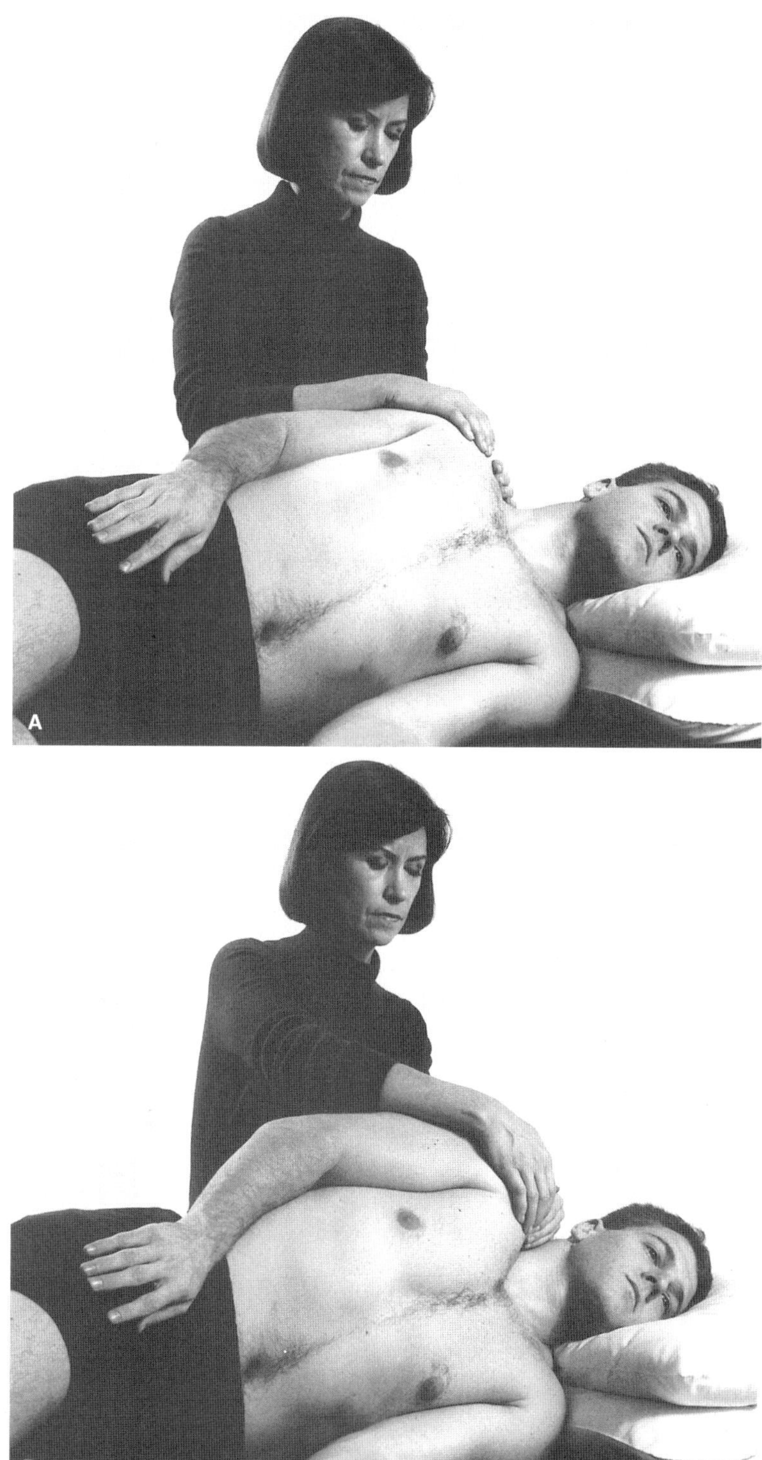

FIGURE 8-1 Scapular anterior elevation.

PURPOSE: Strengthening of levator scapula, serratus anterior, and scalene muscles in diagonal plane of the scapula.

POSITION: Client side lying. Clinician standing behind the client's hips in the line of motion, facing the client's head. Both hands overlapped on the anterior glenohumeral joint and acromion (panel A).

PROCEDURE: Clinician gently takes up the slack, moving the scapula into a depressed position (starting position), and applies quick stretch. Client anteriorly elevates scapula against appropriate resistance. Movement is in a diagonal arc up toward client's nose (panel B).

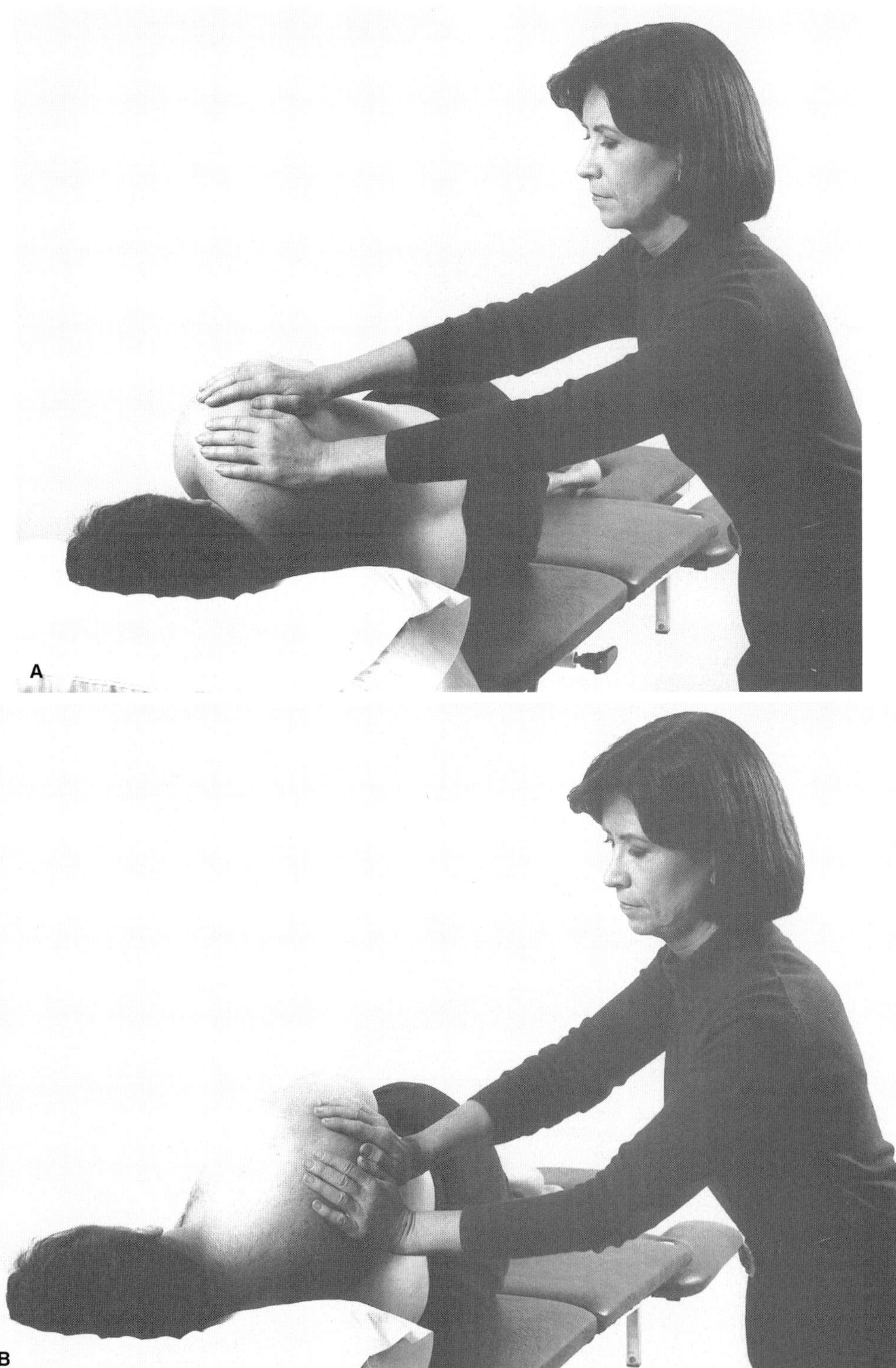

FIGURE 8-2 **Scapular posterior depression.**

PURPOSE: Strengthening of rhomboids and latissimus dorsi muscles in diagonal plane of the scapula.

POSITION: Same as Figure 8-1, *except* manual contacts changed to flat palmed on the middle to lower scapula, along the vertebral border (panel A).

PROCEDURE: Movement is down to the ipsilateral ischial tuberosity (panel B).

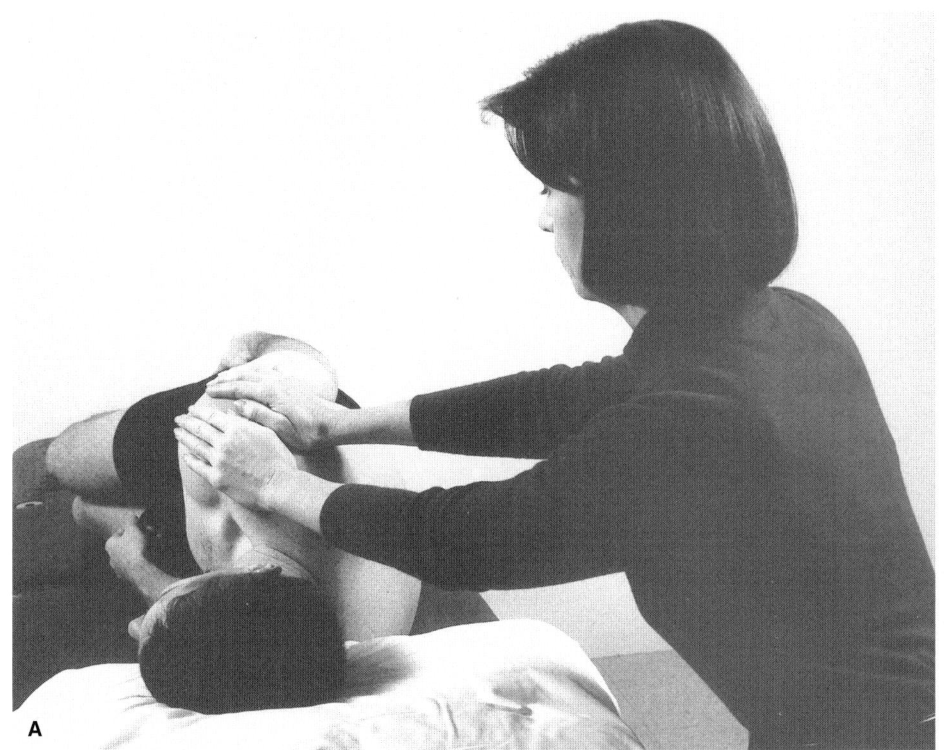

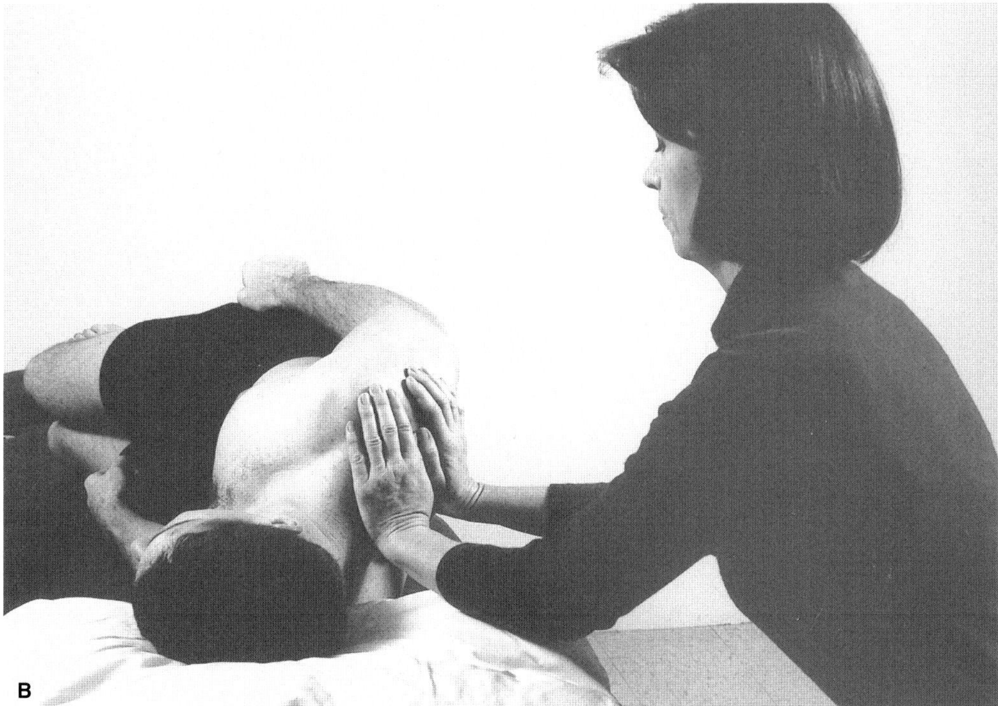

FIGURE 8-3 **Scapular posterior elevation.**

PURPOSE: Strengthening of trapezius and levator scapulae muscles in diagonal plane of the scapula.

POSITION: Client side lying. Clinician standing at client's head, facing the hips. Manual contacts on the distal edge of the upper trapezius, close to the acromion (panel A).

PROCEDURE: Movement is an arc as the client shrugs up toward the ear (panel B).

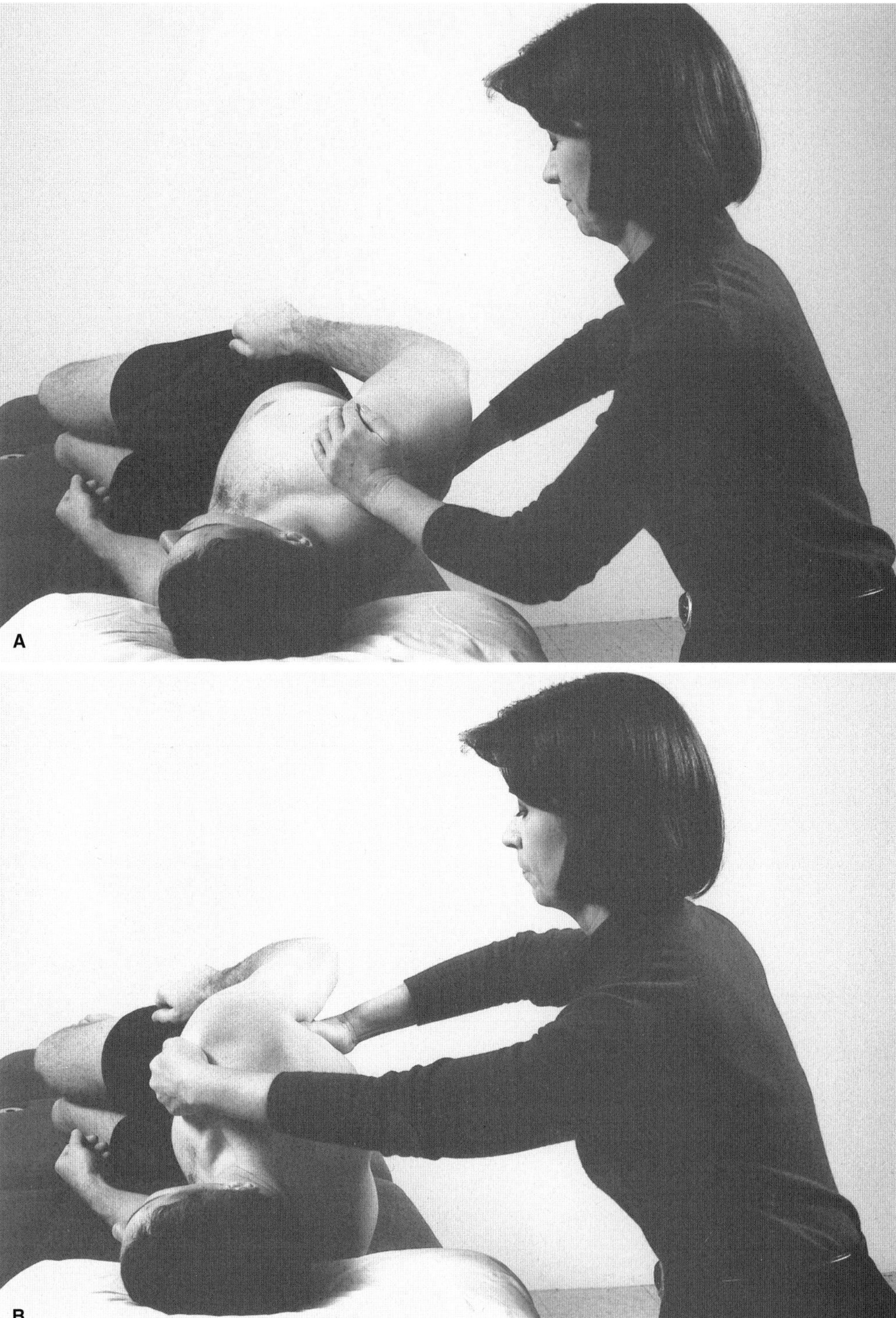

FIGURE 8-4 **Scapular anterior depression.**

PURPOSE: Strengthening of rhomboids and pectoralis minor and major muscles in diagonal plane of the scapula.

POSITION: Same as Figure 8-3, *except* manual contacts moved to either side of the axilla, on the pectoral muscle and coracoid process anteriorly and on the lateral border of the scapula posteriorly (panel A).

PROCEDURE: Client pulls shoulder down toward umbilicus (panel B).

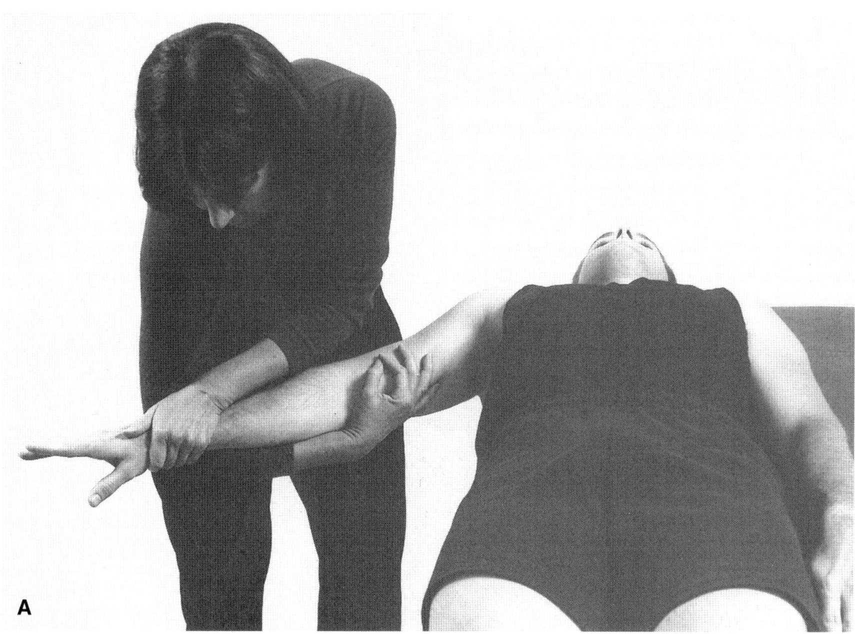

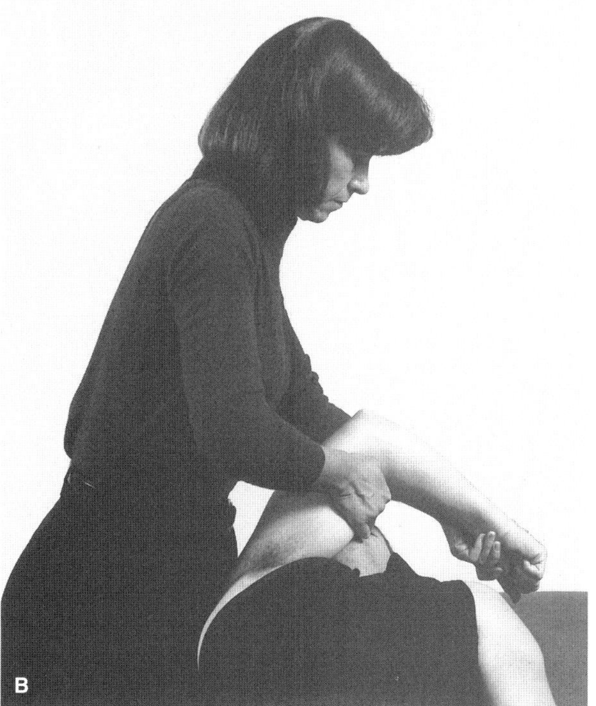

FIGURE 8-5 **Upper extremity: flexion-adduction-external rotation (D1 flexion).**

PURPOSE: Strengthening, ROM, or control of shoulder flexion and adduction, scapular anterior elevation, and wrist flexion. Pattern of choice for initiating rotator cuff activities, because of reduced external rotation and abduction ROM components.

POSITION: Client lying supine. Begins with client's shoulder in slight extension with hand near hip. Clinician standing at client's elbow, facing feet. Distal manual contact on the palm provides most of the traction and rotatory control. Proximal contact can be on the biceps or onto the pectorals (panel A).

PROCEDURE: Client told to "turn and squeeze my hand" then "pull up and across your nose." Clinician pivots toward client's head as the arm moves past. Ends with client's elbow crossing midline around the nose (panel B).

FIGURE 8-6 Upper extremity: extension-abduction-internal rotation (D1 extension).

PURPOSE: Strengthening, ROM, or control of shoulder extension and abduction, scapular depression, internal rotation, and wrist extension.

POSITION: Client lying supine. Clinician standing at client's side near head. Client's arm flexed and adducted. Manual contacts on dorsal surface of the hand (distal) and on posterior surface of the humerus or scapula (proximal) (panel A).

PROCEDURE: Quick stretch, especially in form of traction, applied simultaneously to the hand and shoulder. Client told to "pull wrist up and push your arm down to your side." As arm moves past clinician, traction can be switched to approximation to increase proximal recruitment. Ends with wrist extended and arm at client's hip (panel B).

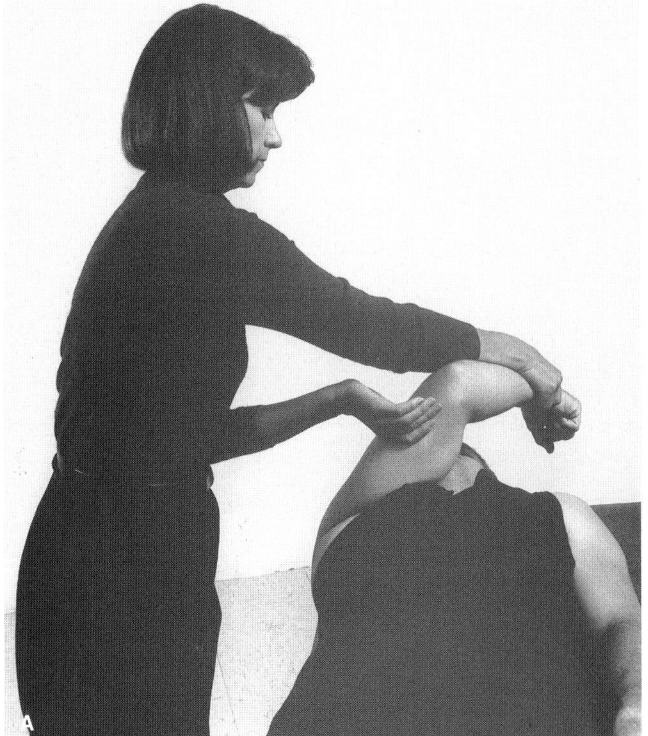

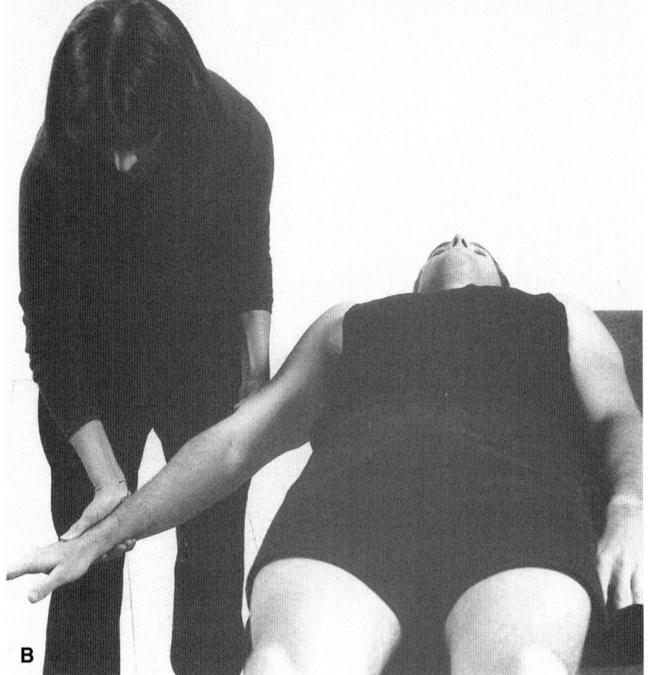

FIGURE 8-7 **Upper extremity: flexion-abduction-external rotation (D2 flexion).**

PURPOSE: Strengthening, ROM, or control of shoulder flexion and abduction, scapular anterior elevation, and wrist extension.

POSITION: Client lying supine. Clinician standing at client's shoulder facing client's feet with a wide base of support in the diagonal of movement. Client's extremity starts from across body, in an elongated, extended position, with elbow crossing the body near hip. Distal manual contact on dorsal hand; proximal contact either on proximal humerus or on scapula to emphasize shoulder and scapular motions (panel A).

PROCEDURE: Clinician takes limb to a fully elongated position, taking up all slack in the muscle groups, and gently applies quick stretch; client told to "pull wrist up and reach." Wrist completes extension before the other components (panel B).

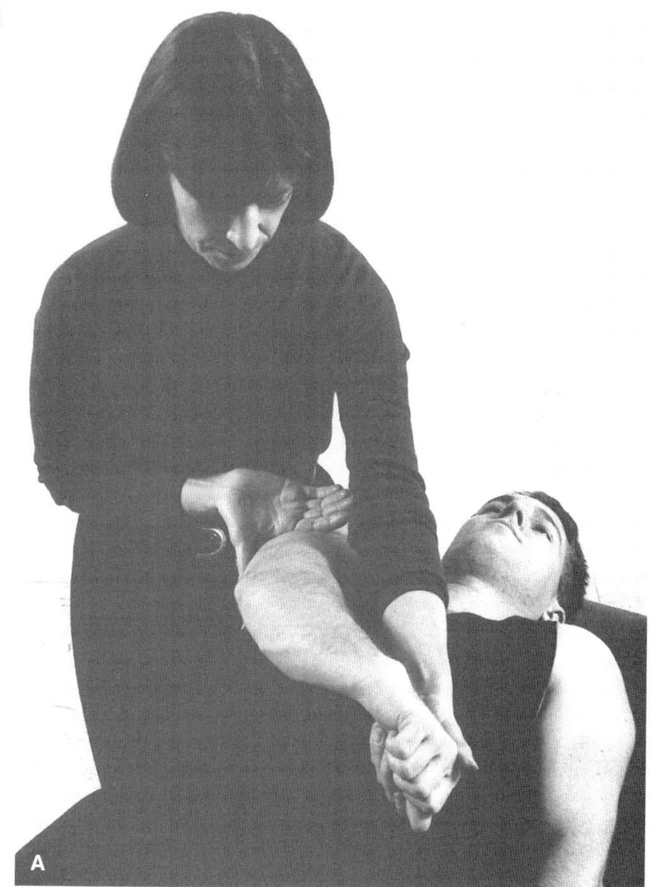
A

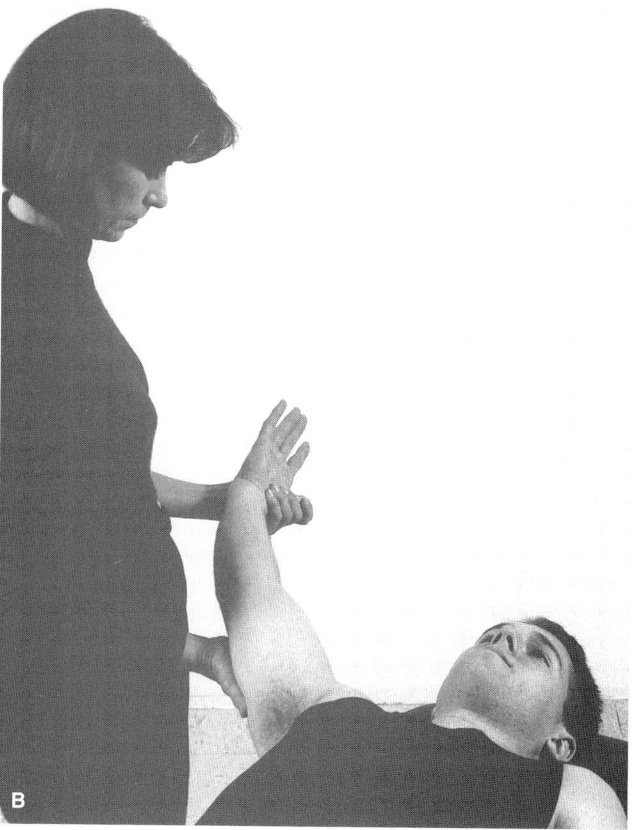
B

FIGURE 8-8 **Upper extremity: extension-adduction-internal rotation (D2 extension).**

PURPOSE: Strengthening, ROM, or control of shoulder extension and adduction, scapular depression, and wrist flexion.

POSITION: Client lying supine. Clinician standing near the client's shoulder. Distal manual contact palm to palm with client (panel A). Proximal contact on pectoral muscles to emphasize recruitment of trunk and scapula or on proximal humerus.

PROCEDURE: Elongation and quick stretch applied; client told to "squeeze and turn your wrist. Now pull down and across." Clinician pivots slightly as the limb passes clinician's center of gravity. Ends in shoulder extension, forearm in pronation, elbow across midline (panel B).

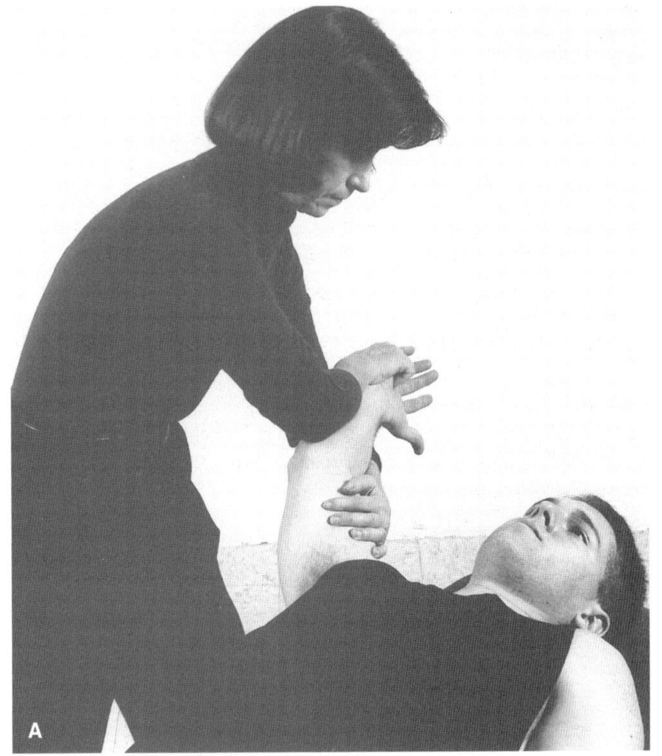
A

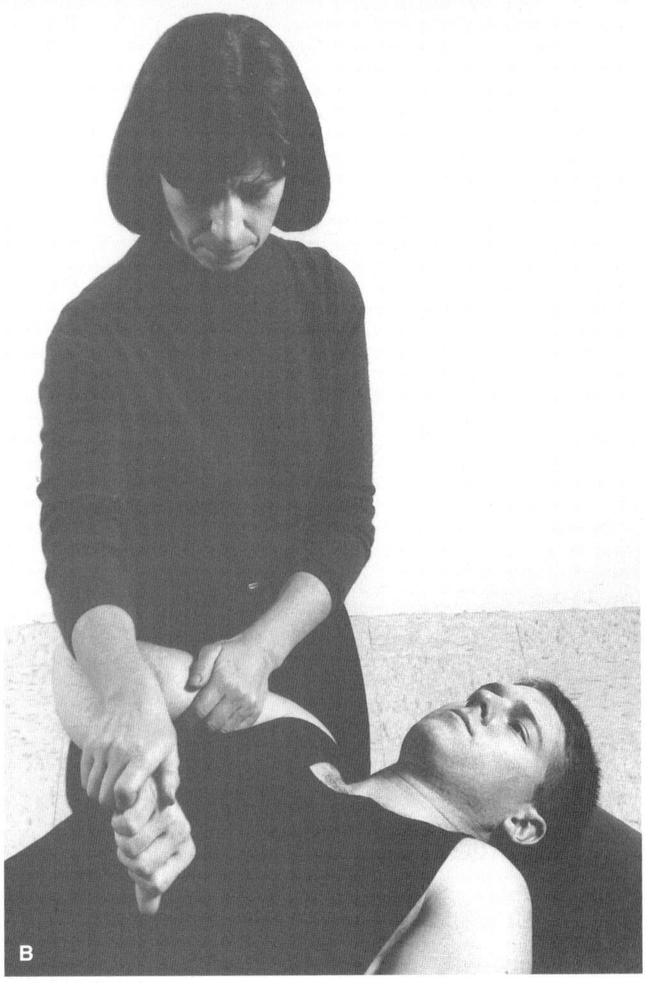
B

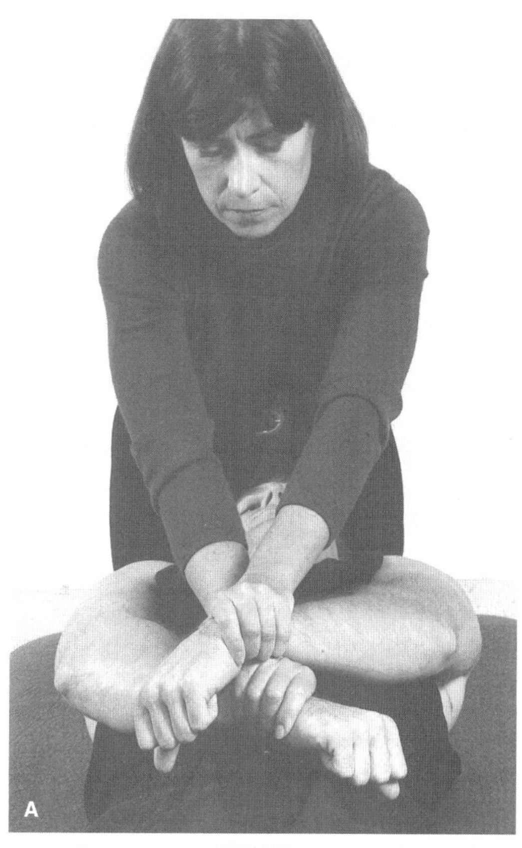

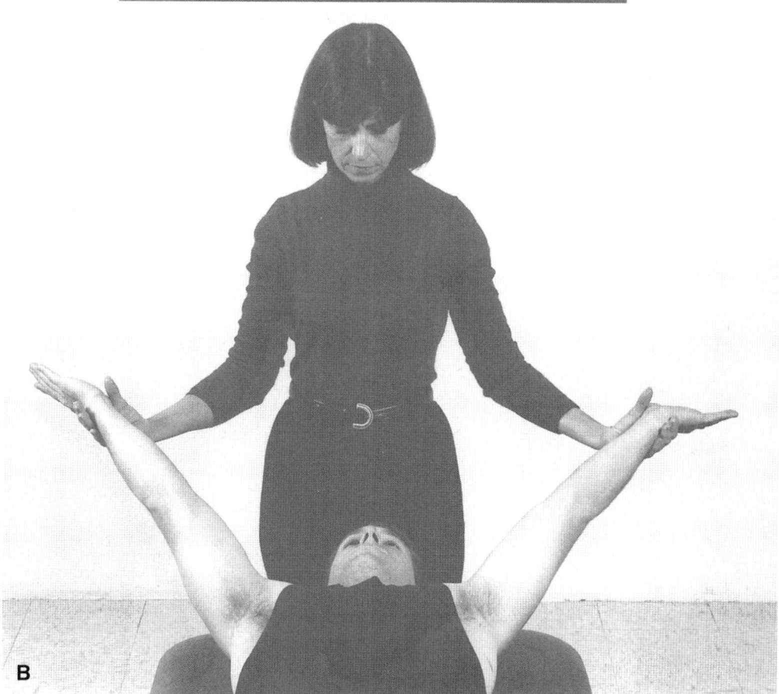

FIGURE 8-9 **Upper extremity: bilateral symmetrical flexion-abduction.**

PURPOSE: Strengthening of shoulder flexion, trunk extension, and control using two strong upper extremities.

POSITION: Client lying supine. Clinician standing at the client's head, arms crossed. Manual contacts on dorsum of wrists (panel A).

PROCEDURE: Client lifts both arms straight overhead against resistance (panel B).

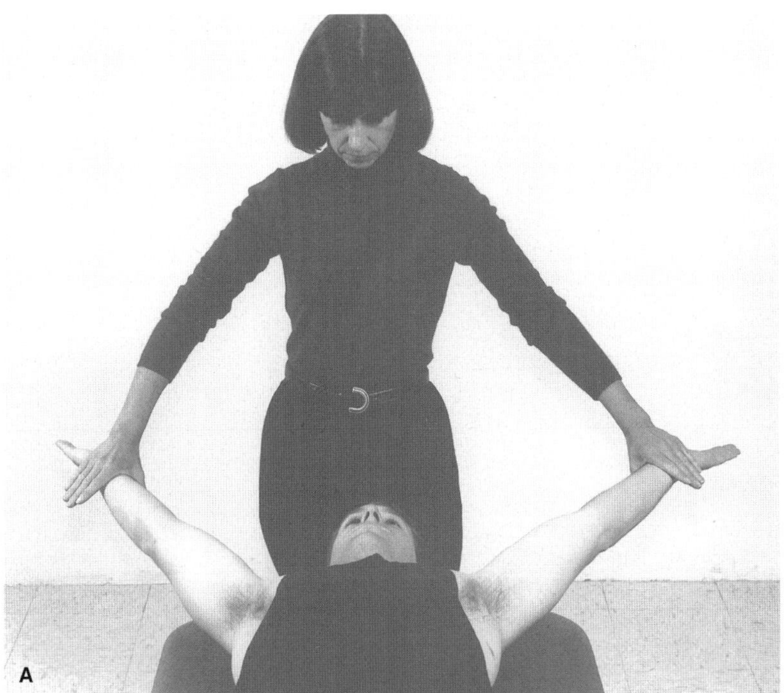

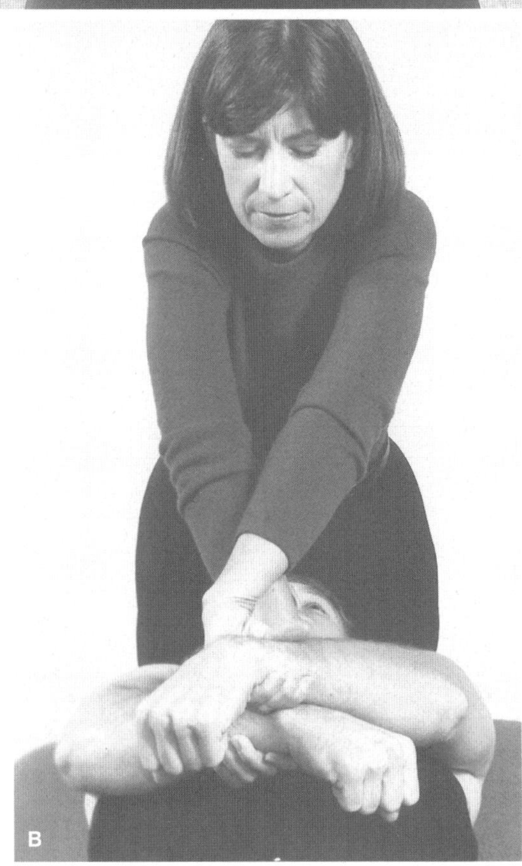

FIGURE 8-10 **Upper extremity: bilateral symmetrical extension-adduction.**

PURPOSE: Strengthening shoulder extension and adduction, upper trunk flexion, and control using two strong upper extremities.

POSITION: Client lying supine. Manual contacts at wrists (panel A).

PROCEDURE: Client told to "squeeze; pull down and across" (panel B).

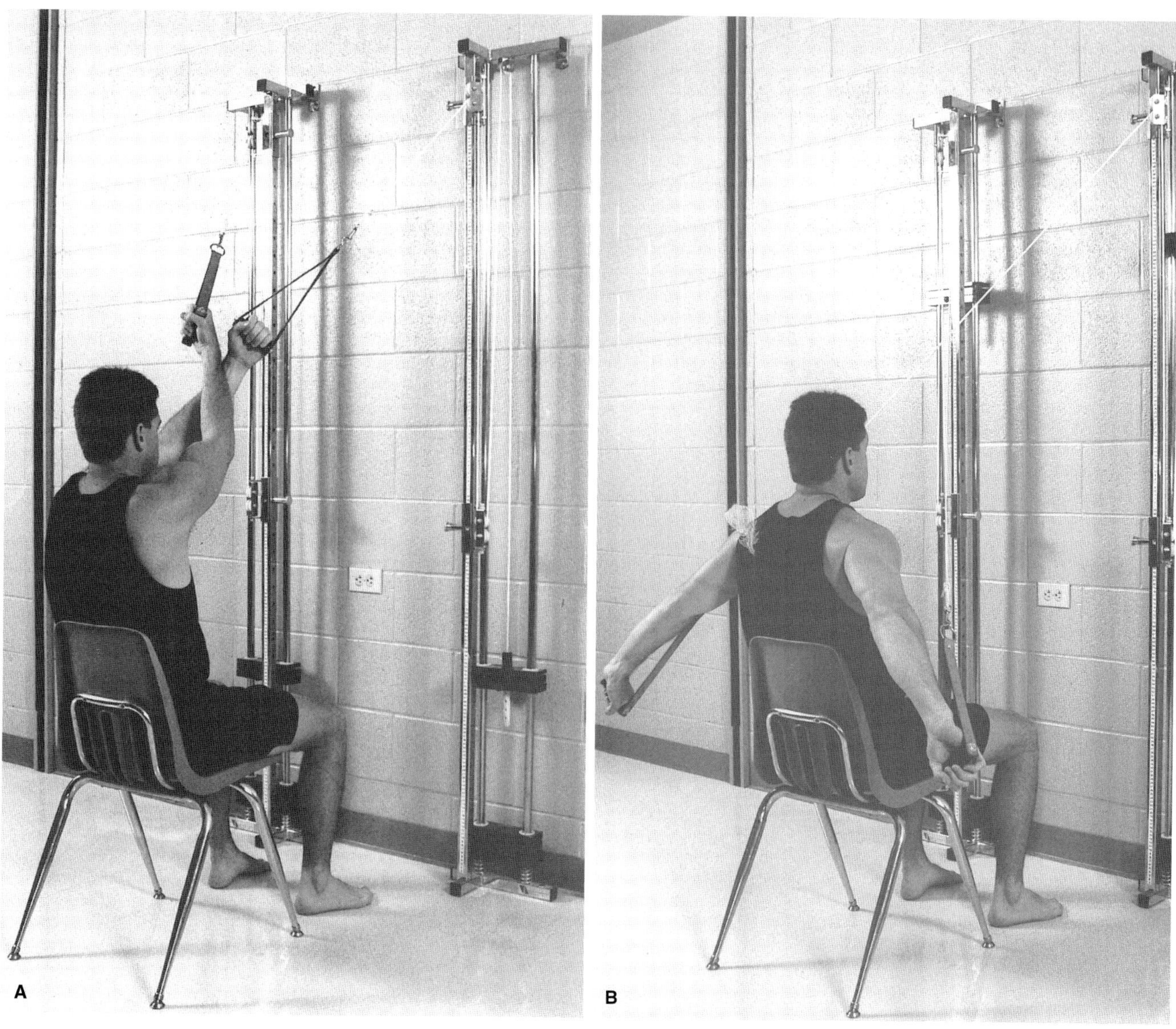

FIGURE 8-11 **Upper extremity: bilateral symmetrical extension-abduction (with pulleys).**

PURPOSE: Strengthening, ROM, or control of shoulder extension, trunk extension, and stabilization.

POSITION: Sitting in chair, client grasps pulley handles with arms crossed, in a position of shoulder adduction, flexion, and external rotation; wrists in flexion and radial deviation (panel A).

PROCEDURE: Client told to "straighten your wrists and pull your arms down to your sides" (panel B).

FIGURE 8-12 Upper extremity: chops.

PURPOSE: Strengthening of trunk flexion; overflow to extremity extensor musculature.

POSITION: Client lying supine. Clinician standing at the end of pattern, so that client chops down to clinician. Client grasping one arm at the wrist. Manual contacts placed distally on dorsal wrist and proximally on scapula or proximal humerus of the abducting (free, nongrasping) arm (panel A).

PROCEDURE: Client told to "tuck your chin and chop down and across to your knees." Head and neck flex, following the leading straight (abducting) arm. Neck motions can be cued with verbal reminders or light, guiding resistance on the forehead. Clinician restrains arm motion until trunk musculature has been activated (panel B).

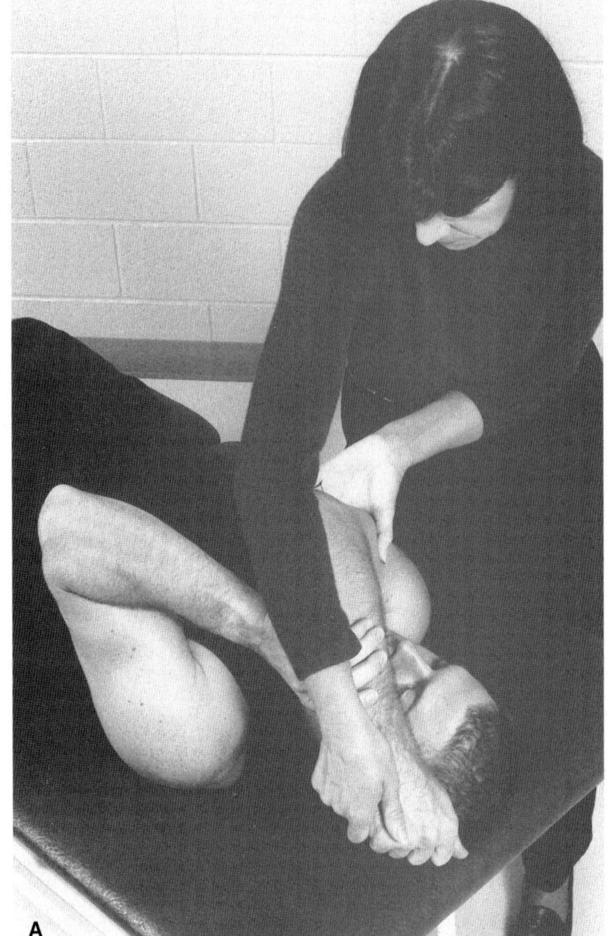

A

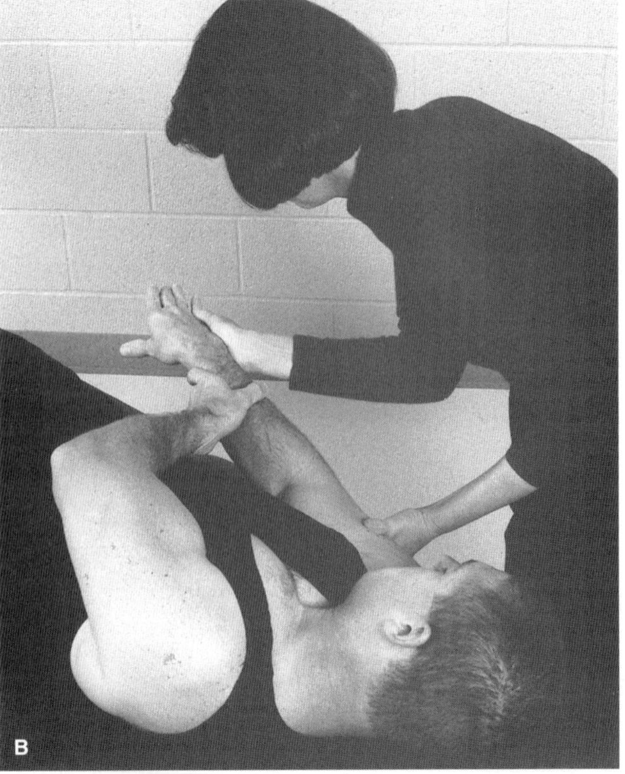

B

FIGURE 8-13 Upper extremity: lifts.

PURPOSE: Facilitate trunk extension, rotation, and lateral bending toward the leading (abducting) arm.

POSITION: Client lying supine. Clinician standing at end of the pattern, so client lifts up to clinician. Lead, abducting arm straight; following limb grasping opposite forearm. Distal manual contact on dorsum of abducting arm; proximal contact on occiput to emphasize neck extension or on scapula (panel A).

PROCEDURE: Client told to "look up and lift your arms up to me" (panel B).

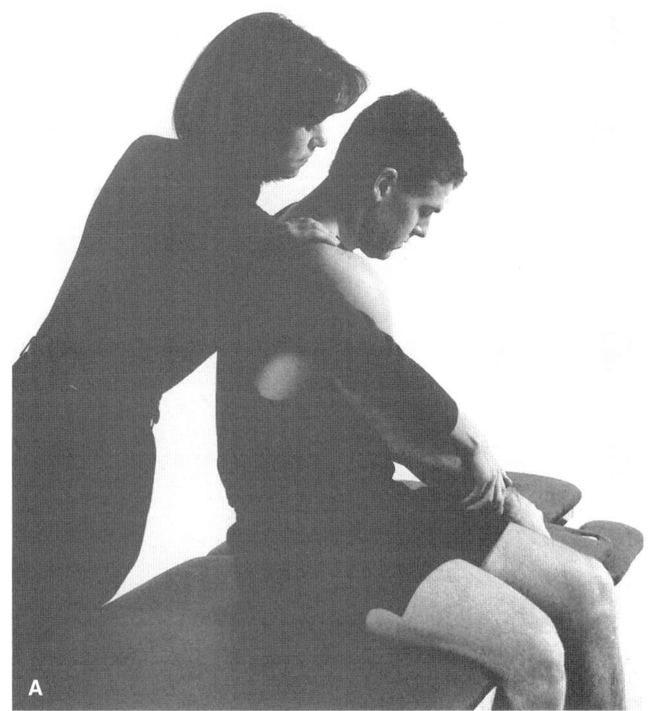
A

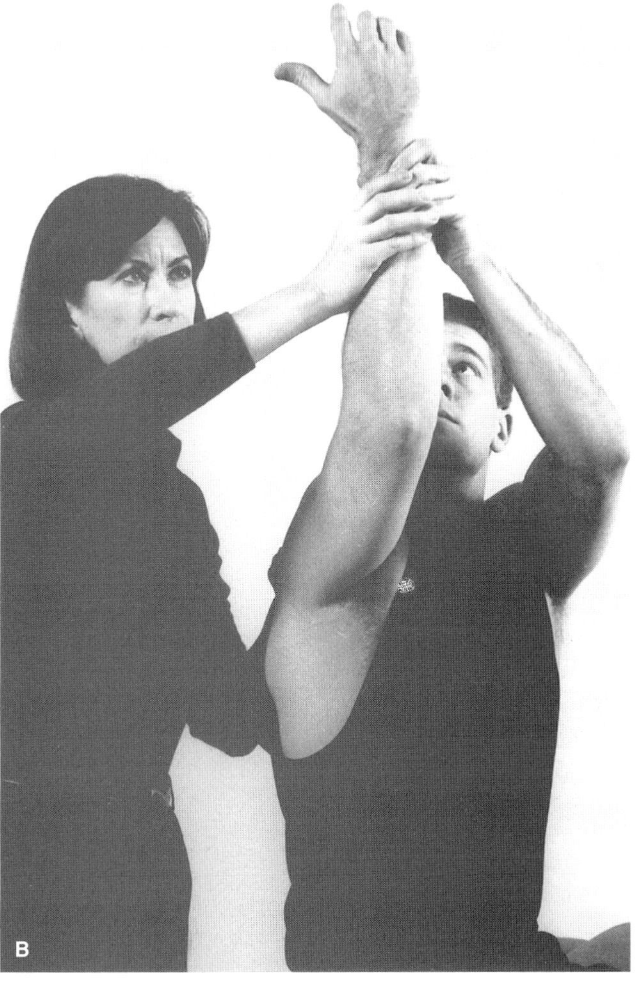
B

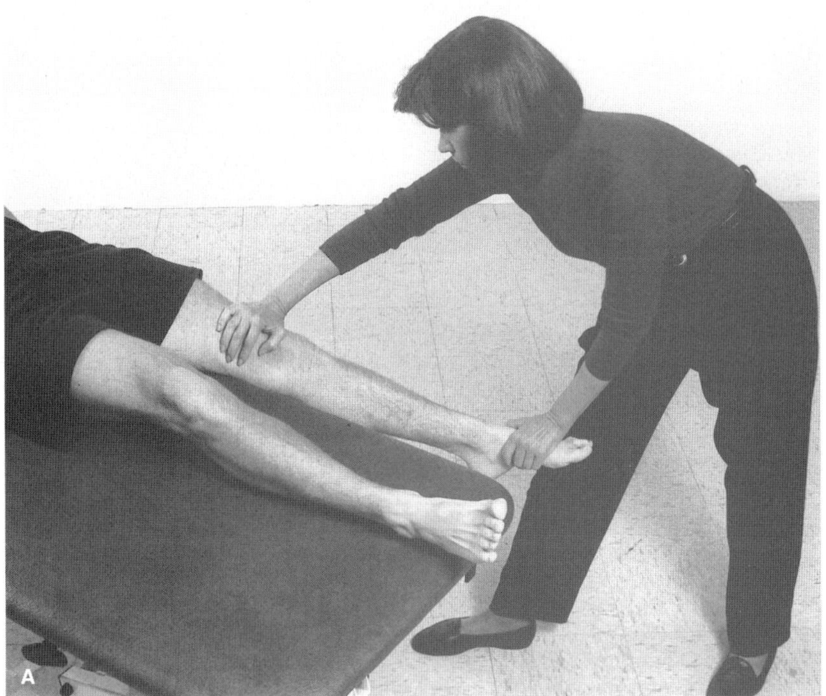

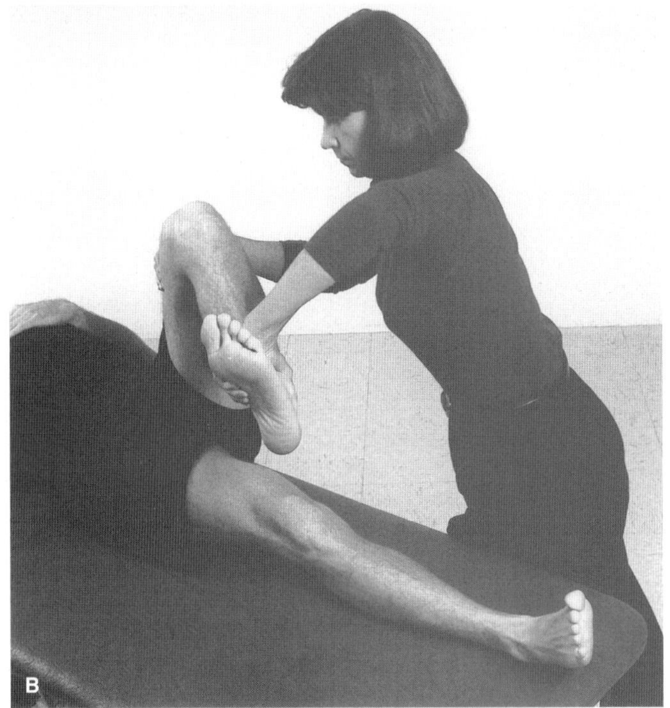

FIGURE 8-14 **Lower extremity: flexion-adduction-external rotation (D1 flexion).**

PURPOSE: Strengthening, ROM, or control of hip flexion, abduction, external rotation, and ankle dorsiflexion and inversion.

POSITION: Client lying supine. Begins with clinician moving limb into an elongated position of hip and knee extension (slightly off the plinth), internal rotation, and ankle plantarflexion with eversion. Manual contacts placed proximally on anterior distal femur and distally on the dorsum of foot (panel A).

PROCEDURE: Corkscrew-like elongation given to entire pattern. Ankle dorsiflexion with inversion initiates motion and provides clinician a handle for traction. As limb moves into flexion, knee and heel cross midline. Knee and ankle both must finish in line, at or slightly across midline (panel B).

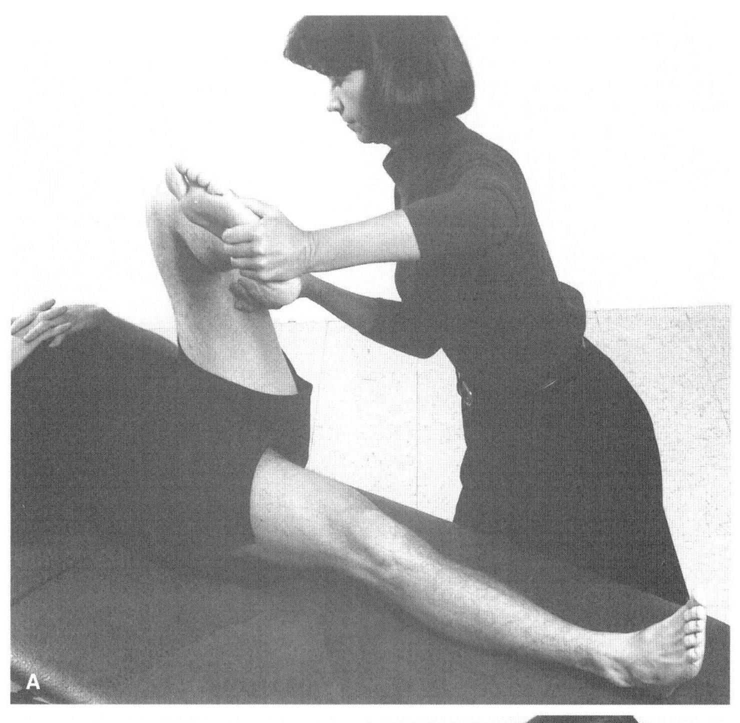

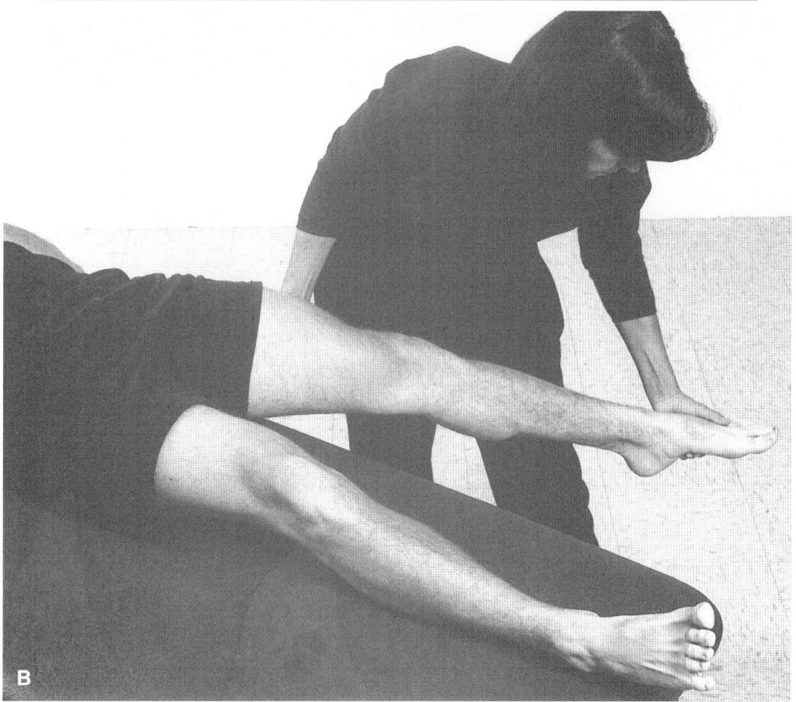

FIGURE 8-15 **Lower extremity: extension-abduction-internal rotation (D1 extension).**

PURPOSE: Strengthening, ROM, or control of hip extension, abduction, internal rotation; and ankle plantar flexion and eversion.

POSITION: Client lying supine. Clinician standing with a wide base of support facing client in line of movement. Client's extremity in a position of hip and knee flexion, full dorsiflexion, and inversion; knee and heel at or slightly across midline. Clinician cupping ball of foot distally and providing proximal contact on hamstrings (panel A).

PROCEDURE: Quick stretch applied simultaneously to hip, knee, and ankle as client told to "point your foot down and kick down and out to me." Ankle plantarflexion and eversion initiate motion, with full hip and knee extension concluding simultaneously (panel B).

FIGURE 8-16 **Lower extremity: flexion-abduction-internal rotation (D2 flexion).**

PURPOSE: Strengthening, ROM, or control of motion of hip flexion, abduction, internal rotation, and ankle dorsiflexion and eversion.

POSITION: Client lying supine. Clinician standing at client's hip, facing feet. Both legs positioned slightly away from clinician, so limb in question begins in an abducted, extended, and externally rotated position. Proximal manual contact on dorsum of foot; distal contact on anterior distal femur just above knee (panel A).

PROCEDURE: Client told to "bring your toes up and out; swing your heel out to me." Ends with heel close to lateral buttock and hip and knee aligned with each other (panel B).

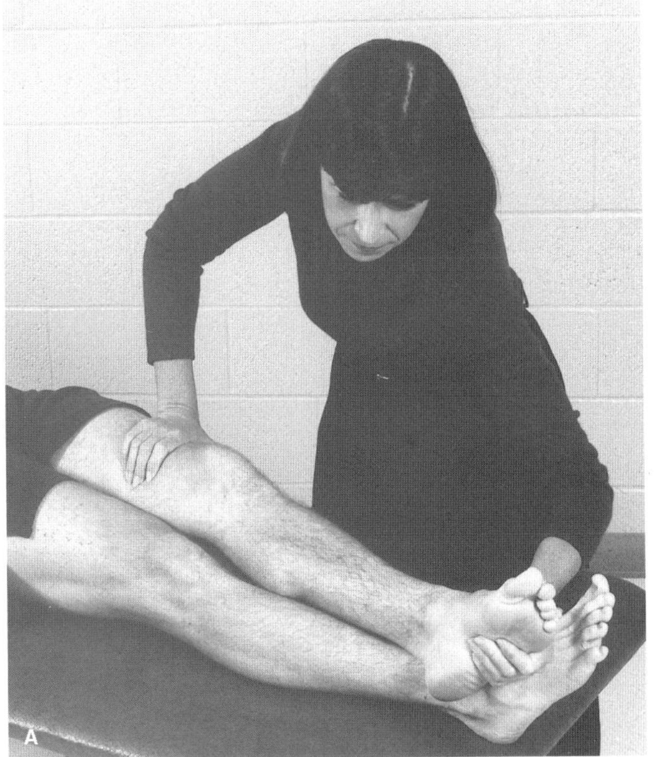
A

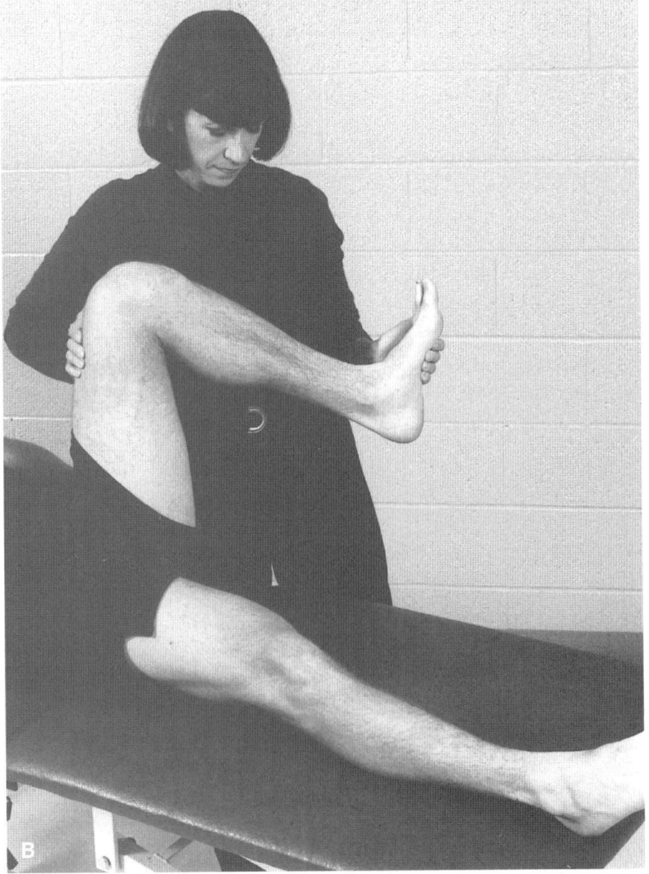
B

FIGURE 8-17 **Lower extremity: extension-adduction-external rotation (D2 extension).**

PURPOSE: Strengthening, ROM, or control of hip extension, adduction, external rotation; ankle plantar flexion and inversion.

POSITION: Client lying supine. Clinician standing in groove, facing client's feet. Manual contacts distally on instep of foot and proximally on medial femur (panel A).

PROCEDURE: Distal motion must come in first, facilitated by quick stretch into flexion. Limb extends with knee finishing across midline (panel B). Clinician may elect to stand at end of pattern to better manually resist extension and adduction.

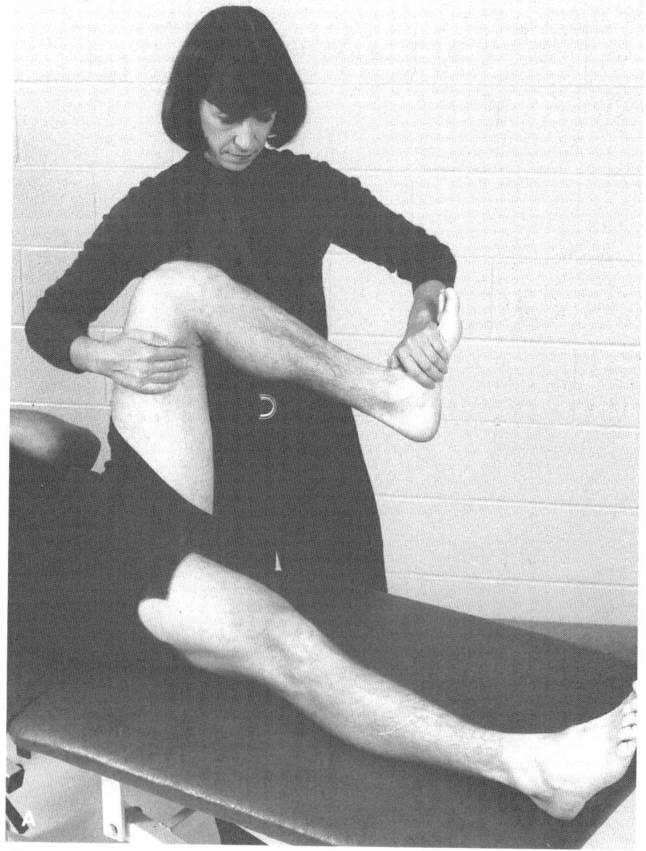

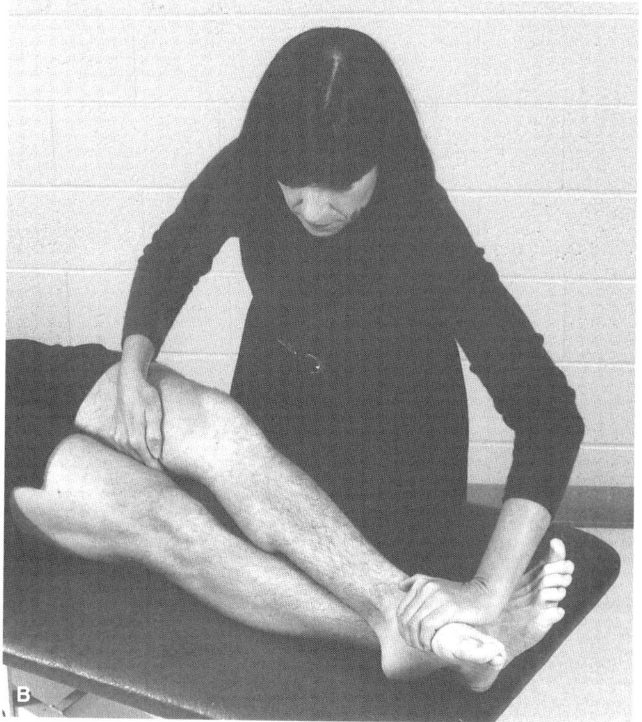

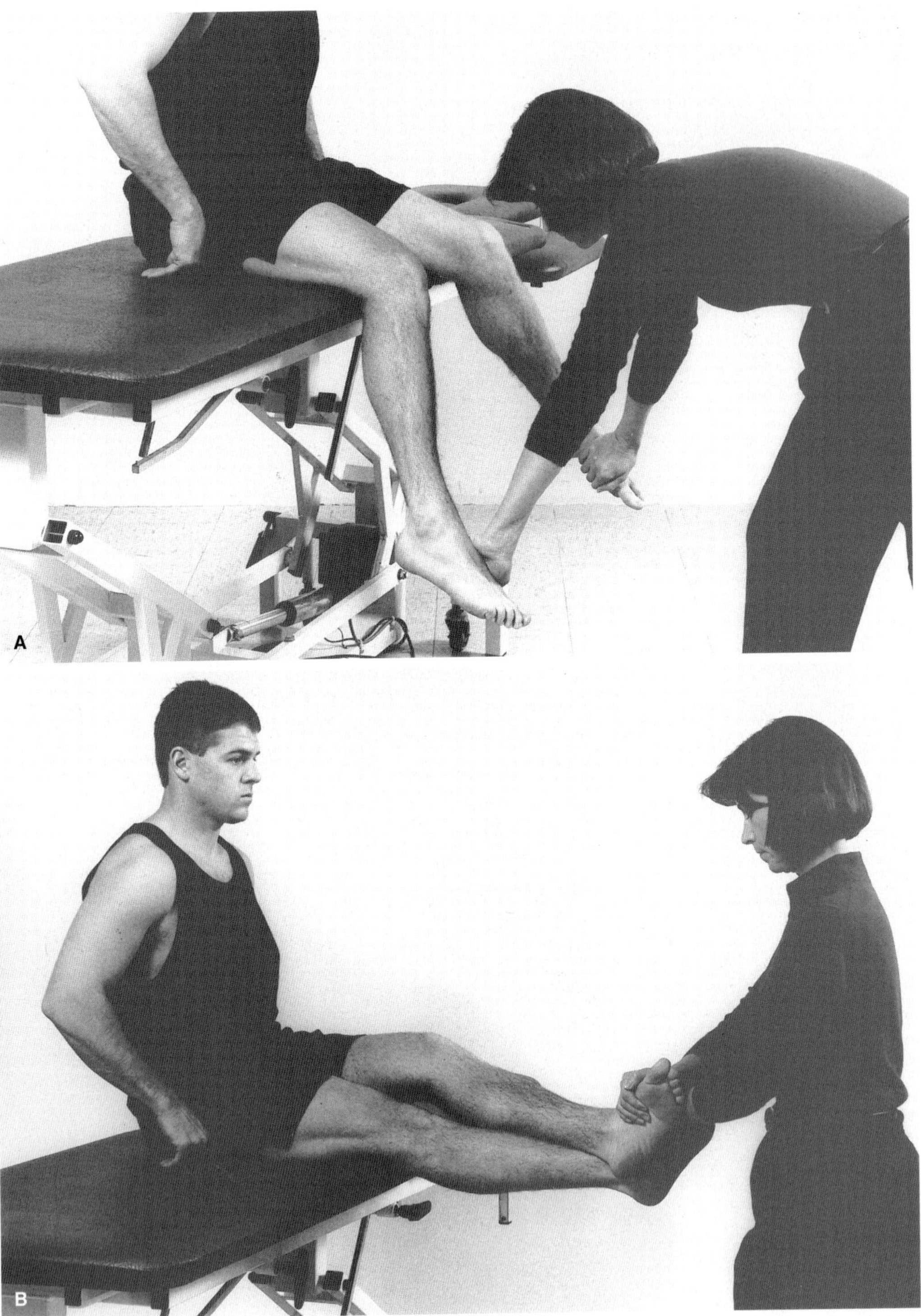

FIGURE 8-18 **Lower extremity: bilateral flexion with knee extension in a sitting position.**

PURPOSE: Strengthening, ROM, or control of knee flexion and extension using advanced lower extremity pattern in sitting.

POSITION: Client sitting with knees flexed and ankles plantarflexed. Clinician standing in front of client centered in middle of both grooves. Manual contacts at dorsal aspect of both feet (panel A).

PROCEDURE: Quick stretch and traction into knee flexion and ankle plantar flexion initiates motion. Ankle dorsiflexion must occur first as client extends both knees. Client told to "lift your toes up and straighten your knees together" (panel B). At end of ROM, clinician switches manual contacts to balls of feet; gentle quick stretch into knee extension initiates motion as client plantarflexes ankle and flexes knees against appropriate resistance.

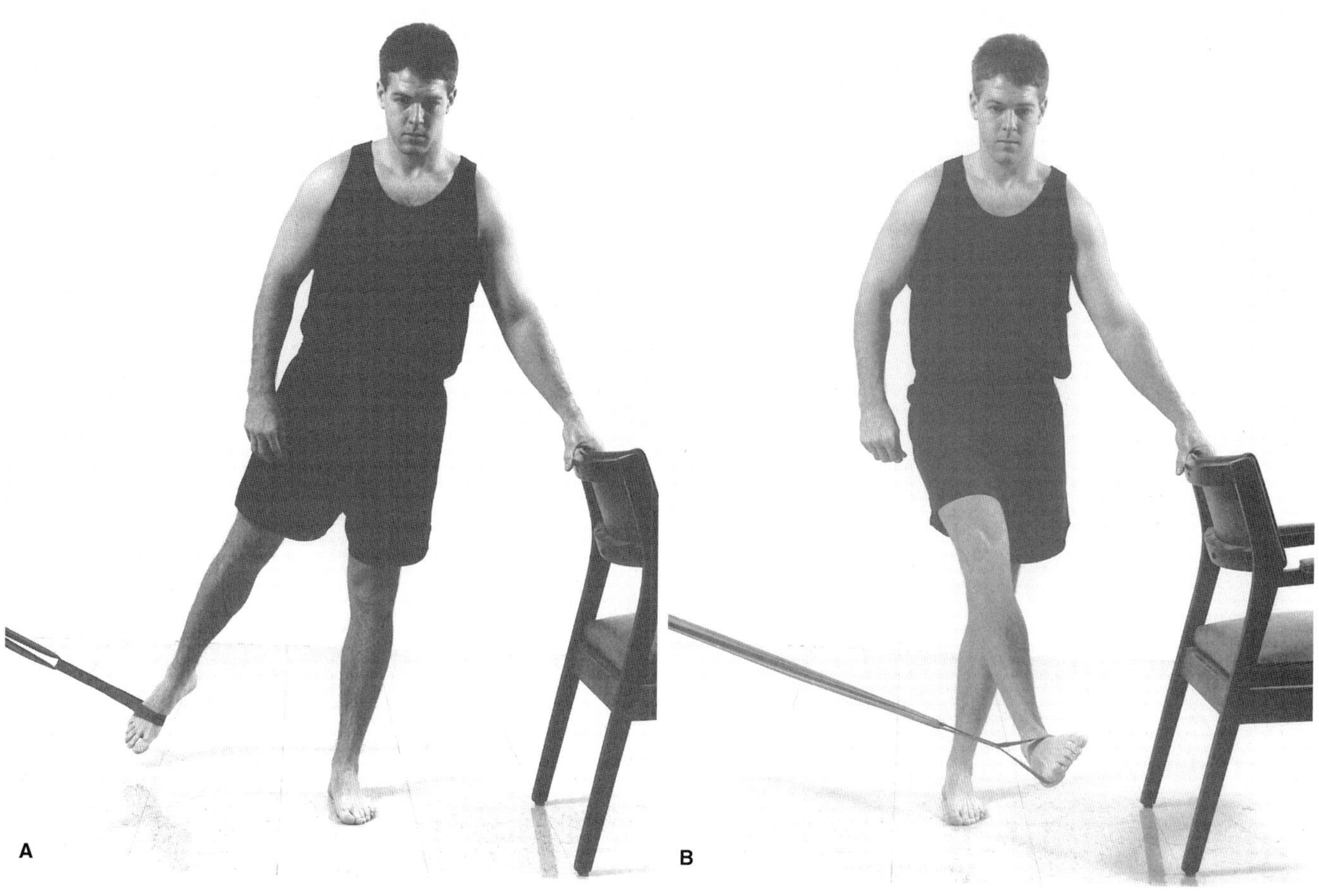

FIGURE 8-19 Elastic tubing for lower extremity (D1 flexion).

PURPOSE: Strengthening, ROM, or control of flexion.

POSITION: Client standing, leg extended and in slight abduction while holding on to chair for balance. End of tubing is hooked around dorsum of flexing extremity (panel A).

PROCEDURE: Client dorsiflexes ankle and flexes extremity up and across body, keeping knee straight (panel B). Eccentric control may be emphasized as client slowly returns extremity to start position against pull of tubing. Pattern simulates kicking a ball.

greatly reduced. Braces may be worn during the pulley program to limit range and protect stability of grafts as needed. Anything done with pulleys in the clinic can be performed with elastic tubing in the home. Examples of setups are shown in Figures 8-19 and 8-20.

■ *Techniques*

All of the PNF patterns and functional movement progressions can be combined with specific techniques to facilitate the stages of movement control: mobility, strength, stability, and skill.[20] The injured individual may require improvement at any or all of these stages. The goal is to combine facilitation, inhibition, strengthening, and relaxation with different types of muscle contractions to achieve specific functional goals. Table 8-4 shows the most common uses for the different techniques. Note that many of the techniques have multiple and overlapping functions.

MOBILITY TECHNIQUES

Often, the first challenge for the injured patient is to appropriately contract the muscle(s) again. **Rhythmic initiation** can help overcoming pain, anxiety, and decreased control and is an effective technique for assisting the initiation of motion. The patient is taken through the complete motion passively, then asked to gradually actively participate with the motion. Eventually, the individual is progressed into a slow reversal technique with the application of guiding and facilitating resistance.

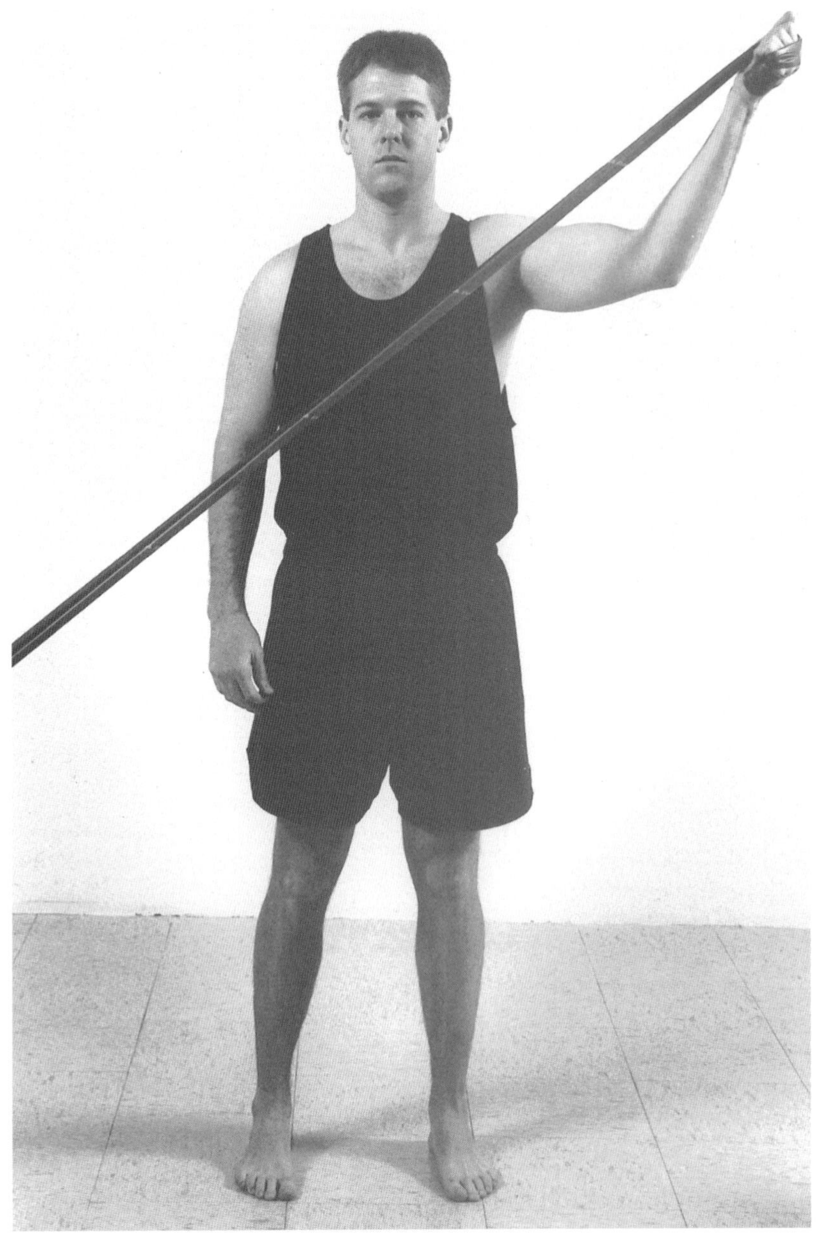

FIGURE 8-20 **Elastic tubing for upper extremity (D2 flexion).**

PURPOSE: Strengthening, ROM, or control of flexion, adduction, and internal rotation in a functional standing position.

POSITION: Standing; client's extremity across body, grasping tubing with shoulder extended, adducted, and internally rotated; elbow pronated and wrist flexed.

PROCEDURE: Client told to "pull wrist up and reach." Pattern simulates throwing a ball.

STRENGTHENING TECHNIQUES

Strengthening is the major focus of most rehabilitation programs. There are distinct advantages for PNF over the use of traditional weight training for strengthening. Manually resisted PNF patterns and activities allow the clinician to more precisely monitor and correct substitutions. The use of normal movement patterns, the emphasis on eccentric control and functional progression, and the ability to vary the speed are additional advantages of PNF over traditional

TABLE 8-4 Summary of PNF Techniques

Mobility
Contract relax[a]
Hold relax[a]
Rhythmic initiation
Strengthening
Slow reversals
Repeated contractions
Timing for emphasis
Rhythmic stabilization
Stability
Alternating isometrics
Rhythmic stabilization
Skill
Timing for emphasis
Resisted progression
Endurance
Slow reversals
Agonist reversals

[a]See Chapter 3.

progressive-resistive programs. Nelson et al.[15] noted better carryover to functional performance measures, including vertical leap and throwing distance, with PNF strengthening activities than with traditional progressive-resistive exercise programs. Furthermore, PNF patterns and principles can be applied to use with equipment. Specific PNF techniques, which can be used to facilitate strengthening, include slow reversals, repeated contractions, timing for emphasis, and agonist reversals.

Slow reversals of reciprocal movement is a high-use technique for applying resistance to increase strength and endurance, teach reversal of movement, and increase coordination. Both directions of a diagonal pattern are performed in a smooth, rhythmical fashion with changes of direction occurring without pause or relaxation. Generally, slow reversals begin with the stronger pattern first, to take advantage of the principle of successive induction. To eliminate lag time when switching directions, the clinician changes the distal manual contact first, provides a new quick stretch, and resists the motion into the opposite direction. The speed, ROM, and quickness of change of direction can be varied to emphasize specific portions of a range or control. Similarly, isometric and eccentric contractions can be superimposed anywhere in the range, at any time. Isometric contractions at the weak point in the range have been shown to increase γ motor neuron recruitment and increase muscle spindle sensitivity, which may be important for enhancing postural stabilizers that may have been overstretched.

Slow reversals are particularly helpful for the patient who is beginning to work on timing and reversals of motion in preparation for sport-specific training, such as throwing or cutting motions. Reversals are rarely slow in daily activities or in sports. The speed of change and type of contraction can be altered constantly in the session to work on neuromuscular control. When focusing on control drills, verbal commands should be kept to a minimum, forcing the individual to rely on tactile and proprioceptive input alone.

Repeated contractions of the weak muscle help facilitate initiation of motion, enhance recruitment, increase active ROM and strength, and offset fatigue. To apply repeated contractions, the clinician fully elongates all the muscles in the pattern, then gives a quick nudge to stretch the muscle further. The patient is told to keep pulling as repeated stretches and resistance are applied, and the limb moves farther toward the end range. Because repeated contractions use quick stretch, their use is contraindicated with joint instability, pain, fracture, or recent surgical procedure.

Timing for emphasis, or **pivots,** blocks the normal timing of muscular contraction to focus on the recruitment, strength, or coordination of a specific muscle group, often in a particular portion of the range. To use this technique effectively, the client must have three things: (1) a strong, stabilizing muscle group; (2) a "handle" or segment onto which the clinician may hold; and (3) a pivot point, or the movement being emphasized. Commonly, the distal or intermediate component is pivoted, but any motion is possible.

For example, consider the use of timing for emphasis for ankle dorsiflexors. Lower extremity flexion against resistance is initiated against manual resistance. At the strongest part of the range, the patient performs an isometric hold of the entire pattern. The clinician applies quick stretch to the dorsiflexors, allowing movement of the dorsiflexors while holding the isometric contraction elsewhere. The pivot on the ankle is repeated two to three times. The activity is finished with quick stretch to the entire pattern to facilitate movement through the entire pattern. This activity can be used in an upright position or in a more functional posture.

The technique of **agonist reversal** is the use of eccentric muscle contractions within a pattern or resisted functional activity to enhance control and strength. The patient is told to keep pulling as the clinician takes the limb back (overpowering the patient) to the original starting position (causing an eccentric contraction). Because the vast majority of high-skill activities have deceleration

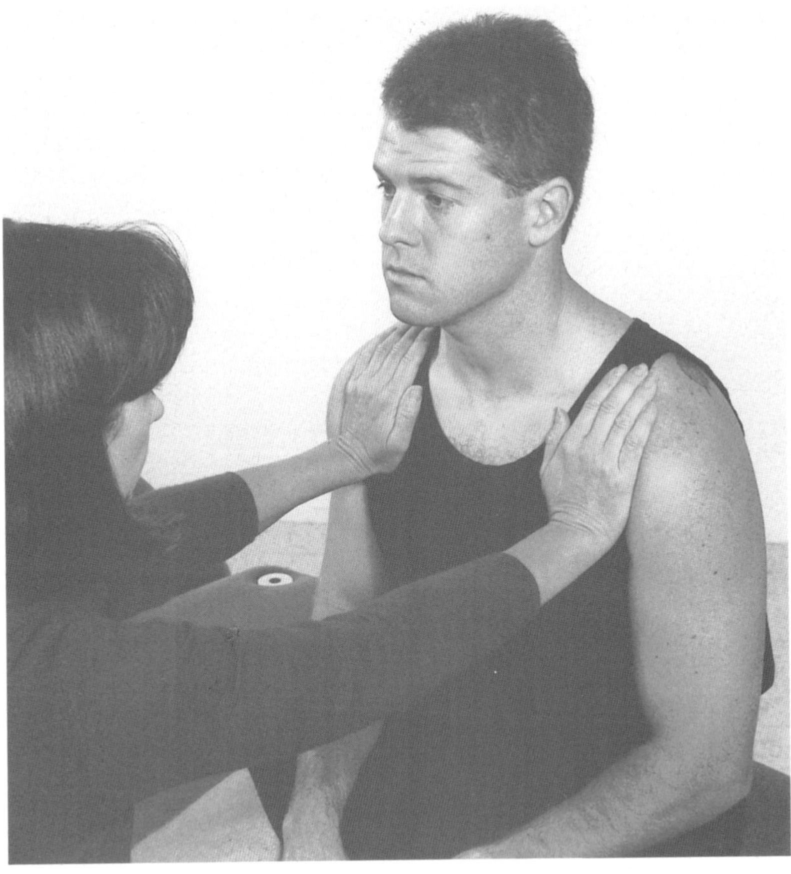

FIGURE 8-21 **Alternating isometrics to trunk flexors in sitting.**

PURPOSE: Activation and strengthening of trunk flexors; overflow and facilitation of hip, knee, and ankle flexor muscles.

POSITION: Client sitting with no back support. Clinician sitting in front of client. Manual contacts with flat hand just inferior to bilateral clavicles.

PROCEDURE: Clinician gradually applies resistance, matching client's effort, so there is little trunk movement. Overflow may result in active movement into hip, knee, and ankle flexor musculature as resistance is built up. Resistance is applied first to one side of trunk (anterior) and then to the other side (posterior).

components, eccentric work is part of essential preparation for functional activities. The most common example is the overhead athlete who must control the deceleration of the arm to avoid excessive stress on supporting noncontractile structures. Agonist reversals can be particularly beneficial for treating tendinitis and patellar tracking disorders.

STABILITY TECHNIQUES

Stability includes both non-weight-bearing isometric muscle stability and dynamic postural activities while weight bearing in proper biomechanical alignment. Techniques frequently used to promote stability include alternating isometrics and rhythmic stabilization.

Alternating isometric contractions is the simplest of these techniques. The clinician provides isometric resistance to the patient in one direction (usually the stronger), telling the patient to "hold, don't let me move you." Resistance is gradually switched to the other direction by moving one hand at a time to the opposite side and telling the patient to switch and hold. No movement of the individual or of the joint should occur (Fig 8-21).

Alternating isometric contractions progress to **rhythmic stabilization,** where an isometric co-contraction for stability is generated around the joint or trunk. This is a bidirectional, rotational technique, with smooth co-contraction in all three planes occurring simultaneously. Manual contacts are placed on opposite sides of the limb or trunk (Figs. 8-22 and 8-23). Isometric rotational resistance is gradually built up, held, then gradually switched to go the other direction. The key to accomplishing smooth change of direction is the use of approximation and the firm, maintained sliding input provided around the joint surface during the transition. The resistance can change directions as many times as is necessary. Most easily used to promote proxi-

FIGURE 8-22 **Rhythmic stabilization to trunk.**

PURPOSE: Stabilization and control of trunk through co-contraction of musculature on both sides of trunk.

POSITION: Client sitting upright with no back support. Clinician sitting in front or behind client with hands on opposite aspects of trunk at inferior clavicle and mid-scapula.

PROCEDURE: Client told to "hold" or "match me" against manual resistance, which attempts to rotate trunk. Resistance is built up slowly over 5 to 10 sec; then held and gradually reduced. To change direction of rotary force, clinician approximates through shoulders, gradually sliding manual contacts from anterior to posterior and visa versa.

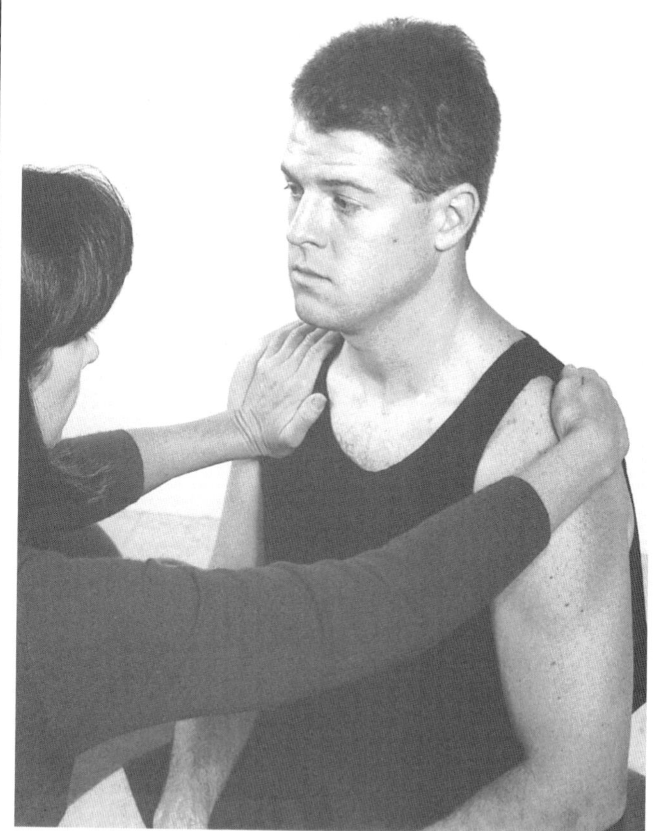

FIGURE 8-23 **Rhythmic stabilization to bilateral upper extremity.**

PURPOSE: Promote co-contraction and stabilization about upper trunk and shoulders; relaxation and ROM.

POSITION: Client lying supine. Clinician standing at head of client. Generally started in mid-ROM or where control is best; may be progressed to other parts of ROM as intervention progresses. Manual contacts on opposite sides of wrist.

PROCEDURE: Client told to "hold" or "match me" against manual resistance, which attempts to flex one arm up and extend the other. Resistance is gradually built up slowly over 5 to 10 sec; then held and gradually reduced. To change direction of force, clinician approximates through extended arms, gradually sliding manual contacts from anterior to posterior and visa versa.

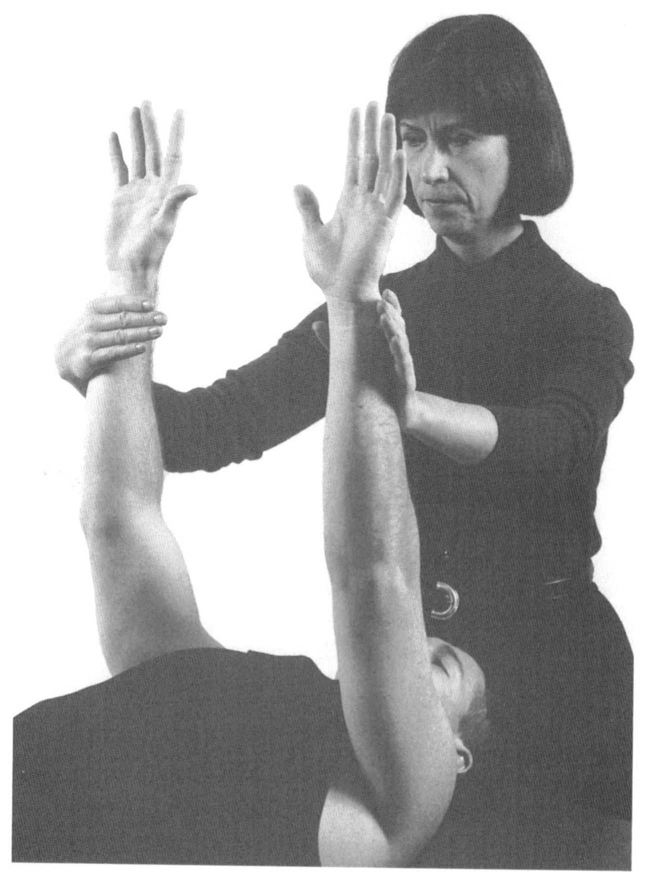

mal trunk control, rhythmic stabilization can be applied to bilateral or even unilateral extremity patterns.

SKILL

An individual performs a variety of activities with consistent and proper timing, sequencing, speed, and coordinated control. Proprioceptive neuromuscular facilitation uses the techniques of resisted progression, normal timing, and timing for emphasis to promote skilled movement. In addition, the techniques of agonist reversals (eccentric contractions) and slow reversals can be used effectively to vary the muscular contractions required within a single exercise session, progressing from isometric to eccentric.

Normal timing enhances the distal to proximal sequence of motions. Stronger, proximal motions are resisted and held back until the desired distal motion is elicited with quick stretch and resistance. The timing may first be enhanced in non-weight-bearing postures and then progressed to upright postures. Skilled performance of movement may also be facilitated by manual resistance, pulleys, or elastic tubing. Examples include resisted gait, braiding, or cutting motions.

CASE STUDY

PATIENT INFORMATION

A 37-year-old female competitive recreational soccer player presented on referral from her orthopedist with a diagnosis of patellar tendinitis and patella-femoral dysfunction. She reported that the morning after the previous week's game she had pain in her left knee accompanied by mild swelling, difficulty ascending and descending stairs, and occasional buckling of the knee when trying to run. She could recall no specific incident or onset of the pain during the game. She also reported occasional crepitus and increased stiffness in the knee after sitting for long periods. She did report a previous medial collateral ligament injury to the same knee in college, which was treated conservatively with good success and return to unbraced competitive play. She was eager to return to her sport.

Examination revealed mild swelling on the inferior-lateral aspect of the patellar tendon region and tenderness to palpation at the inferior pole of the patella. The patellar position was slightly laterally and posteriorly tilted. The range of motion at the knee was limited to 0 to 100° owing to rectus femoris tightness. The hamstrings were tight bilaterally (0 to 70° straight-leg raise). Strength testing indicated left quadriceps strength at 3/5 with a 20° extensor lag; hamstrings were measured at 4/5. Recruitment of the left vastus medialis oblique (VMO) was poor. The strength of all other muscles tested was at 5/5. All ligamentous stability testing noted intact ligaments with no instability present. The examination confirmed the diagnosis made by the physician of patellar tendinitis and patella-femoral syndrome.

LINKS TO

Guide to Physical Therapist Practice* and *Athletic Training Educational Competencies

The patient's diagnosis was consistent with pattern 4E of the *Guide*:[22] "impaired joint mobility, motor function, muscle performance, and range of motion associated with localized inflammation." Included in this diagnostic group is tendinitis, and direct intervention involves "strengthening using resistive exercises."

The therapeutic exercise domain in the *Competencies*[23] refers to treatment of athletes using a variety of techniques. In the teaching objectives listed under this domain, the *Competencies* notes that the athletic trainer, upon graduation from an accredited program, will be able to "describe indications, contraindications, theory and principles for the incorporation and application of various contemporary therapeutic exercises including proprioceptive neuromuscular facilitation (PNF) for muscular strength/endurance, muscle stretching, and improved range of motion." The "demonstration" of these same exercises is also emphasized.

INTERVENTION

Initial intervention was directed at reducing inflammation, regaining full ROM, reducing pain with activity, and independence in a home program. Initial treatment in the clinic included

1. Ice to the affected knee before treatment.
2. Manually resisted contract relax to the hamstrings bilaterally using extension-adduction and extension-abduction patterns in supine.
3. Bilateral lower extremity extension (Fig. 8-18), combined with isometric holds and timing for emphasis at the end range of knee extension (to improve recruitment of VMO and achieve active terminal knee extension).
4. Patellar taping and biofeedback to assist patellar alignment during PNF.
5. Home program: hamstring stretching on an elevated surface using modified contract relax and isometric quad sets.
6. Ice at the end of treatment.

GERIATRIC *Perspectives*

- The specific techniques of PNF, combining diagonal patterns with facilitatory stimuli (tactile contact, resistance, irradiation, approximation, verbal commands, and vision), make the approach useful for promoting strengthening, motor learning, and restoration of motor control in older adults with musculoskeletal and neuromuscular deficits. Research has demonstrated that older adults have decreased response to proprioceptive stimuli, especially if the movement is passive and with small changes in joint angle.[1] Tactile contact and approximation may promote a better feel of the movement pattern for older adults.
- Detection of joint angular movement (the angular threshold) appears to improve with increasing magnitude and speed.[1] Use of PNF diagonals with verbal commands to increase awareness of joint angular movement is an effective intervention for decreasing the angular threshold and promoting motor learning.
- The synergistic recruitment of agonist–antagonist is an appropriate means of incorporating more functional-based strengthening in the rehabilitation for subacute and chronic joint problems. As outlined by Hertling and Kessler,[2] a gradual progression from isometric to eccentric to isotonic muscle strengthening is more likely to demonstrate functional carryover than is rote strengthening. Use of this progression is analogous to promoting stability (holding co-contraction), then grading the stability to allow muscle lengthening, and finally inhibiting the antagonist to allow selective contraction in agonist (controlled mobility). The goal is for the older adult to develop automatic controlled mobility during functional performance.
- Patterns and techniques of PNF are effective for improving isometric, eccentric, and isotonic control in movements requiring control at varied joint angles (small to large ranges). An example of such movement is coming from sit to stand and the control that is needed in flexion to extension of the hip and knee. D1 flexion and D2 extension diagonals combined with techniques such as alternating isometrics and rhythmic stabilization and then progressing to agonist reversal and then to slow reversals and repeated contractions is suggested for assisting the older adult to gain skill in performance of synergistic movements.
- Resistance may be applied using dumbbells, cuff weights, rubber tubing, or items available in the home (cans of soup, bags of dried beans). As suggested for children, clear, precise verbal and written instruction may be necessary and helpful for promoting compliance and understanding in older adults.

1. Schultz AB, Ashton-Miller JA, Alexander NB. Biomechanics of mobility in older adults. In: Hazzard WR, Blass JP, Ettinger WH, et al., eds. Principles of geriatric medicine and gerontology. 4th ed. New York: McGraw-Hill, 1998:131–142.
2. Hertling D, Kessler RM. The knee. In: Hertling D, Kessler RM, eds. Management of common musculoskeletal disorders: physical therapy principles and methods. 3rd ed. Philadelphia: Lippincott-Raven, 1996:315–378.

PROGRESSION

One Week After Initial Treatment

At the time of re-examination, the patient presented with pain-free knee flexion (0 to 115°), with mild complaints of "catching" at end of active full extension. The straight-leg raise increased to 0 to 85°. Quad lag improved to 0 to 10°. The patient reported continued difficulty ascending and descending stairs.

Clinic treatment continued with manually resisted PNF patterns, progressing to unilateral flexion-adduction pattern (D1 flexion) in supine (Fig. 8-14), using slow reversals to increase recruitment and delay fatigue. Standing activities were introduced, including alternating isometrics and rhythmic stabilization to quadriceps and hamstrings using manual resistance. The home program was progressed as follows:

1. Standing lower extremity flexion-adduction with elastic tubing (Fig. 8-19).
2. Partial-range wall squats and slides with knees flexed to a maximum of 20°; emphasis on isometric holds and eccentrics in the closed-chain position.
3. Continue hamstring stretching and patellar taping.
4. Ice after treatment.

Two Weeks After Initial Examination

After two weeks of intervention, examination indicated full knee flexion, and straight-leg range to 95°. No active quadriceps lag was present, and the quadriceps strength tested at 4+/5. The patient reported that she was able to ascend stairs with minimal discomfort and had only mild discomfort with descent. The goal at this time was to continue to strengthen the VMO and begin progression to resistive exercise with in-

PEDIATRIC *Perspectives*

- The principles and patterns of PNF can be, and often are, incorporated into rehabilitation of children with both neuromuscular and musculoskeletal impairments and functional limitations. Proprioceptive neuromuscular facilitation diagonal patterns may be used during development and rehabilitation of athletic skills, because these patterns are similar to the patterns used during sporting motions.
- Interventions of PNF closely parallel the normal sequence of motor behavior acquisition that occurs in children: proximal to distal; stability to mobility. Improvement in all types of motor ability depends on motor learning. Motor learning is enhanced through sensory inputs from multiple systems, including visual, verbal, tactile, and proprioceptive.[1]
- Proprioceptive neuromuscular facilitation techniques use multiple forms of sensory input. Remember that throughout childhood sensory systems are developing and do not demonstrate the same responses as in the adult. Children may not respond like adults in development or rehabilitation of motor ability.
- In younger children, expect less independence for performing complex motor patterns with multiple components (diagonal patterns). This may be owing to attention span or memory and emotional maturity issues. More time may be needed for active assisted or manual resistance treatments for children than for adults. Children may have difficulty adapting an exercise to include tubing, weights, or pulleys. Instruction and feedback in several forms may be necessary (verbal, written, pictorial).

1. Horak FB. Assumptions underlying motor control for neurologic rehabilitation. In: MJ Lister, ed. Contemporary management of motor control problems; proceedings of the II Step conference. Alexandria, VA: Foundation for Physical Therapy, 1991:11–28.

creasing knee motion to prepare for kicking activities and return to play.

Clinic treatment continued with unilateral flexion-adduction pattern with knee extending, using slow reversals and progressing to timing for emphasis on left knee extension, pivoting off the stronger right lower extremity. In addition, the patient performed standing resisted flexion with knee extension to simulate striking a soccer ball; first emphasizing standing on the involved limb, then striking with it.

The home program was progressed to include jogging. If no pain occurred with jogging, the patient was instructed to begin cutting activities. She was told to continue with stretching, strengthening, and ice as needed.

OUTCOMES

Three weeks after initial intervention, the patient called to cancel the next appointment. She reported resolution of pain and return to play without complication.

SUMMARY

- Proprioceptive neuromuscular facilitation is a philosophy of treatment that uses normal diagonal movement patterns, variable resistance and a variety of specific techniques to meet the patient's goals. Basic principles of PNF include the use of specific manual contacts, resistance, and proprioceptive techniques. Optimal resistance is defined as the amount that challenges the patient while still allowing the desired smooth coordinated movement.
- PNF diagonal patterns cross the midline, incorporating all planes of movement, and are similar to many sport-specific movements. Diagonal patterns should be modified according to the structural stability of the joint and extremity. Although primarily a manual technique, PNF patterns and principles are readily applied to the use of equipment for home programs and increased challenge.
- PNF includes methods to increase the ROM (hold relax, contract relax), teach the initiation of movement (rhythmic initiation), increase strength (slow reversals, repeated contractions, timing for emphasis), improve stability (agonist reversals, rhythmic stabilization), and improve skill (resisted progression, normal timing).
- Although an understanding of the philosophy, principles, and techniques of PNF can be gained by reading, skilled application to treatment is best achieved through supervised practice. To best use the information presented here, it is important to practice the techniques and receive feedback from a skilled PNF practitioner.

REFERENCES

1. Kabat H. Central mechanisms for recovery of neuromuscular function. Science 1950;112:23–24.
2. Kabat H. The role of central facilitation in restoration of motor function paralysis. Arch Phys Med 1953;33:521–533.
3. Voss DE, Ionta MK, Myers BJ. Proprioceptive neuromuscular facilitation. 3rd ed. Philadelphia: Harper & Row, 1985.
4. Trueblood PR, Walker JM, Gronley JK. Pelvic exercise and gait in hemiplegia. Phys Ther 1989;69:32–40.
5. Wang RP. Effect of proprioceptive neuromuscular facilitation on the gait of athletes with hemiplegia of long and short duration. Phys Ther 1994;74:1108–1115.
6. Sale DG. Neural adaptation to resistance training. Med Sci Sports Exerc 1988;20(suppl):S135–S145.
7. Bandy WD, Dunleavy K. Adaptability of skeletal muscle: response to increased and decreased use. In: JE Zachazewski, DJ Magee, WS Quillen, eds. Athletic injures and rehabilitation. Philadelphia: Saunders, 1996:55–91.
8. Sherrington C. Integrative activity of the nervous system. New Haven, CT: Yale University Press, 1960.
9. Gordon J. Spinal mechanisms of motor coordination. In: E Kandel, JH Schwartz, TM Jessel, eds. Principles of neural science. 3rd ed. New York: Elsevier, 1991:581–595.
10. Gordon J, Ghez C. Muscle receptors and spinal reflexes: the stretch reflex. In: E Kandel, JH Schwartz, TM Jessel, eds. Principles of neural science. 3rd ed. New York: Elsevier, 1991: 564–580.
11. Engle R. Knee ligament rehabilitation. Clin Manage 1990;10:36–39.
12. Engle RP, Canner GG. Proprioceptive neuromuscular facilitation (PNF) and modified procedure for anterior cruciate ligament (ACL) instability. J Othop Sports Phys Ther 1989;11:230–236.
13. Macefield G, Hagbarth KE, Gorman R, et al. Decline in spindle support to alpha motor neurons during sustained voluntary contractions. J Physiol 1991;440:497–512.
14. Moore MA, Kulkulka CG. Depression of Hoffman reflexes following voluntary contraction and implications for proprioceptive neuromuscular facilitation therapy. Phys Ther 1991;71:321–329.
15. Nelson AG, Chambers RS, McGowan CM, Penrose KW. Proprioceptive neuromuscular facilitation versus weight training for enhancement of muscular strength and athletic performance. J Orthop Sports Phys Ther 1986;7:250–253.
16. Osterling LR, Robertson RN, Troxel RK, Hansen P. Differential responses to proprioceptive neuromuscular (PNF) stretch techniques. Med Sci Sport Exec 1990;22:106–111.
17. Roy MA, Sylvestre, Katch FI, et al. Proprioceptive facilitation of muscle tension during unilateral and bilateral extension. Int J Sports Med 1990;11:289–292.
18. Anderson MA, Foreman TL. Return to competition: functional rehabilitation. In: JE Zachazewski, DJ Magee, WS Quillen, eds. Athletic injures and rehabilitation. Philadelphia: Saunders, 1996: 229–261.
19. Adler SS, Beckers D, Buck M. PNF in practice: an illustrated guide. London: Springer-Verlag, 1993.
20. Sullivan PE, Marcos PD. Clinical decision making in therapeutic exercise. Norwalk, CT: Appleton & Lange, 1995.
21. Paine RM, Voight M. The role of the scapula. J Orthop Sports Phys Ther 1993;18:386–391.
22. American Physical Therapy Association. Guide to physical therapist practice, second edition. Phys Ther 2001;81:1–768.
23. National Athletic Trainers' Association. Athletic training educational competencies. 3rd ed. Dallas: NATA, 1999.

Closed-Kinetic-Chain Exercise and Plyometric Activities

Kevin E. Wilk, PT
Michael M. Reinold, MS, PT

In the rehabilitation of athletic injuries and in sports training, the concept of specificity of training is an important parameter in determining the proper exercise program. The imposed demands during training must mirror those incurred during athletic competition, especially during the advanced phases of the rehabilitation process. In most athletic events, the essential element to enhance performance is the capacity of the muscle to exert maximal force output in a minimal amount of time. Most athletic skills depend on the ability of the muscle to generate force rapidly. To simulate the explosive strength needed in athletics, Verkhoshanski[1] advocated the shock method of training when he introduced the concept of plyometrics in Russia.

Plyometric training was advocated during the 1990s as a form of sports-specific training and rehabilitation training drills in the advanced phases of a rehabilitation program. During many athletic activities—such as playing tennis, throwing a ball, or jumping—the athlete performs a plyometric type of muscular contraction.

It should be noted that before initiation of a plyometric program, closed-kinetic-chain (CKC) drills are required. For example, generally CKC squats or CKC leg press exercises are performed before initiating plyometric jumping drills. Therefore, an integration of CKC and plyometric drills is imperative.

In this chapter, the physiologic rationale and clinical application of both closed-kinetic-chain exercises and plyometric training drills are discussed. In addition, specific exercise drills and their application to patients are presented.

Scientific Basis

CLOSED-KINETIC CHAIN

Terminology

In the past, there has been confusion concerning the clinical use of open-kinetic-chain (OKC) and CKC exercises for rehabilitation. Questions regarding function and safety are frequently brought up when clinicians are deciding which type of exercise to incorporate into a rehabilitation program for a patient. The common assumption that CKC offers a safer, more functional approach to returning the athlete to the premorbid level has helped CKC exercises gain popularity in sports medicine. Although incorporation of both OKC and CKC exercises in rehabilitation protocols may be beneficial to the injured athlete, CKC exercises offer the athlete a dynamic method for increasing neuromuscular joint stability using sport-specific drills. Unfortunately, many clinicians do not have a clear sense of the exact definitions of closed- and open-kinetic-chain exercises.

Originally, kinetic chain terminology was used to describe linkage analysis in mechanical engineering. In 1955, Steindler[2] suggested that the human body could be thought of as a chain consisting of the rigid overlapping segments of the limbs connected by a series of joints. He defined a kinetic chain as a combination of several successfully arranged joints constituting a complex motor unit. Furthermore, he observed that when a foot or hand meets considerable resistance, muscular recruitment and joint motion are different from that observed when the foot or hand is free to move without restriction. Today, most individuals believe CKC exercise takes place when the terminal segment of an appendage is fixed, such as during a squat, leg press, or push-up exercise. Conversely, OKC exercise occurs when the terminal segment is free to move, such as during a seated knee extension exercise or biceps curl maneuver.

Others have defined the open- and closed-chain activities differently. Panaeriello[3] defined CKC activity of the extremity as an activity in which the foot or hand is in contact with the ground or a surface. He emphasized that the body weight must be supported for a closed-kinetic chain to exist.

Although the definitions of OKC and CKC are widely applied in sports medicine, there are numerous exercises and functional activities that do not fall within these concrete delineations. In addition, few exercises can be absolutely classified as an open- or closed-kinetic chain. In fact, most exercises and functional activities, such as running and jumping, involve some combination of open- and closed-kinetic chain succession. In addition, activities in which the distal segment is fixed on an object but the object is moving (e.g., skiing and ice skating) cannot be classified absolutely as closed-kinetic chain. Therefore, limited situations occur when a true CKC effect takes place. Most exercises fall somewhere between a truly fixed CKC and OKC exercise, especially those that involve the upper-extremity kinetic chain.

The conditions that apply to the lower extremity (such as weight-bearing forces) that create a closed-kinetic-chain effect do not routinely occur in the upper extremity. However, because of the unique anatomic configuration of the glenohumeral joint, when the stabilizing muscles contract, a joint compression force is produced that stabilizes the joint, producing much the same effect as a CKC exercise for the lower extremity. Thus, the principles of CKC exercise as explained for the lower extremity may not apply for upper-extremity exercises.[3,4] Lephart and Henry[5] developed a scheme of OKC and CKC exercises for a clinical progression of drills for the shoulder that they termed a "functional classification system" (Tables 9-1 and 9-2).*

Physiologic Basis of Closed-Kinetic-Chain Activities

Closed-kinetic-chain exercises are often chosen over open-kinetic-chain exercises because the clinician wants to stress the joint in a weight-bearing position. Weight-bearing exercises result in joint approximation, which produces stimulation of the articular receptors, whereas length tension changes excite tenomuscular receptors.[6] These mechanoreceptors provide the joint proprioceptive information, which is critical to the dynamic stability of the joint.

Re-establishment of proprioception is an important part of neuromuscular control of the joint. Proprioception arises from activation of afferent neurons located in the joint capsule, ligaments, and surrounding muscles. As will be discussed later in this chapter, muscle spindles and Golgi tendon organs (GTOs) detect change in length and tension of the muscle, respectively. In addition, ligaments and joint capsules contain pacinian corpuscles, Ruffini endings, and GTO-like mechanoreceptors. These mechanoreceptors respond to changes in joint position, velocity, and direction.[5,7]

The joint compression seen with weight bearing facilitates muscular co-contractions of force couples, which provide a dynamic reflex stabilization.[8] Also, CKC exercises rely on the joint musculature to contract concentrically and eccentrically to generate joint mobility and stability farther along the kinetic chain.

Proprioceptive and muscular co-contraction training plays a complementary role in neuromuscular re-education. Adequate intensity and timing of muscular force-couple interaction allows for maximum joint congruency and inherent joint stability. Mechanoreceptors within the static and dynamic structures are cooperatively responsible for the neuromuscular control of the joint when the joint is in a weight-bearing position.

In addition, CKC exercises may also be extremely beneficial in the neuromodulation of pain via the activation of type I and II mechanoreceptors. Therefore, when the client is experiencing significant pain and inflammation, the early initiation of low-level CKC exercises in the acute phase of rehabilitation may be warranted.

PLYOMETRICS

Terminology

Although the term *plyometric* is relatively new, its basic concepts are well established. The roots of plyometric training can be traced to eastern Europe, where it was simply known as jump training or shock training.[1,8] The word *plyometrics* originates from the Greek words *plythein* and *metric*. *Plyo* originates from the Greek word for "more," and *metric* literally means "to measure."[9] The term was first introduced in 1975 by American track coach Fred Wilt.[9]

The practical definition of plyometrics is a quick powerful movement involving a prestretching of the muscle, thereby activating the stretch–shortening cycle of the muscle. Therefore, one purpose of plyometric training is to increase the excitability of the neurologic receptors for improved reactivity of the neuromuscular system. Wilk and Voight[10] referred to this type of muscle training as muscular stretch–shortening exercise drills.

The literature demonstrates that since 1979, many authors have used variations of the Verkhoshanski methodology in an attempt to establish the best stretch–shortening or plyometric training techniques.[8,10–13] There appears to be agreement on the benefits of basic stretch–shortening principles, but controversy exists regarding an optimal training routine.[14,15] Historically, the chief proponents of the plyometrics training approach were in the area of track and field,[16] but recently, authors have discussed programs for baseball,[10,17] football,[18] and basketball.[19] Thus, it appears that plyometric training has become an accepted form of training and rehabilitation in many sports medicine areas.

Adaptation of plyometric stretch–shortening principles can be used to enhance the specificity of training for sports

*Tables 9-1 and 9-2 offer suggestions of OKC and CKC exercises as presented by Lephart and Henry[5] and supported by the authors of this chapter. The editors respectively disagree with the classification of isometric strengthening and PNF (slow reversals) as CKC activities and suggest that they are OKC exercises. But, as appropriately stated by the authors of this chapter, few exercises can be absolutely classified as open or closed, and disagreement will occur.

TABLE 9-1 Open- and Closed-Kinetic-Chain Exercises for the Glenohumeral Joint

Phase	CKC	OKC
Acute	Isometric press-up, push-up, and strengthening; weight bearing shift; axial compression against wall	
Subacute	Resisted wall circles and wall abduction/adduction; slide board; push-ups; PNF[a] slow reversals	Isotonic and isokinetic strengthening
Advanced	Push-ups on balance board; lateral step-ups; shuttle; walking; StairMaster; unilateral weight bearing; plyometric push-ups	Isotonic and isokinetic strengthening; plyometrics; sport-specific training

[a]Proprioceptive neuromuscular facilitation.

that require a maximum amount of muscular force in a minimum amount of time. All movements in competitive athletics involve a repeated series of stretch–shortening cycles.[13,14,16] For example, during the overhead throwing motion, an athlete externally rotates his arm during the cocking phase to produce a stretch on the powerful internal rotator/adductor muscle group. Once the stretch stimulus is completed (full external rotation is achieved), the athlete forcefully accelerates the arm forward into adduction and internal rotation during the acceleration and ball release phases of the throw. Thus the stretch (cocking phase) proceeds the shortening (acceleration, ball release) phases. When an athlete performs a vertical jump, such as to jump to catch a ball or shoot a basketball, she exhibits a stretch–shortening cycle. The athlete first squats or slightly lower herself before jumping. By performing the squatting movement first, a stretch is generated on the plantarflexors, quadriceps, and gluteal muscles. This is the stretch phase of the jump. After the stretch phase is the shortening phase: an explosive push-off that allows the athlete to elevate. Therefore, whether throwing a ball, jumping rope, or swinging a golf club, all the movements involve a stretch–shortening cycle of the muscle.

Consequently, specific exercise drills should be developed to prepare athletes for activities specific to their sport. Plyometric exercise provides a translation from traditional strength training to the explosive movements of various sports. In this chapter, specific examples of plyometric exercise drills are presented for the upper and lower extremity.

Physiologic Basis of Plyometrics

Stretch–shortening exercises use the elastic and reactive properties of a muscle to generate maximum force production. In normal muscle function, the muscle is stretched before it contracts concentrically. This eccentric–concentric coupling (i.e., the stretch–shortening cycle) employs the stimulation of the body's proprioceptors to facilitate an increase in muscle recruitment over a minimum amount of time.

The proprioceptors of the body include the muscle spindle, the GTO, and the joint capsule/ligamentous mech-

TABLE 9-2 Open- and Closed-Kinetic-Chain Exercises for the Scapulothoracic Joint

Phase	CKC	OKC
Acute	Isometric punches, strengthening, and press-ups	Isotonic strengthening
Subacute	Push-ups, military presses, press-ups	Isotonic and isokinetic strengthening; rowing; prone horizontal abduction ($\pm$ external rotation)
Advanced	Neuromuscular control drills: rhythmic stabilization, circles, diagonal patterns	Progression of isotonic strengthening exercises

anoreceptors.[20] Stimulation of these receptors can cause facilitation, inhibition, and modulation of agonist and antagonist muscles.[20,21] Both the muscle spindle and the GTO provide the proprioceptive basis for plyometric training.

The muscle spindle functions mainly as a stretch receptor (Fig. 9-1). The muscle spindle components that are primarily sensitive to changes in velocity are the nuclear bag intrafusal muscle fibers, which are innervated by type Ia phasic nerve fiber. The muscle spindle is provoked by a quick stretch, which reflexively produces a quick contraction of the agonistic and synergistic extrafusal muscle fibers (Fig. 9-2). The firing of the type Ia phasic nerve fibers is influenced by the rate of stretch; the faster and greater the stimulus, the greater the effect of the associated extrafusal fibers. This cycle occurs in 0.3 to 0.5 msec and is mediated at the spinal cord level in the form of a monosynaptic reflex.[20]

The GTO, which is sensitive to tension, is located at the junction between the tendon and muscle both at the origin and at the insertion. The unit is arranged in series with the extrafusal muscle fibers and, therefore, becomes activated with stretch. Unlike the muscle spindle, the GTO has an inhibitory effect on the muscle. Upon activation, impulses are sent to the spinal cord, causing an inhibition of the α-motor neurons of the contracting muscle and its synergists and thus limiting the force produced. It has been postulated that the GTO is a protective mechanism against overcontraction or stretch of the muscle. Because the GTO uses at least one interneuron in its synaptic cycle, inhibition requires more time than monosynaptic excitation by type Ia nerve fibers (Fig. 9-2).[20]

During concentric muscle contraction, the muscle spindle output is reduced because the muscle fibers are either shortening or attempting to shorten. During eccentric contraction, the muscle stretch reflex serves to generate more tension in the lengthening muscle.[22] When the muscle tension increases to a high or potentially harmful level, the GTO fires, generating a neural pattern that reduces the excitation of the muscle. Consequently, the GTO receptors may act as a protective mechanism; but in a correctly carried out plyometric exercise, the reflex arc pathway incorporated with excitation of type Ia nerve fibers overshadows the influence of the GTO.

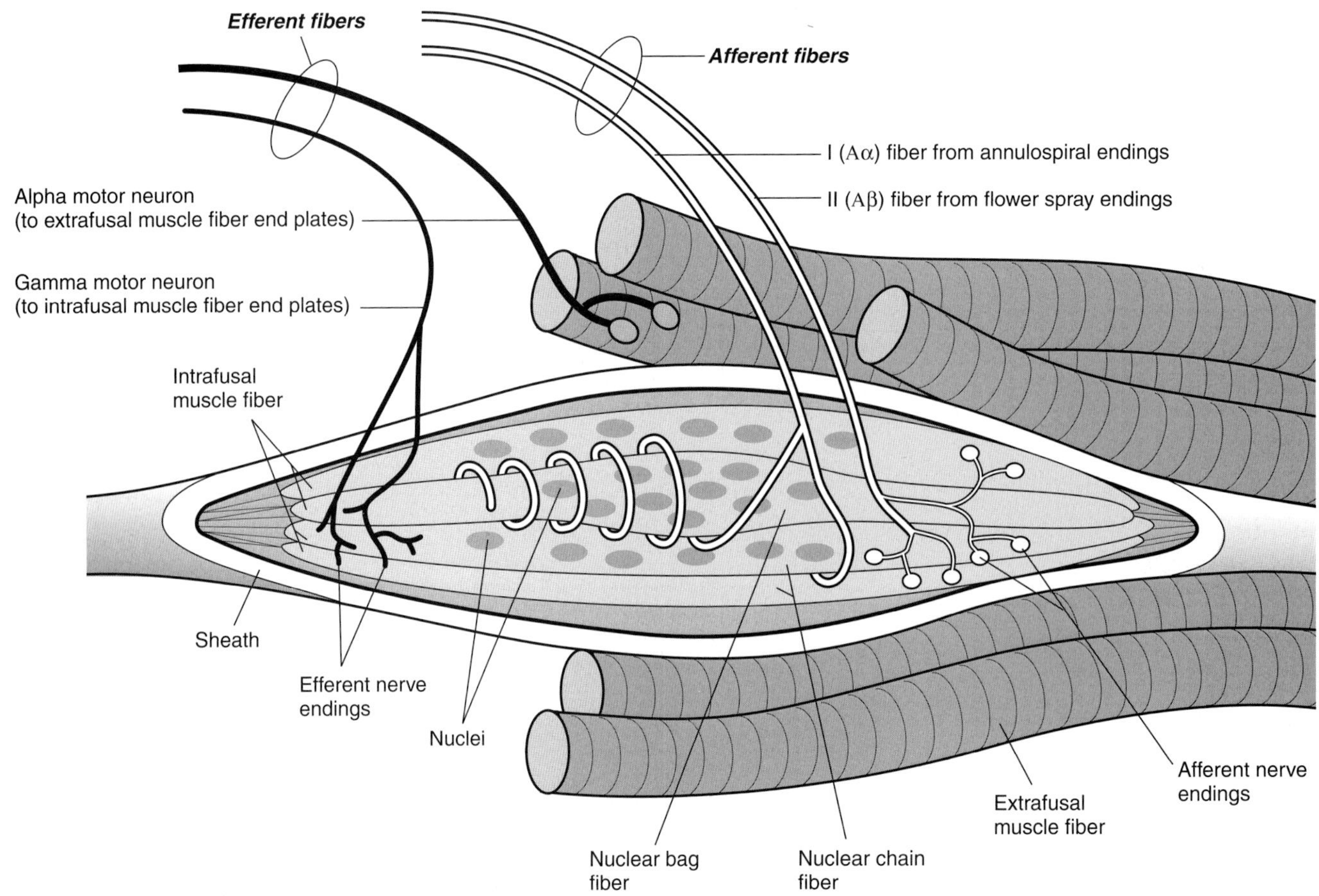

FIGURE 9-1 The muscle spindle.

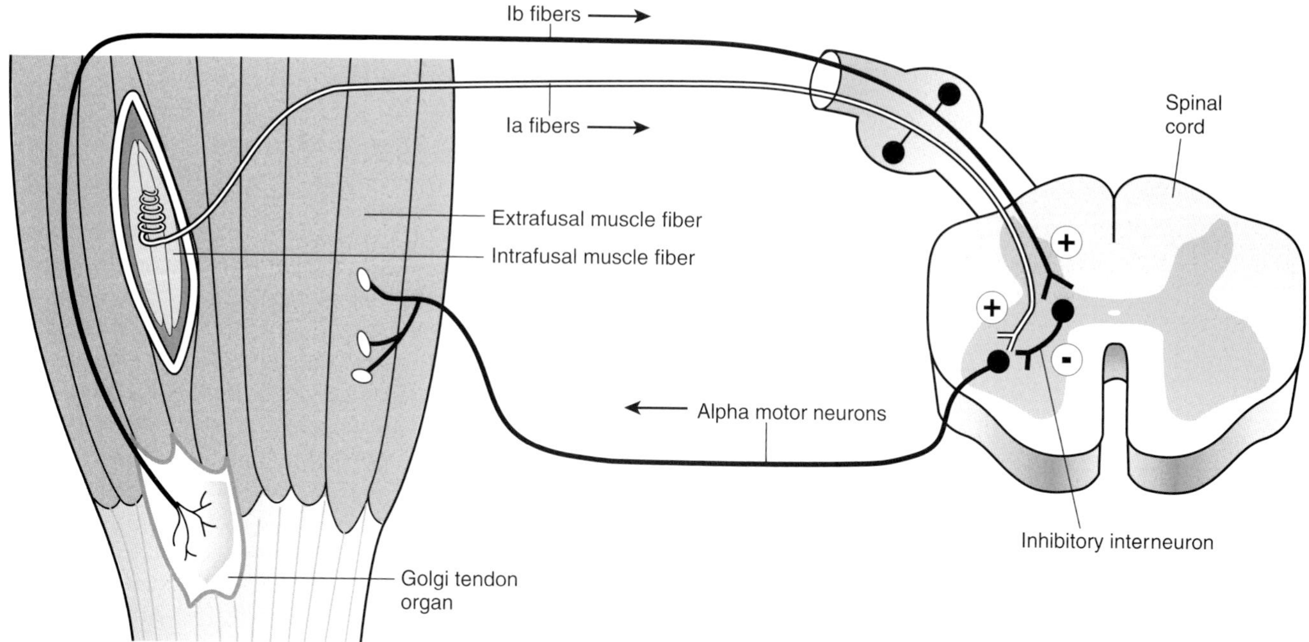

FIGURE 9-2 **Passive stretch reflex.**

In addition to the neurophysiologic stimulus, the positive results of the stretch–shortening exercise can also be attributed to the recoil action of elastic tissues.[13,14,23] Several authors have reported that an eccentric contraction will significantly increase the force generated concentrically as a result of storage of elastic energy.[11,12,23,24] The mechanism for this increased concentric force is the ability of the muscle to use the force produced by the elastic component. During the loading of the muscle that occurs when stretching, the load is transferred to the elastic component and stored as elastic energy. The elastic elements can then deliver increased energy, which is recovered and used for the concentric contraction.[11,23]

The ability of the muscle to use the stored elastic energy is affected by the duration, magnitude, and velocity of stretch. Increased force generated during the concentric contraction is most effective when the preceding eccentric contraction is of short range and performed quickly, without delay.[11,24] The improved or increased muscle performance that occurs by prestretching the muscle is the result of the combined effects of both the storage of elastic energy and the myotatic reflex activation of the muscle.[11,24] The percentage of contribution from each component is not yet known. In addition, the degree of enhanced muscular performance depends on the time between the eccentric and concentric contractions.[14]

Phases of Stretch–Shortening Exercise

Three phases of the plyometric exercise have been described: the setting (stretch) or eccentric phase, the amortization phase, and the concentric (shortening) response phase (Table 9-3). The eccentric, or setting phase, begins when the athlete mentally prepares for the activity and ends when the stretch stimulus is initiated. The advantages of a correct setting phase include increasing the muscle spindle activity by stretching the muscle before activation and mentally biasing the α-motor neuron for optimal extrafusal muscle contraction.[25] The duration of the setting phase is determined by the degree of impulse desired for facilitation of the contraction. With too much or prolonged loading, the elapsed time from eccentric to concentric contraction will prevent optimal exploitation of the stretch–shortening myotatic reflex.[1,26]

The next phase of the stretch–shortening response is amortization. This phase begins as the eccentric contraction starts to wane and ends with the initiation of a concentric force. By definition, it is the electromechanical delay between the eccentric and concentric contractions, during which the muscle must switch from overcoming work to imparting the necessary amount of acceleration in the required direction.[8] Successful training using the stretch–shortening technique relies heavily on the rate of stretch rather than the length of the stretch. If the amortization phase is slow, elastic energy is wasted as heat and the stretch reflex is not activated. The more quickly the individual is able to switch from yielding work to overcoming work, the more powerful the response.

The final period of the stretch–shortening exercise is the concentric response phase. During this phase, the athlete concentrates on the effect of the exercise and prepares for

TABLE 9-3 Phases of Plyometric Exercises

Phase	Description
I	Eccentric: stretch or setting period
II	Amortization: time between eccentric and concentric phases
III	Concentric response: facilitated shortening contraction

initiation of the second repetition. The response phase is the summation of the setting and amortization phases. This stage is often referred to as the resultant or payoff phase, because of the enhanced concentric contraction.[8,15,27,28]

Theoretically, stretch–shortening exercise assists in the improvement of physiologic muscle performance in several ways. Although increasing the speed of the myotatic stretch–reflex response may increase performance, such information has not been documented in the literature. Research does exist to support the idea that the faster a muscle is loaded eccentrically, the greater the concentric force produced.[29] Eccentric loading places stress on the elastic components, thereby increasing the tension of the resultant rebound force.

A second possible mechanism for the increased force production involves the inhibitory effect of the GTO on force production. Because the GTO serves as a protective mechanism limiting the amount of force produced within a muscle, its stimulation threshold becomes the limiting factor. Desensitization of the GTO through a plyometric training program may be possible, which will raise the level of inhibition and ultimately allow increased force production with greater loads applied to the musculoskeletal system.

The last mechanism by which plyometric training may increase muscular performance centers on neuromuscular coordination. The ultimate speed of movement may be limited by neuromuscular coordination. Explosive plyometric training may improve neural efficiency and increase neuromuscular performance. Using the prestretch response, the athlete may better coordinate the activities of the muscle groups. This enhanced neuromuscular coordination could lead to a greater net force production, even in the absence of morphologic change within the muscles themselves (referred to as neural adaptation).[8] In other words, the neurologic system may be enhanced, becoming more automatic.

The implementation of a stretch–shortening program begins with the development of an adequate strength and physical condition base. The development of a greater strength base leads to greater force generation owing to the increased cross-sectional area of both the muscle and the resultant elastic component. Therefore, to produce optimal strength gains and prevent overuse injuries, a structured strengthening program must be instituted before beginning plyometrics.

Clinical Guidelines

Closed-kinetic-chain exercises are often initiated in early phases of rehabilitation to facilitate co-contraction of joint force couples; the use of plyometrics is initiated in advanced stages of rehabilitation in sport-specific exercises. Often used as precursors to the more advanced demands of plyometric training, CKC exercises prepare the joint's ability to establish adequate muscular co-contraction and neuromuscular control to prevent potential overuse injuries.

Many clinicians base their rationale of choosing CKC exercises on the assumptions of increased safety and function. Obvious correlations exist between CKC squatting exercises and functional stopping and CKC step-up and step-down exercises to stair ambulation. Although some exceptions do occur in sports, such as a baseball pitcher's need for OKC proprioceptive exercises, most injured athletes often require the benefits of proprioceptive and neuromuscular rehabilitation observed with CKC exercises.

Weight-bearing during CKC exercises provides joint compression through the summation of ground-reaction forces, long believed to result in increased neuromuscular control and, subsequently, increased joint stability. Dynamic joint stabilization is achieved by co-contraction of the muscles surrounding a joint; lack of this stability often leads to injuries. During sport-specific movements such as running, cutting, and landing from a jump, the athlete relies on muscular co-contraction and eccentric control to dissipate ground-reaction forces. Consequently, athletes with reduced co-contraction and strength imbalances have been shown to have an increase risk of knee ligament injuries.[30] The athlete becomes susceptible to injury when he or she cannot dynamically control the ground-reaction forces muscularly, which places excessive stress on other static tissue, such as ligaments.

For preparing an athlete for competition when dynamic stability is vital to the prevention of injuries, CKC exercises may very well be the best option. But a limitation of CKC exercises is that, if specific muscle weakness is present, other agonistic muscles within the kinetic chain can generate forces to help compensate. In comparison, OKC exercise calls for a more isolated contraction of a muscle or muscle group and, therefore, may best be used for specific muscle strengthening. However, isolated open-chain exercise should be employed in combination with weight-bearing exercises. When an athlete is progressing to plyometric exercises, CKC exercises are used first so that initiation of muscular co-contraction and dynamic stability prepare the healing structures for the increased demands of plyometric exercise.

An integrated approach using both open- and closed-kinetic-chain exercise is recommended; although weight-bearing functional exercises are used in a rehabilitation program more often than isolated joint movements. Weight-bearing exercises are emphasized because such movements produce a greater stabilizing effect on the joint and may diminish ligament strain. Weight-bearing exercise also elicits muscular co-contractions and muscular recruitment in a manner that simulates functional activities. In turn, these activities stimulate mechanoreceptors throughout the kinetic chain. The importance of proprioception training in the rehabilitation program has been well established and cannot be overemphasized (see Chapter 11).

Plyometric exercise trains the neuromuscular system by teaching the system to better accept and apply increased system loads. Using the stretch reflex helps improve the ability of the nervous system to react with maximum speed to the lengthening muscle. The improved stretch reflex allows muscle to contract concentrically with maximal force. Because the plyometric program attempts to modify and retrain the neuromuscular system, the exercise program should be designed with sport specificity in mind.

Closed-kinetic-chain and plyometric exercises are common for lower-extremity rehabilitation, but can also be incorporated into upper-extremity rehabilitation. Athletes often use the upper extremity in an OKC fashion, e.g., when throwing, golfing, shooting a basketball, and performing a tennis stroke. However, some athletes do bear weight on their distal upper extremities, either to protect themselves from a fall or to perform specific sports endeavors (e.g., gymnasts, boxers, football players, and wrestlers). In addition, athletic endeavors such as swimming, throwing, cross-country skiing, and wheelchair propulsion all use principles of rapid opening and closing of the kinetic chain to propel the body or an object through space. Athletes involved in these sports use the upper extremity in much the same way as athletes use the lower extremities when jumping or running. Thus, the theories of enhanced neuromuscular control from CKC exercises and plyometric drills can be applied to the upper extremities.

Both CKC and plyometric exercises have the capacity to condition the upper and lower extremities while being sport specific. Developing intervention protocols that incorporate sport-specific drills not only potentiates the effect of the overall rehabilitation program but may lead to prevention of further athletic injuries.

■ *Techniques*

This section provides the clinician with specific CKC and plyometric drills, programs, and progressions for the upper and lower extremities. We present examples of possible exercises that can be incorporated into the rehabilitation of an injured patient. The demands of each sport should be considered when choosing the most appropriate drills, because the program should be as patient and sport specific as possible.

UPPER EXTREMITY CKC EXERCISE

The clinical use of weight-bearing or axial compression exercises for the upper extremity is based on patient selection and the ultimate goal. The use of weight-bearing exercises for the upper extremity without careful consideration of the biomechanical forces imparted onto the glenohumeral and scapulothoracic joints is not recommended. For example, using push-ups against a wall or on the floor may increase instability in patients with multidirectional instability or posterior instability, because the humeral head translates posteriorly during these exercises, stressing the posterior capsule of the glenohumeral joint. A list of commonly used CKC exercises for the glenohumeral and scapulothoracic joints are presented in Tables 9-1 and 9-2. General guidelines for the progression of CKC exercises for the upper extremity can be found in Table 9-4.

Acute Phase

Glenohumeral Joint

In the acute rehabilitation phase of most glenohumeral joint pathologies (including post-glenohumeral-joint dislocations, subluxations, and rotator-cuff pathologies), the primary goal is to re-establish motion. However, equally as important is the re-establishment of dynamic glenohumeral joint stability and prevention of rotator cuff shutdown. Weight-bearing exercises can be used to promote and enhance dynamic joint stability via the application of various techniques.[31] Often these weight-bearing techniques are employed with the hand fixed and no motion occurring; the resistance is applied either axially or rotationally. These exercises can be used early in the rehabilitation program, because motion is not occurring with heavy resistance, which may irritate the joint.

Therefore, immediately after glenohumeral joint subluxation or dislocation, the injured athlete may perform exercises such as isometric press-up, isometric weight-bearing and weight shifts, and axial compression against a table or wall (Figs. 9-3 to 9.5). These movements produce both joint compression and joint approximation, which should enhance muscular co-contraction about the joint, producing dynamic stability.[31–33] In addition, these exercises may be extremely beneficial in the neuromodulation of pain if the patient is experiencing significant pain and inflammation. These activities are performed with the patient standing or kneeling, placing a proportionate amount of body weight through the hands as tolerated. The patient is instructed to shift his or her weight from side to side, forward to backward, and diagonally on

TABLE 9-4 General Guidelines for Progression of CKC Exercises

Static stabilization ⟶ Dynamic stabilization
Stable surfaces ⟶ Unstable surfaces
Single plane movements ⟶ Multiplane movements
Straight planes ⟶ Diagonal planes
Wide base of support ⟶ Small base of support
No resistance ⟶ Resistance
Rhythmic stabilization ⟶ Resistance throughout range of motion
Fundamental movements ⟶ Dynamic challenging movements
Bilateral support ⟶ Unilateral support
Consistent movements ⟶ Perturbation training

and off of the affected side. These exercises may be progressed to using manual resistance rhythmic stabilization techniques that enhance the recruitment of the musculature involved in the force couples about the glenohumeral joint. These types of weight-bearing and shift exercises can be progressed by having the athlete place his or her feet on a large therapeutic ball (Fig. 9-6) and then on a smaller ball; finally the patient places one hand on top of the other to increase the difficulty.

Hence, the clinician may manually resist the anterior and then posterior musculature via proprioceptive neuromuscular facilitation (PNF) rhythmic stabilization exercises to enhance stabilization of the joint, thereby increasing the efficiency of the musculature involved in the compression of the humeral head within the glenoid (see Fig. 8-23). The muscles on both sides of the joint are referred to as muscular force couples.

Scapulothoracic Joint

Specific exercises can be used for the scapular musculature in much the same fashion as those described for the glenohumeral joint. In the early phases of rehabilitation for a upper-extremity injury, scapular musculature strengthening movements must be integrated into the program. In the acute phase, various movements are used to promote specific musculature activity. Exercises such as an isometric protraction or punching motion with resistance applied to the hand and lateral border of the scapula are excellent for promoting serratus anterior recruitment (Fig. 9-7). Isometric retractions of the scapular muscles may also be integrated into the program to recruit middle trapezius and rhomboid activity. Isometric press-ups can be employed to recruit a co-contraction of the glenohumeral joint and to elicit activity of the latissimus dorsi and teres major (Fig. 9-5).

Subacute Phase

Glenohumeral Joint

In the subacute phase, resistance is applied to the distal segment but some motion is allowed. Examples of these exercises include resisted arm circles against the wall, resisted axial load side-to-side motions either against a wall or on a slide board (see Fig. 12-20), and push-ups. In addition, a multitude of resisted quadruped exercises can be employed during the subacute rehabilitative phase, including manual proximal resistance to the shoulder and pelvis. Resistance can be applied in different amounts to multiple positions in a rhythmic stabilization fashion. This form of exercise can also be progressed to a tripod of the involved extremity or even to a therapeutic ball (see Figs. 12-13, 12-14, and 12-23).

By using weight-bearing exercises, the clinician attempts to enhance dynamic stability while the patient produces a superimposed movement pattern. This activity is a higher level of function than that performed in the acute phase and requires not only dynamic stabilization but also controlled mobility.

Scapulothoracic Joint

In the subacute phase, several CKC exercises, such as push-ups with a plus, military press, and press-ups, are recommended. These exercises are performed to recruit significant muscular activity of the muscles that stabilize the scapula.

Advanced Phase

Glenohumeral Joint

In the advanced phase, the weight-bearing exercises employed are usually high-demand movements that require a tremendous degree of dynamic stability. One example is a push-up with the hands placed on a ball, which produces axial load on the joint but keeps the distal segment

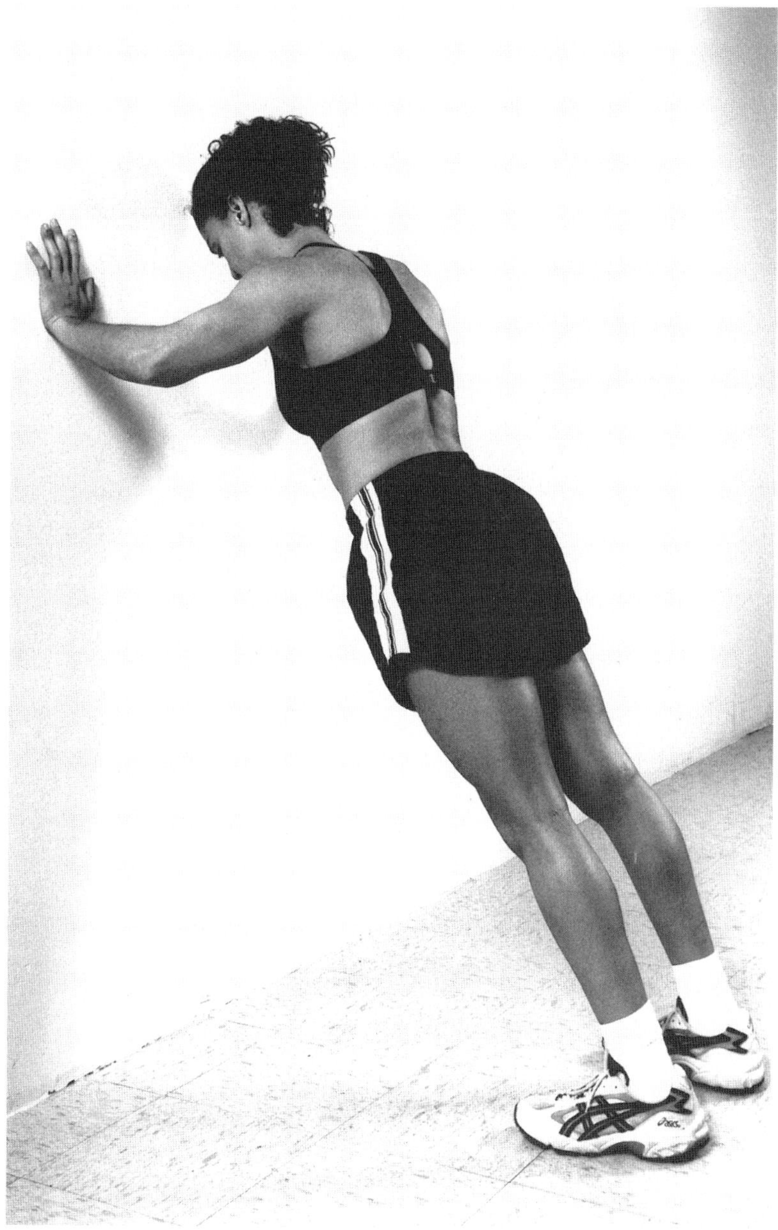

FIGURE 9-3 Axial compression against table or wall—beginning phase.

PURPOSE: CKC exercise to strengthen the muscles of the glenohumeral joint.

POSITION: Client standing with feet away from wall and arms extended against wall.

PROCEDURE: Using arms, clients lowers chest half the distance to wall, keeping hips in (do not allow hips to protrude). Client maintains position 3 to 5 sec.

somewhat free to move (Fig. 9-8). This push-up may be performed on a balance board, on a balance system, or on a movable platform with feet elevated on a therapeutic ball. Other exercises include lateral step-ups using the hands and retrograde or lateral walking on the hands on a treadmill or stair stepper. In this last rehabilitative phase, the exercises are tremendously dynamic and require adequate strength to be carried out properly.

Scapulothoracic Joint

The exercises that may be included in the last, advanced phase of rehabilitation for the scapular musculature were

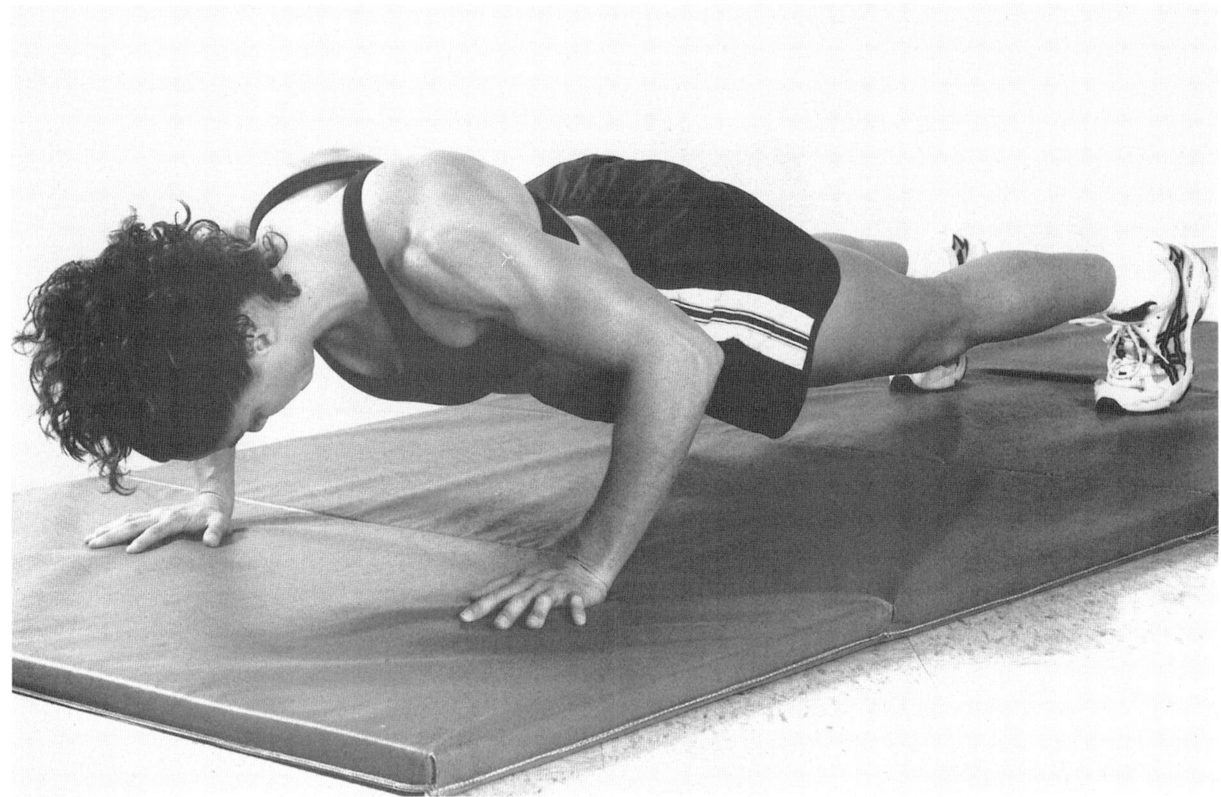

FIGURE 9-4 **Isometric push-up—beginning phase.**

PURPOSE: CKC exercise to strengthen muscles of the glenohumeral joint.

POSITION: Client in push-up position; arms extended.

PROCEDURE: Using arms, client lowers chest half the distance to ground, keeping hips in (do not allow hips to protrude). Client maintains position 3 to 5 sec.

already presented. In addition, a neuromuscular control exercise for the scapular muscles may be used (Fig. 9-9). In this exercise, the involved hand is placed on a table to fix the distal segment, which produces a greater magnitude of scapular activity. The individual is asked to slowly protract and retract and then elevate and depress the scapula to produce a circle or square movement. When these combined movement patterns are performed, tactile stimulus in the form of manual resistance is imparted onto the scapula and then is removed once the athlete produces the motion. The goal of this exercise is to enhance neuromuscular control and isolate dynamic control of the scapular muscles.

LOWER EXTREMITY CKC EXERCISE

The rationale for the use of OKC and CKC exercises for lower extremity rehabilitation is similar to that for upper extremity rehabilitation. Just as not all OKC exercises produce an isolated muscle contraction, not all CKC exercises produce muscular co-contraction of the surrounding musculature. With this in mind, lower-extremity kinetic-chain exercises can be organized into three groups by the muscular activity produced: muscular co-contractions, isolated quadriceps contractions, and isolated hamstring contractions (Table 9-5). Using these categories, the clinician can prescribe exercises based on the desired muscle recruitment pattern.

Closed-kinetic-chain exercise can also be used to develop muscular endurance in the lower extremity. The stair stepper and bicycle are two beneficial and common machines used for developing increased muscular endurance capacity (see Chapter 10) in a closed-kinetic chain, whereas aquatic therapy (see Chapter 13) is extremely valuable for total body muscular conditioning. Numerous exercises involve the closed-kinetic chain and weight bearing for the lower extremity. The clinician must choose the exercises that are most functional and sport specific and must decide if co-contraction or isolated muscle action is indicated for each client. Finally, when particular structures are healing, exercises must be altered based on clinical and biomechanical evidence to avoid stressing those tissues. The clinical guidelines suggested for the progression of the lower extremity are, in

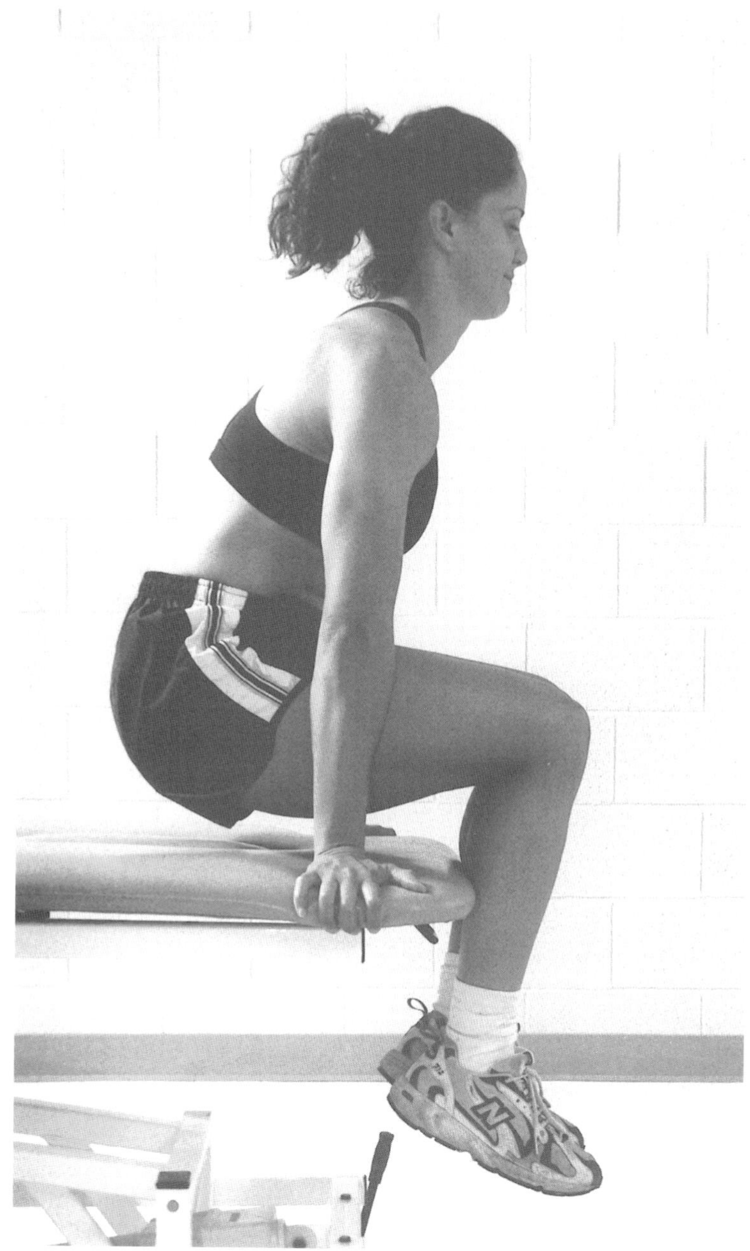

FIGURE 9-5 **Isometric press-up—beginning phase.**

PURPOSE: CKC exercise to strengthen pectoralis major and latissimus dorsi muscles.

POSITION: Client sitting on edge of support surface; hands at sides on support surface.

PROCEDURE: Client presses down with arms, lifting hips off support surface. Client maintains position 3 to 5 sec.

fact, the same as the clinical guidelines for upper-extremity progression and are presented in Table 9-4.

Acute Phase

Closed-kinetic-chain rehabilitation programs can begin in the acute phase. Early goals include re-establishment of motion, dynamic joint stability, and retardation of muscular atrophy (in particular the vastus medialis oblique). The acute phase begins with weight bearing and shifting to provide axial compression and joint approximation, leading to the facilitation of muscular co-contraction and dynamic joint stabilization. Weight-shifting exercises are performed by having the patient stand with bilateral support and shift from side to side and forward to backward,

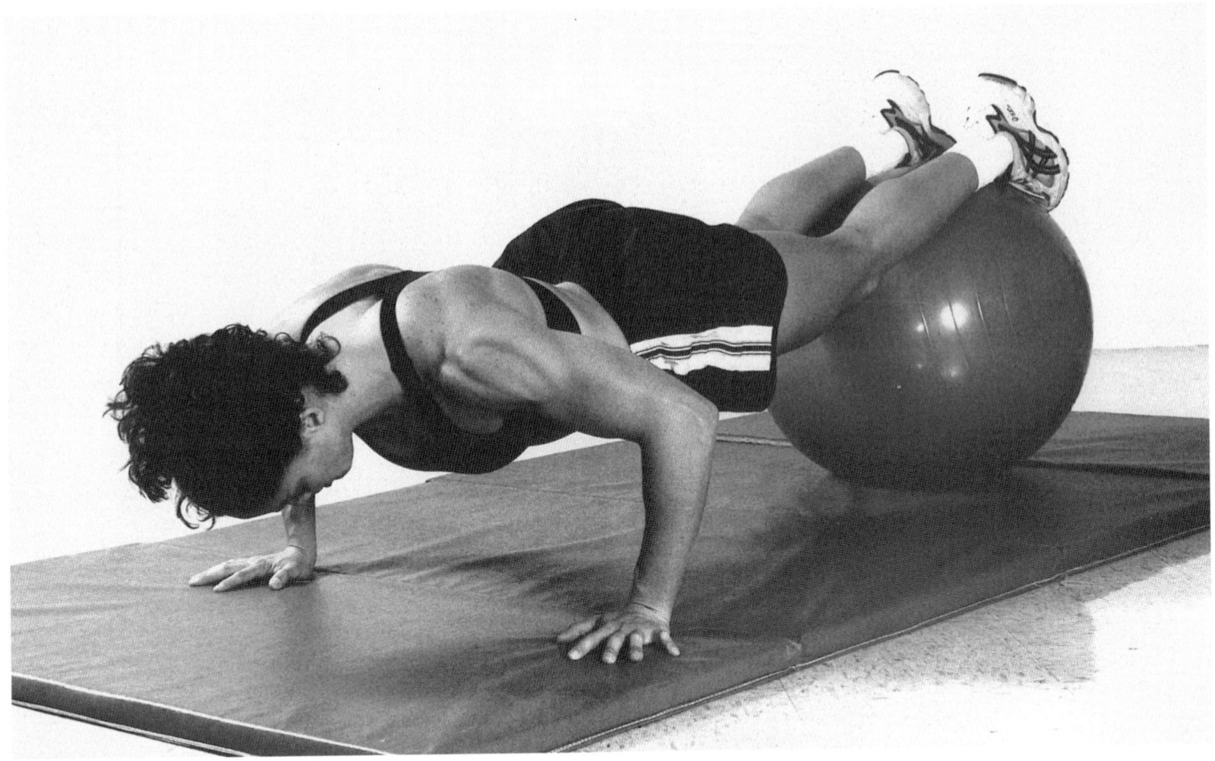

FIGURE 9-6 **Axial compression using therapeutic ball—beginning phase.**

PURPOSE: CKC exercise to strengthen muscles of the glenohumeral joint.

POSITION: Client in push-up position with feet on large therapeutic ball.

PROCEDURE: Using arms, client lowers chest half the distance to ground, keeping hips in (do not allow hips to protrude). Client maintains position 3 to 5 sec.

independently controlling the amount of weight bearing on the involved extremity. Standing mini-squats from 0 to 30° also begin in this stage (Fig. 9-10). As the tissues heal and the patient is able to perform the weight shifting and mini-squats without symptoms, lateral step-ups are initiated onto a step of low intensity; the height of the step controls the intensity of the exercise (Fig. 9-11). Also in the sagittal plane, forward lunges can be initiated if the clinician pays attention to the length and depth of the lunge (Fig. 9-12). Mini-squats are progressed near the end of the acute phase; the client may perform wall slides, if an isolated quadriceps contraction is indicated.

Subacute Phase

The subacute phase progresses the exercises performed in the acute phase. The squat is progressed to a range of 0 to 60° or 75°. The step-up and lunge are progressed to include lateral movements, and exercise-tubing resistance is used. The tubing can be applied from forward, backward, or either side to force the athlete to dynamically stabilize while the tubing produces a weight shifting movement in the direction of application (see Chapter 14).

The initiation of cone drills can begin during the subacute phase. They can be performed forward and laterally and involve the athlete stepping over the cones with a high knee raise and landing with a slightly flexed knee to develop balance and control of joint movements of the hip, knee, and ankle (Fig. 9-13).

Uneven surfaces can also be integrated into the rehabilitation program at this point to increase the demands on the mechanoreceptors. Patients can begin by balancing on foam, then a gym mat, and eventually a wobble board (see Fig. 11-18). As the athlete progresses, dumbbells of different weights can be placed in each hand to offset the athlete's center of gravity. The athlete is then instructed to maintain balance while randomly extending and abducting the arms, which alter the center of gravity.

Advanced Phase

As the athlete progresses to the advanced phase of rehabilitation, increased dynamic stability and an adequate base of strength are necessary to perform the high-demand exercises. Squats and lunges can be performed on an uneven surface with and without manual perturba-

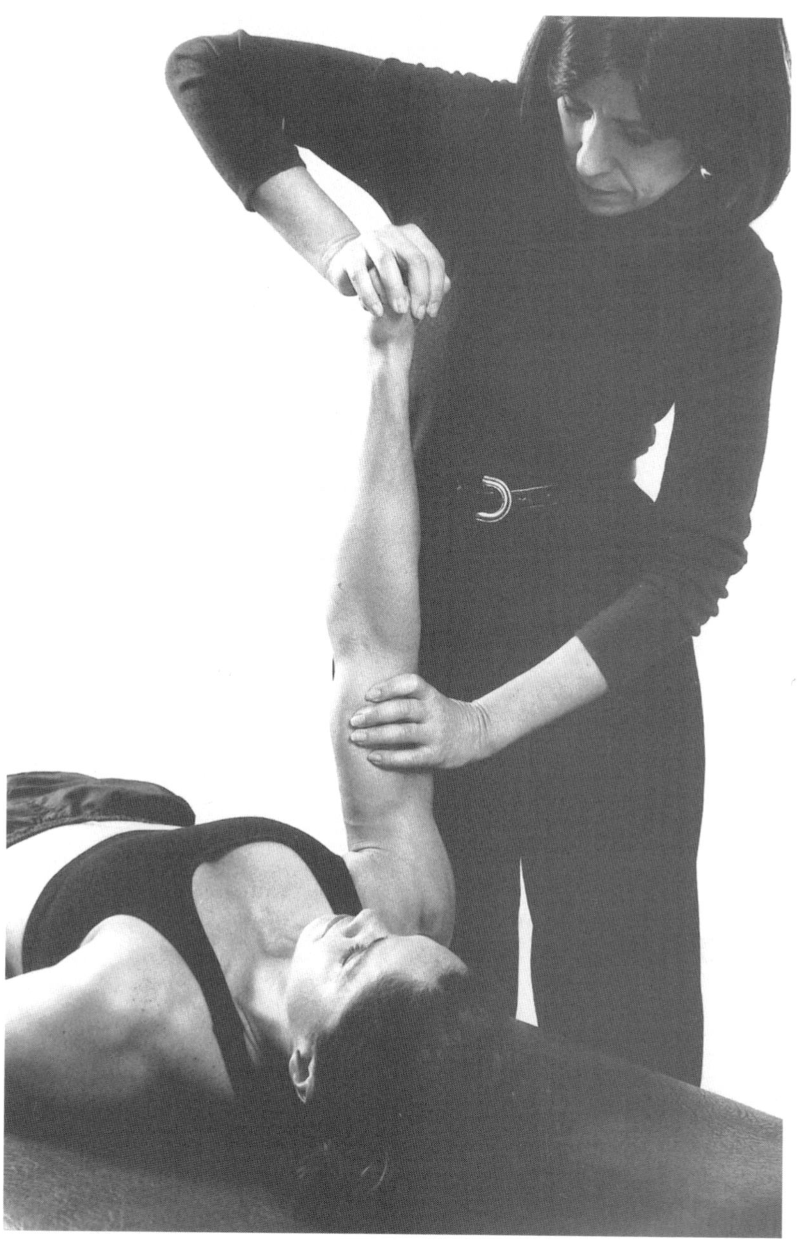

FIGURE 9-7 **Scapular protraction (punches)—beginning phase.**

PURPOSE: CKC exercise to strengthen the serratus anterior muscle.

POSITION: Client lying supine with shoulder flexed 90°; elbow extended; hand in fist.

PROCEDURE: Clinician places one hand at fist and one hand at lateral border of scapula or on upper arm. Clinician isometrically resists client's attempt to punch (keeping elbow extended).

tions to begin training the athlete to respond to quick, unexpected outside forces.

Cone drills can be progressed in intensity (increased speed without deterioration of technique) and duration. Medicine balls can be incorporated into the cone drills and the uneven surface drills. During these drills, the patient must perform the exercise as earlier described but must also catch and throw a ball without deterioration of technique (Fig. 9-14). Progressing to a medicine ball trains the patient to stabilize while loading and unloading external forces.

Functional equipment can be used to further progress the patient. Standing on a slide board develops lateral strength and stability and simulates motions that occur

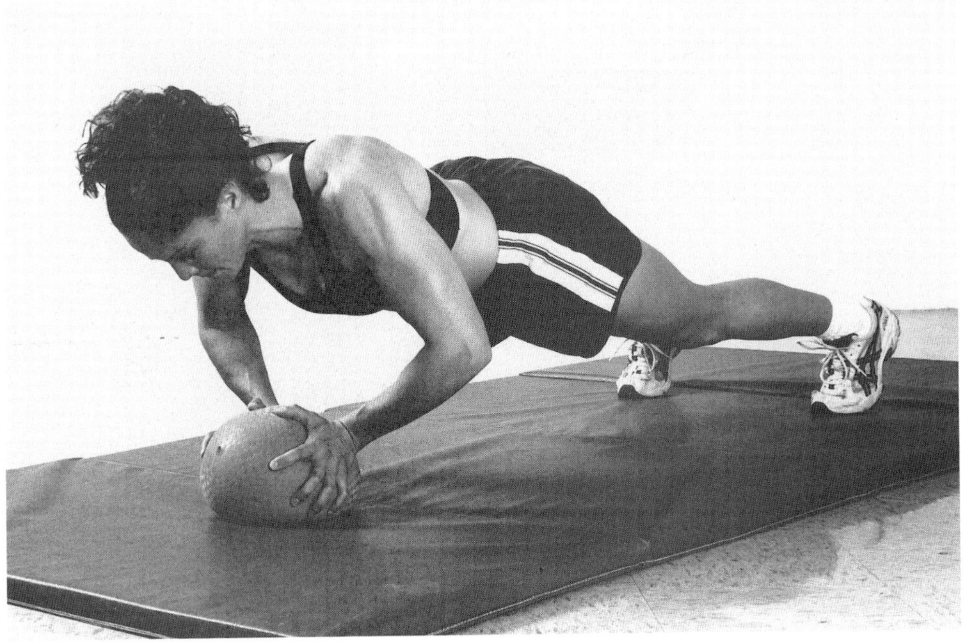

FIGURE 9-8 Push-up with hands placed on ball—advanced phase.

PURPOSE: CKC exercise to strengthen muscles of the scapulothoracic joint.

POSITION: Client in push-up position with hands on ball; arms extended.

PROCEDURE: Using arms, client lowers chest half the distance to ball, keeping hips in (do not allow hips to protrude). Client maintains position 3 to 5 sec.

FIGURE 9-9 Neuromuscular control exercises—advanced phase.

PURPOSE: CKC exercise to enhance neuromuscular control and isolate dynamic control of scapular muscles.

POSITION: Client side lying, with hand on support surface to fix distal segment.

PROCEDURE: Client slowly protracts/retracts and elevates/depresses scapula (proximal segment) to produce a circular motion. Clinician alternates between manual resistance and no resistance.

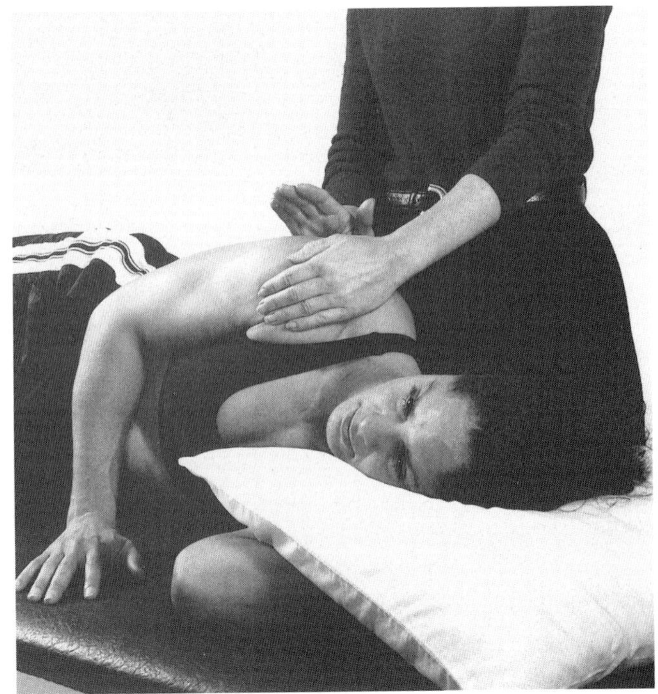

TABLE 9-5 Muscle Recruitment Patterns of Lower-Extremity CKC Activities

Class	Exercises
Muscular co-contractions	Vertical squats (0–30°)
	Lateral lunges with knee flexed to 30°
	Slide board (including Fitter)
	Balance drills with knee flexed to 30°
Quadriceps contractions	Wall squats
	Leg press (45–90°)
	Lateral step-ups
Hamstring contractions	Retrograde stair machines
	Squats > 45°
	Front lunges onto box

frequently in sports such as hockey (Fig. 11-19). Increase the challenge on the slide board by asking the athlete to perform upper-extremity exercises while incorporating dynamic lower-extremity side-to-side activities to facilitate the development of balance and agility. The slide board can be used to train quadriceps, hamstring, and gastrocnemius muscular co-contraction.

UPPER EXTREMITY PLYOMETRIC DRILLS

As noted, the implementation of the stretch–shortening program begins with the development of an adequate strength and physical condition base. A sample upper extremity stretch–shortening exercise program is presented to illustrate its clinical applications. The program is organized into four groups: warm-up exercises, throwing movements, trunk exercises, and wall exercises (Table 9-6). General suggestions for progressing the program are presented in Table 9-7.

Warm-Up

Warm-up exercises are designed to provide the body (especially the shoulder, arm, and trunk) an adequate physiologic preparation before beginning a plyometric program. An active warm-up should facilitate muscular performance by increasing blood flow, muscle and core temperatures, speed of contraction, oxygen use, and nervous system transmission. The first three warm-up exercises—trunk rotations (Fig. 9-15), trunk side bends, and wood chops (Fig. 9-16)—use a 9-lb medicine ball. Some warm-up exercises are performed with exercise tubing and include internal and external rotation movements of the shoulder with the arm in 90° of shoulder abduction and 90° of elbow flexion to simulate the throwing position. Finally, push-ups with both hands on the ground can enhance the warm-up period. Athletes should perform two to three sets of 10 repetitions each of these warm-up exercises before beginning the exercise session.

Throwing Movement

Throwing movement stretch–shortening exercises attempt to isolate the muscles and muscle groups necessary for throwing. These exercises are performed in combined movement patterns similar to the throwing motion. Beginning drills are throwing movement plyometrics using a 4-lb Plyoball (Integrated Functional Products, Dublin, CA). The first drill is a two-hand overhead soccer throw (Fig. 9-17), followed by a two-hand chest pass (Fig. 9-18). These exercises can be performed with a partner or with the use of a spring-loaded bounce-back device called the Plyoback (Integrated Functional Products).

In addition, several of the stretch–shortening drills require exercise tubing. The first movement involves stretch–shortening movement for the external rotators in which the athlete brings the tubing back into external rotation and holds that position for 2 sec (Fig. 9-19). The athlete then allows the external rotator musculature to release the isometric contraction, allowing the tubing to pull the arm into internal rotation. Thus the external rotators eccentrically control the movement. Once the arm reaches full internal rotation (horizontal), the external rotators contract concentrically to bring the tubing back into external rotation. This constitutes one stretch–shortening repetition.

Similar movements are performed for the internal rotators and for proprioceptive neuromuscular facilitation diagonal patterns, including D2 flexion and D2 extension of the upper extremity (see Figs. 8-7 and 8-8).

FIGURE 9-10 **Standing mini-squats—beginning phase.**

PURPOSE: CKC exercise to strengthen muscles of the lower extremity.

POSITION: Client standing; hands on support surface for balance control.

PROCEDURE: Client performs small (mini) squat from 0 to 30° of knee flexion.

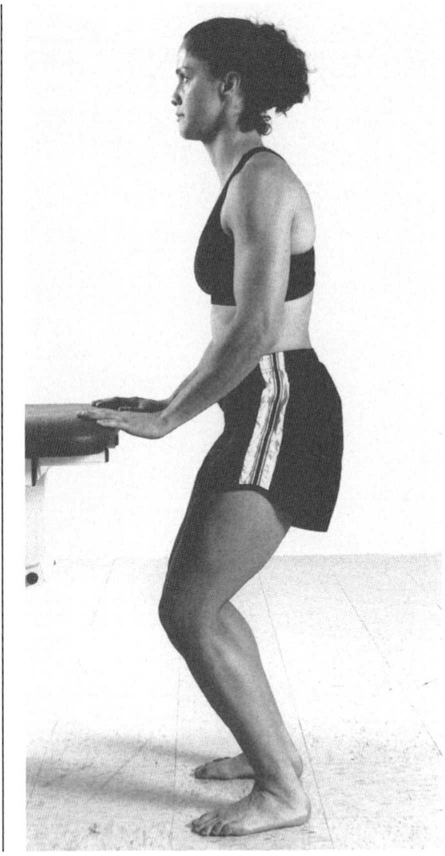

FIGURE 9-11 **Lateral step-ups—beginning phase.**

PURPOSE: CKC exercise to strengthen muscles of the lower extremity.

POSITION: Client standing with one foot on top of stool.

PROCEDURE: Client slowly extends hip and knee of extremity on stool to lift body up on stool. Client then slowly lowers body to floor.

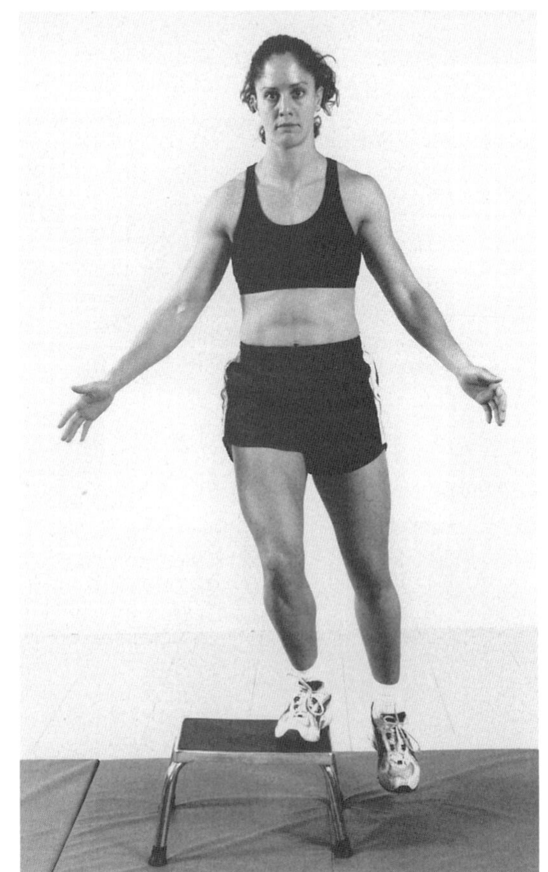

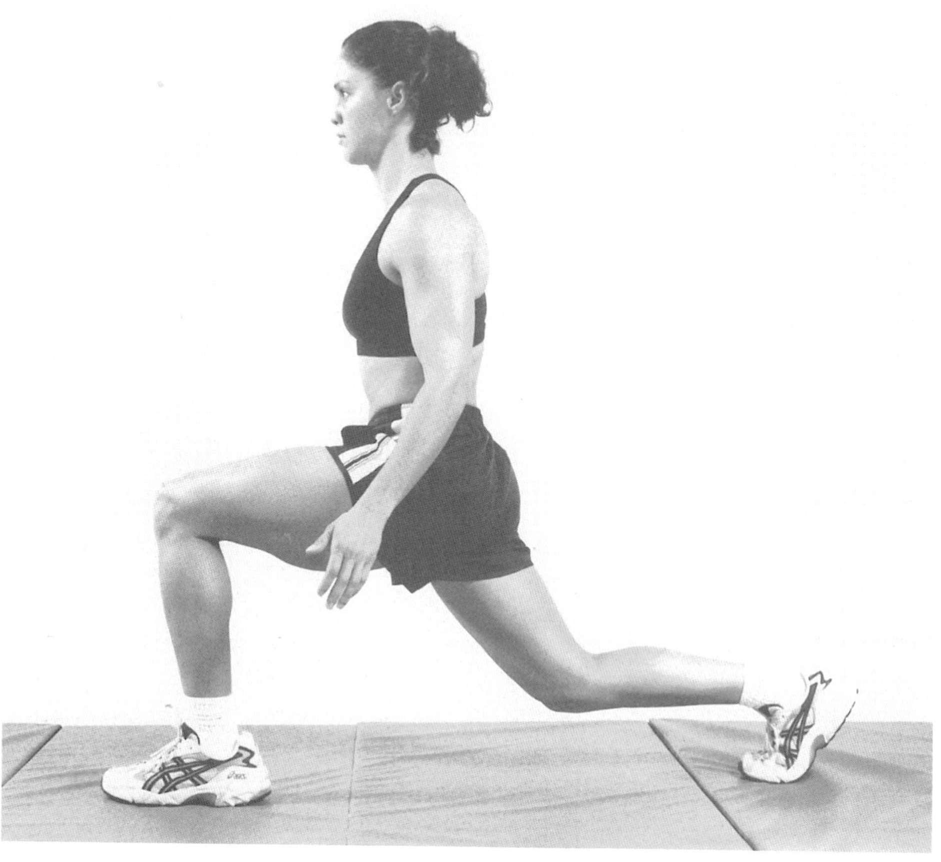

FIGURE 9-12 **Lunges—beginning phase.**

PURPOSE: CKC to strengthen muscles of the lower extremity.

POSITION: Client standing with feet together.

PROCEDURE: Client takes a step forward, lowering body until forward knee flexes to 90°. Client maintains position 1 to 2 sec and then returns to starting position.

The stretch–shortening technique can also be performed for the elbow flexors using exercise tubing.

Push-ups to enhance the strength of the serratus anterior, pectoralis major, deltoid, triceps, and biceps musculature can also be incorporated into the program. Push-ups can be advanced to a plyometric exercise by using the assistance of a clinician, performing push-ups against a wall (Fig. 9-20), and using a 6- to 8-in. box and the ground in a depth-jump-training manner (Fig. 9-21). Two to four sets of six to eight repetitions of all of these exercise drills are performed two to three times weekly.

Another group of exercises or drills uses a 2-lb medicine ball or Plyoball and a wall, which allows the athlete the opportunity to perform plyometric medicine ball drills. Using a 2-lb pound medicine ball, the athlete can perform a one-handed plyometric baseball throw (Fig. 9-22). To further challenge the athlete, exercises can be performed in the kneeling position to eliminate the use of the lower extremities and increase the demands on the trunk and upper extremities. A commonly used exercise drill is called wall dribbling. The athlete quickly dribbles a 2-lb ball against a wall, making a half circle. This drill is usually performed for a specific time period, e.g., 30 to 120 sec.

The purpose of the stretch–shortening throwing exercises is to provide the athlete with advanced strengthening exercises that are more aggressive and at a higher exercise level than a simple isotonic dumbbell exercise program. A stretch–shortening programs can implemented only after the patient has undergone a strengthening program for an extended period of time and has a satisfactory clinical examination.

Trunk Exercises

Two groups of stretch–shortening drills for trunk strengthening purposes emphasize the abdominal and trunk extensor muscles. Exercises in this group include medicine ball sit-ups, sit-ups with rotation, and sit-ups with throws (Fig. 9-23). Trunk exercise drills are performed two to

FIGURE 9-13 **Cone drills—intermediate phase.**

PURPOSE: CKC exercise to develop balance and control the joint movements of hip, knee, and ankle.

POSITION: Client standing. Two to three cones lined up 6 to 8 in. apart.

PROCEDURE: Using exaggerated high knees (hip flexion), client steps over cones.

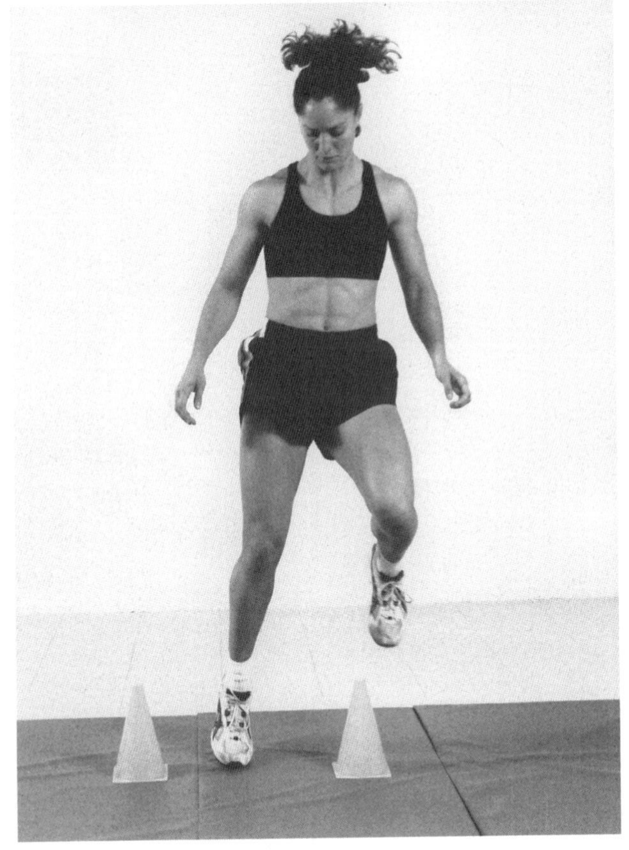

FIGURE 9-14 **Cone drills with medicine ball throws—advanced phase.**

PURPOSE: CKC exercise to develop balance and control the joint movement of hip, knee, and ankle and to train client to stabilize lower extremity while loading and unloading external forces.

POSITION: Client standing. Two to three cones lined up 6 to 8 in. apart.

PROCEDURE: Using exaggerated high knees (hip flexion), client steps over cones while catching and throwing a ball.

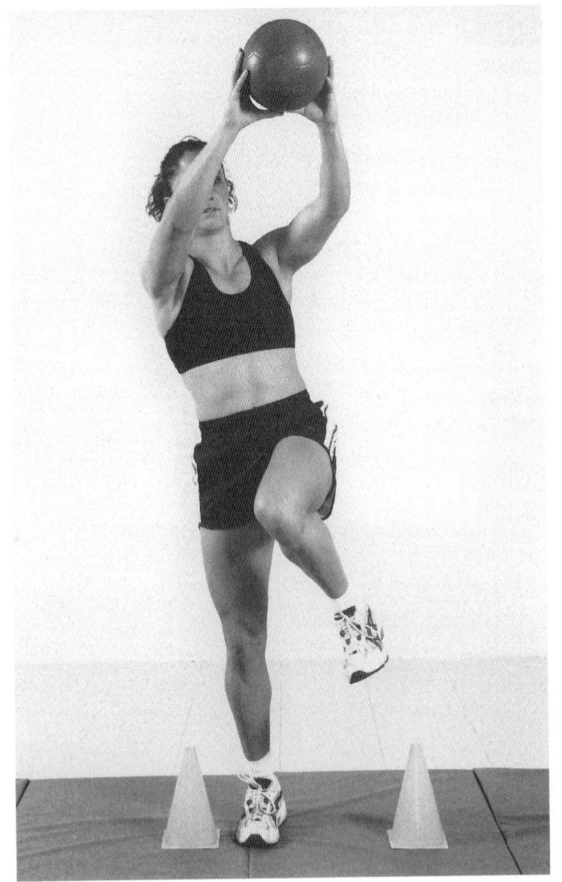

TABLE 9-6 Upper-Extremity Plyometric Program

Group	Exercises
Warm-up	Trunk rotation with medicine ball
	Side bends
	Wood chops
	Push-ups
	Internal and external shoulder rotation with tubing (90° abduction)
Throwing movements	Two-hand chest pass
	Two-hand soccer throw
	Internal and external shoulder rotation with tubing (90° abduction; fast speed)
	One-hand baseball throw
Trunk exercises	Sit-ups with medicine ball
	Sit-ups with rotation
	Sit-ups with throws and rotation
Wall exercises	Two-hand overhead soccer throw
	Two-hand chest pass
	One-hand baseball throw (standing; kneeling)
	One-hand wall dribble
	Multiple jumps

three times a week for three to four sets of six to eight repetitions. Performing trunk exercises is extremely important for the overhead athlete.

LOWER EXTREMITY PLYOMETRIC DRILLS

Implementation criteria of plyometric exercises for the lower extremity follow the same guidelines as those the upper extremity. Lower extremity plyometric drills can be divided into four different categories: warm-up, jump drills, box drills, and depth jumps (Table 9-8). Sport-specific drills should always be chosen to enhance the rehabilitation of the injured athlete. The clinician should observe the techniques of jumping and should stress correct posture, minimum side to side and forward to backward deviations, landing with toe-heel motion, landing with slightly flexed knees, and instant preparation for subsequent jumps. As the athlete progresses and the plyometric drills become more advanced, drills should concentrate on developing strength and power. As the patient masters proper technique, the focus shifts to quality, distance, height, or speed of jumping, depending on the goals of the athlete.

TABLE 9-7 General Guidelines for Progression of Lower-Extremity Plyometric Activities

Two-hand drills → One-hand drills
Bilateral drills → Unilateral drills
Light Plyoball → Heavy Plyoball
Movements close to body → Movements away from body
Single-joint movements → Multiple-joint movements
Straight planes → Diagonal planes
Single planes → Multiple planes
Specific drills → Sport-specific drills

Chu[34] suggested counting the number of foot contacts as a measure of frequency when using plyometrics for the lower extremity. A range of 60 to 100 foot touches per training session is considered appropriate for the beginner; 100 to 150, for the intermediate exerciser; and 150 to 200, for the advanced exerciser.

Warm-Up

As with any plyometric training program, an adequate warm-up is essential to avoid overuse injuries. Warm-up begins with stretching the lower extremities, followed by light running. Running can be progressed to include skipping, lateral side shuffles, backward running, and carioca drills.

Jumps

Jump drills begin with basic hops in place on both extremities (double-ankle hop) using full ankle range of motion for hopping momentum. This activity can be progressed to performing the exercise on one extremity (single-ankle hops). These exercises are of low intensity, and the client should focus on technique and amortization phase length. It is essential for the athlete to develop the proper recoil from each jump to minimize the length of the amortization phase. Squat jumping involves dropping into a squat position before jumping with maximal extension of the lower extremities (Fig. 9-24). Tuck jumps begin with a slight squat; then the athlete brings both knees up to the chest and holds until extending to land in a vertical position (Fig. 9-25). The vertical and tuck jumps should focus on the production of power; they require a period of recovery between jumps.

The 180° jumps begin with a two-footed jump; the patient rotates 180° in midair, holding the landing, and then

FIGURE 9-15 **Trunk rotation.**

PURPOSE: Warm-up exercise for upper extremity before plyometric drills.

POSITION: Client standing, holding medicine ball in both hands in front with elbows extended.

PROCEDURE: Client rotates trunk to right and to left keeping ball in front of body with elbows extended. It is important to pause at each extreme of rotation before rotating in opposite direction.

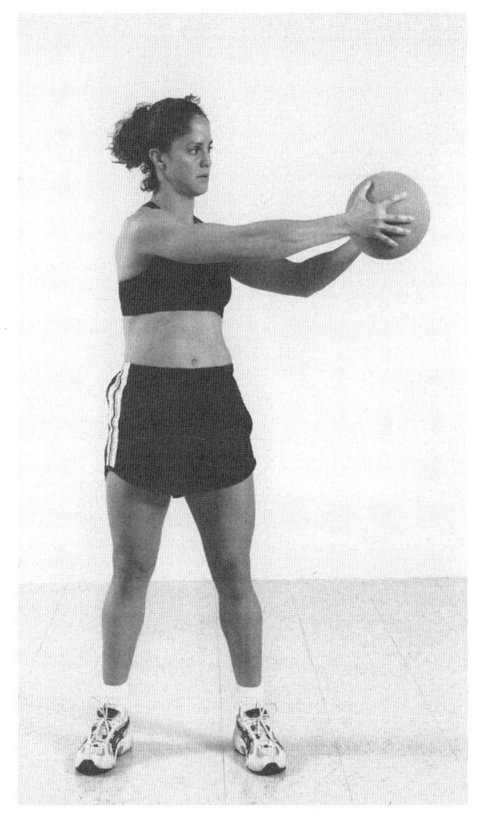

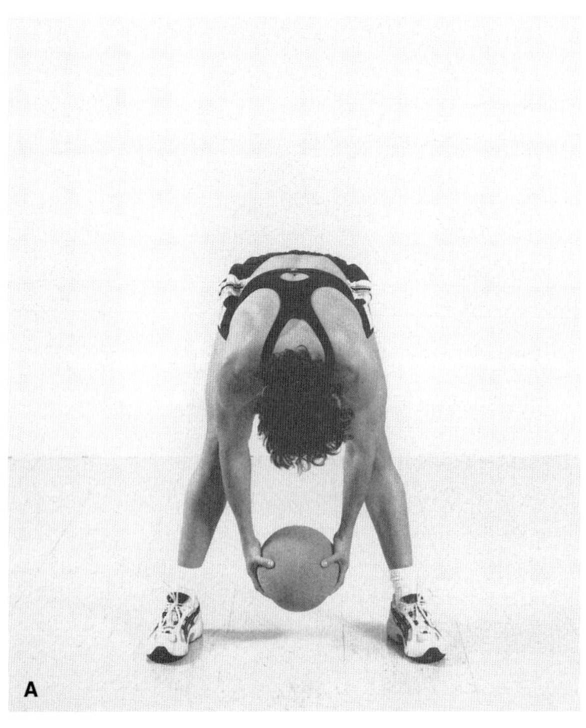

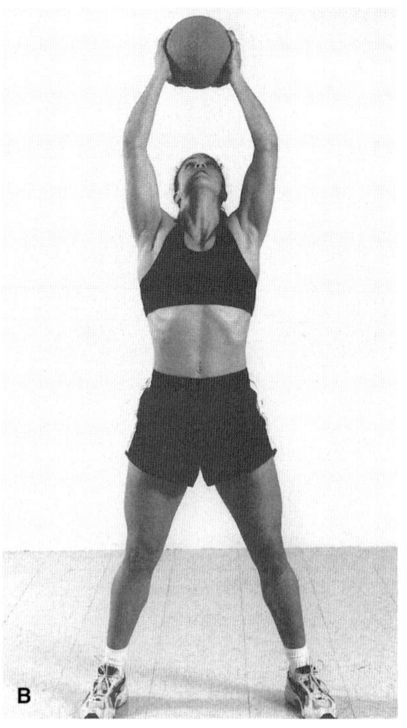

FIGURE 9-16 **Wood chops.**

PURPOSE: Warm-up exercise for upper extremity before plyometric drills.

POSITION: Client standing, holding medicine ball in both hands in front with elbows extended.

PROCEDURE: Client forward bends, pauses at full trunk flexion (panel A), and then extends spine fully while raising ball overhead (panel B). It is important to pause at each extreme of flexion and extension.

FIGURE 9-17 **Two-hand overhead soccer throw.**

PURPOSE: Plyometric drill to facilitate movement patterns similar to throwing motion.

POSITION: Client standing and holding medicine ball with both hands behind head.

PROCEDURE: Client takes one step forward and throws ball with both hands.

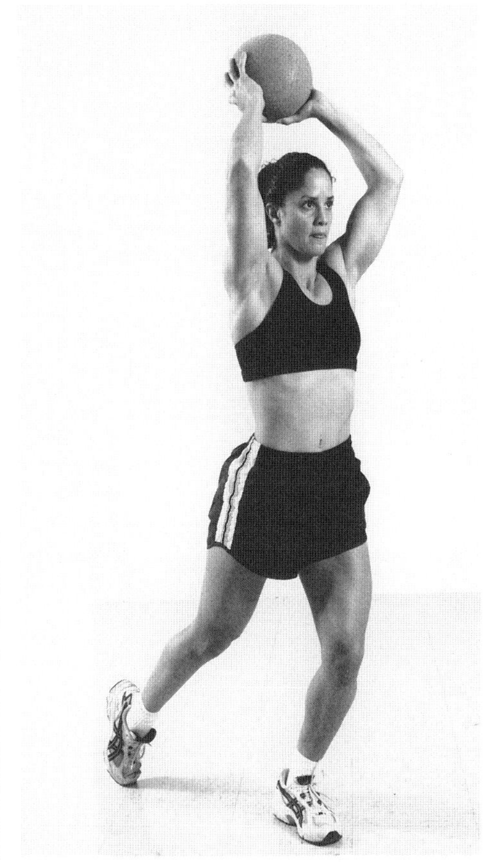

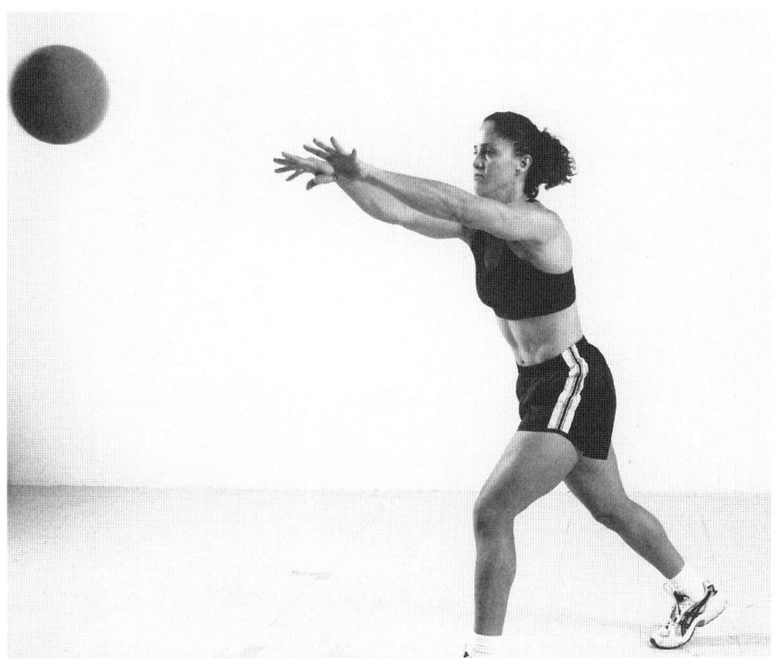

FIGURE 9-18 **Two-hand chest pass.**

PURPOSE: Plyometric drill to facilitate movement patterns similar to throwing motion.

POSITION: Client standing and holding medicine ball in both hands against chest.

PROCEDURE: Client takes one step forward and extends elbows, throwing ball by pushing with both hands.

FIGURE 9-19 External rotation with elastic tubing—throwing movement.

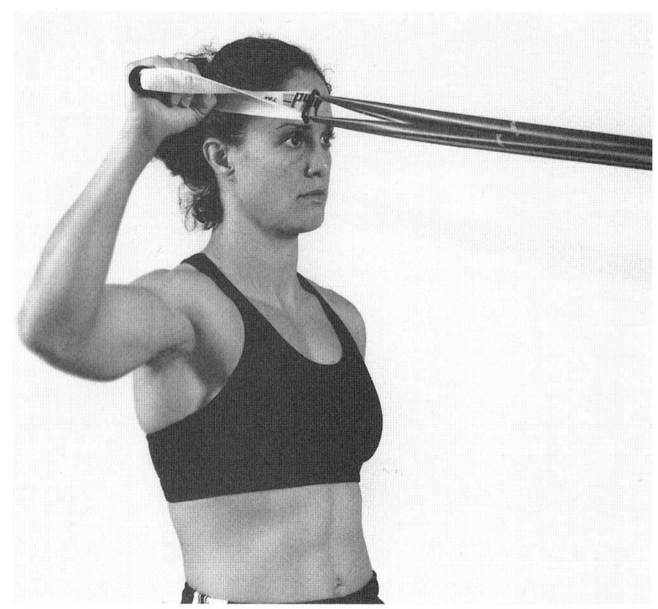

PURPOSE: Plyometric drill to facilitate stretch–shortening activities for external rotator muscles.

POSITION: Client standing and facing elastic tubing, which is attached to the wall at eye level, shoulder in 90° abduction and neutral external and internal rotation. Client holding elastic tubing.

PROCEDURE: Client pulls tubing back into external rotation (concentric contraction), holds position for 2 sec (isometric contraction), and then releases external rotator muscles to allow tubing to pull arm into internal rotation (eccentric contraction).

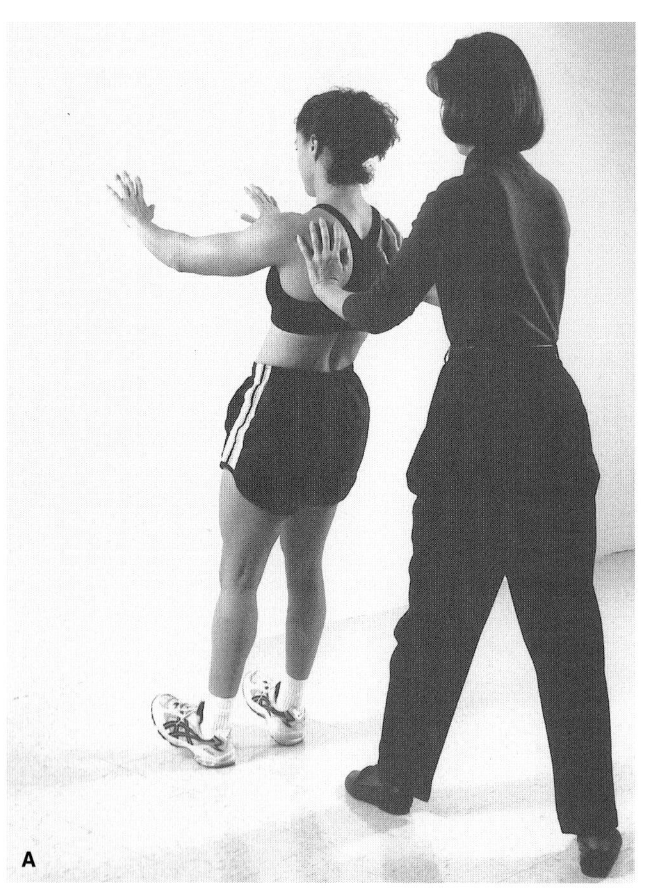

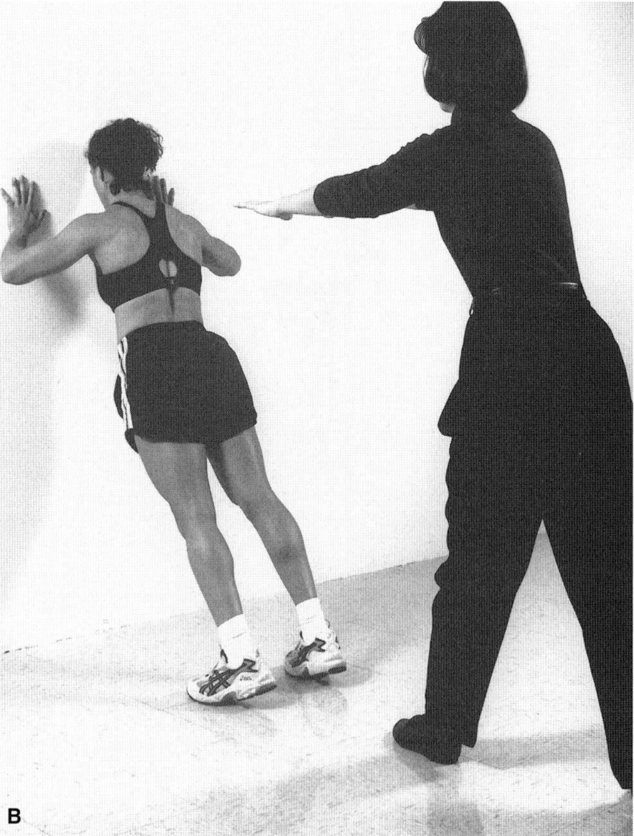

FIGURE 9-20 Plyometric push-ups on wall—advanced phase.

PURPOSE: Plyometric drill to strengthen muscles of the glenohumeral and scapulothoracic joint.

POSITION: Client standing with feet 8 to 10 in. from wall with hands in push-up position against wall. Clinician standing behind client.

PROCEDURE: Keeping feet in place, client pushes body from wall by extending arms (concentric contraction). Clinician catches patient, and pushes patient back toward the wall (panel A). Patient catches body against wall with hands (eccentric contraction) (panel B) and immediately pushes away again (concentric contraction)

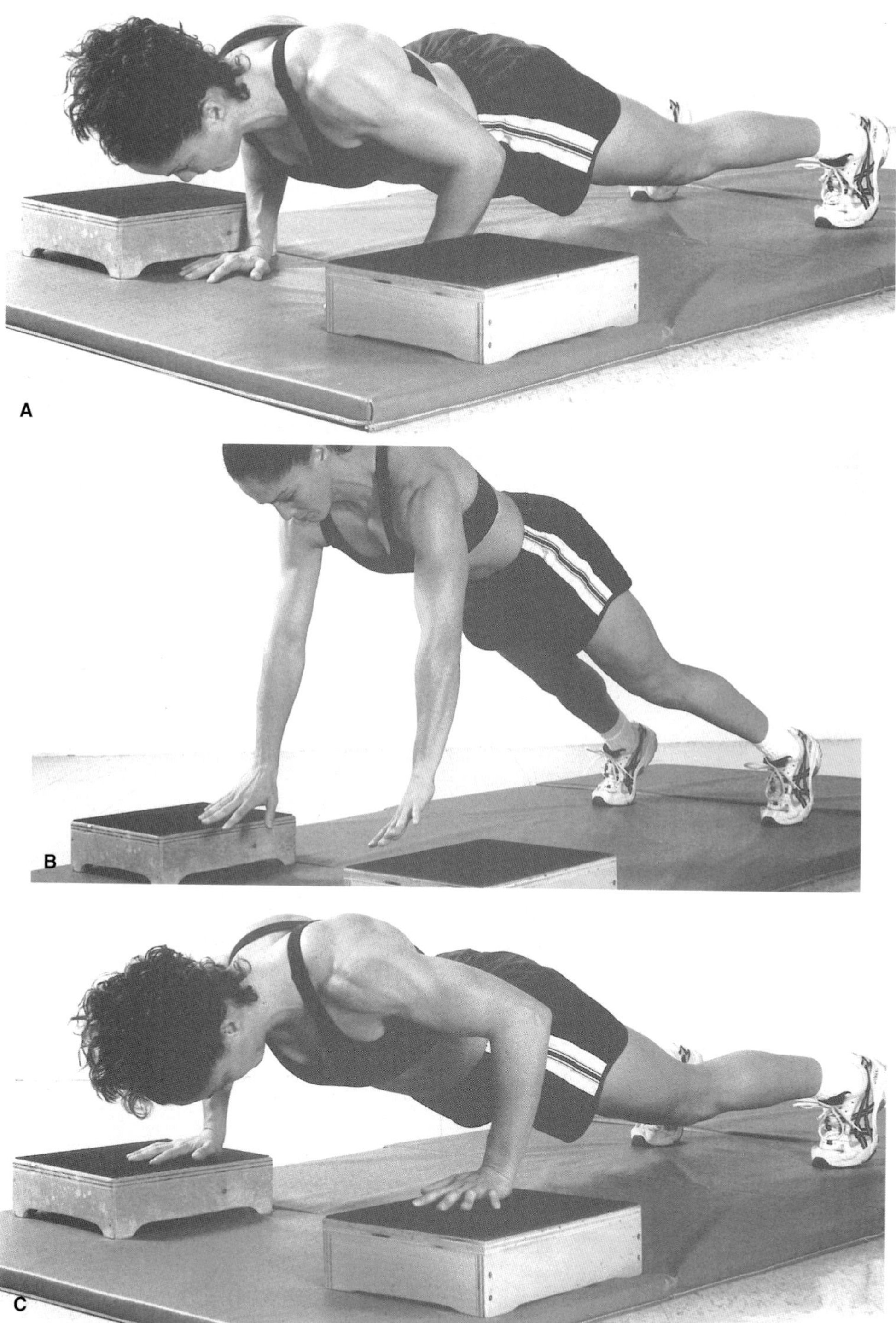

FIGURE 9-21 **Plyometric push-ups with boxes—advanced phase.**

PURPOSE: Plyometric drills to strengthen muscles of the glenohumeral and scapulothoracic joint.

POSITION: Client in push-up position between two 6- to 8-in.-high boxes (panel A).

PROCEDURE: From the support surface, client pushes with arms hard enough to lift body from ground (concentric contraction) (panel B). When high enough off ground, client moves upper extremity slightly laterally and catches body with hands on boxes (eccentric contraction) (panel C). Client then pushes off boxes to lift body from boxes (concentric contraction) and catches body on support surface (eccentric contraction).

FIGURE 9-22 One-handed plyometric baseball throw on wall—throwing movement.

PURPOSE: Plyometric drills to facilitate stretch–shortening activities for external rotator muscles.

POSITION: Client standing directly in front of wall with shoulder in 90° abduction and full external rotation and elbow in 90° flexion. Client holding small medicine ball in one hand.

PROCEDURE: Client repeatedly internally rotates shoulder to throw (concentric exercise) ball against wall and catches ball as it returns from wall (eccentric contraction).

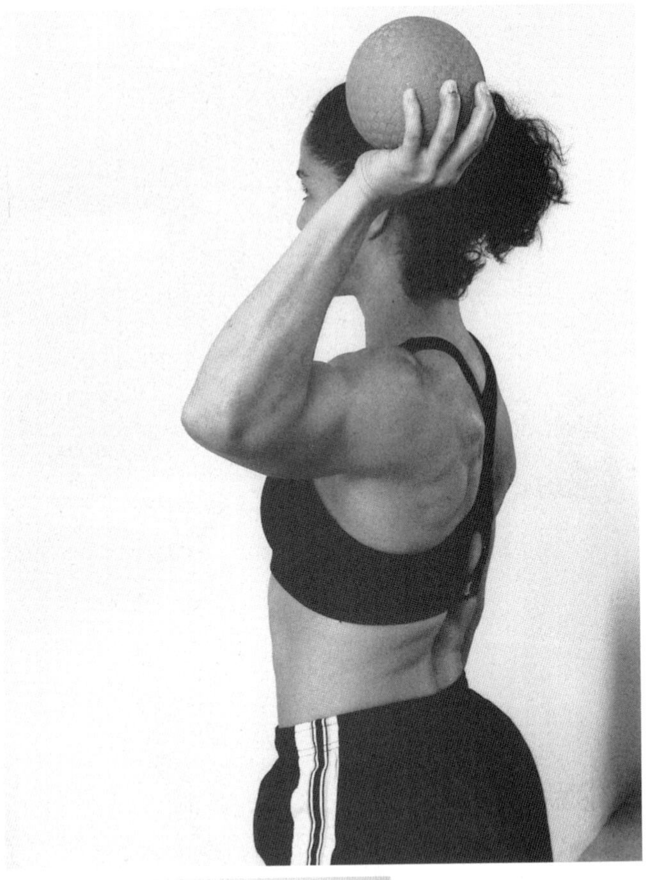

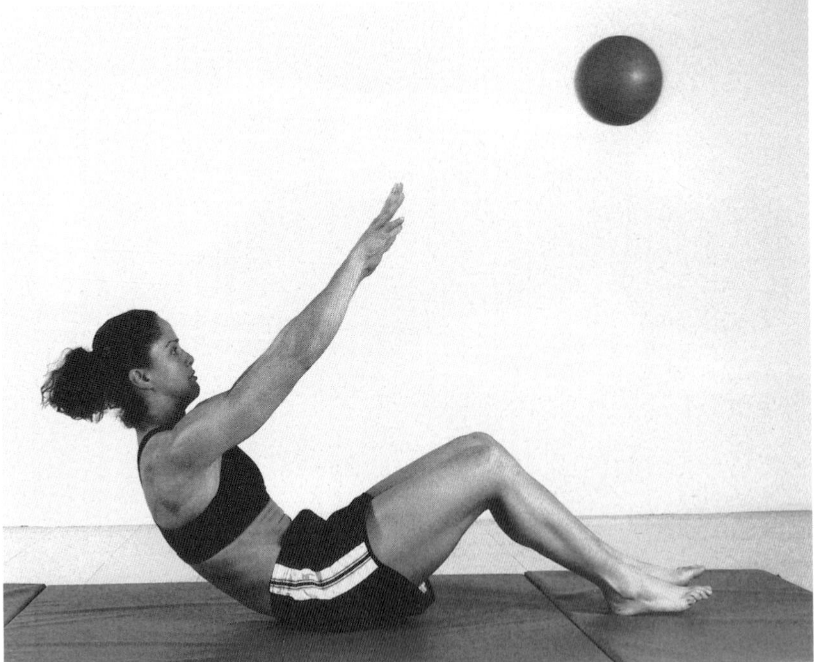

FIGURE 9-23 Sit-up with throw—trunk.

PURPOSE: Strengthen abdominal muscles.

POSITION: Client lying supine with knees flexed, holding medicine ball in both hands overhead.

PROCEDURE: Client sits up and simultaneously throws ball with overhead soccer throw.

TABLE 9-8 Lower-Extremity Plyometric Program

Group	Exercises
Warm-up	Stretching of lower-extremity muscles
	Running
	Skipping
	Lateral side shuffles
	Backward running
	Carioca
Jump drills	Double-ankle hops
	Single-ankle hops
	Squat jumps
	Vertical jumps
	Tuck jumps
	180° jumps
	Agility jumps
Box drills	Front jumps
	Lateral jumps
	Multiple jumps
Depth jumps	Forward jumps
	Squat depth jumps

reverses direction. Cones or tape on the floor can be used for multiple forward, lateral, diagonal, or zigzag jumps and hops on one or two limbs (called agility jumps) (Fig. 9-26). The athlete is instructed to jump as quickly as possible to the cone or tape. One of the most important aspects of plyometric training is the landing after the jump. A soft landing is strongly encouraged, and the patient is told to land as light as a feather. The soft landing aids in controlling ground-reaction forces.

Box Jumps

Box jumps (aerobic benches can be used) begin with basic front and lateral box jumps (Fig. 9-27). The athlete begins on level ground and jumps onto a box of prescribed height. To do box push-off drills, the patient faces a box and puts one foot on it. Then the patient extends the lower extremity that is on the box, achieving maximal height and landing on top of the box. The patient returns to the original position. The patient can alternate the lower extremities, working each one in turn. Lateral push-off drills can also be incorporated.

Multiple box jumps can be performed in the forward or lateral direction, with the athlete jumping up onto the box, down from the box, and then back up to another box (Fig. 9-28). In addition, turns can be added (Fig. 9-29). Box drills can be progressed from low intensity to high intensity by adjusting the height of the box. Furthermore, the individual can be progressed from performing the exercise on two legs to performing it on one extremity.

Depth Jumps

Box jumps are progressed to include depth jumps. Depth jumps from atop a box use the athlete's potential energy to vary the ground-reaction forces produced during landing. The simplest form of depth jumping involves the athlete stepping from the top of a box and landing flexed and holding the landing (Fig. 9-30). The athlete should not jump from the box but rather step off the edge of the box so the exercise can be reliably reproduced at different prescribed heights.

Once the proper landing technique is learned and tolerated by the patient, depth jumps can be followed by a maximal vertical jump, recoiling as rapidly as possible after absorbing the impact. The athlete recoils after landing and jumps up from landing as rapidly as possible to decrease the amortization phase. A squat depth jump

FIGURE 9-24 **Squat jumps.**

PURPOSE: Plyometric drill to strengthen lower extremity muscles.

POSITION: Client in squat position.

PROCEDURE: From squat position (panel A), client jumps vertically as high as possible (concentric contraction) (panel B). Upon landing, client absorbs shock into squat (eccentric contraction). Repeat.

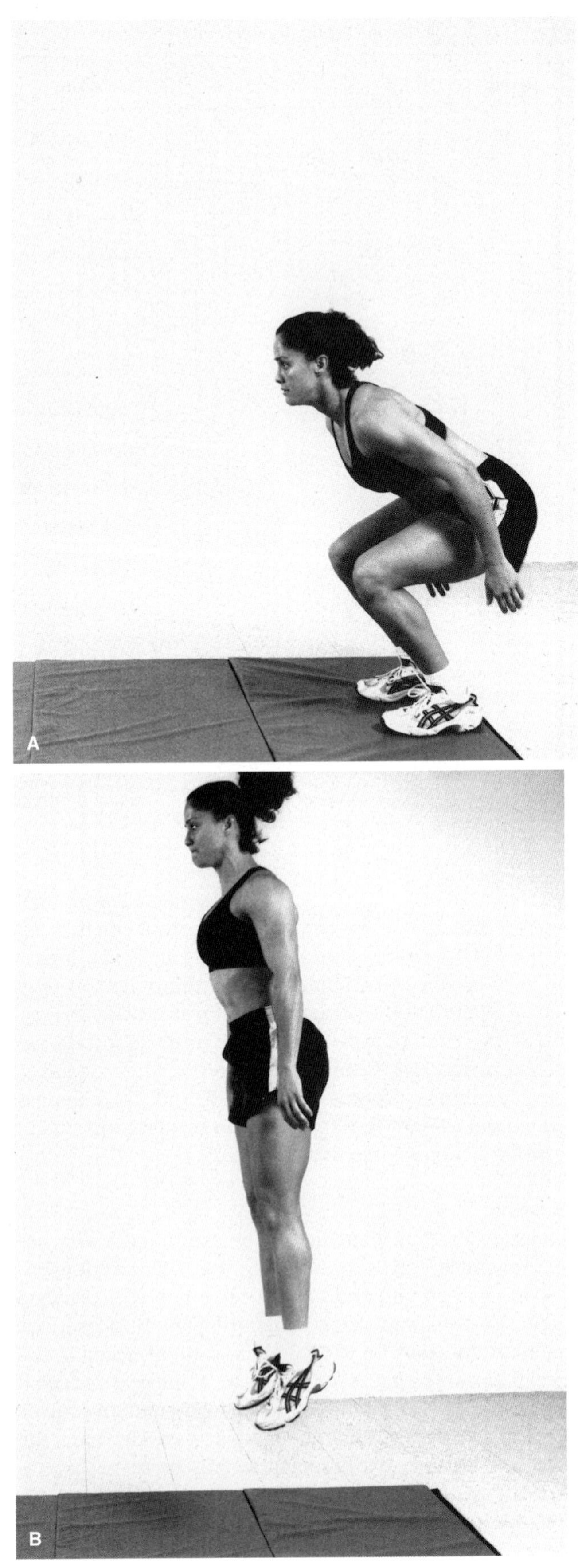

FIGURE 9-25 **Tuck jumps.**

PURPOSE: Plyometric drill to strengthen lower extremity muscles.

POSITION: Client standing.

PROCEDURE: Client jumps vertically as high as possible (concentric contraction). During jump, client brings both knees up to chest and holds briefly (accentuation of concentric contraction). Client absorbs shock on landing (eccentric contraction). Repeat.

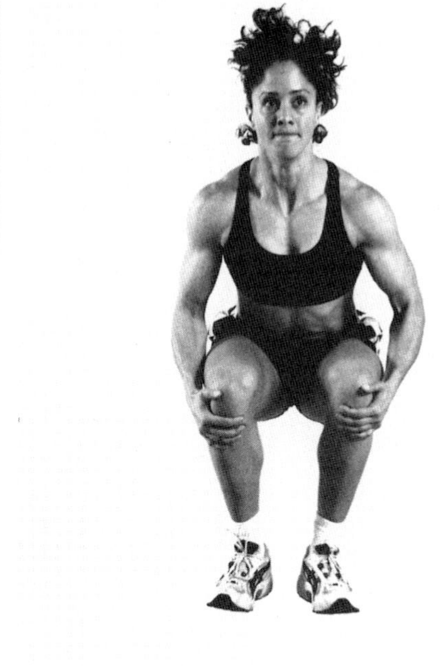

FIGURE 9-26 **Agility jumps.**

PURPOSE: Plyometric drill to enhance agility.

POSITION: Client standing; tape on floor marks four quadrants.

PROCEDURE: Client quickly jumps from one quadrant to the next quadrant, jumping as quickly as possible and landing lightly.

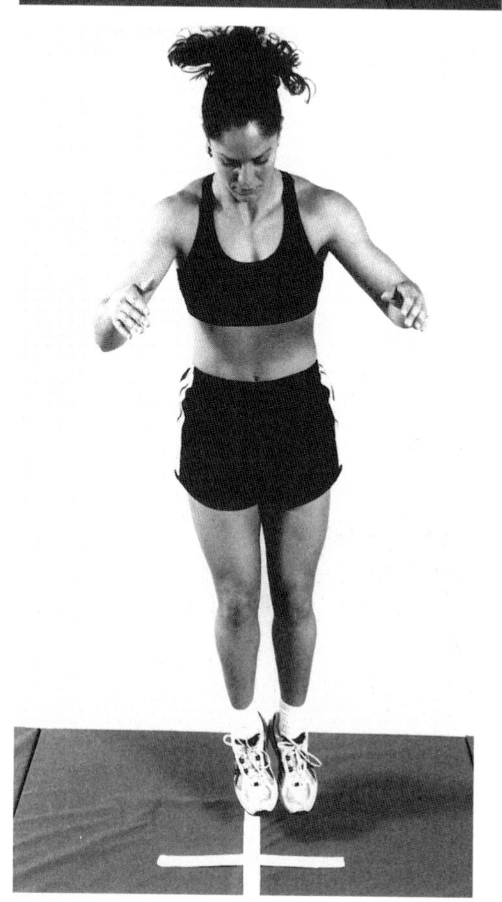

FIGURE 9-27 **Front box jumps.**

PURPOSE: Plyometric drills to facilitate stretch–shortening of lower-extremity muscles.

POSITION: Client standing and facing box.

PROCEDURE: Facing box, client jumps up to land on box (concentric contraction). After landing (eccentric contraction), client immediately jumps from box back to floor (concentric contraction). Repeat.

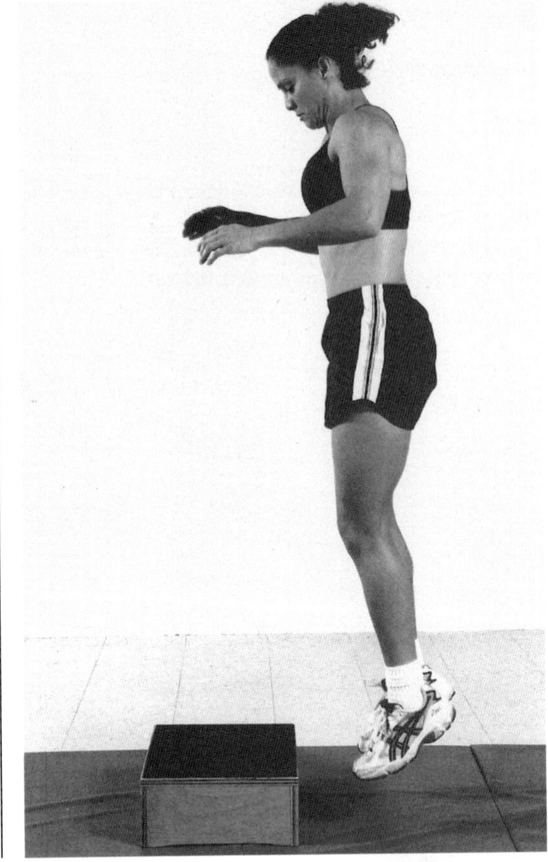

FIGURE 9-28 **Multiple box jumps.**

PURPOSE: Plyometric drills to facilitate stretch–shortening of lower-extremity muscles.

POSITION: Client standing between two boxes but not facing either box.

PROCEDURE: Facing same direction during entire drill, client jumps laterally up to land on first box (concentric contraction). After landing (eccentric contraction), patient immediately jumps back to floor (concentric contraction). Patient lands on ground (eccentric contraction) and immediately jumps laterally to land on second box (concentric contraction), then immediately jumps back to the original position (concentric contraction).

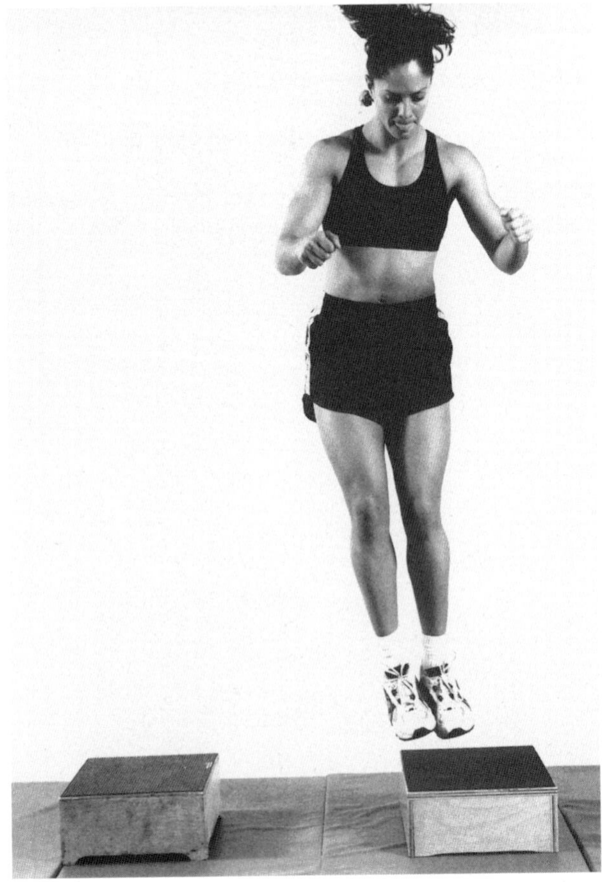

FIGURE 9-29 Multiple box jumps with turns.

PURPOSE: Plyometric drills to facilitate stretch–shortening for lower-extremity muscles.

POSITION: Client standing between two boxes but not facing either box.

PROCEDURE: Client jumps up and simultaneously turns to land on first box (concentric contraction). After landing (eccentric contraction), patient immediately jumps from box while turning in original direction (concentric contraction). Client lands on ground (eccentric contraction) and immediately jumps and simultaneously turns toward second box (concentric contraction). Client lands on second box (eccentric contraction), then immediately jumps from box and turns back to original position (concentric contraction).

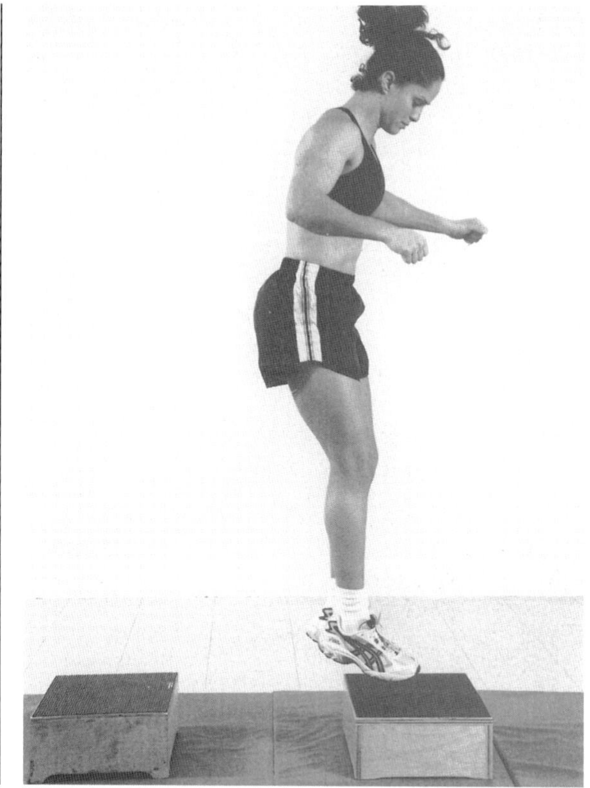

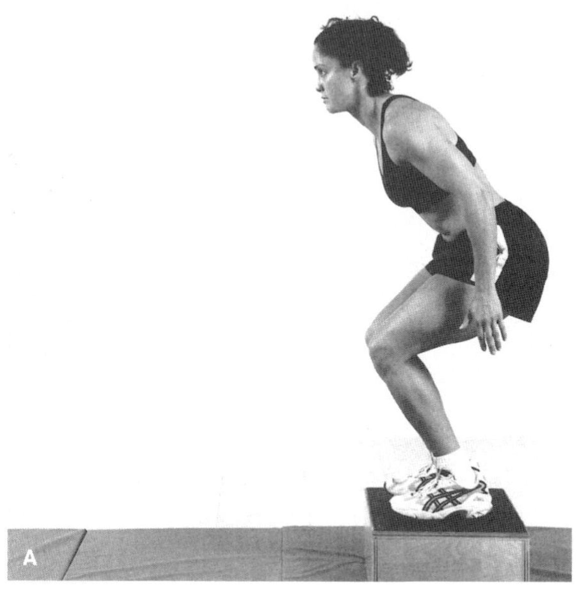

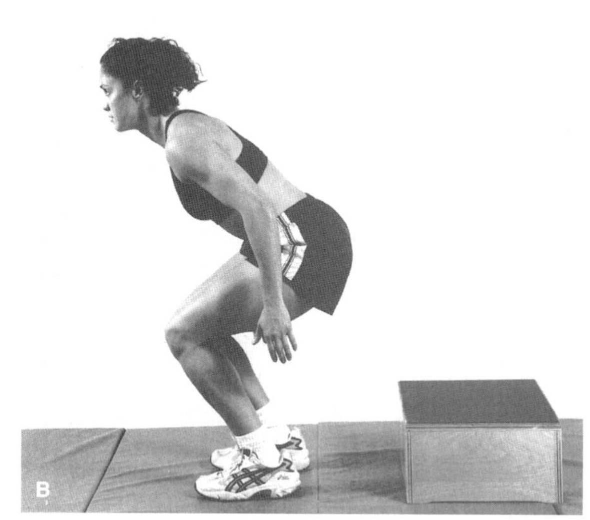

FIGURE 9-30 Depth jumps.

PURPOSE: Plyometric drills to facilitate stretch–shortening for lower-extremity muscles.

POSITION: Client standing on top of box.

PROCEDURE: Client steps off edge of box (should not jump) (panel A) and sticks the landing in a squat position (eccentric contraction) (panel B).

NOTE: The exercise can end in squat position or client can jump up out of squat position (concentric contraction). For added difficulty, client can jump (concentric contraction) and land on second box (eccentric contraction).

begins with the athlete stepping off a box and landing in a squat position, followed by a quick explosion out of the squat and again landing in a squat position. For added difficulty, the athlete can land on a second box.

PROGRESSION

Plyometric exercises for the lower extremity can be progressed by adding weight (using medicine balls), altering the height of box drills and depth jumps, and jumping from and landing on uneven surfaces. Each progression stresses the athlete's force production, eccentric control of landing, and modulation of proprioceptive input. In addition, all plyometric exercises can be progressed by advancing the activity from two legs to one leg for a very aggressive plyometric exercise program.

PRECAUTIONS: PLYOMETRICS

Contraindications to performing upper and lower extremity plyometric exercises include acute inflammation or pain, immediate postoperative pathology, and gross instabilities. The most significant contraindication to an intense stretch–shortening exercise program is for individuals who have not been involved in a weight-training program. Intense stretch–shortening exercise programs are intended to be advanced strengthening programs for the competitive athlete to enhance athletic performance and are not recommended for the recreational athlete. Athletes appear to exhibit the greatest gain from a well-designed plyometric program. The clinician should be aware of the adverse reactions secondary to this form of exercise, such as delayed-onset muscular soreness. In addition, it should be noted that this form of exercise should not be performed for an extended period of time, because of the large stresses that occur during exercise. More appropriately, stretch–shortening exercise is used during the first and second preparation phases of training, using the concept of periodization (see Chapter 5).

CASE STUDY

PATIENT INFORMATION

The patient was an 18-year-old male who played high school football and ran track. He injured his knee during football practice while he was trying to block a lineman. He reported that his left knee was planted when he felt the knee pop and shift out of place. He stated that pain was immediate and he was unable to walk without limping.

The athlete presented to the clinic 1 day after injury. Examination indicated an antalgic flexed knee gait and moderate joint effusion. He was able to perform a straight leg raise with 0° extension. Active range of motion (ROM) was 0 to 116° and 0 to 146° for the involved and noninjured knees, respectively. The Lachman's test was positive.

Examination was consistent with a diagnosis of sprain to the anterior cruciate ligament (ACL). The athlete was referred to an orthopedic surgeon, who recommended autogenous bone–patellar tendon–bone ACL reconstruction.

LINKS TO *Guide to Physical Therapist Practice* and *Athletic Training Educational Competencies*

According to the *Guide*,[15] pattern 4D relates to the diagnosis of this patient. The pattern is described as "impaired joint mobility, motor function, muscle performance, and range of motion associated with other connective tissue dysfunction" and includes sprains of the knee and leg. Direct intervention includes "strengthening and power, including plyometric," exercises and "neuromuscular education and reeducation." No specific reference is made to CKC exercises.

In the therapeutic exercise domain, the *Competencies*[36] refers to treatment of athletes using a variety of techniques. In the teaching objectives listed under this domain, the *Competencies* indicates that the athletic trainer, upon graduation from an accredited program, will be able to "describe indications, contraindications, theory and principles for the incorporation and application of various contemporary therapeutic exercises including closed chain and plyometrics." The document also emphasizes the demonstration of these same exercises.

INTERVENTION

One Week Postsurgery

One week after surgery, the athlete returned, demonstrating a slight antalgic gait without assistive devices. He reported using the continuous passive motion machine (CPM) machine on his ACL-reconstructed knee (see Fig. 2-33). He presented with moderate joint effusion; pain was rated at 1/5; ROM was 0 to 100° and 0 to 142° for the involved and noninvolved knees, respectively.

Initial goals included decreasing swelling, obtaining full passive knee extension, and obtaining 110° of flexion. Intervention consisted of the following home exercise program:

1. Discontinue use of CPM.
2. Heel props: 10 min every hour (while lying supine, patient props prop heel up on towel roll and places weight over the anterior knee to promote increased extension).

GERIATRIC *Perspectives*

- Functional assessment of older adults should include examination of specific CKC task performance requiring integration of dynamic multijoint motion and incorporating concentric, eccentric, and isometric muscle activity.[1] Examination of task performance in dynamic movements involves the whole individual and his or her interaction with the environmental aspects of the tasks (e.g., the height of steps or other surface). Functional tests to examine CKC control may include bilateral stance with knee flexion, unilateral stance with knee flexion, and bilateral and unilateral balance reactions and equilibrium responses when standing with eyes open and closed.[1]
- Older adults need to perform exercises directed toward gains in function and independence. Independent performance of activities of daily living (ADLs) require that the lower extremities function in closed-chain tasks.[1] Examples of such ADLs are dressing oneself and toileting.
- Strengthening programs should include both CKC and OKC (Chapter 6) exercises to maximize physical performance.[2] Closed-chain exercises emphasize control while the distal end is fixed, whereas open-chain exercises improve control when the distal end is free moving. A good example of such interaction between closed- and open-chain exercise is walking, in which the cyclic movement requires that the distal point of contact alternate between fixed and free.
- Because older adults are more prone to falls in challenging postural tasks, special attention should be given to the placement of the center of mass (Chapter 12) and the placement of the foot during CKC exercise. In addition, the exercise should be performed slowly with control and with external support, as needed for safety.
- With the exception of the older athlete, plyometrics may not be the optimal choice for rehabilitation of the aged. Movements requiring quick power and rapid muscle reactivity should be used with caution because of age-related changes in muscle tissue.

1. Scott KF. Closed kinetic chain assessment: rehabilitation of improved function in the older patient. Top Geriatr Rehabil 1995;11:1–5.
2. Judge JO. Resistance training. Top Geriatr Rehabil 1993;8:38–50.

3. Prone hangs with weight: 10 min every hour.
4. Wall slides and heel slides: three times a day (Fig. 2-14).
5. Patellar mobilization (Fig. 4-27).

Two Weeks Postsurgery

At 2 weeks after surgery, the athlete reported that his knee had improved daily and he worked on his home exercises daily. He presented with normal gait but still rated his pain at 1/5. A mild effusion was present. Range of motion was 0 to 126° for the reconstructed knee.

The goals at this point were to maintain full extension, control swelling, increase flexion, and begin early strengthening. The home exercise program was updated to include the following:

1. Standing mini-squats from 0 to 30° (Fig. 9-10).
2. Forward step-ups.
3. Stationary bicycle (Fig. 10-5).
4. Continue wall slides and prone hangs.

One Month Postsurgery

One month postsurgery, the athlete stated that his knees continued to improve and he rated his reconstructed knee at 60%. He presented with normal gait, mild effusion, and no reports of pain. Range of motion was 0 to 135°.

Goals were to achieve full flexion ROM and to progress to more advanced strengthening activities. The program at this stage was as follows:

1. Progress squat to a range of 0 to 60°.
2. Progress step-up to include forward and lateral movements (Fig. 9-11).
3. Forward lunges (Fig. 9-12).
4. Initiation of balance activities (Figs. 11-11 and 11-12).
5. Continue bicycle.

Two Months Postsurgery

Examination at the 2-month follow-up indicated that ROM was equal bilaterally. The home exercise program consisted of the following:

PEDIATRIC *Perspectives*

- Plyometrics can be used to train children in fun, play-related movements such as hopscotch and bouncing activities.[1] Use of plyometrics during rehabilitation is determined by the needs of the patient for his or her chosen activity.[1] Children who are not competitive athletes may engage in many common activities that do not require aggressive plyometric training. Take into account the patient's age, experience, maturity, and attention span when considering use of plyometrics.[1] Lack of sufficient attention span may contraindicate the use of plyometrics in rehabilitation of children.
- In children, as in adults, the muscles of postural support must be strong enough to withstand the stresses of plyometric training. When using plyometrics, the training level and muscular conditioning base of the participant must be taken into account. For children who are essentially "untrained" and who lack basic muscular strength, endurance, and neuromuscular coordination, low-intensity CKC and plyometric activities may be at top limit of intervention methods. Examples of low-intensity exercises that may be used are single-leg squats and jump/play activities. Use discretion and close supervision when requiring medium-intensity skills.[2] It is probably wise to avoid high-intensity and large vertical dimensions when using plyometrics with most children.
- It is common for children to lack coordination, which suggests the need to pay attention to proper technique during training. Ongoing supervision during plyometric programs used with children is essential. Be certain that children's performances are routinely evaluated and that youngsters are able to demonstrate mastery of a skill before given clearance to move to the next level of difficulty in a program.
- Concentric strengthening may be preferable as children develop mature muscles (see "Pediatric Perspectives" in Chapter 5) and bones. Therefore, good judgment must be used when prescribing CKC and plyometric exercises to children; both interventions have significant eccentric muscle actions, even at low levels.
- For highly trained child athletes, plyometrics may be a requisite for complete return to function. For example, a young female gymnast must be able to perform many complex CKC and plyometric movements of both the upper and lower extremities. To complete a well-designed functional progression, sport-specific movements should be incorporated into the rehabilitation via both CKC and plyometric exercises.

1. Chu D. Jumping into plyometrics. Champaign, IL: Leisure, 1992.
2. Albert M. Eccentric muscle training in sports and orthopedics. New York: Churchill-Livingston, 1995.

1. Continue bicycle
2. Continue closed-chain step-ups, mini-squats, and lunges.
3. Begin closed-chain cone drills (Fig. 9-13).
4. Begin calf raises.
5. Step machine (Fig. 10-7).
6. Open-chain hamstring curls with weight.

Three Months Postsurgery

At 3 months, the athlete reported that he continued to improve and feel stronger. He also reported no problem with the home exercise program. Isokinetic examination indicated that the left quadriceps strength was 70% of the right. The exercise program was revised as follows:

1. Jogging
2. Plyometric program: warm-up exercises (jogging; hamstring, quadriceps, and gastrocnemius stretching; Figs. 3-7 to 3-10, 3-17), double-ankle jumps, and tuck jumps (Fig. 9-25).
3. Open-chain quadriceps strengthening (see Fig. 6-18).
4. Continue closed-chain exercise program.

Four Months Postsurgery

After 4 months, the patient was progressing well. The home exercise program was revised as follows:

1. Continue open-chain strengthening.
2. Continue plyometric program.
3. Single-ankle jumps
4. Box jumps (Figs. 9-27 to 9-29).
5. Continue jogging program.

Five Months Postsurgery

At the 5-month follow-up the patient reported no problems with any activities during the previous month. Functional testing using a one-legged hop for distance and a one-legged vertical hop indicated no deficit in the injured knee. The goal at this point was to prepare the athlete to return to full activities and competition. The home exercise program was progressed to include running and agility drills with his football coach. In addition, the athlete was instructed to perform depth jumps two times per week (Fig. 9-30).

OUTCOME

Examination at the end of 6 months indicated no deficits in the left knee. The athlete was cleared to participate in all activities. He completed an uneventful season in football and track the following year.

SUMMARY

- When designing a rehabilitation program for a patient, the clinician must consider the patient's goals and functional demands. Based on these desired goals the clinician can begin to formulate a rehabilitation program.
- An integrated program that uses both open- and closed-kinetic exercises is the most appropriate plan. There are unique advantages to each form of exercise, and the clinician should carefully consider them when developing a program. Plyometrics are designed to provide a functional form of exercise just before the initiation of sport-specific training. They are an excellent from of training for the competitive athlete.

REFERENCES

1. Verkhoshanski Y. Depth jumping in the training of jumpers. Track Technique 1983;51:1618–1619.
2. Steindler A. Kinesiology of the human body under normal and pathological conditions. Springfield, IL: Thomas, 1955.
3. Panariello RA. The closed kinetic chain in strength training. Natl Strength Condition Assoc J 1991;13:29–33.
4. Dillman CJ, Murray TA, Hindermeister RA. Biomechanical differences of open and closed chain exercises with respect to the shoulder. J Sport Rehabil 1994;3:228–238.
5. Lephart SM, Henry TJ. The physiological basis for open and closed kinetic chain rehabilitation for the upper extremity. J Sport Rehabil 1996;5:71–87.
6. Clark FJ, Burgess PR. Slowly adapting receptors in cat knee joint. Can they signal joint angle? J Neurophysiol 1975;38:1448–1463.
7. Lephart SM, Pincivero JR, Giraldo JL, Fu FH. The role of proprioception in the management and rehabilitation of athletic injuries. Am J Sports Med 1997;25:130–137.
8. Voight M, Draovitch P. Plyometrics. In: M Albert, ed. Eccentric muscle training in sports and orthopedics. New York, Churchill Livingston, 1991:45–73.
9. Wilt F. Plyometrics, what it is and how it works. Athl J 1975;55: 76–90.
10. Wilk K, Voight M. Plyometrics for the shoulder complex. In: J Andrews, K Wilk, eds. The athlete's shoulder. New York: Churchill Livingston, 1993:543–566.
11. Bosco C, Komi P. Potentiation of the mechanical behavior of the human skeletal muscle through prestretching. Acta Physiol Scand 1979;106:467–472.
12. Bosco C, Tarkka J, Komi P. Effects of elastic energy and myoelectric potentiation of triceps surca during stretch-shortening cycle exercise. Int J Sports Med 1982;2:137–141.
13. Cavagna G. Elastic bounce of the body. J Appl Physiol 1970;29: 29–82.
14. Cavagna G, Disman B, Margarai R. Positive work done by previously stretched muscle. J Appl Physiol 1968;24:21–32.
15. Chu D. Plyometric exercise. Natl Strength Condition Assoc J 1984;6:56–62.
16. Blattner S, Noble L. Relative effects of isokinetic and plyometric training on vertical jumping performance. Res Q 1979;50:583–588.
17. Gambetta V, Odgers S, Coleman A, Craig T. The science, philosophy, and objectives of training and conditioning for baseball. In: J Andrews, B Zarins, K Wilk, eds. Injuries in baseball. Philadelphia: Lippincott-Raven, 1998:533–536.
18. Arthur M, Bailey B. Complete conditioning for football. Champaign, IL: Human Kinetics, 1998:165–237.
19. Hewett T, Riccobene J, Lindenfeld T. The effect of neuromuscular training on the incidence of knee injury in female athletes: a prospective study. Am J Sports Med 1999;27:699–706.
20. Gordon J, Ghez C. Muscle receptors and spinal reflexes: the stretch reflex. In: E Kandel, JH Schwartz, TM Jessell, eds. Principles of neural science. 3rd ed. New York: Elsevier, 1991:564–580.
21. Knott M, Voss D. Proprioceptive neuromuscular facilitation. New York: Harper & Row, 1968.
22. Komi P, Buskirk E. Effects of eccentric and concentric muscle conditioning on tension and electrical activity of human muscle. Ergonomics 1972;15:417–422.
23. Cavagna G, Saibene F, Margaria R. Effect of negative work on the amount of positive work performed by an isolated muscle. J Appl Physiol 1965;20:157–160.
24. Assmussen E, Bonde-Peterson F. Storage of elastic energy in skeletal muscle in man. Acta Physiol Scand 1974;91:385–392.
25. Eldred E. Functional implications of dynamic and static components of the spindle response to stretch. Am J Phys Med 1967; 46:129–140.
26. Komi P, Bosco C. Utilization of stored elastic energy in leg extensor muscles by men and women. Med Sci Sports Exerc 1978; 10:261–265.
27. Chu D. The language of plyometrics. Natl Strength Condition Assoc J 1984;6:30–31.
28. Voight M. Stretch-strengthening: an introduction to plyometrics. Orthop Phys Ther Clin North Am 1992;1:243–252.
29. Lundin P. A review of plyometric training. Natl Strength Condition Assoc J 1985;7:65–70.
30. Barratta R, Solomonow M, Zhou B. Muscular coactivation: the role of the antagonist musculature in maintaining knee stability. Am J Sports Med 1998;16:113–122.
31. Wilk K, Arrigo C. Current concepts in the rehabilitation of the athletic shoulder. J Orthop Sports Phys Ther 1993;18:364–378.
32. Davies G, Dickoff-Hoffman S. Neuromuscular testing and rehabilitation of the shoulder complex. J Orthop Sports Phys Ther 1993;18:449–458.
33. Wilk KE, Arrigo CA, Andrews JR. The stabilizing structures of the glenohumeral joint. J Orthop Sports Phys Ther 1997;15:364–379.
34. Chu D. Jumping into plyometrics. Champaign, IL: Human Kinetics, 1992.
35. American Physical Therapy Association. Guide to physical therapist practice, second edition. Phys Ther 2001;81:1–768.
36. National Athletic Trainers' Association. Athletic training educational competencies. 3rd ed. Dallas: NATA, 199

CHAPTER

Principles of Aerobic Conditioning

Janet Bezner, PT, PhD

The positive influence of exercise on general health and well-being has been hypothesized and studied with great interest by most of the world. Throughout Western history, dating back to and probably starting with Hippocrates (the father of preventative medicine), exercise has been recommended to improve health and physical function and to increase longevity.[1,2] Conversely, the notion that sedentary individuals tend to contract illness more readily than those who are active has been observed and documented since at least the 16th century.[2] In the 19th and 20th centuries, these ideas led to the creation of physical education curricula; the study of exercise physiology as a science; and maturation of the literature regarding exercise, including clarification of the many terms used to describe movement of the body.[2]

Caspersen et al.[3] defined physical activity as any bodily movement produced by skeletal muscles that results in energy expenditure. Exercise is a type of physical activity that is planned, structured, repetitive, and purposely aimed at improving physical fitness. Physical fitness is a set of attributes that people have or achieve and includes components of health-related (cardiorespiratory endurance, body composition, muscular endurance, muscular strength, flexibility) and athletic-related skills.[3] Being physically fit, therefore, enables an individual to perform daily tasks without undue fatigue and with sufficient energy to enjoy leisure-time activities and to respond in an emergency situation, if one arises. A primary activity used to achieve physical fitness is cardiorespiratory endurance training, whereby one performs repetitive movements of large muscle groups fueled by an adequate response from the circulatory and respiratory systems to sustain physical activity and eliminate fatigue.[2] Cardiorespiratory endurance training is the ability of the whole body to sustain prolonged exercise.[4]

Another term for cardiorespiratory endurance training is aerobic training, indicating the role of oxygen in the performance of these types of activities. The highest rate of oxygen that the body can consume during maximal exercise is termed aerobic capacity.[4] Maximal oxygen uptake ($\dot{V}o_2max$) is considered the best measurement of aerobic capacity and, therefore, cardiorespiratory endurance and fitness.[4]

The literature contains convincing evidence that the regular performance of cardiorespiratory endurance activities reduces the risk of coronary heart disease and is associated with lower mortality rates in both older and younger adults.[2,5,6] Despite this evidence, recent surveys of exercise trends in the United States illustrate that approximately 15% of U.S. adults perform vigorous physical activity (three times per week for at least 20 min) during leisure time, 22% partake in sustained physical activity (five times per week for at least 30 min) of any intensity during leisure time, and 25% of adults perform no physical activity in leisure time.[2] Adolescents and young adults (ages 12 to 21) are similarly inactive and approximately 50% regularly participate in vigorous physical activity.[2]

Owing to the widespread prevalence of physical inactivity among the U.S. population, the U.S. Public Health Service created goals for exercise participation in the *Healthy People 2000*[7] and the *Healthy People 2010*[8] documents, aimed at improving the quality of and increasing the years of healthy life. In addition, the U.S. Department of Health and Human Services (DHHS), the Centers for Disease Control and Prevention (CDC), the National Council on Physical Fitness and Sports (NCPFS), and the American College of Sports Medicine (ACSM) recommend that all adults should accumulate 30 min or more of moderate-intensity physical activity on most, and preferably all, days of the week.[2,9] Toward that end, clinicians have an opportunity to contribute to the overall well-being of the patients and clients served by prescribing meaningful exercise programs based on the most contemporary scientific evidence. The scientific basis of aerobic training is presented in this chapter, along with guidelines for prescribing and supervising aerobic exercise.

■ *Scientific Basis*

ENERGY SOURCES USED DURING AEROBIC EXERCISE

The performance of aerobic exercise requires readily available energy sources at the cellular level. Ingested food (composed of carbohydrate, fat, and protein) is converted to and stored in the cell as adenosine triphosphate (ATP), the body's basic energy source for cellular metabolism and the performance of muscular activity. Each energy source has a unique route, whereby ingested food is converted to ATP. Adenosine triphosphate is produced by three methods, or metabolic pathways.[4] To base an exercise prescription on sound scientific principles, understanding and differentiation of the fuel sources and metabolic pathways are paramount.

Fuel Sources

Carbohydrates (including sugars, starches, and fibers) are the preferred energy source for the body and are the only fuel capable of being used by the central nervous system (CNS). In addition, carbohydrate is the only fuel that can be used during anaerobic metabolism. Carbohydrates are converted to glucose and stored in muscle cells and the liver as glycogen; 1200 to 2000 kcal of energy can be stored in the body. Each gram of carbohydrate ingested produces approximately 4 kcal of energy.[4]

Fat can also be used as an energy source and forms the body's largest store of potential energy; the reserve is about 70,000 kcal in a lean adult.[4] Fat is generally stored as triglycerides. Before triglycerides can be used for energy, they must be broken down into free fatty acids (FFAs) and glycerol; FFAs are used to form ATP by aerobic oxidation. The process of triglyceride reduction (lipolysis) requires significant amounts of oxygen; thus carbohydrate fuel sources are more efficient than fat fuel sources[10] and are preferred during high-intensity exercise. Each gram of fat produces 9 kcal of energy.

Protein is used as an energy source in cases of starvation or extreme energy depletion and provides 5 to 10% of the total energy needed to perform endurance exercise. It is not a preferred energy source under normal conditions.[4] Each gram of protein produces approximately 4 kcal of energy.

Metabolic Pathways

ATP–Phosphocreatine System

The first pathway for production of ATP is anaerobic, meaning that it does not require oxygen to function (although the pathway can occur in the presence of oxygen). This pathway is called the ATP-phosphocreatine (PCr; or creatin phosphate) system.[4] Phosphocreatine is a high-energy compound like ATP, that replenishes ATP in a working muscle, extending the time to fatigue by 10 to 20 sec.[10] Thus, energy released as a result of the breakdown of PCr is not used for cellular metabolism but to prevent the ATP level from falling. One molecule of ATP is produced per molecule of PCr. This simple energy system can produce 3 to 15 sec of maximal muscular work[4] and requires an adequate recovery time, generally three times longer than the duration of the activity.

Glycolytic System

The production of ATP during longer bouts of activity requires the breakdown of food energy sources. In the glycolytic system, or during anaerobic glycolysis, ATP is produced through the breakdown of glucose obtained from the ingestion of carbohydrates or from the breakdown of glycogen stored in the liver. Anaerobic glycolysis, which also occurs without the presence of oxygen, is much more complex than the ATP-PCr pathway, requiring numerous enzymatic reactions to breakdown glucose and produce energy. The end product of glycolysis is pyruvic acid, which is converted to lactic acid in the absence of oxygen. The net energy production from each molecule of glucose used is two molecules of ATP, and each molecule of glycogen yields three molecules of ATP.

Although the energy yield from the glycolytic system is small, the combined energy production of the ATP-PCr and glycolytic pathways enables muscles to contract without a continuous oxygen supply, thus providing an energy source for the first part of a high-intensity exercise until the respiratory and circulatory systems catch up to the sudden increased demands placed on them. Furthermore, the glycolytic system can provide energy for only a limited time, because the end product of the pathway, lactic acid, accumulates in the muscles and inhibits further glycogen breakdown, eventually impeding muscle contraction.[4]

Oxidative System

The production of ATP from the breakdown of fuel sources in the presence of oxygen is termed aerobic oxidation, or cellular respiration. This process occurs in the mitochondria, which are the cellular organelles conveniently located next to myofibrils, the contractile elements of individual muscle fibers. The oxidative production of ATP involves several complex processes, including aerobic glycolysis, the Krebs cycle, and the electron transport chain.[4]

Carbohydrate, or glycogen, is broken down in aerobic glycolysis, in a similar manner as the breakdown of carbohydrate in anaerobic glycolysis. But in the presence of oxygen, pyruvic acid is converted to acetyl coenzyme A (acetyl CoA), which can then enter the Krebs cycle, producing two molecules of ATP. The end result of the Krebs cycle is the production of carbon dioxide and hydrogen ions, which enter the electron transport chain, undergo a series of reactions, and produce ATP and water. The net ATP production from aerobic oxidation is 39 molecules of ATP from 1 molecule of glycogen, or 38 molecules of ATP from 1 molecule of glucose.[4]

Therefore, the presence of oxygen enables significantly more energy to be produced and results in the ability to perform longer periods of work without muscle contraction being impeded from the buildup of lactic acid. Figure 10-1 summarizes and compares the energy-production capabilities of the three metabolic pathways.[11]

SELECTION OF METABOLIC PATHWAY AND FUEL SOURCE DURING EXERCISE

High-intensity, brief-duration exercise (efforts of < 15 sec) generally relies on stored ATP in the muscle for energy and employs the ATP-PCr pathway. High-intensity, short-duration exercise (efforts of 1 to 2 min) relies on the anaerobic pathways, including the ATP-PCr and glycolysis systems for the provision of ATP. Both of these types of exercise use carbohydrate or glucose as a fuel source.[4]

Submaximal exercise efforts use carbohydrate, fat, and protein for energy. Low-intensity exercise (< 50% of maximal oxygen consumption) performed for long duration uses both FFA and carbohydrate fuel sources within the aerobic oxidative pathway to produce ATP.[10] In the presence of an abundant supply of oxygen, as exercise duration increases or intensity decreases, the body will use more FFAs than carbohydrates for ATP production. During work loads of moderate to heavy intensity (> 50% of maximal oxygen consumption), carbohydrates are used more than FFAs for ATP production. As the workload approaches maximal exercise capacity, the proportion of FFA oxidation decreases and that of carbohydrate oxidation increases. Above maximal levels, exercise is anaerobic and can be performed for only a short time.[10] As noted, protein participates as an energy source only in extremely deficient situations (starvation) and minimally during endurance exercise.[4]

To summarize, carbohydrate is the preferred fuel source for supplying the body with energy in the form of ATP during exercise. Exercise can occur anaerobically, via the ATP-PCr or anaerobic glycolysis pathways, or aerobically, via the aerobic oxidative pathway. The oxidative pathway has the greatest ATP yield and enables exercise to continue for prolonged periods without the fatigue caused by lactic acid buildup. To support the aerobic needs of prolonged exercise, numerous changes occur in the cardiovascular and respiratory systems, which are discussed next.

NORMAL RESPONSES TO ACUTE AEROBIC EXERCISE

Numerous cardiovascular and respiratory mechanisms aimed at delivering oxygen to the tissues contribute to the ability to sustain exercise aerobically. To examine an individual's response to exercise, it is important to understand the normal physiologic changes that occur as a result of physical activity. The following sections outline the changes expected during aerobic exercise and are considered normal responses.[4,10–12]

Heart Rate

Heart rate (HR) is measured in beats per minute. A linear relationship exists between HR and the intensity of exercise, indicating that as workload or intensity increases, HR increases proportionally. The magnitude of increase in HR is influenced by many factors, including age, fitness level, type of activity being performed, presence of disease, medications, blood volume, and environmental factors (e.g., temperature and humidity).[4]

Stroke Volume

The volume, or amount, of blood (measured in milliliters) ejected from the left ventricle per heart beat is termed the

FIGURE 10-1 Energy production capabilities of the three metabolic pathways.

This figure depicts the actions and interactions of the ATP-phosphocreatine, glycolytic, and oxidative metabolic pathways. High-intensity, brief duration exercise is fueled by the ATP-phosphocreatine pathway, whereas high-intensity, short duration exercise relies on the glycolytic pathway, both of which are anaerobic. The aerobic oxidative pathway provides energy for muscular contraction during prolonged exercise of low to moderate intensity.

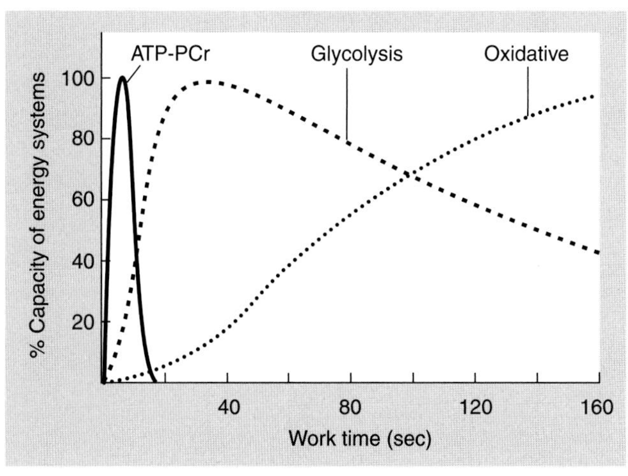

stroke volume (SV). As workload increases, SV increases linearly up to approximately 50% of aerobic capacity, after which it increases only slightly. Factors that influence the magnitude of change in SV include ventricular function, body position, and exercise intensity.[4]

Cardiac Output

The product of HR and SV is cardiac output ($\dot{Q}$), or the amount of blood (measured in liters) ejected from the left ventricle per minute. Cardiac output increases linearly with workload owing to the increases in HR and SV in response to increasing exercise intensity. Changes in $\dot{Q}$ depend on age, posture, body size, presence of disease, and level of physical conditioning.[4]

Arterial–Venous Oxygen Difference

The amount of oxygen extracted by the tissues from the blood represents the difference between arterial blood oxygen content and venous blood oxygen content and is referred to as the arterial–venous oxygen difference (a − vO_2 difference; measured in milliliters per deciliter). As exercise intensity increases, a − vO_2 difference increases linearly, indicating that the tissues are extracting more oxygen from the blood; creating a decreasing venous oxygen content as exercise progresses.[4]

Blood Flow

The distribution of blood flow (measured in milliliters) to the body changes dramatically during acute exercise. When at rest, 15 to 20% of the cardiac output goes to muscle, but during exercise 80 to 85% is distributed to working muscle and shunted away from the viscera. During heavy exercise, or when the body starts to overheat, increased blood flow is delivered to the skin to conduct heat away from the body's core, leaving less blood for working muscles.[4]

Blood Pressure

The two components of blood pressure (BP)—systolic (SBP) and diastolic (DBP) pressure (measured in milliliters of mercury)—respond differently during acute bouts of exercise. To facilitate blood and oxygen delivery to the tissues, SBP increases linearly with workload. Because DBP represents the pressure in the arteries when the heart is at rest, it changes little during aerobic exercise, regardless of intensity. A change in DBP from a resting value of < 15 mm Hg is considered a normal response. Both SBP and DBP are higher during upper-extremity aerobic activity than during lower-extremity aerobic activity.[4]

Pulmonary Ventilation

The respiratory system responds to exercise by increasing the rate and depth of breathing to increase the amount of air exchanged (measured in liters) per minute. An immediate increase in rate and depth occurs in response to exercise and is thought to be facilitated by the nervous system and initiated by the movement of the body. A second, more gradual, increase occurs in response to temperature and blood chemical changes as a result of the increased oxygen use by the tissues. Thus, both tidal volume (the amount of air moved in and out of the lungs during regular breathing) and respiratory rate increase in proportion to the intensity of exercise.[4]

ABNORMAL RESPONSES TO AEROBIC EXERCISE

Individuals with suspected cardiovascular disease, or any other type of disease that may produce an abnormal response to exercise, should be appropriately screened and tested before the initiation of an exercise program (discussed in greater detail later in this chapter). Abnormal responses may also occur in individuals without known or documented disease. Routine monitoring of exercise response is important and can be used to evaluate the appropriateness of the exercise prescription and as an indication that further diagnostic testing is indicated. In general, responses that are inconsistent with the normal responses described previously are considered abnormal. Of the parameters described, HR and BP are most commonly examined during exercise. Examples of abnormal responses to aerobic exercise are the failure of the HR to rise in proportion to exercise intensity, the failure of the SBP to rise during exercise, a decrease in the SBP of 20 mm Hg during exercise, and an increase in the DBP of 15 mm Hg during exercise.[11] The clinician should be able to recognize other signs and symptoms of exercise intolerance, which are presented in Table 10-1.

Knowledge of the normal and abnormal physiologic and symptom responses to exercise will enable the clinician to prescribe and monitor exercise safely and confidently and to minimize the occurrence of untoward events during exercise. Regular exposure to aerobic exercise re-

TABLE 10-1 Signs and Symptoms of Exercise Intolerance
Angina: chest, left arm, jaw, back, or lower neck pain or pressure
Unusual or severe shortness of breath
Abnormal diaphoresis
Pallor, cyanosis, cold and clammy skin
CNS symptoms: vertigo, ataxia, gait problems, or confusion
Leg cramps or intermittent claudication
Physical or verbal manifestations of severe fatigue or shortness of breath

Reprinted with permission from American College of Sports Medicine. Resource manual for guidelines for exercise testing and prescription. 3rd ed. Baltimore: Williams & Wilkins, 1998.

sults in changes to the cardiovascular and respiratory systems that can also be examined by monitoring basic physiologic variables during exercise.

CARDIOVASCULAR AND RESPIRATORY ADAPTATIONS TO AEROBIC CONDITIONING

The documented benefits of aerobic exercise are a result of the adaptations that occur in the oxygen-delivery system with the performance of regular activity. These adaptations, considered chronic changes, enable more efficient performance of exercise and affect cardiorespiratory endurance and fitness level.

Cardiovascular Adaptations

Factors involving the heart that adapt in response to a regular exercise stimulus include heart size, HR, SV, and $\dot{Q}$. The weight and volume of the heart and the thickness and chamber size of the left ventricle increase with training. As a result, the heart pumps out more blood per beat (SV) and the force of each contraction is stronger. With training, the left ventricle is more completely filled during diastole, increasing stroke volume (at rest as well as during submaximal and maximal exercise) and plasma blood volume.

Changes in the HR include a decreased resting rate and a decreased rate at submaximal exercise levels, indicating that the individual can perform the same amount of work with less effort after training. Maximal HR typically does not change as a result of training. The amount of time it takes for the HR to return to resting after exercise decreases as a result of training and is a useful indicator of progress toward better fitness. Since $\dot{Q}$ is the product of HR and SV ($\dot{Q}$ = HR × SV), no change occurs at rest or during submaximal exercise because HR decreases and SV increases. However, owing to the increase in maximum SV, maximum $\dot{Q}$ increases considerably.[4,11]

Adaptations also occur to the vascular system, including blood volume, blood pressure, and blood flow changes. Aerobic training increases overall blood volume, primarily because of an increase in plasma volume. The increase in blood plasma results from an increased release of hormones (antidiuretic and aldosterone) that promote water retention by the kidney and an increase in the amount of plasma proteins (namely albumin). A small increase in the number of red blood cells may also contribute to the increase in blood volume. The net effect of greater blood volume is the delivery of more oxygen to the tissues.

Resting blood pressure changes seen with training are most noteworthy in hypertensive or borderline hypertensive patients, in whom aerobic training can decrease both SBP and DBP by 10 mm Hg. During the performance of submaximal and maximal exercise, little change, if any, occurs in blood pressure as a result of training. Several adaptations are responsible for the increase in blood flow to muscle in a trained individual, including greater capillarization in the trained muscles, greater opening of existing capillaries in trained muscles, and more efficient distribution of blood flow to active muscles.[4,11]

Respiratory Adaptations

The capacity of the respiratory system to deliver oxygen to the body typically surpasses the ability of the body to use oxygen, thus the respiratory component of performance is not a limiting factor in the development of endurance. Nevertheless, adaptations in the respiratory system do occur in response to aerobic training. The amount of air in the lungs, represented by lung volume measures, is unchanged at rest and during submaximal exercise in trained individuals. However, tidal volume, the amount of air breathed in and out during normal respiration, increases during maximal exercise. Respiratory rate (RR) is lower at rest and during submaximal exercise and increases at maximal levels of exercise. The combined increase in tidal volume and RR during maximal exercise of trained individuals produces a substantial increase in pulmonary ventilation, or the process of movement of air into and out of the lungs.

Pulmonary ventilation at rest is either unchanged or slightly reduced and during submaximal exercise is slightly reduced after training. The process of gas exchange in the alveoli, or pulmonary diffusion, is unchanged at rest and at submaximal exercise levels but increases during maximal exercise owing to the increased blood flow to the lungs and the increased ventilation, as noted. These two factors create a situation that enables more alveoli to participate in gas exchange and more oxygen perfuses into the arterial system during maximal exercise. Finally, $a-vO_2$ difference increases at maximal exercise in response to training as a result of increased oxygen distraction by the tissues and greater blood flow to the tissues, owing to more effective blood distribution.[4,11]

Aerobic Capacity Adaptations

The net effect of these cardiovascular and respiratory adaptations on aerobic capacity is an increase in $\dot{V}O_2$max as a result of endurance training. When $\dot{V}O_2$ is measured in Lm, it is termed *absolute* VO_2max, whereas when it is in ml/kg/min, it is *relative* $\dot{V}O_2$max because it is relative to body weight. A typical training program performed at 75% of $\dot{V}O_2$max (described in a later section), three times per week, at 30 min per session, over the course of 6 months can improve $\dot{V}O_2$max by 15 to 20% in a previously sedentary individual. Resting $\dot{V}O_2$max is either unchanged or slightly increased after training, and submaximal $\dot{V}O_2$ is either unchanged or slightly reduced, representing more efficiency.[4]

PSYCHOLOGICAL BENEFITS OF TRAINING

In addition to a myriad of cardiovascular, respiratory, and metabolic improvements that occur after aerobic training, psychological benefits have been documented, although these effects are less well understood. An overall assessment of the literature indicates that depression, mood, anxiety, psychological well-being, and perceptions of physical function and well-being improve in response to the performance of physical activity.[2,13] The finding that exercise can decrease symptoms of depression and anxiety is consistent with the fact that individuals who are inactive are more likely to have depressive symptoms than are active individuals. Improvements in depression and mood have been found in populations with and without clinically diagnosed psychological impairment and in those with good psychological health, although the literature is less conclusive in this specific area.

A number of factors have been postulated to explain the beneficial effects of aerobic training on psychological function, including changes in neurotransmitter concentrations, body temperature, hormones, cardiorespiratory function, and metabolic processes as well as improvement in psychosocial factors such as social support, self-efficacy, and stress relief. Further research is needed to verify the potential contribution of changes in these factors to improvement in psychological function.[2]

Despite the inability to explain why psychological parameters improve in response to training, the effect on overall quality of life is positive.[14,15] This improvement in quality of life has been demonstrated in individuals with and without disease,[16–19] including patients with coronary heart disease who are obese[20] and elderly,[21] patients with chronic heart failure,[22] patients who have undergone coronary bypass graft surgery,[23] and patients with multiple sclerosis[24] and cancer.[25]

HEALTH-RELATED BENEFITS TO EXERCISE

The observed improvement in quality of life in individuals who participate in regular exercise is achieved from quantities of exercise considered to produce health-related (vs. fitness-related) benefits. Fitness-related benefits result in significant changes in physical fitness level, as measured by cardiorespiratory endurance and body composition changes. Specific recommendations for fitness-related changes usually include vigorous, continuous activities with a focus on the specific parameters of exercise (intensity, mode, duration, frequency). Health-related benefits can be achieved through the performance of moderate intensity, intermittent activity with a focus on the accumulated amount of activity performed.[9] Documented health-related benefits from the performance of regular exercise are presented in Table 10-2.[9,11]

Although improvement in fitness level is a worthwhile goal and results in health-related benefits, exercise to achieve health-related benefits appears to be easier for most people to incorporate into their lifestyle and thus provides a valuable exercise option.[26–28] The specific parameters necessary to achieve both fitness- and health-related benefits of aerobic exercise are presented later in this chapter.

TABLE 10-2 Health-Related Benefits from Performance of Regular Exercise

Decreased fatigue
Improved performance in work- and sports-related activities
Improved blood lipid profile
Enhanced immune function
Improved glucose tolerance and insulin sensitivity
Improved body composition
Enhanced sense of well-being
Decreased risk of coronary artery disease, cancer of the colon and breast, hypertension, non-insulin-dependent diabetes mellitus, osteoporosis, anxiety, and depression

From Pate RR, Pratt M, Blair SN, et al. Physical activity and public health. JAMA 1995;273:402–407; and American College of Sports Medicine. Resource manual for guidelines for exercise testing and prescription. 3rd ed. Baltimore: Williams & Wilkins, 1998.

Clinical Guidelines

SCREENING AND SUPERVISION OF EXERCISE

Screening

Before the initiation of an exercise program, individuals should be examined to ensure safety, minimize risks, maximize benefits, and optimize adherence.[11] Preparticipation assessment should include an examination of readiness to participate in exercise, health history (including coronary artery disease risk factors), and health behaviors.

The ACSM[29] created guidelines delineating who should be medically examined before participation in vigorous exercise (defined as intensity > 60% $\dot{V}O_2max$). Clients who do *not* require medical evaluation include asymptomatic apparently healthy women under the age of 50 and men under the age of 40 who have fewer than two coronary artery disease (CAD) risk factors (family history of CAD, cigarette smoker, hypertension, hypercholesterolemia, diabetes mellitus, sedentary lifestyle).[29] The definition of asymptomatic in relation to screening for participation in exercise is presented in Table 10-3.[29]

Asymptomatic apparently healthy men and women, regardless of age or CAD risk factor status, who wish to begin a moderate exercise training program (defined as intensity between 40 and 60% $\dot{V}O_2max$) do not need a medical examination. For individuals who do not require medical

TABLE 10-3 Definition of an Asymptomatic Individual

No pain in the chest, neck, jaws, or other areas that suggest ischemia
No shortness of breath at rest or with mild exertion
No dizziness or syncope
No orthopnea
No ankle edema
No palpitations or tachycardia
No intermittent claudication
No known heart murmur
No unusual fatigue or shortness of breath with usual activities

Reprinted with permission from American College of Sports Medicine. Guidelines for exercise testing and prescription. 5th ed. Media, PA: Williams & Wilkins, 1995.

evaluation, preparticipation screening can be performed using a self-report questionnaire, such as the Physical Activity Readiness Questionnaire (PAR-Q) (Fig. 10-2).[11,29,30] Based on the answers to the seven questions on the PAR-Q, individuals between the ages of 15 and 69 can either appropriately participate in exercise or be referred to a physician for further evaluation before beginning an exercise program. All individuals who fall outside of the boundaries described should be referred to a physician for medical examination before participating in exercise training.

The clinician should study the client's health history to identify known diseases and symptoms that might indicate the presence of disease and, therefore, require modification of the exercise prescription. Specific diseases and conditions that should be noted because of their association with CAD include cardiovascular and respiratory disease, diabetes, obesity, hypertension, and abnormal blood lipid levels.[11]

Also relevant from the client's history are the individual's health behaviors, typically included in the assessment of social habits.[31] Alcohol and drug use, cigarette smoking, diet content, current activity level, and eating disorders should be reviewed, because these factors may affect exercise prescription. Other factors that may affect the exercise prescription are medications, personality/behavior, and pregnancy and breast-feeding status.[11]

Supervision

A thorough screening or medical examination is critical for determining which individuals may require supervision during exercise.[29] Apparently healthy individuals do not require supervision during the performance of aerobic exercise, but individuals with two or more risk factors for CAD or who have documented CAD should be supervised during exercise. Supervision is also recommended for clients with cardiorespiratory disease.[29]

GRADED EXERCISE TESTING

The development of an appropriate and useful exercise prescription for cardiorespiratory endurance depends on an accurate examination of $\dot{V}O_2max$, which is most commonly achieved through the performance of a graded exercise test (GXT). Exercise tests can be maximal, in which clients perform to their physiologic or symptom limit, or submaximal, in which an arbitrary stopping or limiting criterion is used.

Maximal Graded Exercise Tests

The most important characteristics of a maximal GXT are a variable or graded workload that increases gradually and a total test time of 8 to 12 min.[29] In addition, individuals undergoing maximal GXT testing are usually monitored with an electrocardiogram (ECG).

The direct measurement of $\dot{V}O_2max$ involves the analysis of expired gases, which requires special equipment and personnel and is costly and time-consuming.[29] However, $\dot{V}O_2max$ can be estimated from prediction equations after the client exercises to the point of volitional fatigue, or it can be estimated from submaximal tests. For most clinicians, maximal exercise testing is not feasible, because of the special equipment required and the ECG monitoring, although it is the most accurate test of aerobic capacity. Furthermore, it is recommended that maximal GXT be reserved for research purposes, testing patients with specific diseases, and for evaluating athletes.[11] Therefore, submaximal testing is most commonly used, especially for low-risk, apparently healthy individuals. Clinicians who wish to conduct maximal graded exercise testing are referred to resources provided by the ACSM.[11,29]

Submaximal Graded Exercise Tests

Submaximal exercise tests can be used to estimate $\dot{V}O_2max$ because of the linear relationship between HR and $\dot{V}O_2$ and between HR and workload.[11] That is, as workload or $\dot{V}O_2$ increases, HR increases in a linear, predictable fashion. Therefore, $\dot{V}O_2max$ can be estimated by plotting HR against workload for at least two exercise workloads and extrapolating to the age-predicted maximum HR (220 − age).[29] The assumptions used for submaximal testing are presented in Table 10-4.

Failure to meet these assumptions fully, which is usually the case, results in errors in the predicted $\dot{V}O_2max$. Therefore, $\dot{V}O_2max$ measured by submaximal tests is less accurate than that measured by maximal tests. Submaximal tests are appropriately used to document change over time in response to aerobic training and, given the time and money saved, are clinically useful.

The ACSM[29] provides recommendations for physician

Physical Activity Readiness
Questionnaire - PAR-Q
revised 1994

PAR-Q & YOU

(A Questionnaire for People Aged 15 to 69)

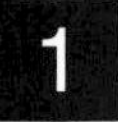

Regular physical activity is fun and healthy, and increasingly more people are starting to become more active every day. Being more active is very safe for most people. However, some people should check with their doctor before they start becoming much more physically active.

If you are planning to become much more physically active that you are now, start by answering the seven questions in the box below. If you are between the ages of 15 and 69, the PAR-Q will tell you if you should check with your doctor before you start. If you are over 69 years of age, and you are not used to being very active, check with your doctor.

Common sense is your best guide when you answer these questions. Please read the questions carefully and answer each one honestly.

YES	NO	
_____	_____	1. Has your doctor ever said that you have a heart condition <u>and</u> that you should only do physical activity recommended by a doctor?
_____	_____	2. Do you feel pain in your chest when you do physical activity?
_____	_____	3. In the past month, have you had chest pain when you were not doing physical activity?
_____	_____	4. Do you lose your balance because of dizziness or do you ever lose consciousness?
_____	_____	5. Do you have a bone or joint problem that could be made worse by a change in your physical activity?
_____	_____	6. Is your doctor currently prescribing drugs (for example, water pills) for blood pressure or heart condition?
_____	_____	7. Do you know of *any other reason* why you should not do physical activity?

2

If you answered YES to any questions:

Talk to your doctor by phone or in person BEFORE you start becoming much more physicaly active or BEFORE you have a fitness appraisal. Tell your doctor about the PAR-Q and which questions you answered YES.

- You may be able to do any activity you want—as long as you start slowly and build up gradually. Or, you may need to restrict your activities to those which are safe for you. Talk with your doctor about the kinds of activities you wish to participate in and follow his/her advice.
- Find our which community programs are safe and helpful to you.

If you answered NO to all questions:

If you answered NO honestly to all PAR-Q questions, you can be reasonably sure that you can:

- start becoming much more physically active—begin slowly and build up gradually. This is the safest and easiest way to go.
- take part in a fitness appraisal—this is an excellent way to determine your basic fitness so that you can plan the best way for you to live actively.

Delay becoming much more active:

- if you are not feeling well because of temporary illness such as a cold or a fever—wait until your feel better; or
- if you are or may be pregnant—talk to your doctor before you start becoming more active.

3

Please note:

1. If your health changes so that you then answer YES to any of the above questions, tell your fitness or health professional. Ask whether you should change your physical activity plans.
2. Informed Use of the PAR-Q: The Canadian Society for Exercise Physiology, Health Canada, and their agents assume no liability for persons who undertake physical activity, and if in doubt after completing this questionnaire, consult your doctor prior to physical activity.
3. If the PAR-Q is being given to a person before he or she participates in a physical activity program or fitness appraisal, this section may be used for legal or administrative purposes.

I have read, understood and completed this questionnaire. Any questions I had were answered to my full satisfaction

Name ______________________________

Signature ______________________________ Date ______________

Signature of Parent ______________________________ Witness ______________

or Guardian (for participants under the age of majority)

You are encouraged to copy the PAR-Q but only if you use the entire form.

Supported by HealthCanada
Sante Canada

FIGURE 10-2 **The Physical Activity Readiness Questionnaire.**

The Physical Activity Readiness Questionaire (PAR-Q) can be used to screen individuals 15 to 69 years old prior to participation in a moderate intensity exercise program. It was developed to identify those individuals for whom physical activity might be contraindicated or who need further medical evaluation prior to participation in exercise.

TABLE 10-4 Assumptions for Using Submaximal Testing to Estimate $\dot{V}O_2max$

The workloads used are reproducible
HR is allowed to reach a steady state at each stage of the test
Age-predicted maximum HR is uniform (220 − age), with a prediction error of 10–15%
A linear relationship exists between HR and oxygen uptake
Mechanical efficiency is the same for everyone ($\dot{V}O_2$ at a given work rate)

Data from American College of Sports Medicine. Resource manual for guidelines for exercise testing and prescription. 3rd ed. Baltimore: Williams & Wilkins, 1998; and American College of Sports Medicine. Guidelines for exercise testing and prescription. 5th ed. Media, PA: Williams & Wilkins, 1995.

supervision during GXT. For women under the age of 50 and men under the age of 40 who are without risk factors or symptoms (as defined previously), physician supervision for maximal and submaximal testing is not deemed necessary. Clients in these age ranges who have two or more risk factors but no symptoms or disease can undergo submaximal testing without physician supervision. Physician supervision during submaximal and maximal testing is recommended for any individual who has CAD or symptoms of CAD. Finally, physician supervision is recommended for maximal testing of men over the age of 40 and women over the age of 50 who have two or more risk factors for CAD but no symptoms. Therefore, clinicians can safely perform submaximal testing of any aged client who is symptom or disease free (as defined by ACSM).[29]

Numerous testing protocols have been published and are available for submaximal exercise testing. Because of the requirement of reproducible workloads, treadmills, bicycle ergometers, and stepping protocols are most commonly used. Test selection should be based on safety concerns; staff familiarity with and knowledge of the testing protocol; equipment availability; and client goals, abilities, and conditions (such as orthopedic limitations).

Bicycle Ergometer

A common bicycle ergometer test is the Åstrand-Ryhming protocol.[29] This test involves a single 6-min stage, and workload is based on sex and activity status:

Unconditioned females: 300 to 450 kg/min (50 to 75 W).
Conditioned females: 450 to 600 kg/min (75 to 100 W).
Unconditioned males: 300 to 600 kg/min (50 to 100 W).
Conditioned males: 600 to 900 kg/min (100 to 150 W).

Individuals pedal at 50 revolutions/min and HR is measured during the 5th and 6th min. The two HR measures must be within 5 beats of each other and the HR must be between 130 and 170 beats/min for the test to be completed. If the HR is < 130 beats/min, the resistance should be increased by 50 to 100 Ws and the test continued for another 6 min. The test may be terminated when the HR in the 5th and 6th min differs by no more than 5 beats and is between 130 and 170 beats/min. The average of the 2 HR, obtained during the 5th and 6th minutes is calculated, and a nomogram is used to estimate $\dot{V}O_2max$.[29] The value determined from the nomogram is multiplied by a correction factor to account for age of the client (Fig. 10-3; Table 10-5).

For example, an unconditioned 40-year-old female performed the test at a resistance of 75 W (450 kg/min) and attained a HR in the 5th min of 150 beats/min and a HR in the 6th min of 154 beats/min. Thus the average HR used in the nomogram (Fig. 10-3) is 152 beats/min. To use the nomogram, place the left end of a straightedge along the line for women with a pulse rate of 152 beats/min (left side of the figure). The right end of the straightedge is now lined up at the appropriate workload for this woman: 450 kg/min. The point at which the straightedge crosses the $\dot{V}O_2max$ line indicates the client's estimated $\dot{V}O_2max$: 2.0 L/min. The estimated $\dot{V}O_2max$ (2.0 L/min) is then corrected for age by multiplying by 0.83 (Table 10-5) to yield a $\dot{V}O_2max$ of 1.66 L/min for this client.

Treadmill

Submaximal treadmill tests are also used to estimate $\dot{V}O_2max$.[29] A single-stage submaximal treadmill test was developed for testing low-risk clients. The test involves beginning with a comfortable walking pace between 2.0 and 4.5 mph at 0% grade for a 2- 4-min warm-up designed to increase the HR to within 50 to 75% of the age-predicted (220 − age) maximum HR, followed by 4 min at 5% grade at the same self-selected walking speed. Heart rate is measured at the end of the 4-min stage, and $\dot{V}O_2max$ is estimated using the following equation:

$$\dot{V}O_2max\ (\text{mL/kg/min}) = 15.1 + [21.8 \times \text{speed (mph)}] \times [0.327 \times \text{HR (beats/min)}] - [0.263 \times \text{speed} \times \text{age (years)}] + [0.00504 \times \text{HR} \times \text{age}] + [5.98 \times \text{sex}]$$

where sex is given a value of 0 for females and 1 for males.

Step

Step tests were developed to test large numbers of individuals expeditiously and represent another mode of submaximal exercise testing. Several protocols have been developed, but only one is presented here.[32] The Queens College Step Test requires a 16.25-in. step (similar to the height of a bleacher).[32,33] Individuals step up and down to a 4-count rhythm:

Count 1: client places one foot on the step.
Count 2: client places the other foot on the step.
Count 3: the first foot is brought back to the ground.
Count 4: the second foot is brought down.

FIGURE 10-3 The Åstrand-Rhyming nomogram.

A nomogram used to calculate aerobic capacity (VO_{2max}) from pulse rate during submaximal work. Knowledge of the pulse rate, sex, and work load of a client allows the clinician to determine absolute VO_{2max}. VO_{2max} values obtained from the nomogram should be adjusted for age by a correction factor (Table 10-5).

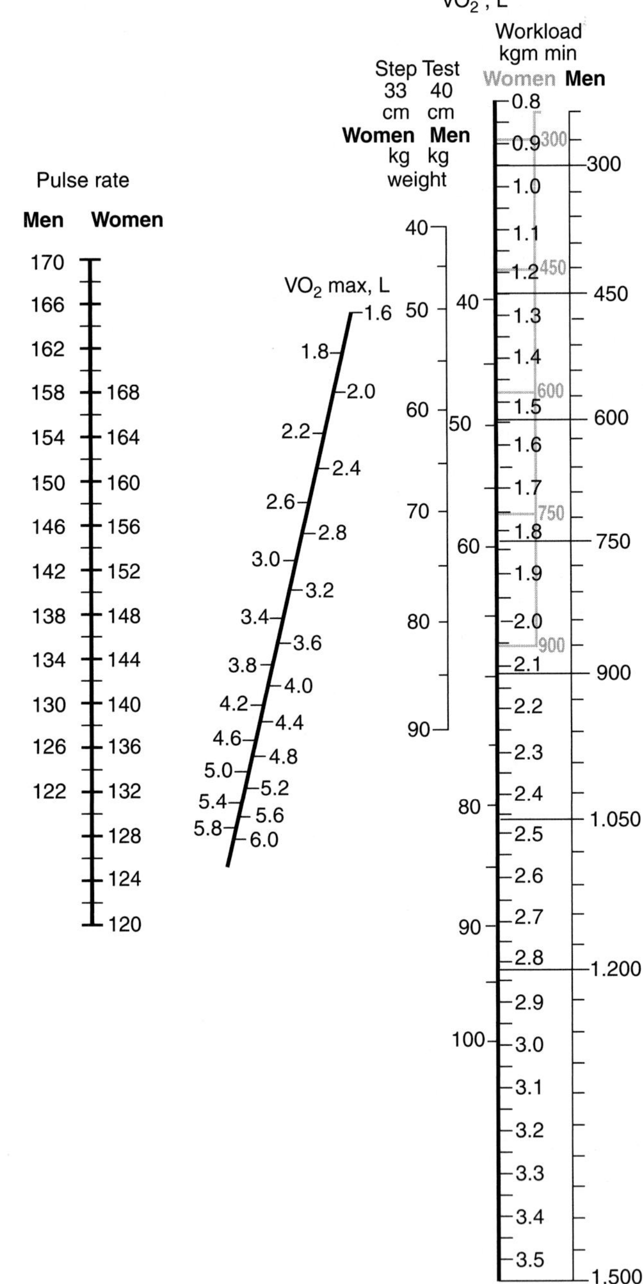

A metronome helps maintain the prescribed stepping beat. Females step for 3 min at a rate of 22 steps/min, and males step for 3 min at a rate of 24 steps/min. After 3 min, a recovery 15-sec pulse is measured, starting 5 sec into recovery, while the client remains standing. The pulse rate obtained is converted to beats per minute by multiplying by four. This value is termed the recovery HR. The following equations are then used to estimate $\dot{V}O_2max$:

$$\text{Females: } \dot{V}O_2max\ (\text{mL/kg/min}) = 65.81 - [0.1847 - \text{recovery HR (beats/min)}]$$

$$\text{Males: } \dot{V}O_2max\ (\text{mL/kg/min}) = 111.33 - [0.42 \times \text{recovery HR (beats/min)}]$$

Field

Field tests refer to exercise testing protocols that are derived from events performed outside, or '"in the field." These tests are submaximal tests and, like the step test, are more practical for testing large groups of people. Field tests are appropriate when time and equipment are limited and for examining individuals over the age of 40. Although variety of field tests exist, only the Cooper 12-min test and the 1-mile walk test are presented.[33]

In the Cooper 12-min test, individuals are instructed to

TABLE 10-5 Correction Factor for Age for Astrand-Rhyming Nomogram

Age	Correction Factor
15	1.10
25	1.00
35	0.87
40	0.83
45	0.78
50	0.75
55	0.71
60	0.68
65	0.65

Reprinted with permission from American College of Sports Medicine. Guidelines for exercise testing and prescription. 5th ed. Media, PA: Williams & Wilkins, 1995.

cover the most distance possible in 12 min, preferably by running, although walking is acceptable. The distance covered in 12 min is recorded and $\dot{V}O_2max$ is estimated according to the following equation:

$$\dot{V}O_2max\ (mL/kg/min) = 35.97 \times (\text{total miles run}) - 11.29$$

The 1-mile walk test is another option in the submaximal field test category.[34] Individuals walk 1 mile as fast as possible, without running. The average HR for the last 2 min of the walk is recorded by a heart rate monitor. If a HR monitor is not available, a 15-sec pulse can be measured immediately after the test is completed. $\dot{V}O_2max$ is estimated from the following equation:

$$\dot{V}O_2max\ (mL/kg/min) = 132.85 - [0.077 \times \text{body weight (lb)}] - [0.39 \times \text{age (years)}] + [6.32 \times \text{sex}] - [3.26 \times \text{elapsed time (min)}] - [0.16 \times \text{HR (beats/min)}]$$

where sex is scored 0 for females and 1 for males.

Monitoring

All clients should be closely monitored during exercise test performance. Vital signs should be examined before, during each stage or workload of the test, and after the test for 4 to 8 min of recovery.[11] In addition, a rating of perceived exertion (RPE) is commonly used to monitor exercise tolerance.[35] Rating of perceived extertion refers to the "degree of heaviness and strain experienced in physical work as estimated according to a specific rating method"[35] and indicates overall perceived exertion. The Borg RPE scale is shown in Table 10-6.[35] In addition, individuals should be monitored for signs and symptoms of exercise intolerance.

TABLE 10-6 Rating of Perceived Exertion

Rating	Description
6	None at all
7	Extremely light
8	
9	Light
10	
11	Light
12	
13	Somewhat hard
14	
15	Hard (heavy)
16	
17	Very hard
18	
19	Extremely hard
20	Maximal

Reprinted with permission from American College of Sports Medicine. The recommended quantity and quality of exercise for developing and maintaining cardiorespiratory and muscular fitness in healthy adults. Med Sci Sports Exerc 1990;22:265–274.

The guidelines for stopping an exercise test are presented in Table 10-7.[29]

Summary—Graded Exercise Testing

Exercise testing serves several important functions. Maximal testing can be used to screen for the presence of CAD and to directly measure $\dot{V}O_2max$ in situations that require accuracy (research, athletic performance). Submaximal exercise testing is less accurate than maximal testing but is useful for establishing a baseline before initiating an exercise training program, for documenting improvement as a response to training, for motivating a client to adopt an exercise habit, and for formulating an exercise prescription based on physiologic parameters specific to the client.

Techniques: Exercise Prescription

An individualized exercise prescription has five components: intensity, duration, frequency, mode, and progression of activity. When possible, the exercise prescription should be based on an objective examination of the client's

TABLE 10-7 Guidelines for Cessation of GXT

Onset of angina or angina-like symptoms
A significant drop (20 mm Hg) in SBP or a failure of the SBP to rise with an increase in exercise intensity
Excessive rise in SBP $>$ 260 mm Hg or DBP $>$ 115 mm Hg
Signs of poor perfusion: lightheadedness, confusion, ataxia, pallor, cyanosis, nausea, cold or clammy skin
Failure of HR to increase with increased exercise intensity
Noticeable change in heart rhythm
Client asks to stop
Physical or verbal manifestations of severe fatigue
Failure of the testing equipment

Reprinted with permission from American College of Sports Medicine. Guidelines for exercise testing and prescription. 5th ed. Media, PA: Williams & Wilkins, 1995.

should be based on an objective examination of the client's response to exercise. A primary objective of an exercise prescription is to assist in the adoption of regular physical activity as a lifestyle habit; thus, the clinician should take into consideration the behavioral characteristics, personal goals, and exercise preferences of the client.[29] Furthermore, the exercise prescription should function to improve physical fitness, reduce body fat, and improve cardiorespiratory endurance, depending on the specific goals of the individual. Clinicians should recognize that a thorough exercise prescription should include activities that address all elements of health-related physical fitness (cardiorespiratory endurance, body composition, muscular endurance, strength, and flexibility); however, this chapter focuses only on cardiorespiratory endurance.

INTENSITY

Exercise intensity indicates how much exercise should be performed or how hard the client should exercise and is typically prescribed on the basis of maximal HR (HR_{max}), HR reserve, $\dot{V}O_2max$, or RPE. Prescribing exercise intensity using HR is considered the preferred method, because of the correlation between HR and stress on the heart and because it is easy to monitor during exercise.[4] One method of prescribing exercise is to use a percentage of HR_{max}, either directly determined by a graded exercise test or estimated on the basis of the age-predicted maximum HR (220 − age). The training range should be between 60 and 90% of HR_{max}.[29]

A second method for prescribing exercise involves the use of the HR reserve, or the Karvonen formula:

$$\text{HR reserve} = (HR_{max} - HR_{rest}) \times (\text{training range}) + HR_{rest}$$

where the training range is a value between .50 to .85, selected by the clinician.

If exercise is prescribed based on $\dot{V}O_2max$, 50 to 85% is also used as a training range. If RPE is the base, the prescribed exercise intensity is within the range of 12 to 16 (Table 10-6). The RPE is especially useful for prescribing intensity for individuals who are unable to take their pulse or when HR is altered because of the influence of medication. The use of RPE should be considered an adjunct to monitoring HR in all other individuals.[29]

Selection of an appropriate training range, as opposed to a specific training value, has been recommended to provide greater flexibility in the exercise prescription while ensuring that a training response will be achieved.[4] For example, a client who is starting out on an exercise program might be given a target HR at the lower end of the range (e.g., between 60 and 70% of HR_{max}), instead of being told to keep the target HR at 90% of HR_{max}. Health-related benefits can be realized at lower intensities, and thus lower intensities may be appropriate if the goal of exercise is to improve health instead of fitness.[36]

DURATION

The length of time spent exercising is described by the component of duration. The optimal duration recommended for aerobic training is between 20 and 30 min per session of exercise.[4,29] For individuals who are unable to perform 20 min of continuous exercise, discontinuous exercise can be prescribed. That is, several 10-min bouts can be performed, for example, until the client can tolerate 20 to 30 min of continuous exercise. Duration can be progressed up to 60 min of continuous activity.[29]

Duration should also include warm-up (5 to 15 min) and a cool-down (5 to 10 min) activities in addition to the aerobic component. The warm-up slowly increases the HR and respiratory rate and will reduce muscle soreness. The warm-up can include gentle stretching activities and low-intensity training using the mode selected for aerobic conditioning.[4] An appropriate cool-down can be accomplished by gradually reducing the intensity of the endurance activity and continuing beyond the duration of the training period at a low level. Stretching activities are also appropriate as part of the cool-down and enhance flexibility.

FREQUENCY

A second time-related component of exercise prescription is frequency, or how often exercise should be performed. The optimal frequency for most individuals is 3 to 5 times per week.[4,29] Clients should begin a program at 3 to 4 times per week and progress to 5 times. Individuals with low functional capacities can perform daily or twice daily exercise, because the total amount of exercise (considering intensity, duration, and frequency) is low.[29]

Clinicians should consider the interaction of intensity, duration, and frequency for clients who are not capable of meeting the minimal criteria. These factors are also important for clients who exceed the suggested limits of exercise because of the increased risk for musculoskeletal injury as a result of overtraining.

MODE

The question of which activity to perform is addressed by the component of mode in the exercise prescription. Generally, the greatest improvement in aerobic capacity is achieved through rhythmical activities that involve the large muscle groups, such as walking, running, hiking, cycling, rowing, and swimming.[29] A wide variety of activities can be prescribed to improve cardiorespiratory endurance, but it has been suggested that unfit individuals start out with activities that can be maintained at a constant intensity, such as cycling and treadmill walking. Once a basic level of fitness has been obtained, activities with variable intensity, such as team and individual sports and dancing, can be prescribed.[4,29]

Consideration should also be given to potential orthopedic stresses produced by the selected mode.[29] For example, an obese client might reap greater benefits and a decreased risk of injury with a non-weight-bearing activity (cycling, water aerobics) than with a weight-bearing activity (walking, running). Individuals are more likely to engage in activities they enjoy and have access to; fortunately, there is a wide variety of modes available to enhance compliance with the exercise prescription.

Figures 10-4 to 10-10 illustrate aerobic activities commonly performed on equipment that meet the criteria for appropriate exercise. These exercises involve large muscle groups; are appropriate for enhancing cardiovascular fitness if proper guidelines for intensity, duration, and frequency are followed; and can be used in a clinical setting. The purpose of each activity is to increase aerobic capacity. The client should be able to perform the exercise at a level based on previous activity and tolerance to stress. Compliance is enhanced if the client finds the exercise enjoyable. The procedure for each exercise is based on the intensity, duration, frequency, and progression that the clinician prescribes for the client. The client is thus provided with an individualized exercise prescription and treatment plan for safely and efficiently increasing aerobic capacity.

FIGURE 10-4 Recumbent bicycle.

ADVANTAGES: Seat is more comfortable compared to a traditional bicycle; back support provides a more upright spine posture; relatively quiet to operate; easy to monitor/measure vital signs during use; safer than a traditional bicycle due to wider base of support and ease of mounting and dismounting.[11]

DISADVANTAGES: Local muscle fatigue in the lower extremities may limit performance; difficult to elevate heart rate to target range due to the more supine position required on the recumbent bicycle compared to a traditional bicycle or other modes of upright exercise.

FIT: Seat position should be adjusted to allow 15-20 degrees of knee flexion when the lower extremity is in the most outstretched position on the pedal and the ankle is at 90 degrees of dorsiflexion.

(Courtesy of Lifefitness, Franklin Park, IL.)

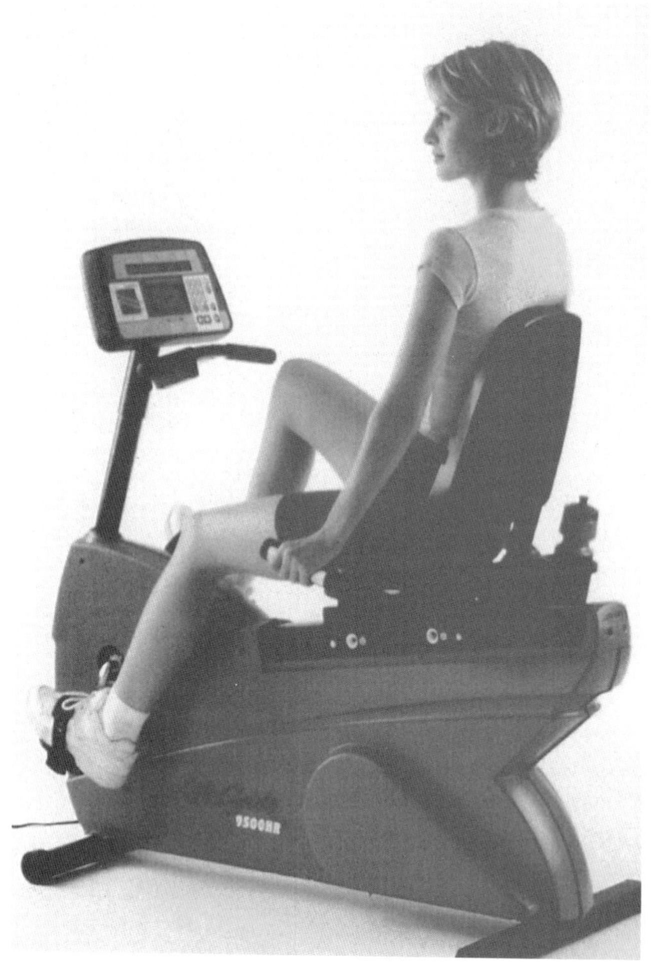

FIGURE 10-5 **Stationary bicycle.**

ADVANTAGES: Allows non-weight bearing exercise, no impact Relatively quiet to operate; easy to monitor/measure vital signs during use; requires little time/effort for habituation.

DISADVANTAGES: Local muscle fatigue in the lower extremities may limit performance; difficult to elevate heart rate to target range due to muscle fatigue limitation; not all clients are familiar with or experienced with bicycling; no weight bearing achieved.

FIT: Seat position should be adjusted to allow 15-20 degrees of knee flexion when the foot is in the lowest position on the pedal and the ankle is in 90 degrees of dorsiflexion.

(Courtesy of Lifefitness, Franklin Park, IL.)

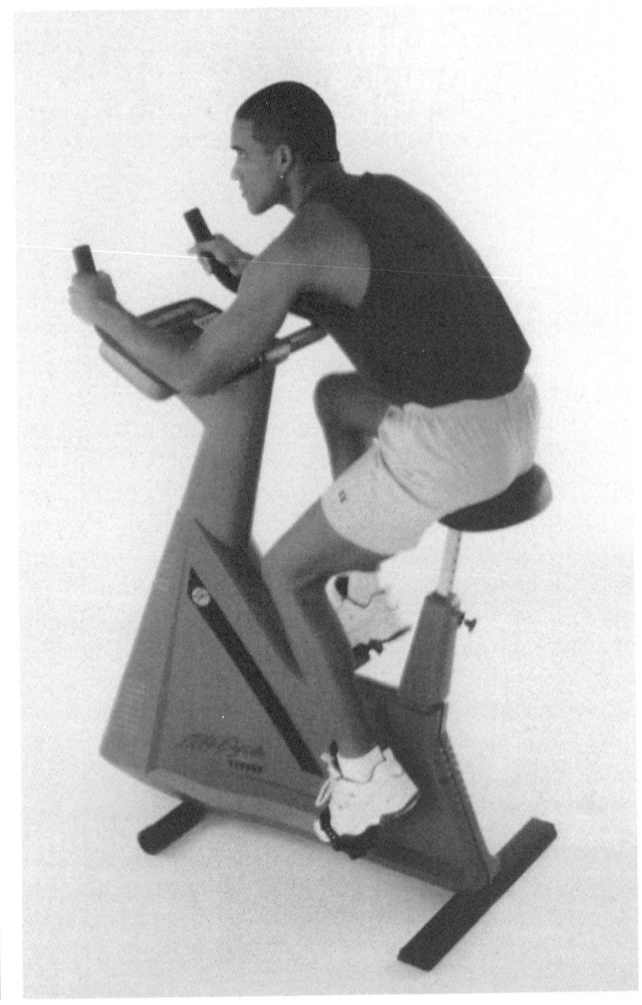

FIGURE 10-6 **Nu-Step recumbent stepper.**

ADVANTAGES: Large seat provides a comfortable form of sitting activity; the motion of stepping is familiar to most clients, so habituation is minimal; provides a low-impact form of activity; safer than a traditional stair climber due to wider base of support and ease of mounting and dismounting; utilizes all four limbs so is considered a total body exercise and clients can easily achieve target heart rate.

DISADVANTAGES: No weight bearing achieved; may be difficult to measure vital signs due to involvement of upper extremities during exercise.

FIT: Seat should be adjusted to allow slight knee flexion when lower extremity is in the most extended position.

(Courtesy of Lalonde & Co, Ann Arbor, MI.)

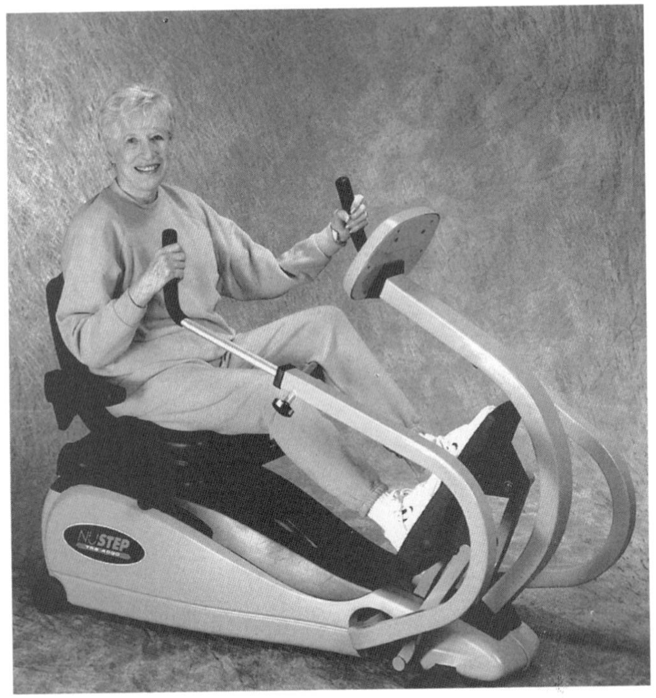

FIGURE 10-7 **Stair-climber.**

ADVANTAGES: The motion of stepping is familiar to most clients, so habituation is minimal; provides weight-bearing; provides a low-impact form of activity; occupies less space than most other types of equipment.

DISADVANTAGES: May aggravate or cause a knee problem due to stress on knee joints; posture on the equipment should be carefully scrutinized due to tendency for users to adopt poor postures and rely too much on upper extremities for support; somewhat difficult to mount, requires good balance.

(Courtesy of Lifefitness, Franklin Park, IL.)

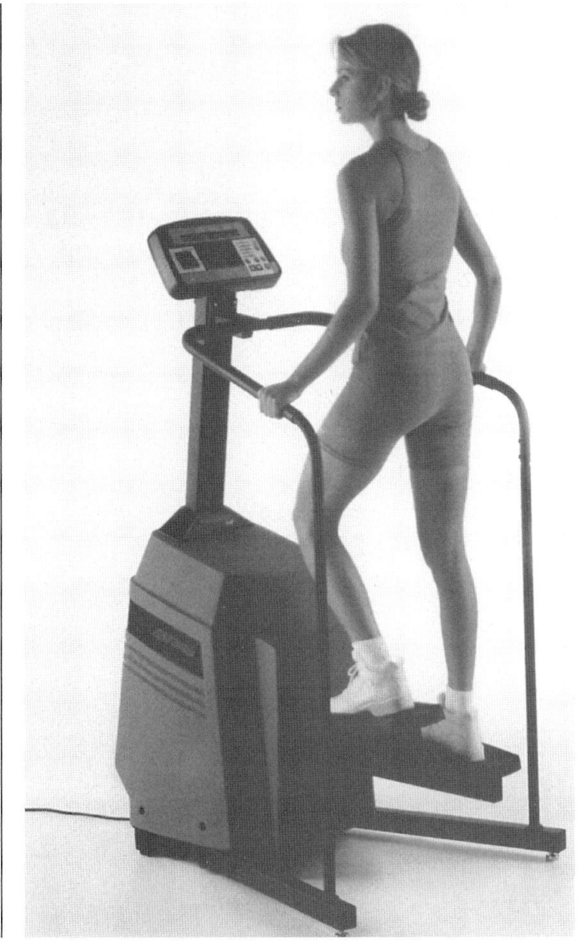

FIGURE 10-8 **Treadmill.**

ADVANTAGES: Walking/running are familiar activities for most clients, so requires minimal habituation; provides weight bearing; uses large lower extremity muscles that require less energy, enabling heart rate to be elevated and kept in the target range without local muscle fatigue; easy to adjust intensity (speed and/or elevation).

DISADVANTAGES: Weight bearing exercise may be difficult for obese clients or for those with orthopedic limitations; requires a lot of space; expensive; difficult to monitor/measure vital signs when clients walk fast or run; tends to makes significant noise when in use (making it difficult to hear blood pressure.

(Courtesy of Lifefitness, Franklin Park, IL.)

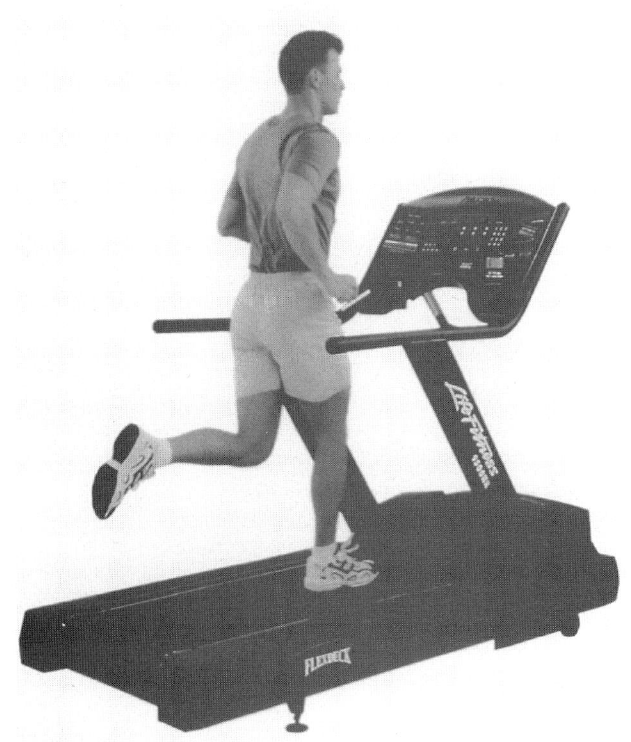

FIGURE 10-9 **Total Body System.**

ADVANTAGES: Utilizes all four limbs so is considered a total body exercise and clients can easily achieve target heart rate; low impact.

DISADVANTAGES: Requires greater coordination than other modes of activity so takes client longer to habituate; requires greater floor space than other pieces of equipment; difficult to monitor/measure vital signs due to involvement of upper extremities during exercise; difficult to mount/dismount.

(Courtesy of Lifefitness, Franklin Park, IL.)

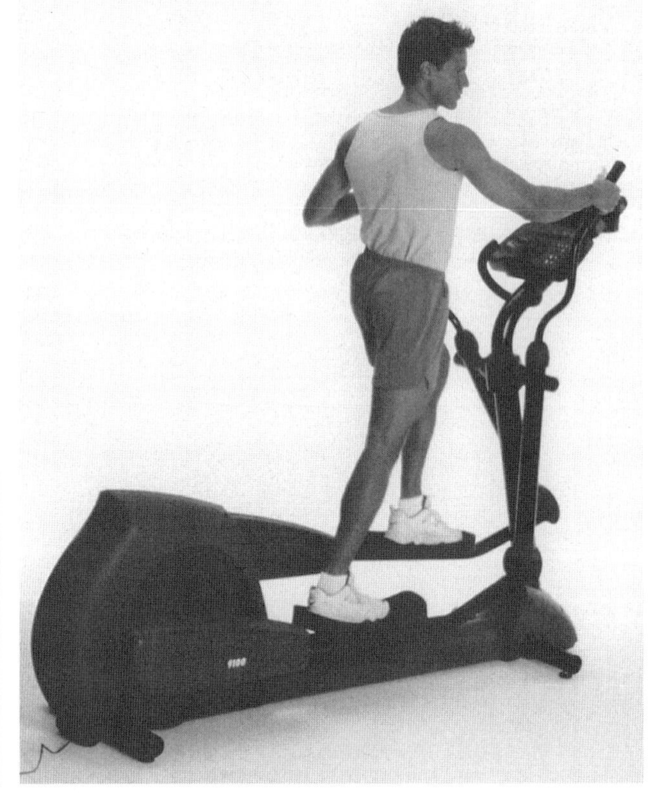

FIGURE 10-10 **Upper Body Ergometer.**

ADVANTAGES: Eliminates lower extremities for those with significant lower extremity impairments, while providing a mechanism to perform aerobic exercise; easy to mount/dismount; relatively quiet to operate.

DISADVANTAGES: Local muscle fatigue limits performance; lower heart rates are achieved due to the use of smaller muscles; unfamiliar for most clients so requires greater habituation time; difficult to monitor/measure vital signs during activity.

FIT: Seat should be adjusted to allow slight elbow flexion during maximum upper extremity extension while back maintains contact with seat; seat height should be adjusted so that client shoulder height is even with the axis of the arm crank.

(Courtesy of Henley Healthcare, Sugar Land.)

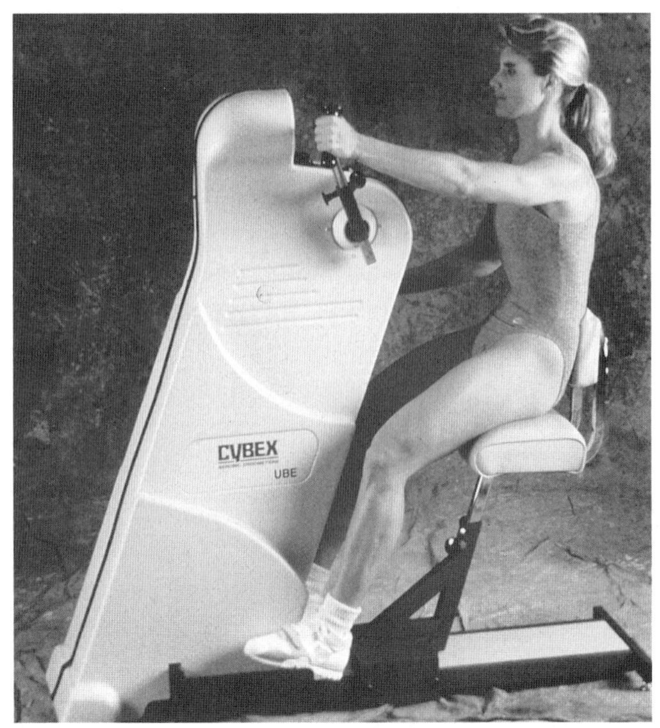

PROGRESSION

The final component of the exercise prescription is progression, or how the program changes over time. An aerobic exercise program may progress through a series of stages: initiation, improvement, and maintenance.

Initiation Stage

The initiation stage is designed to enable the individual to slowly adapt to the exercise program and lasts 3 to 6 weeks.[12,29] The parameters of the prescription are set at low ranges, so that exercise is prescribed at 40 to 60% of HR reserve or $\dot{V}O_2$max (RPE of 11 to 12), duration is set between 15 and 40 min per session, and frequency is prescribed for three times per week on nonconsecutive days, up to six times per week. Individuals who are not experienced with exercise or who have lower aerobic capacities should begin at the low end of the ranges provided (e.g., 40% of HR reserve, 15 min per session, three times per week). Clients who have experience with exercise or who have higher aerobic capacities can begin at the higher end of the ranges.

Improvement Stage

Progression to the improvement stage is recommended when the client can perform the exercise prescription independently at a frequency of five to six sessions per week for a duration of 30 to 40 min for 2 weeks without signs of musculoskeletal overuse or excessive fatigue.[11] Progression continues during the improvement stage, but at a faster rate than in the initiation stage.[29] This stage lasts 4 to 5 months and involves increases in intensity to the higher ranges (60 to 85% HR reserve or $\dot{V}O_2$max) and consistent increases in duration to 20 to 30 min continuously.

Because intensity and duration interact and depend on each other, only one parameter should be increased per exercise session.[11] For example, if intensity is increased, duration should be decreased so the training volume (intensity × duration × frequency) does not increase more than 10% per week. When intensity is held constant, duration should be increased by no more than 5 to 10 min per session.[11]

Although these general guidelines are helpful, the client's objective and subjective training responses should most heavily influence training progression.[11] Signs and symptoms of inappropriately paced progression include inability to complete an exercise session, decreased interest in training, increased HR and RPE values at the same workload, and increased complaints of aches and pains.[37] Adjustments in the rate of progression should be made for age and deconditioning because of the increased time required for adaptation in the elderly and deconditioned.[29] Together, the initiation and improvement stages should take about 6 months and result in a 5 to 30% increase in aerobic capacity.[11,36]

Maintenance Stage

During the maintenance stage of training, further improvement in aerobic capacity is minimal and the focus is on maintaining the fitness level, diversifying the mode, and enjoying exercise as a lifetime habit.[11] It is important to realize that fitness level will decrease about 50% within 4 to 12 weeks if a maintenance program is not performed, indicating the importance of prescribing activities that are similar in energy cost to the activities performed during the improvement stage.

Activity diversification is, therefore, suggested to decrease boredom and increase enjoyment, decrease the potential for overuse injuries, add competition to the program if desired, and explore new interests.[11,28] For example, a client who was new to exercise and began a training program with treadmill walking or with a cycling program because of the ability to carefully control and monitor workload could participate in water exercise or soccer during the maintenance stage. Additional physical activities can substitute for activities performed in the earlier stages, so that the total training volume stays the same to maintain aerobic conditioning. Individuals training for competition, which usually occurs during the maintenance stage, can diversify training on non-competition days to decrease overuse, rotate muscle groups to spread out stresses, and maintain the cardiovascular fitness.[11]

It is also appropriate to review training goals, repeat exercise testing, and establish new goals during the maintenance stage so that the participant will be more likely to continue exercising as a regular habit. The documented success of programs designed to encourage the adoption of a regular exercise habit is similar to the success of changing other health-related behaviors, such as cessation of smoking and weight reduction. Approximately 50% of clients who initiate such health-related behaviors reach the maintenance stage.[38]

Compliance

Factors that best predict exercise dropout (or noncompliance) are related to the client, program, and other characteristics. Personal characteristics that predict dropout are smoking, sedentary leisure time, sedentary occupation, Type A personality, blue-collar occupation, overweight or overfat, poor self-image, depressed, anxious, and a poor credit rating.[39] Program factors that predict dropout include inconvenient time or location, excessive costs, high-intensity, lack of variety, solo participation, lack of positive feedback, inflexible goals, and poor leadership. Additional factors that have been identified to predict dropouts are lack of spouse support, inclement weather, excessive job travel, injury, medical problems, and job change or move. These factors in sum indicate clinicians should develop specific strategies to enhance compliance with the exercise prescription.[40] Table 10-8 lists some of these strategies.

The use of behavior change theories to enhance the

TABLE 10-8 Suggested Strategies for Enhancing Compliance with the Exercise Prescription

Minimize musculoskeletal injuries by adhering to the principles of exercise prescription
Encourage group participation or exercising with a partner
Emphasize a variety of modes of activities and enjoyment in the program
Incorporate behavioral techniques and base the prescription on theories of behavior change
Use periodic testing to document progress
Give immediate feedback to reinforce behavior changes
Recognize accomplishments
Invite the client's partner to become involved and support the training program
Ensure that the exercise leaders are qualified and enthusiastic

Reprinted with permission from Franklin BA. Program factors that influence exercise adherence: practical adherence skills for the clinical staff. In: RK Dishman, ed. Exercise adherence. Champaign, IL: Human Kinetics, 1988:237–258.

adoption of exercise has recently received increased attention in the literature, specifically the application of the "stages of change" model.[28,39,41–43] The model posits that individuals cycle along a continuum of behavioral change from precontemplation (no intention to make a change), to contemplation (considering a change), to preparation (beginning to make changes), to action (actively engaging in the new behavior), to maintenance (sustaining the change over time).[42] Researchers have shown that pre-exercise identification of the client's stage can be used to target an intervention approach that will enhance movement toward maintenance.[42] Assessment of the stage is easily accomplished via a five-item questionnaire; one item represents each stage (Table 10-9).

Once the stage is identified, the intervention can be tailored to enhance compliance and movement toward maintenance. For example, an individual in the contemplation stage is not quite ready for an exercise prescription. Efforts in this stage should focus on providing information about the costs and benefits of exercise, strategies to increase activity within the present lifestyle, and the social benefits of activity. Clients in the preparation stage benefit most from a thorough examination and exercise prescription. And clients in the action or maintenance stage benefit from learning about strategies to prevent relapse, making exercise enjoyable, and diversifying the exercise prescription to include more variety. Given the difficulty most people encounter when changing health-related behaviors, it seems prudent to use documented behavior change theories when possible, such as the stages of change model.

SUMMARY—EXERCISE PRESCRIPTION

A scientifically based exercise prescription includes the elements of intensity, duration, frequency, mode, and progression. The program is individualized, based on ob-

TABLE 10-9 Questionnaire to Determine the Stage of Change of a Client

Stage	Question
Precontemplation	"I presently do not exercise and do not plan to start exercising in the next 6 months"
Contemplation	"I presently do not exercise, but I have been thinking about starting to exercise within the next 6 months"
Preparation	"I presently get some exercise, but not regularly"
Action	"I presently exercise on a regular basis, but I have begun doing so only within the past 6 months"
Maintenance	"I presently exercise on a regular basis and have been doing so for longer than 6 months"

Reprinted with permission from Marcus BH, Simkin LR. The stages of exercise behavior. J Sports Med Phys Fitness 1993;33:83–88.

jective data obtained from a thorough examination and on psychosocial factors unique to the client. Compliance with an exercise prescription is most likely achieved when the prescription meets the needs and goals of the individual and is based on recognized scientific principles and theoretical models.

CASE STUDY

PATIENT INFORMATION

A 46-year-old female presented 10 weeks after an arthroscopic repair of the right medial meniscus. A review of her history revealed hypercholesterolemia for 1 year and a hysterectomy 4 years earlier. The patient was currently taking 30 mg atorvastatin once a day (cholesterol lowering medication). Immediately after the surgery, the patient underwent a knee rehabilitation program; the knee pain resolved, and she was discharged with all goals achieved. Now that she was pain free, her goals were to start exercising again to decrease her cholesterol levels, to stay healthy, and to decrease her body weight by 20 lb. The health history examination revealed no family history of CAD; no smoking, alcohol, or drug use; and no eating disorders. The patient had been on a low-fat diet since her diagnosis of hypercholesterolemia.

The physical examination revealed that she was 5 ft. 4 in. (1.65 m) tall, weighed 160 lb (72.7 kg), and had a body mass index, [BMI; calculated as weight (kg) divided by height (m^2)] of 27 kg/m^2. The patient's resting vital signs were HR = 86; BP = 132/80; and RR = 16. Her right knee showed 0° extension and 120° flexion, manual muscle testing revealed 5/5 hamstrings strength and 4+/5 quadriceps strength, and her hips and ankles were within the normal limits for range of motion and strength bilaterally. The patient's gait was without deviation. She rated her pain as 0/10, except after significant walking or standing, which she rated as a 2/10. She had returned to work full time and was independent in activities of daily living. The patient completed the PAR-Q and answered yes to questions 5 and 6 (Fig. 10-2).

LINKS TO

Guide to Physical Therapist Practice* and *Athletic Training Educational Competencies

The primary pattern from the *Guide*[31] that applies to this patient is pattern 4I. This pattern is described as "impaired joint mobility, motor function, muscle performance, and range of motion associated with bony or soft tissue surgery." Meniscal repairs are included within this pattern, which lists aerobic endurance activities under the specific direct interventions. A secondary pattern for this patient is pattern 6A: "primary prevention/risk factor reduction for cardiopulmonary disorders," because she has hypercholesterolemia, a risk factor for CAD. Aerobic conditioning activities are also included as a specific direct intervention in pattern 6A.

The therapeutic exercise domain in the *Competencies*[44] refers to treatment of athletes using a variety of techniques. In the teaching objectives listed under this domain, the *Competencies* indicates that the athletic trainer, upon graduation from an accredited program, will be able to "describe indications, contraindications, theory and principles for the incorporation and application of various contemporary therapeutic exercises including cardiovascular exercise including the use of stationary bicycle, upper extremity ergometer, treadmill, stair climbing, etc." The demonstration of these aerobic activities is also emphasized.

INTERVENTION

The patient returned to the clinic under her earlier prescription for knee rehabilitation. Because of her age and sex, PAR-Q results, and presence of one (hypercholesterolemia) and possibly two (sedentary lifestyle) risk factors for CAD, the referring physician was contacted to discuss whether the patient required further medical screening before commencing an exercise program. After a discussion with the primary-care physician, it was determined that she should undergo a submaximal GXT with supervision and monitoring, followed by 1 week of supervised exercise training. If the client was symptom-free during the supervised exercise period, an independent exercise program could be prescribed.

Because the client was 10 weeks postsurgery and was unconditioned, the Astrand-Rhyming bicycle ergometer submaximal GXT was selected and administered. She completed 6 min of exercise at a workload of 450 kg/min (as recommended for unconditioned females) with a HR at both the 5th and 6th minute of 130 beats/min. Using the nomogram (Fig. 10-3), the clinician plotted a line from a HR of 130 beats/min (for females) to a workload of 450 kg/min (for females); the line crossed the $\dot{V}O_2max$ line at 2.8 L/min. Using the correction factor for her age (Table 10-5), the adjusted estimated $\dot{V}O_2max$ for the patient was 2.2 L/min.

The clinician then converted the absolute $\dot{V}O_2max$ to the relative $\dot{V}O_2max$:

$$(2.2 \text{ L/min} \times 1000 \text{ mL/L}) \div 72.7 \text{ kg (weight)} = 30.3 \text{ mL/kg/min}$$

According to Table 10-10, which shows the normal $\dot{V}O_2max$ values adjusted by age and sex, the patient fell within the normal range (32 ± 21 mL/kg/min).

GERIATRIC Perspectives

- A thorough and systematic approach to prescribing an appropriate exercise session is essential if the intervention is to be effective. A detailed history of exercise, lifestyle, and barriers to exercise should be obtained. Christmas and Andersen[1] provided a helpful review of the benefits of exercise in older adults along with guidelines for prescription and recommendations for improving compliance.
- Research indicates that exercise capacity, as measured by $\dot{V}O_2max$, declines with aging. However, some disagreement exists concerning the amount of the decline, which is generally reported to be 0.5 to 1.0 mL/kg/min per year.
- Healthy older adults can tolerate endurance training at relatively intense levels (85% HR reserve) without a significant increase in rates of injury. In addition, some studies have demonstrated health benefits for older adults involved in low- to moderate-intensity training (50% HR reserve).[2]
- Maximal HR declines with age and exhibits a sex difference. However, the sex difference appears to be related to the greater percent of body fat in older women than in older men.[3] Although age is the single most important factor associated with a decline in maximal HR, other factors that affect exercise performance are mode of exercise, level of fitness, and motivation.[1,4] Maximal HR has been determined to be lower for bicycle ergometry and swimming than for the treadmill. Older individuals may hesitate to exert maximal effort owing to constraints related to poor muscle tone, cardiopulmonary disease, and musculoskeletal problems (e.g., arthritis).
- Various simple, objective measurements may help determine whether maximal effort was performed: patient appearance and breathing rate, Borg scale, age-predicted HR, and SBP.[5] The Borg scale uses a numeric indicator (on a scale of 6 to 20 or 0 to 10) and corresponding descriptor (very, very light to very, very hard) and has been found to correlate with the percentage of maximal HR during exercise. Resting SBP may rise an average of 35 mm Hg over the adult lifespan, and is thought to be associated with a loss of elasticity in the major blood vessels. Higher resting SBP is associated with higher peak blood pressure during exercise.[6]
- Normal responses to acute aerobic exercise may be altered by certain cardiovascular medications. For instance, nonselective β-blockers may decrease the heart rate and metabolic response to acute exercise. Individuals on this, and similar, antihypertensive medication should be supervised and instructed in exercise safety.[7]
- To safely conduct exercise testing in older adults with disabilities or balance precautions, Smith and Gilligan[8] proposed a modification of the step test. The modified chair-step test is performed while sitting and includes incremental stages to increase the cardiovascular demands.

1. Christmas C, Andersen RA. Exercise and older patients: guidelines for the clinician. J Am Geriatr Soc 2000;48:318–324.
2. Hazzard WR, Blass JP, Ettinger WH, et al. Principles of geriatric medicine and gerontology. 4th ed. New York; McGraw-Hill, 1998.
3. Hollenberg M, Long HN, Turner D, Tager IB. Treadmill exercise testing in an epidemiological study of elderly subjects. J Gerontol Bio Sci 1998;53A:B259–B267.
4. Londeree BR, Moeschberger ML. Influence of age and other factors on maximal heart rate. J Cardiac Rehab 1984;4:44–49.
5. Froelicher VF. Manual of exercise testing. St. Louis: Mosby-Year Book, 1994.
6. Shephard RJ. Aging, physical activity, and health. Champaign, IL: Human Kinetics, 1997.
7. Gordon NF, Duncan JJ. Effect of beta-blockers on exercise physiology: implications for exercise training. Med Sci Sports Exerc 1991;23:668–676.
8. Smith EL, Gilligan C. Physical activity prescription for the older adult. Physician Sportsmed 1983;11:91–101.

According to the stages of change model, this patient was in the preparation stage, meaning that she was ready to adopt a regular exercise habit and was ready for an exercise prescription for guidance. According to recent guidelines, the BMI of 27 kg/m^2 classified the patient as overweight (BMI $<$ 25 = normal; 25 to $<$ 30 = overweight; 30+ = obese).[45] Because the patient was overweight and considering her goals, the clinician thought a lower-intensity, longer-duration program would be an appropriate prescription to decrease the risk of musculoskeletal injury and maximize weight loss. The recommended weight loss goal was to lose 1 to 2 lb per week through nutrition changes and exercise.[11] Because she had already adopted a low-fat diet, the exercise program was thought to assist in her goal to lose weight.

Because the patient reported knee pain after walking, the exercise program was initially prescribed on the bicycle. The program was to be progressed to walking as her knee and fitness level allowed. The initial prescription was as follows.

PEDIATRIC *Perspectives*

- Many physiologic differences in the cardiac, circulatory, and respiratory systems exist among the child, adolescent, and adult. In the child, as in the adult, HR and cardiac output increase as work intensity increases.[1] However, compared to the adult, the child's heart rate is higher and SV lower, and total cardiac output is somewhat lower at a given workload.[2]
- Children are less mechanically efficient than adults and, therefore, lose more energy than adults when performing the same activity at the same intensity.[1] Children demonstrate a $a-vO_2$ difference and increased blood flow to exercising muscle than adults. This suggests an improved oxygen delivery system in children that compensates for lower cardiac output.[1]
- Because of smaller body mass, children have lower absolute values for aerobic capacity.[2,3] Small children demonstrate lower SBP and DBP than adolescents, both of which are lower than the adult.[1,2] Boys have higher peak SBP than age-matched girls.[1]
- When exercising, children breathe more frequently (greater ventilatory equivalent) than adults at any level of oxygen uptake.[2]
- Special concern must be taken with children who exercise in hot environments. Children have a relatively poorer ability to dissipate heat during exercise than adults.[1,3] Children generate more metabolic heat per unit body size, have lower sweating rates, and slower onset of sweating related to rise in core temperature than do adults. From a practical standpoint, exercise levels should be reduced for children exposed to hot environments and additional time should be allowed for acclimatization compared to adults.[2]
- During weight-bearing exercise (running, walking) the oxygen uptake of children is 10 to 30% higher than of adults at a designated, submaximal pace.[2]
- Evidence exists that cardiac hypertrophy results from endurance training in children.[2,3] It is currently unclear whether the aerobic system in children will adapt with training, because it is difficult to distinguish the effects of growth and maturation from those of training.[1,2] Training seems to have less effect on children under the age of 10; however, improved performance may be related to improved mechanical efficiency, increased anaerobic capacity, and training effects that occur during free play.[2]
- When initiating a program for children, be creative with fitness activities. Suggestions include fitness-based games and activities that are fun. As children age, progress to intramural and local league sports.[4]
- The ACSM guidelines for children in grades 3 and above recommend base training of 30 min accumulated exercise throughout the day in segments of at least 10 min each, progressing to 60 to 120 min (accumulated) for athletic performance.[4]

1. Thein LA. The child and adolescent athlete. In: JE Zachezewski, DJ Magee, WS Quillen, eds. Athletic injuries and rehabilitation. Philadelphia: Saunders, 1996:933–958.
2. McArdle WD, Katch FI, Katch VL. Exercise physiology. 4th ed. Baltimore: Williams & Wilkins, 1996.
3. Bar-Or R. Pediatric sports medicine for the practitioner: from physiologic principles to clinical applications. New York: Springer-Verlag, 1983.
4. American College of Sports Medicine. ACSM's guidelines for exercise testing and prescription. 3rd ed. Baltimore: Williams & Wilkins, 1998.

TABLE 10-10 Normal Values of $\dot{V}o_2max$ (mL/kg/min) Uptake at Different Ages by Sex

Age	Male	Female
20–29	43 (± 22)	36 (± 21)
30–39	42 (± 22)	34 (± 21)
40–49	40 (± 22)	32 (± 21)
50–59	36 (± 22)	29 (± 22)
60–69	33 (± 22)	27 (± 22)
70–79	29 (± 22)	27 (± 22)

Reprinted with permission from American College of Sports Medicine. Resource manual for guidelines for exercise testing and prescription. 3rd ed. Baltimore: Williams & Wilkins, 1998.

Intensity: Using the Karvonen equation and 40 to 60% as the beginning HR range, the target HR was calculated as follows:

$$\text{Target HR at 40\% HR reserve} = [(HR_{max} - HR_{rest}) \times 0.4] + HR_{rest} = [(174 - 86) \times 0.4] + 86 = 121 \text{ beats/min}$$

$$\text{Target HR at 60\% HR reserve} = [(HR_{max} - HR_{rest}) \times 0.6] + HR_{rest} = [(174 - 86) \times 0.6] + 86 = 139 \text{ beats/min}$$

Thus, the training HR range was set at 121 to 139 beats/min. The clinician referred to the patient's submaximal GXT to determine the workload required to reach the target HR range. The patient achieved a HR of 135 at a workload of 450 kg/min of resistance on the bicycle ergometer. Therefore, the initial workload was set at that level and the HR was monitored to determine whether resistance should be increased or decreased. The RPE was also used to monitor intensity, at an initial level of 12 to 13.

Duration: After a 10-min warm-up (5 min of gentle ROM and stretching exercises and 5 min of no-load work on the bicycle), the patient was asked to pedal for 15 to 20 min, increasing 5 min per week to the goal of 30 to 40 min. The session ended with a 3-min cool-down on the bike at no load and 5 to 10 min of stretching.

Frequency: The patient was told to exercise three times per week the first week in the clinic where she could be supervised. She was progressed to five times per week, as tolerated.

Mode: Stationary bicycle ergometer (Fig. 10-5).

The initial goals of the program were to become independent in pulse-taking and monitoring of exercise, perform the exercise prescription independently, and progress to exercising at 450 kg/min for 35 to 40 min for four to five times per week by week 4.

The patient experienced no signs or symptoms of exercise intolerance during week 1 of supervised exercise and was able to complete the exercise as prescribed. She was given a home program, and was asked to return in 3 weeks.

PROGRESSION

Four Weeks After Initial Examination

At re-examination after week 4, she was exercising on the bicycle at 450 kg/min for 35 min continuously four to five times per week. The program was modified by increasing the target HR range to 60 to 70% of HR reserve, or 139 to 147 beats/min (RPE = 13 to 14). To meet this intensity, the patient had to set a higher workload on the bicycle (500 to 600 kg/min). The duration was initially decreased to 20 min to offset the increase in intensity, and she was instructed to increase the duration 5 min per week until she reached 40 min. The frequency was continued at three to five times per week.

Three Months After Initial Examination

At the 3-month follow-up, the patient reported that she successfully completed the training program on the bicycle over the previous 2 months and was currently exercising three to five times per week at 500 to 600 kg/min for 40 min. The patient noted that she was spending approximately 1 hr for each exercise session and wished to maintain the same time frame. She felt that she could add walking to her program on alternate days to increase overall energy expenditure. The patient was told to use her HR as a guide and to start out walking 20 min at a fast enough speed to put her HR into the training range of 139 to 147 beats/min (RPE = 13 to 14). She was instructed to increase duration no more than 5 min per week. The patient was scheduled for a return examination in 3 months, when a repeat GXT would be performed to examine progress.

Six Months After Initial Examination

At the 6-month re-examination, the client weighed 146 lb (66.36 kg) and her resting HR was 78. She had been exercising five to six times per week: three on the bicycle and two to three walking. She was able to increase her target HR into the prescribed range by cycling at 600 kg/min and by walking as fast as she could.

A follow-up submaximal test was performed. The Astrand Rhyming bicycle ergometer protocol was repeated. This time the client completed 6 min of exercise at a workload of 600 kg/min with a resulting HR at both the 5th and 6th minute of 138 beats/min. Using the nomogram (Fig. 10-3), the clinician plotted a line from a HR of 138 beats/min (for females) to a workload of 600 kg/min (for females); the line crossed the $\dot{V}o_2max$ line at 3.0 L/min. Using the correction factor for her age (Table 10-5), the clinician determined the patient's adjusted estimated $\dot{V}o_2max$ to be 2.3 L/min.

The clinician then converted her absolute $\dot{V}o_2max$ to a relative $\dot{V}o_2max$:

$$(2.3 \text{ L/min} \times 1000 \text{ ml/L}) \div 66.36 \text{ kg (weight)} = 35.2 \text{ mL/kg/min}$$

The client's predicted $\dot{V}O_2max$ had increased approximately 15% over the 6-month training period and she had lost approximately 15 lb.

OUTCOME

Strategies to reinforce the adoption of regular exercise were discussed with the patient, who revealed her intention to continue exercising regularly. She had established a relationship with a neighbor with whom she walked, and she was satisfied using the stationary bicycle because it was at home and convenient. A new exercise prescription was provided using an intensity of 70 to 80% HR reserve (145 to 155 beats/min), which would require a resistance of between 600 and 750 kg/min on the bicycle ergometer. The patient had met her initial goals, except she had lost only 15 lb. She was, however, confident that with continued exercise she would lose the remaining 5 lb and maintain her weight at that level.

SUMMARY

- Significant evidence exists to support the recommendation that adults should participate in regular physical activity. Although recent evidence suggests that moderately intense activities provide important health-related benefits (including efforts to adopt a more active lifestyle),[27,28] improvements in aerobic conditioning are achieved through careful examination of cardiorespiratory endurance capacity and exercise prescription. A method to generate safe and effective exercise prescriptions was presented, based on an understanding of the following concepts.

- The primary energy sources used during aerobic exercise are carbohydrate and fat. High-intensity, brief-duration exercise relies on the ATP-PCr metabolic pathway; high-intensity, short-duration exercise relies on the ATP-PCr and anaerobic glycolysis pathways; and submaximal-intensity, long-duration exercise relies on the oxidative pathway.
- Normal responses to acute aerobic exercise include increased HR, SV, $\dot{Q}$, $a-vO_2$, SBP, and pulmonary ventilation in response to an increasing workload. The distribution of blood flow shifts to provide increased blood to the working muscles, and DBP changes little during acute exercise. Abnormal responses include signs and symptoms of exercise intolerance.
- Adaptations to chronic exercise include increased heart size, increased SV at rest, decreased resting and submaximal HR and RR, increased overall blood volume, increased blood flow to the muscles, and an increased $\dot{V}O_2max$. Psychological benefits of training include improvements in depression, mood, anxiety, well-being, and perceptions of physical function.
- Specific guidelines were presented for the screening and supervision of GXT and exercise sessions based on age, sex, and the presence of risk factors for CAD. Submaximal graded exercise testing can be used to establish a baseline of aerobic fitness before participation in an aerobic training program and from which to establish an exercise prescription. Submaximal tests include bicycle ergometer tests, treadmill tests, and field tests.
- An individualized exercise prescription should include parameters for intensity, duration, frequency, and mode. Progression should include an initiation stage of 3 to 6 weeks, an improvement stage of 4 to 5 months, and a maintenance stage aimed at the adoption of a lifetime exercise habit.

REFERENCES

1. Berryman JW. Out of many, one. A history of the American College of Sports Medicine. Champaign, IL: Human Kinetics, 1995.
2. U.S. Department of Health and Human Services. Physical activity and health: a report of the surgeon general. Atlanta: Centers for Disease Control and Prevention, 1996.
3. Caspersen CJ, Powell KE, Christenson GM. Physical activity, exercise, and physical fitness: definitions and distinctions for health-related research. Public Health Rep 1985;100:126–131.
4. Wilmore JH, Costill DL. Physiology of sport and exercise. 2nd ed. Champaign, IL: Human Kinetics, 1999.
5. Blair SN, Kohl HW, Paffenbarger RS, et al. Physical fitness and all-cause mortality. JAMA 1989;262:2395–2401.
6. Paffenbarger RS, Hyde RT, Wing AL. Physical activity and physical fitness as determinants of health and longevity. In: C Bouchard, RJ Shephard, T Stephens, eds. Physical activity, fitness, and health: international proceedings and consensus statement. Champaign, IL: Human Kinetics, 1994:33–48.
7. Public Health Service. Healthy people 2000: national health promotion and disease prevention objectives [DHHS Pub. No. (PHS) 91-50212]. Washington DC: DHHS, 1990.
8. U.S. Department of Health and Human Services. Healthy people 2010 objectives: draft for public comment. http://web.health.gov/healthypeople/2010. Accessed Nov 11, 1999.
9. Pate RR, Pratt M, Blair SN, et al. Physical activity and public health. JAMA 1995;273:402–407.
10. Hasson SM. Clinical exercise physiology. St. Louis: Mosby, 1994.
11. American College of Sports Medicine. Resource manual for guidelines for exercise testing and prescription. 3rd ed. Baltimore: Williams & Wilkins, 1998.
12. Berne RM, Levy MN. Cardiovascular physiology. 7th ed. St. Louis: Mosby, 1997.
13. McAuley E. Physical activity and psychosocial outcomes. In: C Bouchard, RJ Shephard, T Stephens, eds. Physical activity, fitness, and health: international proceedings and consensus statement. Champaign, IL: Human Kinetics, 1994:551–568.
14. Caspersen CJ, Powell KE, Merritt RK. Measurement of health status and well-being. In: C Bouchard, RJ Shephard, T Stephens, eds. Physical activity, fitness, and health: international proceedings and consensus statement. Champaign, IL: Human Kinetics, 1994:180–202.
15. Rejeski WJ, Brawley LR, Shumaker SA. Physical activity and health-related quality of life. Exerc Sport Sci Rev 1996;24:71–108.
16. McMurdo MET, Burnett L. Randomised controlled trial of exercise in the elderly. Gerontology 1992;38:292–298.
17. Ruuskanen JM, Ruoppila I. Physical activity and psychological well-being among people aged 65 to 84 years. Age Ageing 1995;24:292–296.
18. Woodruff SI, Conway TL. Impact of health and fitness-related behavior on quality of life. Soc Ind Res 1992;25:391–405.
19. Norris R, Carroll D, Cochrane R. The effects of aerobic and anaerobic training on fitness, blood pressure, and psychological stress and well-being. J Psychosomatic Res 1990;34:367–375.
20. Lavie CJ, Milani RV. Effects of cardiac rehabilitation, exercise training, and weight reduction on exercise capacity, coronary risk factors, behavioral characteristics, and quality of life in obese coronary patients. Am J Cardiol 1997;79:397–401.
21. Lavie CJ, Milani RV. Effects of cardiac rehabilitation and exercise training programs in patients, 75 years of age. Am J Cardiol 1996;78:675–677.
22. Kavanagh T, Myers MG, Baigrie RS, et al. Quality of life and cardiorespiratory function in chronic heart failure: effects of 12 months aerobic training. Heart 1996;76:42–49.
23. LeFort SM, Hannah TE. Return to work following an aquafitness and muscle strengthening program for the low back injured. Arch Phys Med Rehabil 1994;75:1247–1255.
24. Petajan JH, Gappmaier E, White AT, et al. Impact of aerobic training on fitness and quality of life in multiple sclerosis. Ann Neurol 1996;39:432–441.
25. Smith SL. Physical exercise as an oncology nursing intervention to enhance quality of life. Oncol Nurs Forum 1996;23:771–778.
26. Manson JE, Hu FB, Rich-Edwards JW, et al. A prospective study of walking as compared with vigorous exercise in the prevention of coronary heart disease in women. N Engl J Med 1999;341:650–658.
27. Andersen RE, Wadden TA, Bartlett SJ, et al. Effects of lifestyle activity vs structured aerobic exercise in obese women. JAMA 1999;281:335–340.
28. Dunn AL, Marcus BH, Kampert JB, et al. Comparison of lifestyle and structured interventions to increase physical activity and cardiorespiratory fitness. JAMA 1999;281:327–334.
29. American College of Sports Medicine. Guidelines for exercise testing and prescription. 5th ed. Media, PA: Williams & Wilkins, 1995.
30. American Association of Cardiovascular and Pulmonary Rehabilitation. Guidelines for cardiac rehabilitation and secondary prevention programs. 3rd ed. Champaign, IL: Human Kinetics, 1999.
31. American Physical Therapy Association. Guide to physical therapist practice, second edition. Phys Ther 2001;81:1–768.
32. McArdle WD, Katch FI, Pechar GS, et al. Reliability and interrelationships between maximal oxygen intake, physical work capacity and step-test scores in college women. Med Sci Sports Exerc 1972;4:182–186.

33. Maud PJ, Foster C. Physiological assessment of human fitness. Champaign, IL: Human Kinetics, 1995.
34. Kline GM, Porcari JP, Hintermeister R, et al. Estimation of $\dot{V}O_2$ max from a one-mile track walk, gender, age, and body weight. Med Sci Sports Exerc 1987;19:253–259.
35. Borg G. Borg's perceived exertion and pain scales. Champaign, IL: Human Kinetics, 1998.
36. American College of Sports Medicine. The recommended quantity and quality of exercise for developing and maintaining cardiorespiratory and muscular fitness in healthy adults. Med Sci Sports Exerc 1990;22:265–274.
37. Lehmann M, Foster C, Keul J. Overtraining in endurance athletes: a brief review. Med Sci Sports Exerc 1993;25:854–862.
38. Dishman RK. Exercise adherence. Champaign, IL: Human Kinetics, 1988.
39. Cardinal BJ. The stages of exercise scale and stages of exercise behavior in female adults. J Sports Med Phys Fitness 1995;35: 87–92.
40. Franklin BA. Program factors that influence exercise adherence: practical adherence skills for the clinical staff. In: RK Dishman, ed. Exercise adherence. Champaign, IL: Human Kinetics, 1988: 237–258.
41. Marcus BH, Simkin LR. The stages of exercise behavior. J Sports Med Phys Fitness 1993;33:83–88.
42. Marcus BH, Rakowski W, Rossi JS. Assessing motivational readiness and decision making for exercise. Health Psychol 1992;11: 257–261.
43. Marcus BH, Rossi JS, Selby VC, et al. The stages and processes of exercise adoption and maintenance in a worksite sample. Health Psychol 1992;11:386–395.
44. National Athletic Trainers' Association. Athletic training educational competencies. 3rd ed. Dallas: NATA, 1999.
45. National Heart, Lung, and Blood Institute. Clinical guidelines on the identification, evaluation, and treatment of overweight and obesity in adults. Bethesda, MD: National Institutes of Health, June 1998.

SECTION

Special Consideration in Therapeutic Exercise

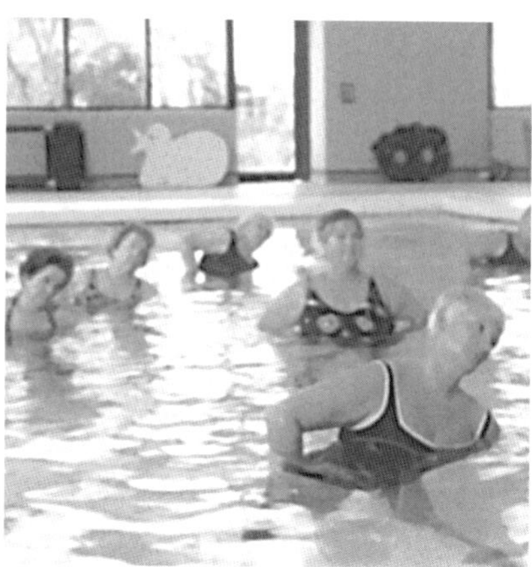

Balance Training

Bridgett Wallace, PT

Balance is essential for individuals to move about their environment and successfully carry out daily activities. Although the definition of balance and its neural mechanisms have changed over the years, this chapter will focus on the systems theory.[1] The systems model focuses on a dynamic interplay between various systems by integrating both motor and sensory strategies to maintain static and dynamic balance. This integration is a complex process that depends on (1) sensory inputs, (2) sensorimotor integration by the central nervous system (CNS), and (3) postural responses.[2] Since about 1980, the literature has expanded on the systematic approach to postural stability for developing more clinical tests and a better understanding of balance. Specifically, this chapter focuses on much of the pioneering work by Nashner.[3,4] The information is presented from a systematic approach to balance that includes biomechanical factors, sensory organization, and coordination of postural movements (musculoskeletal components).

■ Scientific Basis

BIOMECHANICAL COMPONENTS OF BALANCE

Balance is the process of controlling the body's center of gravity over the support base or, more generally, within the limits of stability, whether stationary or moving. Balance can be divided into static and dynamic balance. Static balance refers to an individual's ability to maintain a stable antigravity position while at rest by maintaining the center of gravity within the available base of support. Dynamic balance involves automatic postural responses to the disruption of the center of gravity position.[1]

Base of Support

The base of support is defined as the area within the perimeter of the contact surface between the feet and the support surface.[4] In normal stance on a flat surface, the base of support is almost square. Although a tandem stance (standing with one foot in front of the other, heel touching toe) and walking extend the length of the person's support surface, the width is narrow. When the support base becomes smaller than the feet (tandem) or unstable, the base of support is decreased and the individual's stability is reduced.

Limits of Stability

To maintain balance in standing, the center of gravity must be kept upright within specific boundaries of space, referred to as limits of stability. Thus limits of stability can be defined as the greatest distance a person can lean away from the base of support without changing that base.[5] Limits of stability allow individuals to overcome the destabilizing effect of gravity by performing small corrective sways in the anterior-posterior (AP) dimension as well as laterally. The limits of stability for a normal adult who is standing upright is approximately 12° AP and 16° laterally.[3] These limits of stability are sometimes illustrated by a "cone of stability." If sway occurs outside the cone, a strategy must be used to restore balance. Figure 11-1 demonstrates the limits of stability boundaries during standing, walking, and sitting.[3]

Center of Gravity

The center of gravity is defined as the central point within the limits of stability area.[4] When a normal person stands upright, the center of gravity is centered over the base of support provided by the feet. A centralized center of gravity allows the individual's sway boundaries to be as large as the stability limits. On the other hand, a person with an abnormal center of gravity will not be as stable within the limits of stability. The relationships among the limits of stability, the sway envelope, and the center of gravity are shown in Figure 11-2.[3]

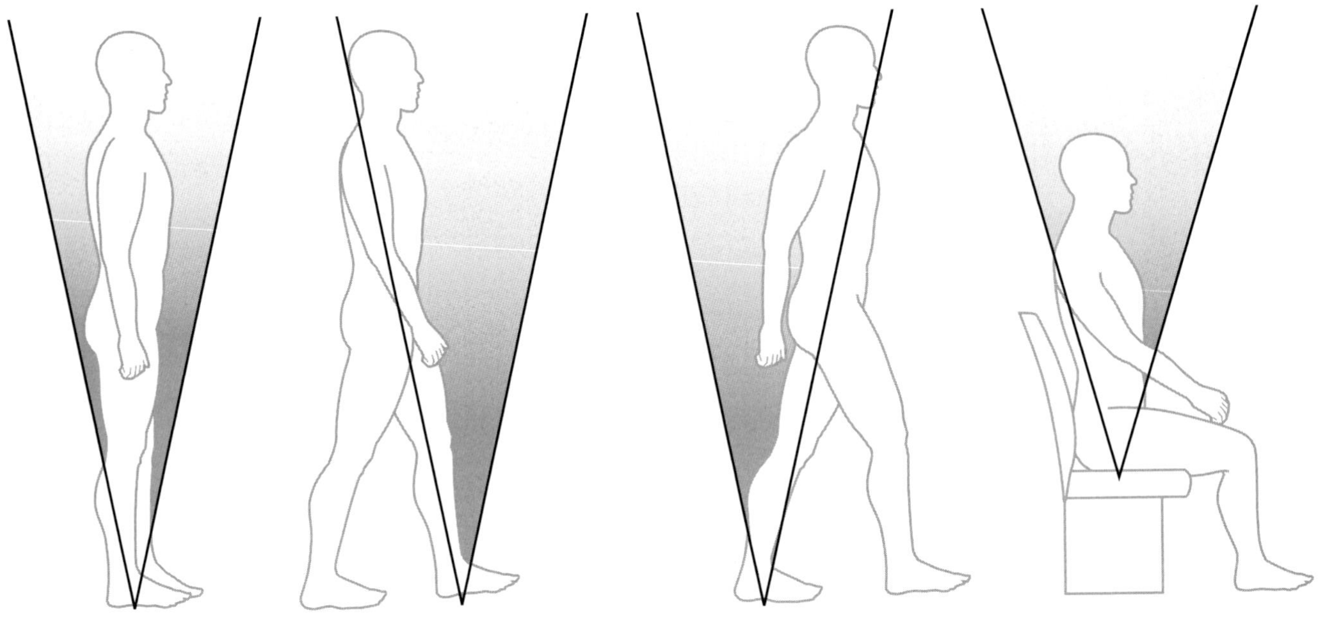

FIGURE 11-1 **Boundaries of the limits of support during standing, walking, and sitting.**

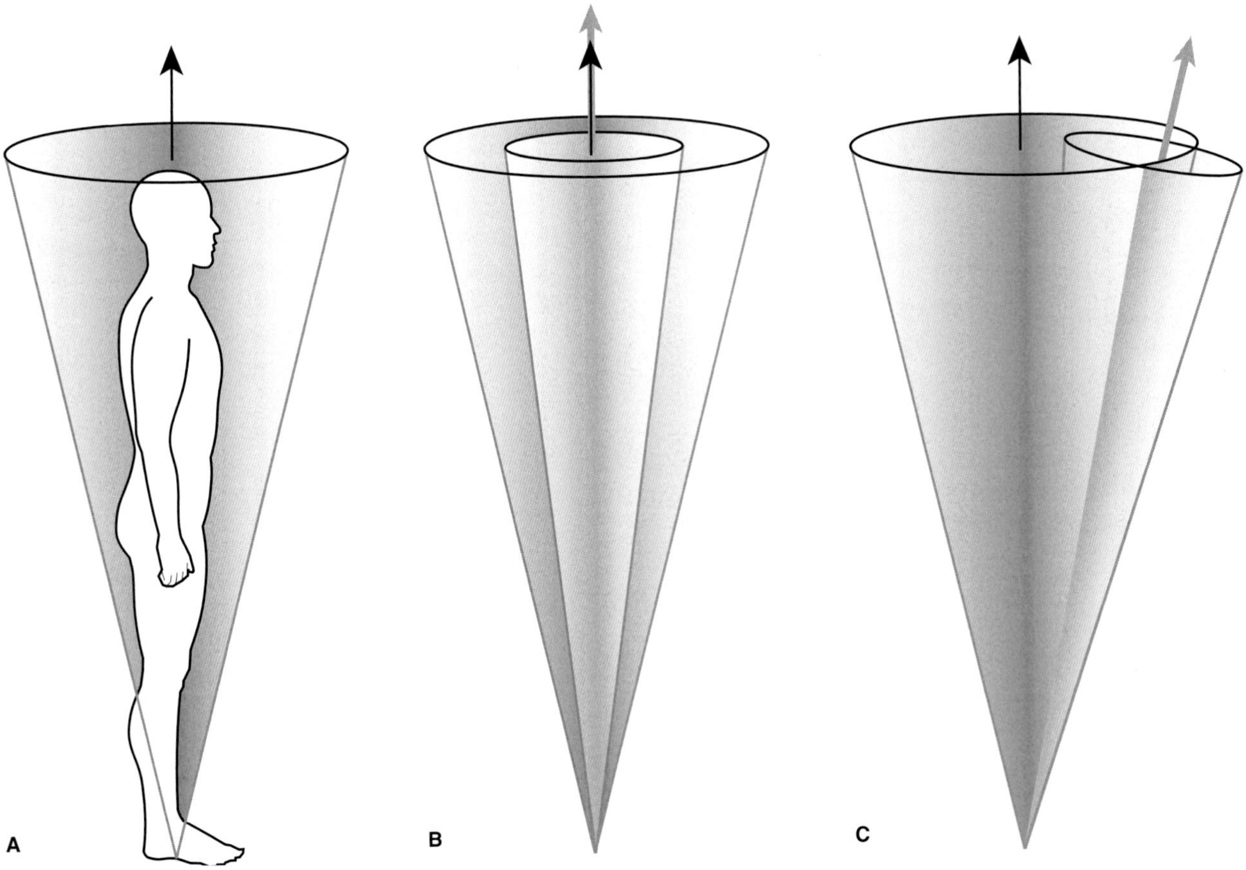

FIGURE 11-2

A. Relationship among the limit of support, the sway envelope, and the center of gravity alignment. **B.** The center of gravity alignment centered within the limit of support. **C.** An offset center of gravity (leaning forward) requires the individual to make an adjustment to maintain balance.

From a biomechanical standpoint, postural stability is the angular distance between the center of gravity and the limits of stability.[3] Therefore, a person's static postural alignment and the dynamic sway affect his or her stability.

SENSORY COMPONENTS OF BALANCE

Balance requires accurate information from sensory input, effective processing by the CNS, and appropriate responses of motor control.[2] Therefore, imbalance can occur from neuropathy, involvement of the CNS, and decreased muscle strength. Proper examination of each component is critical for determining a client's underlying problem and the appropriate treatment plan.

Sensory Organization

The CNS relies on information from three sensory systems: proprioception, visual, and vestibular. No single system provides all the information. Each system contributes a different, yet important, role in maintaining balance. The ability of the CNS to select, suppress, and combine appropriate inputs under changing environmental conditions is called "sensory organization."[6]

Proprioception inputs provide information about the orientation of the body and body parts relative to each other and the support surface. Information is received from joint and skin receptors, deep pressure, and muscle proprioception.[6,7] Proprioception cues are the dominant inputs for maintaining balance when the support surface is firm and fixed.[6,8] Visual inputs provide an individual information about the physical surroundings relative to the position and movement of the head. Visual cues are particularly important when proprioceptive inputs are unreliable.[6,9]

Vestibular inputs provide both a sensory and a motor function to the individual. The sensory component of the vestibular system measures the angular velocity and linear acceleration of the head and detects the position of the head relative to gravity.[6] The motor component, however, uses motor pathways for postural control and coordinated movement. One mechanism within the vestibular motor system is the vestibulospinal reflex. The vestibulospinal reflex initiates a person's appropriate body movements to maintain an upright posture and to stabilize the head and trunk.[10,11] The vestibulo-ocular reflex, on the other hand, stabilizes vision during head and body movements, thus allowing for accurate dynamic vision.[6,10] Because the system has sensory and motor components, the vestibular system plays an important role in balance. This system is dominant when a conflict exists between proprioceptive and visual cues and for postural stability during ambulation.[6,7]

Examination of Sensory Organization

These three sensory inputs (proprioceptive, visual, and vestibular) provide the individual with redundant information regarding orientation. This redundancy allows normal individuals to select, suppress, or combine the appropriate inputs to maintain balance under changing environmental conditions.[3] Nashner[3,4] pioneered technologic advances for examining appropriate sensory integration. One such advancement is known as computerized dynamic posturography, which examines sensory and motor components of the postural control system. The two protocols of this system are the sensory organization test (SOT), which isolates and compares the three sensory inputs, and the movement coordination test (MCT), discussed later in this chapter. A less-sophisticated test for examining the sensory and motor components of balance is the clinical test for sensory interaction and behavior (CTSIB).

Sensory Organization Test

The SOT protocol is used to examine the relative contribution of vision, vestibular, and proprioceptive inputs to the control of postural stability when conflicting sensory input occurs (Fig. 11-3). Postural sway can be examined under six increasingly challenging conditions (Fig. 11-4). Baseline sway is recorded in quiet standing with the eyes open. The reliance on vision is then examined by asking the patient to close the eyes. A significant increase in sway or loss of balance suggests an over-reliance on visual input.[3,12]

Sensory integration is also examined when the surrounding visual field moves in concert with sway (sway-referenced vision), creating inaccurate visual input. The patient is then retested on a support surface that moves with sway (sway-referenced support), thereby reducing the quality and availability of proprioceptive input for sensory integration. With the eyes open, vision and vestibular input contribute to the postural responses. With the eyes closed, vestibular input is the primary source of information, because proprioceptive input is altered. The most challenging condition includes sway-referenced vision and sway-referenced support surface.[3,12]

Clinical Test for Sensory Interaction and Balance

A less-sophisticated tool for examining sensory organization is the CTSIB, also known as the "foam and dome."[10,12] The CTSIB requires the patient to maintain standing balance under six different conditions (Fig. 11-5). During the first three conditions, the individual stands on a firm surface for 30 sec with eyes open, eyes closed, and while wearing a "dome" to produce inaccurate visual cues. The individual repeats these tasks while standing on a foam surface. The tester uses the first condition as a baseline for comparing sway under the other conditions.[10,12]

MUSCULOSKELETAL COMPONENTS OF BALANCE

Many muscles are involved in the coordination of postural stability. This section focuses on key muscle groups and joint actions involved in balance and automatic postural reactions.

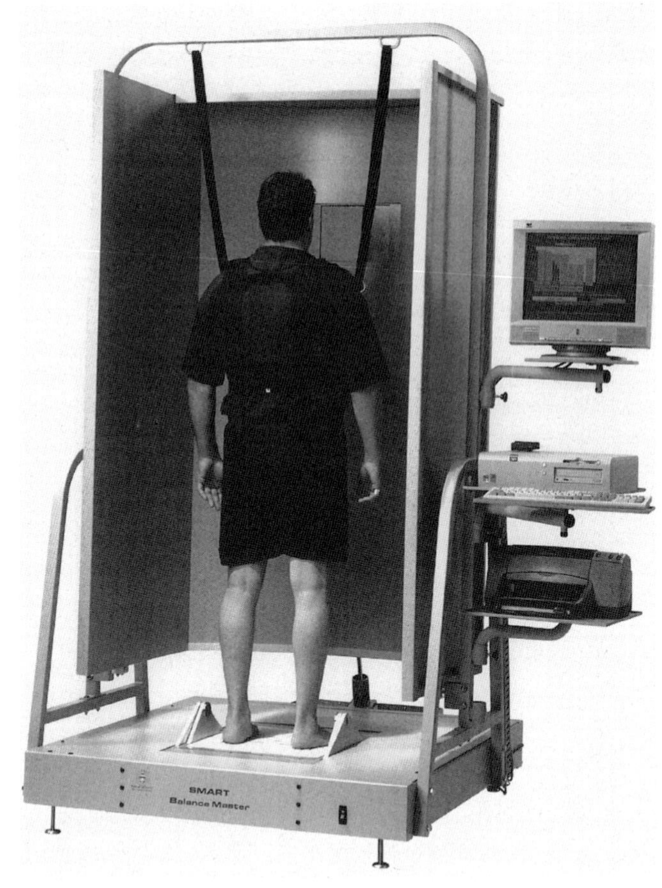

FIGURE 11-3 The SOT performed on a SMART Balance Master.

A type of computerized posturography. Postural sway is examined under six increasingly challenging conditions illustrated in Figure 11-4.

(Courtesy of Neurocom International, Inc., Clackamas, OR.)

Key Muscle Groups

Figure 11-6 shows the major muscle groups that control the body's center of gravity during standing.[4] Postural stability primarily depends on coordinated actions between the trunk and the lower extremities. The motions around the hip, knee, and ankle include joint-specific muscle actions and indirect, inertial forces of neighboring joints.[2–4] Therefore, the anatomic classification of a muscle may differ from the functional classification. For example, the anatomic classification of the tibialis anterior muscle is dorsiflexion. In walking, however, the functional classification of the tibialis anterior is knee flexion, even though no insertion of this muscle occurs at the knee. As the ankle dorsiflexes, the lower leg begins to move forward during gait and inertia causes the thigh to lag behind, resulting in knee flexion.

By the same inertial interactions, the gastrocnemius muscle is defined as an ankle extensor (plantarflexion) and a knee flexor anatomically, but it functionally acts as a knee extensor in standing. The anatomic actions of the quadriceps muscle are hip flexion and knee extension, but it indirectly acts as ankle plantarflexion (extensors). The direct actions of the hamstring muscles are hip extension and knee flexion, but they have an indirect effect on ankle dorsiflexion (flexors).[3,4] These actions are summarized in Table 11-1.[3]

Automatic Postural Reactions

To maintain balance, the body must make continual adjustments. Most of what is currently known about postural control is based on stereotypical postural strategies activated in response to AP perturbation or displacement.[3,10] Horak and Nashner[13] described three primary strategies used for controlling AP sway: ankle, hip, and stepping (Figs. 11-7 to 11-9). These strategies adjust the body's center of gravity so that the body is maintained within the base of support, preventing the loss of balance or falling. Several factors determine which strategy is the most effective response to a postural challenge: speed and intensity of the displacing forces, characteristics of the support surface, and magnitude of the displacement of the center of mass.

The responses an individual makes during sudden perturbations are called automatic postural reactions.[4,13] These responses occur before voluntary movement and after reflexes, yet are similar to both. Automatic postural movements are like reflexes because they respond quickly and are relatively similar among individuals. However, like

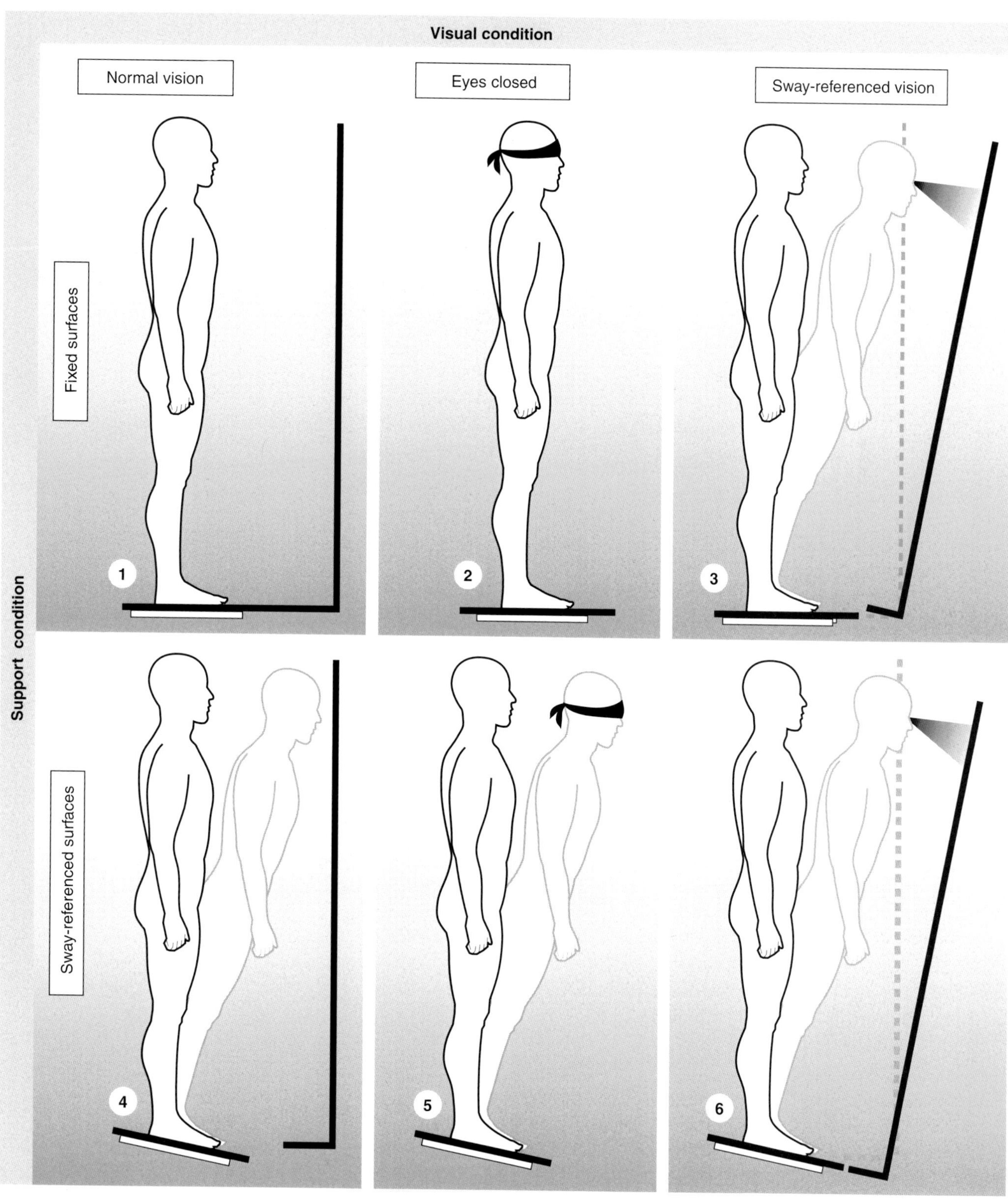

FIGURE 11-4 **Six balance testing conditions.**

(Courtesy of Neurocom International, Inc., Clackamas, OR.)

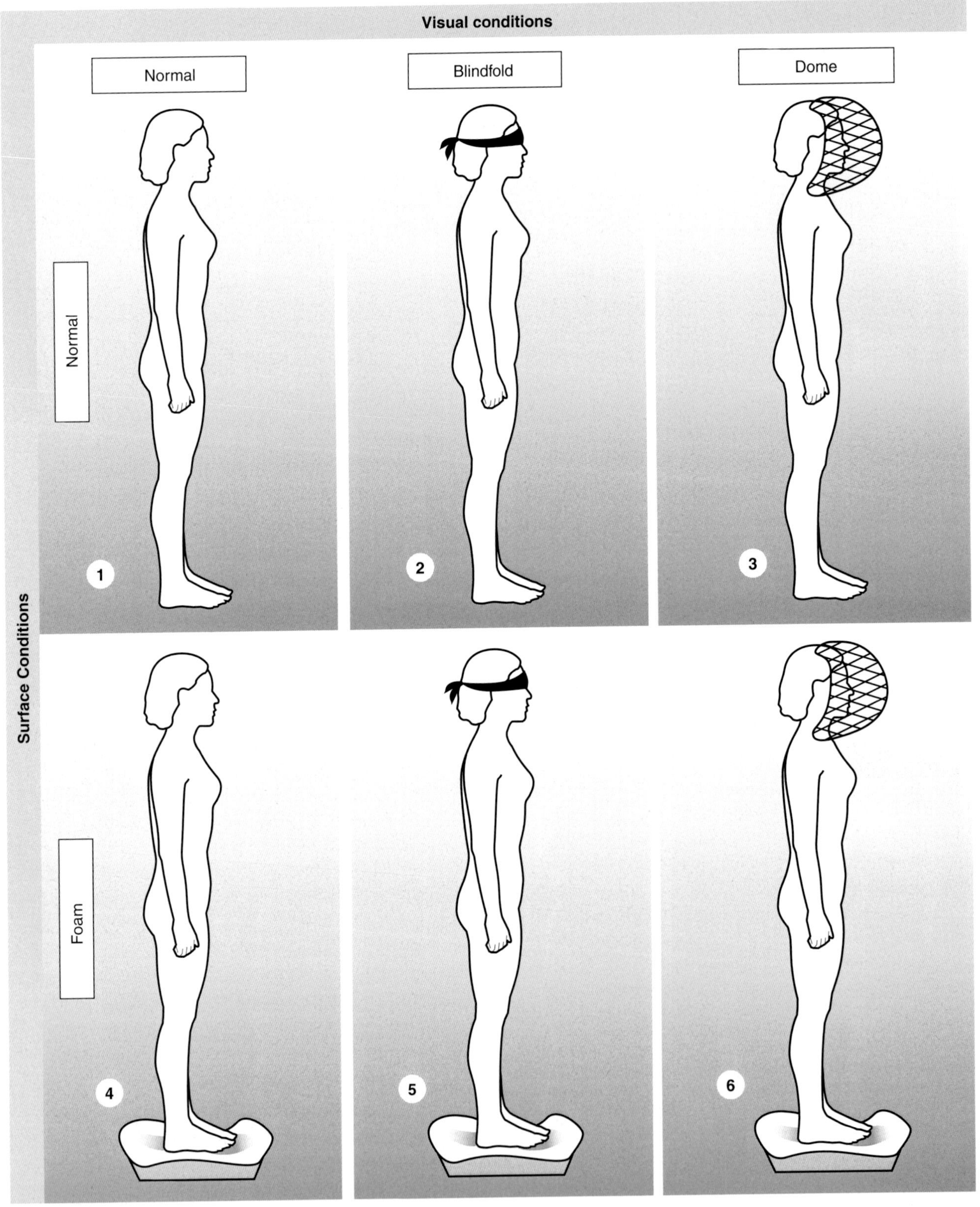

FIGURE 11-5 **The CTSIB.**

(Courtesy of Neurocom International, Inc., Clackamas, OR.)

FIGURE 11-6 Key muscle groups that control the center of gravity when standing.

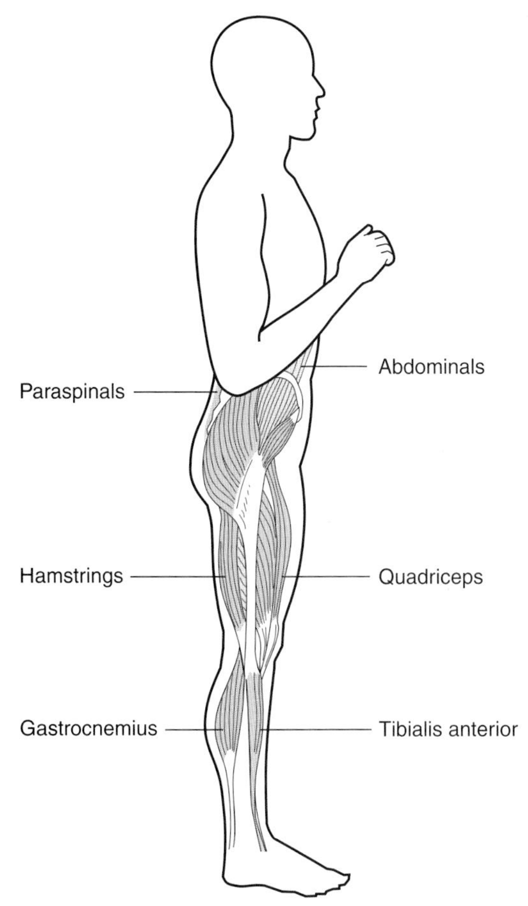

voluntary movements, they primarily depend on coordination responses between the lower trunk and the leg muscles.[4,14]

These responses can be thought of a class of functionally organized responses that activate muscles to bring the body's center of mass into a state of equilibrium.[3] Each of the strategies has reflex, automatic, and volitional components, which interact to match the response to the challenge. Table 11-2 compares reflexes, automatic postural responses, and voluntary movement.[4] To prevent a fall after a sudden perturbation or to maintain balance during locomotion, the healthy individual responds with appropriate muscular actions, called postural strategies.

Ankle Strategy

Small disturbances in the center of gravity can be compensated by motion at the ankle (Fig. 11-7). The ankle strategy repositions the center of mass after small displacements owing to slow-speed perturbations, which usually occur on a large, firm, supporting surface. The

TABLE 11-1 Anatomic and Functional Classification of Muscles Involved in Balance Movements

	Extension		Flexion	
Joint	Anatomic	Functional	Anatomic	Functional
Hip	Paraspinals Hamstrings	Paraspinals Quadriceps	Abdominal Quadriceps	Abdominal Hamstrings
Knee	Quadriceps	Gastrocnemius	Hamstrings, gastrocnemius	Tibialis anterior
Ankle	Gastrocnemius	Quadriceps	Tibialis anterior	Hamstrings

FIGURE 11-7 Ankle strategy.

STRATEGY USED: Center of mass is repositioned after small, slow-speed pertubation.

EXAMPLE: Posterior sway of the body is counteracted by tibialis anterior muscles pulling the body anterior.

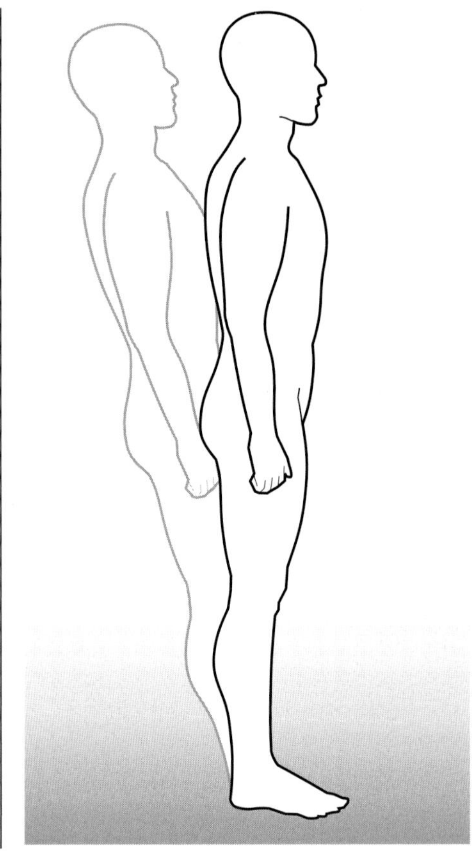

FIGURE 11-8 Hip strategy.

STRATEGY USED: Center of mass is repositioned using rapid, compensatory hip flexion or extension to redistribute body weight.

EXAMPLE: Hip flexion and extension in response to standing on a bus that is rapidly accelerating.

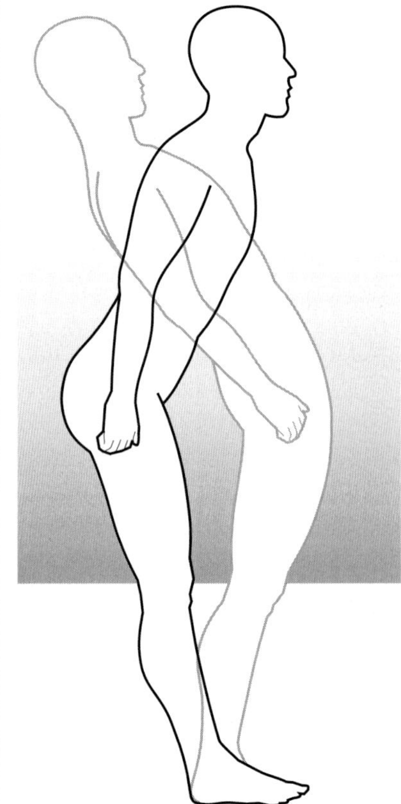

FIGURE 11-9 **Stepping strategy.**

STRATEGY USED: Center of mass can only be repositioned by taking a step to enlarge the base of support. New postural control is then established.

EXAMPLE: Stumbling on an unexpectedly uneven sidewalk.

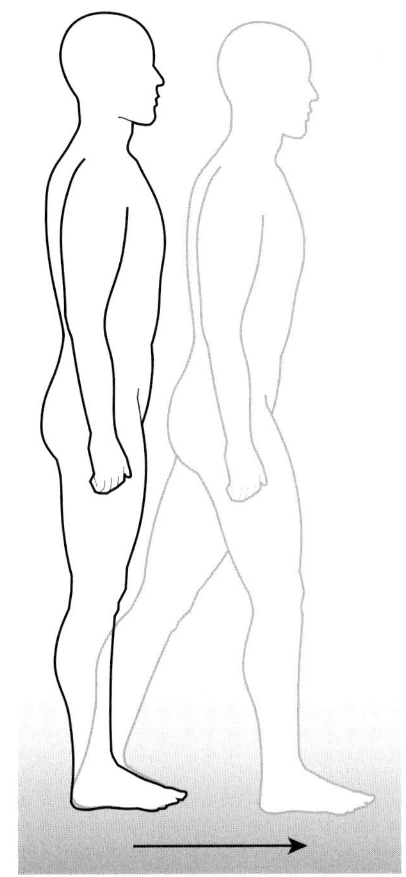

oscillations around the ankle joint with normal postural sway are an example of the ankle strategy. Anterior sway of the body is counteracted by gastrocnemius muscle activity, which pulls the body posterior. Conversely, posterior sway of the body is counteracted by contraction of the anterior tibialis muscles, which pulls the body anterior.

Hip Strategy

If the disturbance in the center of gravity is too great to be counteracted by motion at the ankle, the patient will use a hip or stepping strategy to maintain the center of gravity within the base of support. The hip strategy uses a rapid compensatory hip flexion or extension to redistribute the body weight within the available base of sup-

TABLE 11-2 **Properties of the Three Movement Systems**

Property	Reflex	Automatic	Voluntary
Mediating pathway	Spinal cord	Brainstem, subcortical	Brainstem, subcortical
Mode of activation	External stimulus	External stimulus	Self-stimulus
Response properties	Localized to point of stimulus; highly stereotypic	Coordinated among leg and trunk muscles; stereotypic but adaptable	Unlimited variety
Role in posture	Regulate muscle forces	Coordinate movements across joints	Generate purposeful behaviors
Onset time	Fixed at 35–40 msec	Fixed at 85–95 msec	Varies 150+ msec

port when the center of mass is near the edge of the sway envelope (Fig. 11-8). The hip strategy is usually employed in response to a moderate or large postural disturbance, especially on an uneven, narrow, or moving surface. For example, the hip strategy is often used while standing on a bus that is rapidly accelerating.

Stepping Strategy

When sudden, large amplitude forces displace the center of mass beyond the limits of control, a step is used to enlarge the base of support and redefine a new sway envelope (Fig. 11-9). New postural control can then be reestablished. An example of the stepping strategy is the uncoordinated step that often follows a stumble on an unexpectedly uneven sidewalk.

Examination of Automatic Postural Movements

Automatic postural movements can be analyzed at a range of velocities and directions using the MCT (Fig. 11-10). As noted, the MCT is the second protocol of computerized dynamic posturography. This test requires the patient to maintain standing balance as the support surface repeats various unexpected displacements. Testing includes changing magnitudes of forward and backward displacements as well as tilts of toes up and toes down.[2,3] Diener et al.[14] noted that automatic postural reactions in normal individuals were proportional to the size of the perturbation; hence, the forward and backward translations of the MCT vary in magnitude (small, medium, and large).

Clinical Guidelines

BIOMECHANICAL DEFICITS

When inputs are impaired, such as with inadequate range of motion (ROM) or weakness in the lower extremities, the postural control system receives distorted information. This inaccurate information can result in a malaligned center of gravity within the stability limits, which causes altered movement and increases the risk of falling. For example, if the center of gravity is offset to the left, just a small amount of sway in that direction (left) will cause the individual to exceed the limits of stability. Once this happens, the individual must step or use external support to prevent a fall.

FIGURE 11-10 The MCT.

A type of computerized posturography. Test requires patient to maintain standing balance as support surface tilts the toes up and down and displaces patient forward and backward.

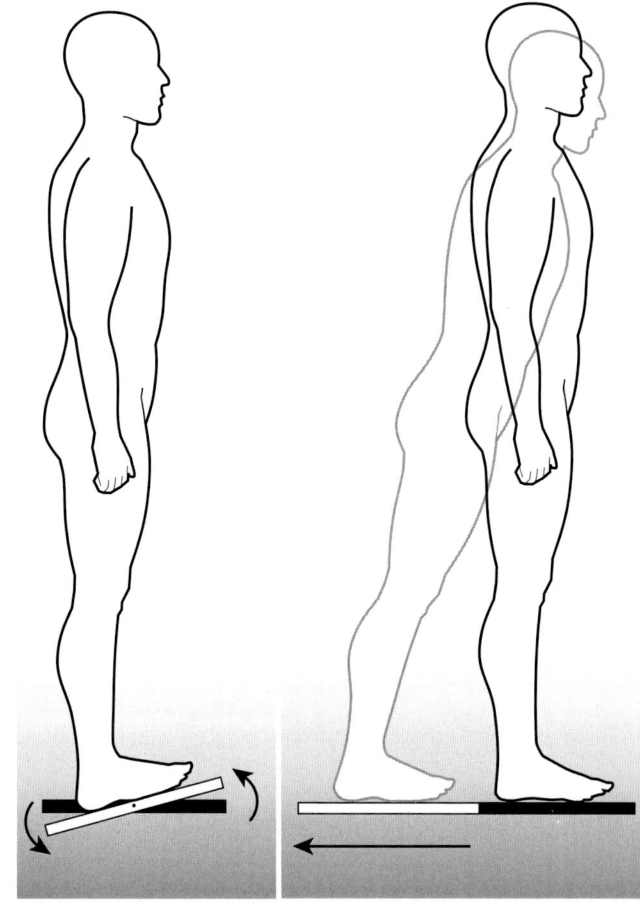

Pain can decrease the patient's normal stability limits. If a patient has knee pain with full weight bearing, he or she compensates by leaning away from the affected side. Thus the patient develops an offset center of gravity, and movement patterns are compromised.

SENSORY DEFICITS

Lack of balance is usually multifactorial; however, examination for sensory organization provides valuable information. Once the deficit or deficits have been appropriately identified, the clinician can design a specific treatment plan to improve the impaired sensory system or can teach the patient compensatory strategies. For example, a patient with neuropathy has impaired proprioceptive cues, but could compensate by using an assistive device and depending more on visual and vestibular cues.[1] Increasing the use of the remaining sensory systems is crucial for this patient. In contrast, a person who suffers from an inner-ear disorder may have impaired use of vestibular cues for balance.[1] Treatment should focus on decreasing the intact sensory systems (visual and proprioception), allowing the vestibular system to adapt.

Balance impairment with neurologic involvement can be much more complex. For example, the client may have impaired use of individual sensory systems (e.g., decreased proprioception and visual deficits) along with impaired central processing of the sensory organization mechanisms.[1,15] Treatment should focus on improving the use of individual sensory systems and teaching the client strategies to optimize sensory selection.

MUSCULOSKELETAL DEFICITS

Ankle strategies require adequate ROM and strength in the ankles and intact proprioception for the individual to adequately sense the support base. Muscle weakness and decreased ROM also limit the use of hip strategies, but proprioception input is not as critical.[7] However, more recent studies have shown that individuals who suffer from vestibular loss are unable to use hip strategies, although their ability to use ankle strategies is unaffected.[7,16]

Postural stability not only requires adequate strength and ROM from the musculoskeletal system but also the ability of the CNS to adequately generate these forces. For instance, abnormal muscle tone (hypertonicity and hypotonicity) may limit the individual's ability to recruit muscles required for balance. Impaired coordination of postural strategies can also be a problem. Deficits in these areas are seen with neurologic involvement such as stroke, head injury, and Parkinson disease.[1,17]

Treatment of musculoskeletal problems includes strengthening and ROM exercises, techniques to correct abnormal tone (facilitation or inhibition), and various coordination activities to improve timing of postural reactions. The following section focuses on major points of clinical application for biomechanical, sensory, and musculoskeletal deficits.

■ *Techniques*

BIOMECHANICAL FACTORS

A malaligned center of gravity decreases one's limits of stability, compromising normal movement patterns. As noted, these biomechanical deficits can be a result of inadequate ROM, decreased strength, pain, swelling, and joint instability. Treatment includes appropriate modalities such as ice, heat, massage, and mobilization (chapter 4). Range of motion (chapter 2), stretching (chapter 3), and strengthening (chapters 5 to 9) exercises are also used. Refer to the appropriate chapter for more information.

SENSORY ORGANIZATION TRAINING

The postural control system depends on the demands of the individual's activity and the surroundings; therefore, treatment needs to be task and environmental specific. Sensory systems respond to environmental changes, so exercises should focus on isolating, suppressing, and combining the different inputs under different conditions. To isolate a patient's proprioceptive inputs, visual cues must be removed (eyes closed) or destabilized. Visual inputs are destabilized when the patient moves his or her eyes and head together in a variety of planes (horizontal, vertical, diagonal), decreasing gaze stability. Prism glasses and moving visual fields are also used to produce inaccurate cues for orientation.[1] During all of these exercises, the patient is asked to stand on a firm, stable surface to optimize proprioceptive inputs. This technique is particularly important for visually dependent patients.

To stimulate vestibular inputs, the patient's reliance on visual and somatosensory cues need to be reduced simultaneously. The patient's level of function determines the difficulty of the task. For example, Patient A may be able to decrease surface cues only by changing from her normal stance (feet apart and eyes open on a firm surface) to a stance with feet together and eyes closed on a firm surface. Patient B's exercises, on the other hand, may require him to stand on a foam surface with feet together and eyes closed. Regardless of the sensory deficit, activities should require the patient to maintain balance under progressively more difficult static and dynamic activities.[1,18]

MUSCULOSKELETAL EXERCISES

As discussed, sensory systems respond to environmental changes, whereas the musculoskeletal system responds more to task constraints. The goal of treatment is to optimize the patient's use of movement strategies for improving postural stability under changing conditions.

Static balance skills can be initiated once the individual is able to bear weight on the lower extremity. The general progression of static balance activities is to progress from bilateral to unilateral and from eyes open to eyes closed. The logical progression of balance training to destabilizing proprioception is from a stable surface and to an unstable surface, such as a mini-trampoline or balance board. As joint position changes, dynamic stabilization must occur for the patient to maintain control on the unstable surface.

The patients should initially perform the static balance activities while concentrating on the specific task (position sense and neuromuscular control) to facilitate and maximize sensory output. As the task becomes easier, activities to distract the patient's concentration (catching a ball or performing mental exercises) should be incorporated into the training program. These distraction activities help facilitate the conversion of conscious to unconscious motor programming.

Techniques to Improve Ankle Strategies

To improve ankle strategies, the patient should perform the exercises on a broad stable surface, concentrating on AP sway. The patient maintains slow, small sways while standing on a firm surface to minimize the use of hip strategies. Examples of activities that can be used to facilitate and improve ankle strategies are presented in Figures 11-11 to 11-14.

FIGURE 11-11 **One-foot standing balance.**

PURPOSE: Facilitate and improve ankle strategies.

POSITION: Client standing with feet shoulder width apart on firm surface.

PROCEDURE: Client lifts right leg off ground and establishes balance on left leg.

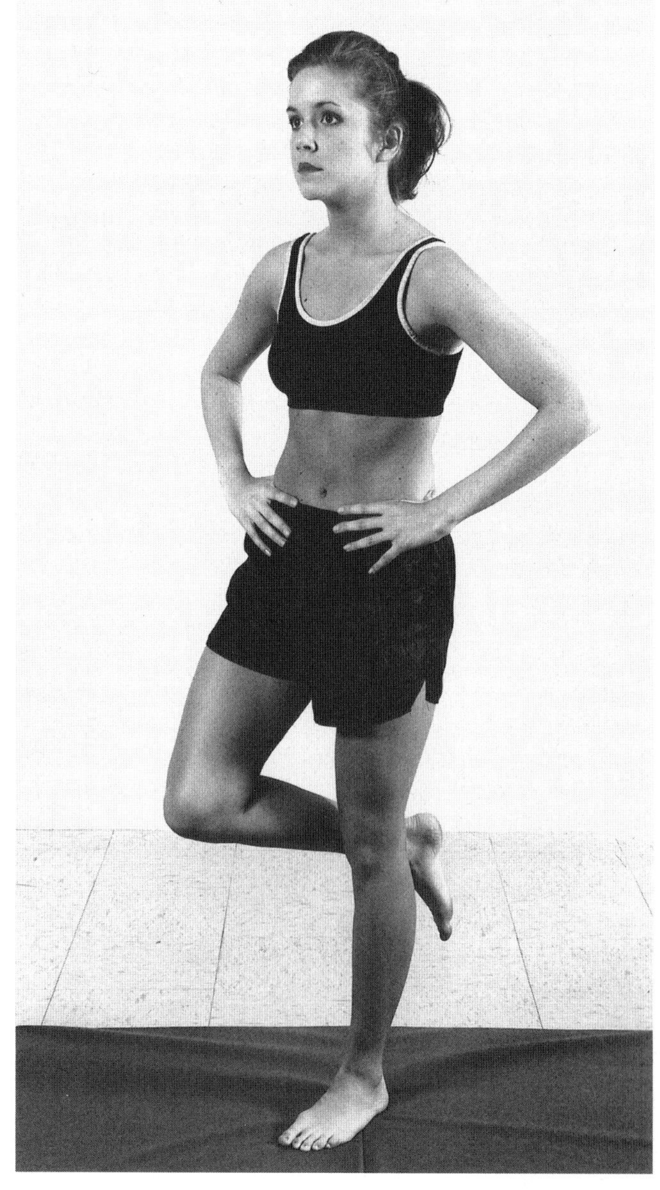

FIGURE 11-12 **One-foot standing balance with hip flexion.**

PURPOSE: Facilitate and improve ankle strategies.

POSITION: Client standing with feet shoulder width apart on firm surface.

PROCEDURE: Client lifts right leg off ground and establishes balance on left leg. The client flexes right hip and knee.

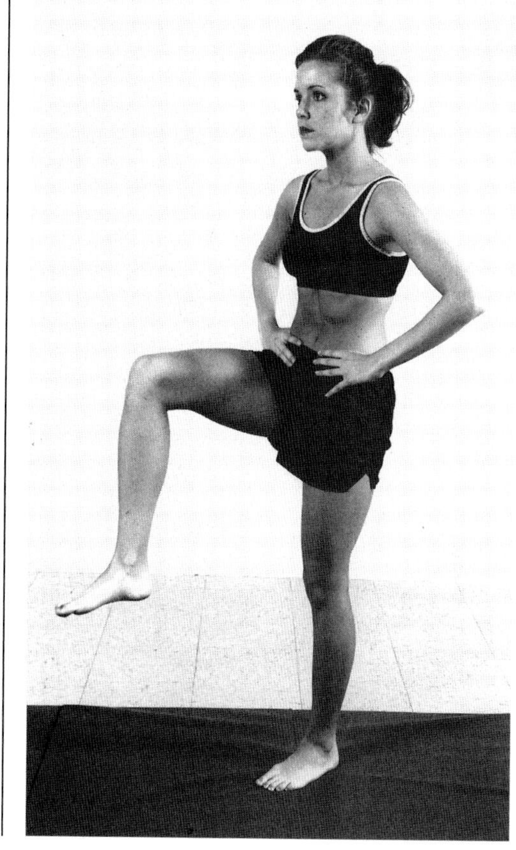

FIGURE 11-13 **One-foot standing balance using weights in diagonal pattern.**

PURPOSE: Facilitate and improve ankle strategies.

POSITION: Client standing with feet shoulder width apart on firm surface.

PROCEDURE: Client lifts right leg off ground and establishes balance on left leg. Then client lifts lightweight dumbbell in diagonal pattern from right hip to left shoulder and then from left hip to right shoulder.

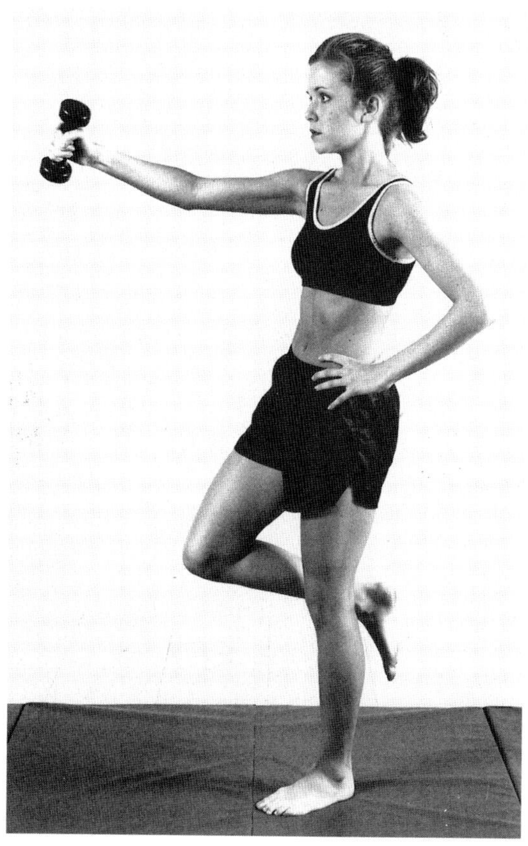

FIGURE 11-14 One-foot standing balance while playing catch.

PURPOSE: Facilitate and improve ankle strategies.

POSITION: Client standing with feet shoulder width apart on firm surface.

PROCEDURE: Client lifts right leg off ground and establishes balance on left leg. Clinician gently tosses ball to client, who catches it.

NOTE: Initially, ball should be thrown near client's body.

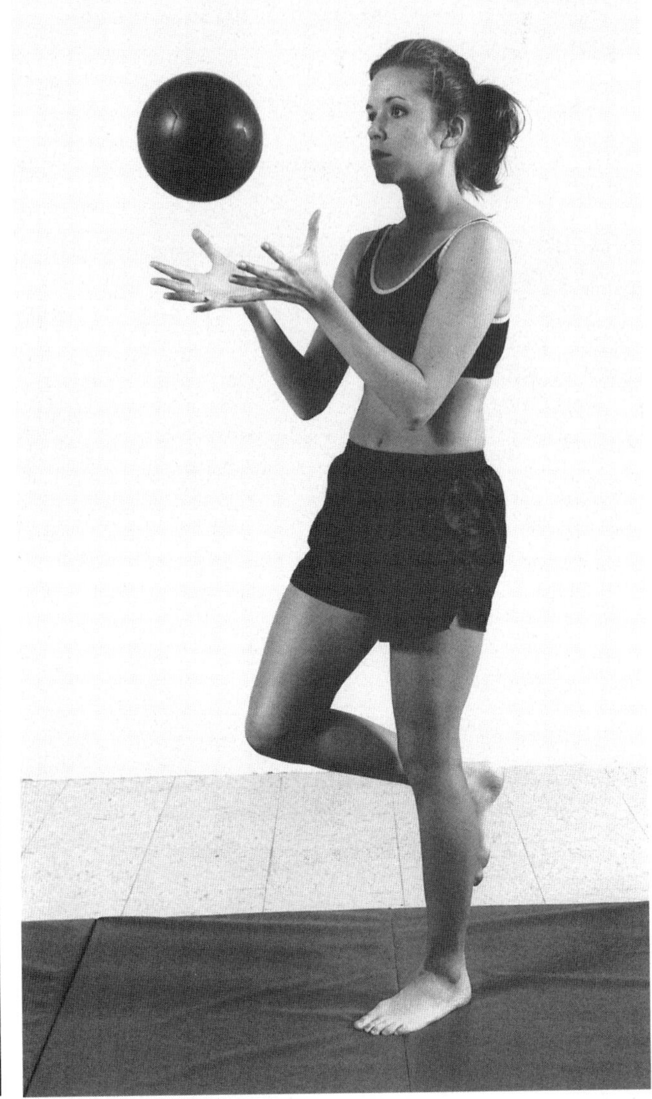

Techniques to Improve Hip Strategies

Exercises to improve the use of hip strategies should be performed on unstable surfaces and at high sway frequencies. These exercises exceed the capabilities of ankle strategies and usually result in movement and adjustments of the trunk. Figures 11-15 to 11-21 demonstrate exercises that can be used to improve hip strategies.

Techniques to Improve Stepping Strategies

Stepping strategies are used once the stability limits have been exceeded. Although stepping strategies are normal reactions for preventing a fall, many patients avoid this pattern and prefer to reach for external support. Reaching for support is especially common in elderly patients, who are proprioceptive and hip dependent. Patients should practice step-ups (Fig. 11-22), step-downs (forward and lateral), and step-overs (also called carioca and braiding) (Fig. 11-23) to help with stepping strategies. To make the training more difficult, the patient can increase the speed at which the step-overs are performed.

A particularly helpful technique is the push and nudge. For example, the patient stands with feet together. The clinician's hands are placed on the patient's shoulders, offering support. The patient maintains an upright posture and leans forward into the clinician's hands until the limit of stability is reached. The clinician—without warning—removes the support, forcing the patient to step to prevent a fall (Fig. 11-24). This exercise can be performed in all directions (anterior, posterior, and lateral).

FIGURE 11-15 **One-foot standing balance with forward bending.**

PURPOSE: Facilitate and improve hip strategies.

POSITION: Client standing with feet shoulder width apart on firm surface.

PROCEDURE: Client lifts right foot off ground and establishes balance on left leg. Then client bends forward as far as possible while maintaining balance.

NOTE: Modifications include bending backward and to each side.

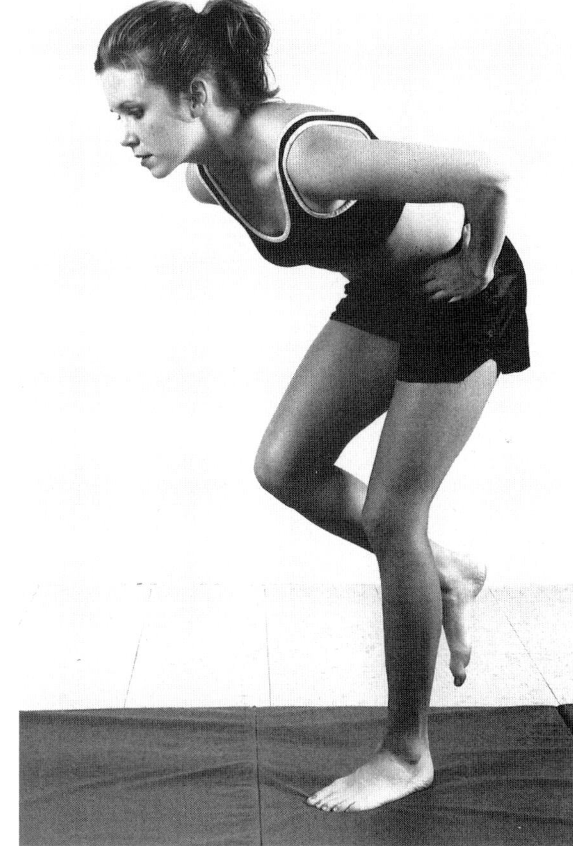

FIGURE 11-16 **One-foot standing balance while playing catch.**

PURPOSE: Facilitate and improve hip strategies.

POSITION: Client standing with feet shoulder width apart on firm surface.

PROCEDURE: Client lifts right foot off ground and establishes balance on left leg. Clinician throws ball to client, who catches it and throws ball back to clinician. Clinician gradually shifts direction and angle of ball toss so that client must reach away from body.

NOTE: Ball should be thrown so that patient must reach away from body.

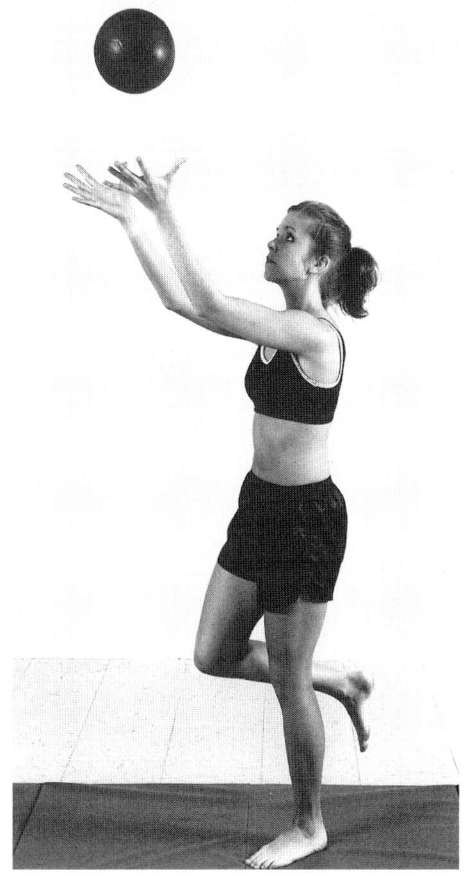

FIGURE 11-17 **One-foot standing balance on mini-trampoline.**

PURPOSE: Facilitate and improve hip strategies.

POSITION: Client standing with feet shoulder width apart on mini-trampoline.

PROCEDURE: Client lifts right foot off ground and establishes balance on left leg (panel A).

NOTE: Activity can be progressed to a more difficult level by asking patient to catch and throw a ball while standing on one leg on mini-trampoline (panel B).

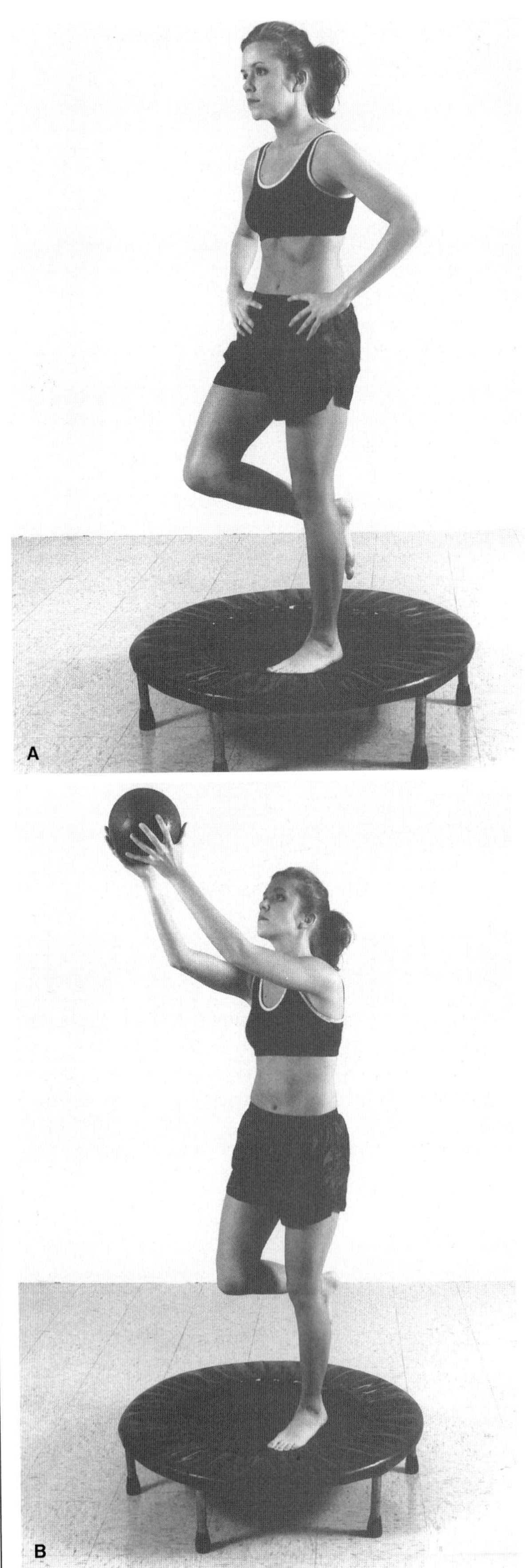

FIGURE 11-18 Two-foot standing balance on rocker (balance) board.

PURPOSE: Facilitate and improve hip strategies.

POSITION: Client standing with feet shoulder width apart on rocker board.

PROCEDURE: Client establishes balance with both feet remaining on rocker board while attempting to keep all surfaces of board off ground.

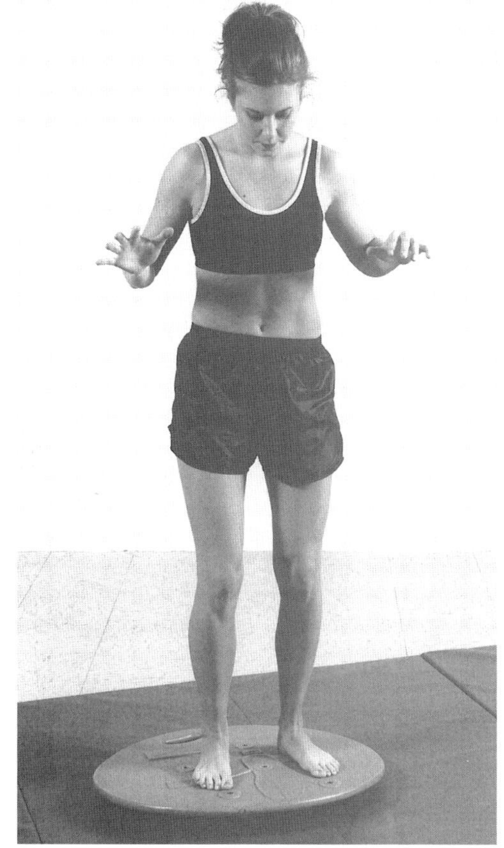

FIGURE 11-19 Two-foot standing balance on sliding board.

PURPOSE: Facilitate and improve hip strategies.

POSITION: Client standing with feet shoulder width apart on sliding board.

PROCEDURE: Client establishes balance with both feet remaining on sliding board while attempting to shift weight at hips to move sliding piece laterally back and forth on base.

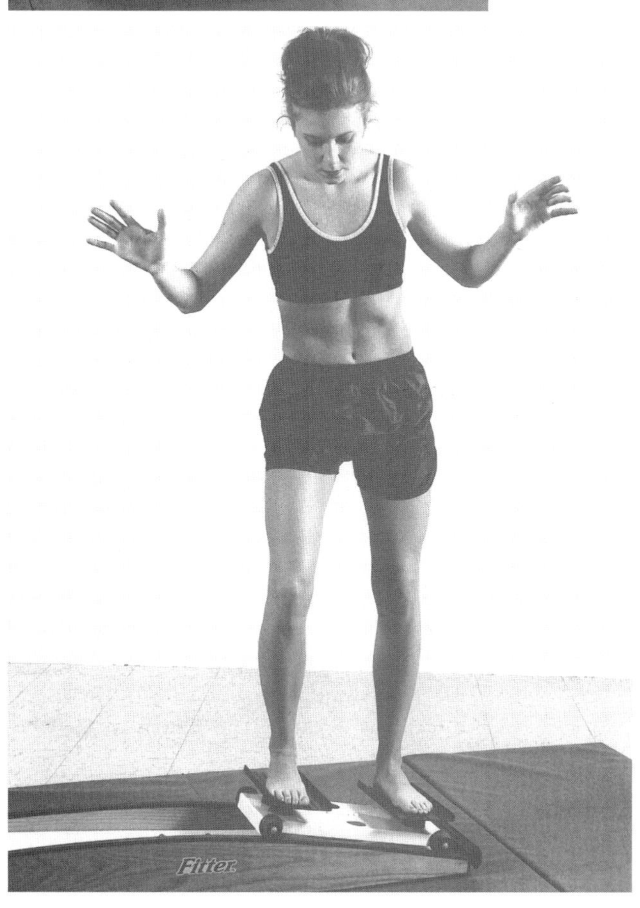

FIGURE 11-20 **Two-foot standing balance in surfer position on foam roller.**

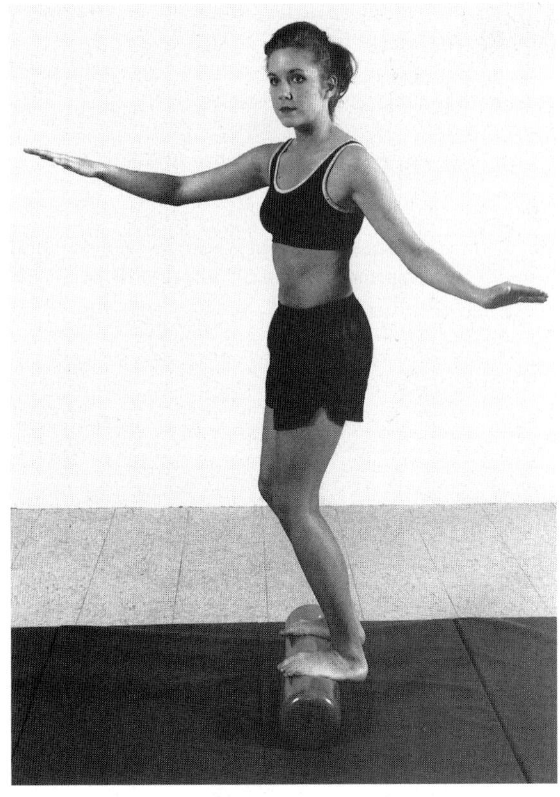

PURPOSE: Facilitate and improve hip strategies.

POSITION: Client standing with feet shoulder width apart on foam roller.

PROCEDURE: Client establishes and maintains balance with one foot in front of the other, assuming a surfer position.

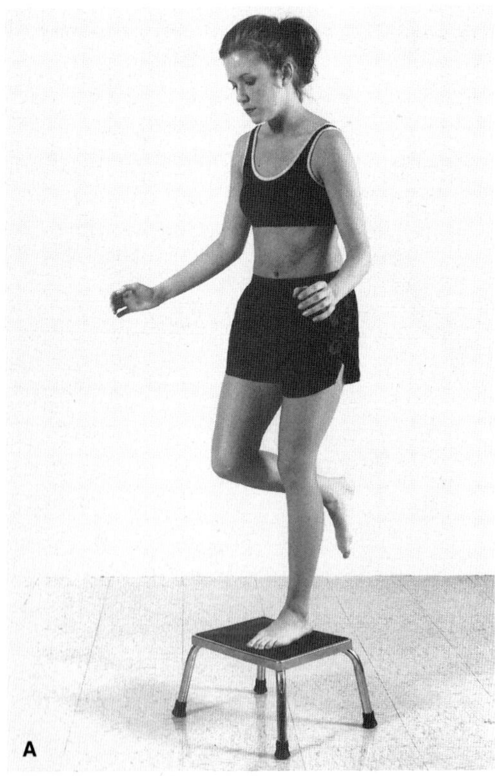

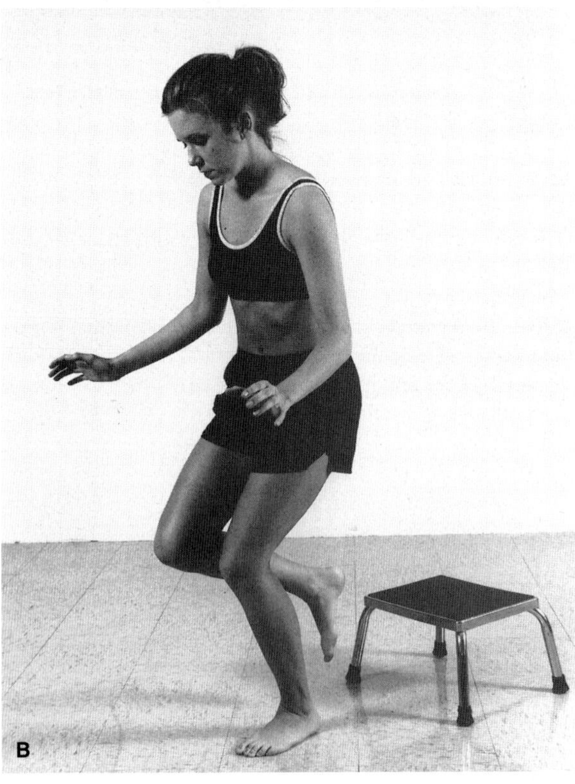

FIGURE 11-21 **One-foot hop from stool.**

PURPOSE: Facilitate and improve hip strategies.

POSITION: Client standing on one foot on top of foot stool (panel A).

PROCEDURE: Client establishes balance, hops down from stool, and maintains balance (panel B).

FIGURE 11-22 Forward step-up on stool.

PURPOSE: Facilitate and improve stepping strategies.

POSITION: Client standing with feet shoulder width apart facing step stool.

PROCEDURE: Client maintains balance while stepping up onto stool with lead foot and then brings up trailing foot. Client reverses process, stepping down.

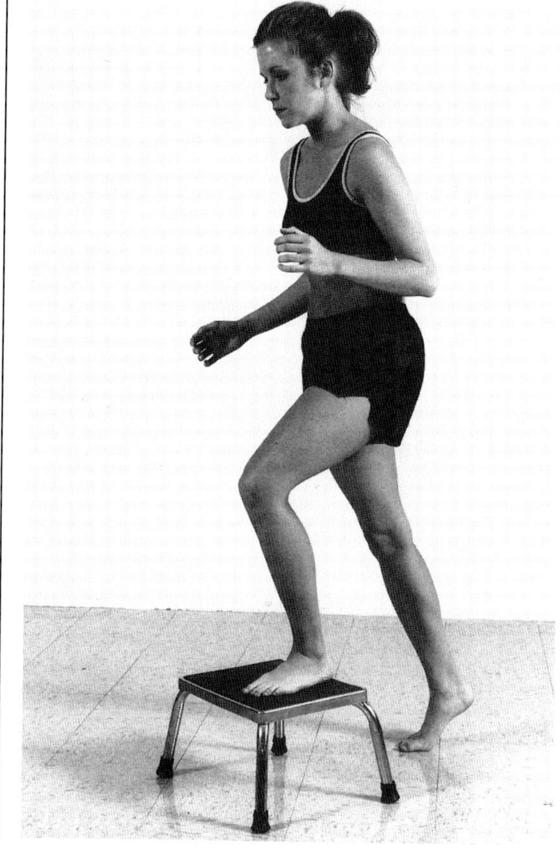

FIGURE 11-23 Slow and controlled step-overs.

PURPOSE: Facilitate and improve stepping strategies.

POSITION: Client standing with feet shoulder width apart on firm surface.

PROCEDURE: Client crosses one leg over in front of the other and slowly steps in a controlled movement.

NOTE: This technique can be progressed to faster controlled movements.

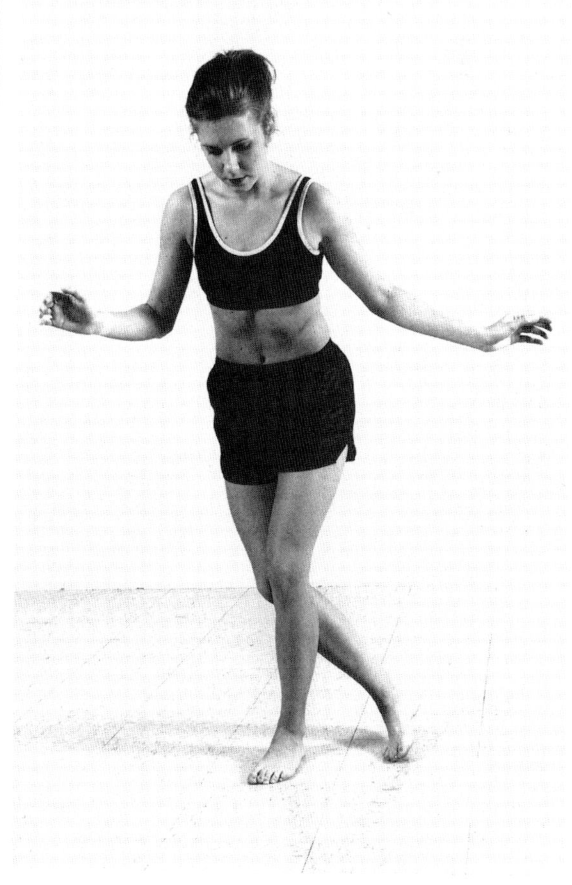

FIGURE 11-24 Push and nudge in anterior direction.

PURPOSE: Facilitate and improve stepping strategies.

POSITION: Client standing with feet shoulder width apart on firm surface. Clinician places hands on client's shoulders.

PROCEDURE: Client leans forward into clinician's support as far as balance allows (panel A). Clinician quickly removes support, forcing client to compensate by taking a step (panel B).

NOTE: Clinician may change direction of support to posterior or lateral.

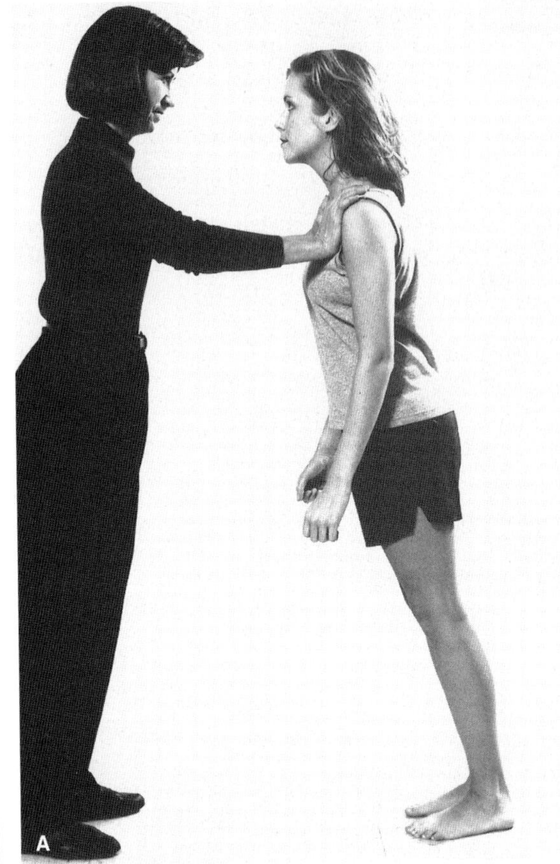

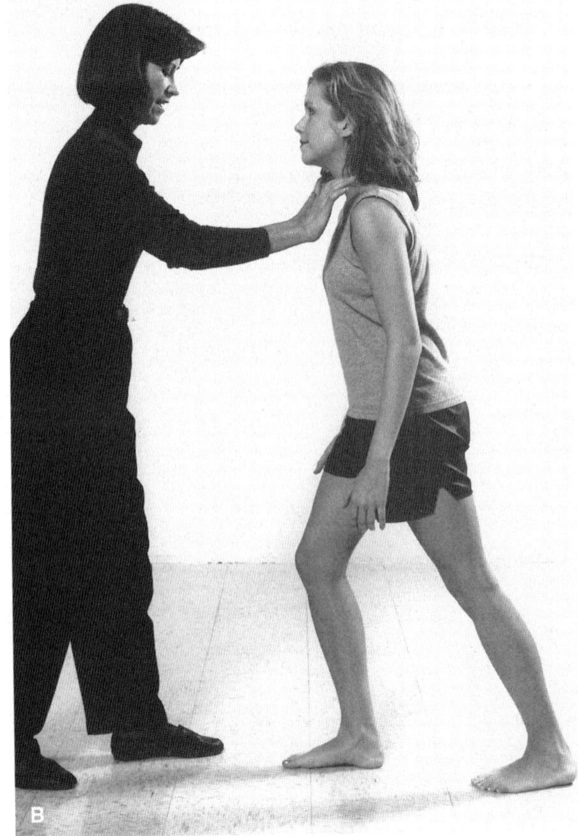

CASE STUDY

PATIENT INFORMATION

Patient was a 43-year-old male who had left ankle pain and edema. The patient reported that he "twisted" his left ankle two days before the appointment while stepping off a ladder onto uneven ground. He complained of moderate lateral ankle pain and had been unable to walk without limping since his injury.

Examination revealed that the patient presented with localized swelling and pain over the lateral aspect of the ankle. The patient's strength with eversion and plantarflexion was 4/5, secondary to pain with resistance. He was particularly tender to palpation of the anterior talofibular ligament. All ankle laxity tests were negative. Based on these finding, the patient was diagnosed with a first-degree inversion ankle sprain.

LINKS TO

Guide to Physical Therapist Practice* and *Athletic Training Educational Competencies

According to the *Guide*,[19] pattern 4D relates to the diagnosis of this patient. The pattern is described as "impaired joint mobility, muscle performance, and range of motion associated with connective tissue dysfunction" and includes ligamentous sprain. Tests and measures of this diagnosis include quantification of static and dynamic balance. Anticipated goals are improving balance through direct intervention using "balance and coordination training" and "posture awareness training."

The *Competencies*[20] refers to treatment of athletes using a variety of techniques. In the teaching objectives, the document indicates that the athletic trainer, upon graduation from an accredited program, will be able to "describe indications, contraindications, theory and principles for the incorporation and application of various contemporary therapeutic exercises including exercises to improve dynamic joint stability, neuromuscular coordination, postural stability, and proprioception." Demonstration of these exercises is also emphasized.

INTERVENTION

The physician instructed the patient to use ice, wear a compression wrap, elevate the leg, and rest for the first 48 hr. The patient was instructed in the following home exercise program, and was told to perform it in the morning and evening.

1. Stretch the Achilles tendon, using a towel for assistance: three repetitions, each held 20 sec.
2. Active plantarflexion, dorsiflexion ROM, and circumduction of the ankle: 20 repetitions (see Fig. 2-16).
3. Pick up objects (e.g., marbles) one at time and place them in a container: 20 repetitions.

PROGRESSION

Two Weeks After Initial Examination

The patient reported that he was able to complete the home exercise program without pain and with minimal swelling. His chief complaints were a mild limp when walking that worsened when he was fatigued and instability when walking on uneven surfaces. Further examination using computer assisted technology showed decreased limits of stability (75% of normal to the left, including AP planes) and decreased weight bearing on the left in 60° to 90° squats.

In the clinic, treatment consisted of stretching, riding a bicycle (see Fig. 10-5), walking on the treadmill (see Fig. 10-8) in all directions (forward, backward, sidestepping), and using a rocker (balance) board (Fig. 11-18). The patient's home program was advanced as follows:

1. Resistive ankle exercise with tubing in all directions (see Fig. 6-19).
2. Continue stretching.
3. Step-ups and step-downs (Fig. 11-22).
4. Squats (Fig. 9-10).
5. Toe-raises while standing.
6. Balance activities on balance and sliding boards (Figs. 11-18 and 11-19).

OUTCOMES

Four weeks after the initial examination, the patient had no complaints of pain. His primary goal was to return to playing basketball on the weekends. On re-examination the clinician noted no significant swelling and a strength of 5/5 (using manual muscle test). Computerized testing revealed a normal center of gravity and normal limits of stability. The patient was discharged from intervention. He was told to continue with his home exercise program, except the tubing exercises were discontinued and jogging and jump roping were added.

SUMMARY

- Balance is a complex process of controlling the body's center of gravity over the base of support, whether the individual is stationary or moving. Balance requires

GERIATRIC Perspectives

- Under circumstances of low-task demand, age-related changes in postural control (control of balance and coordination) are minimal through age 70. With advancing age, anatomic and physiologic changes occur in biomechanical capabilities that affect static and dynamic balance, such as decline in proprioceptive, vestibular, and visual responses; decrease in muscle mass; increase in postural sway; slowing of motor reaction time; and alterations in central control of balance.
- In addition, the sensing threshold for postural stimuli is affected by age, resulting in increased muscle onset latencies. Compared to younger adults, older adults require 10 to 30 msec longer to volitionally develop the same levels of ankle torque or to begin to take a step to recover balance after a disturbance.[1]
- The visual system is a major contributor to balance, giving the older individual information on location in space and the environment. However, vision is affected by aging and may provide distorted or inaccurate information.[2] In addition, corrective lenses (e.g., bifocals) tend to blur images from the ground or in the distance.
- The number of vestibular neurons and the size of the nerve fibers decrease with aging.[3] With increasing age over 40, a slow reduction in the number of myelinated nerve fibers is evident. By age 70+, a loss of 40 to 50% may be noted compared to younger adults.[4]
- Synergist motor responses responsible for restoration of balance after a disturbance are also affected by aging, resulting in altered muscle activation sequences, agonist-antagonist stiffness (co-contraction), slowed postural responses, and use of disordered postural strategies.[5] In response to a small disturbance, older adults will generally use a hip strategy rather than an ankle strategy typically observed in young adults.
- Research has determined that restoration of balance is not a fixed reflexive response to disturbance but rather is a multifactorial event involving interaction of the body (musculoskeletal and neuromuscular), the magnitude of the disturbance, and the attentional demands placed on the older individual by the environment.[6–8]
- Older adults are at greater risk of experiencing an injurious fall requiring hospitalization. Therefore, all examinations of adults over age 60 should include a balance screening (functional reach test[9]) and falls risk assessment (Elderly Fall Screening Test[10]).

1. Stelmach GE, Populin L, Muller F. Postural muscle onset and voluntary movement in the elderly. Neurosci Lett 1990;117:188–193.
2. Simoneau M, Teasdale N, Bourdin C, et al. Aging and postural control: postural perturbations caused by changing visual anchor. J Am Geriatr Soc 1999;47:235–241.
3. Spirduso WW. Balance, posture, and locomotion. In: WW Spirduso, ed. Physical dimensions of aging. Champaign, IL: Human Kinetics, 1995:155–184.
4. Rees TS, Duckert LG, Carey JP. Auditory and vestibular dysfunction. In: WR Hazard, JP Blass, WH Ettinger, et al., eds. Principles of geriatric medicine and gerontology. 4th ed. New York: McGraw-Hill, 1998:617–632.
5. Woollacott MH. Changes in posture and voluntary control in the elderly: research findings and rehabilitation. Top Geriatr Rehabil 1990;5:1–11.
6. Maylor EA, Wing AM. Age differences in postural stability are increased by additional cognitive demands. J Gerontol Psychol Sci 1996;51B:P143–P154.
7. Shumway-Cook A, Woollacott MH. Attentional demands and postural control: the effect of sensory context. J Gerontol Med Sci 2000:55A;M10–M16.
8. Brown L, Shumway-Cook A, Woollacott MH. Attentional demands and postural recovery: the effects of aging. J Gerontol Med Sci 1999;54A:M165–M171.
9. Duncan PW, Weiner DK, Chandler J, Studenski S. Functional reach: a new clinical measure of balance. J Gerontol Med Sci 1990;45:M192–M197.
10. Cwikel JG, Fried AV, Biderman A, Galinsky D. Validation of a fall-risk screening test, the Elderly Fall Screening Test (EFST), for community-dwelling elderly. Disability Rehabil 1998;20:161–167.

accurate information from sensory input, effective processing by the CNS, and appropriate responses of motor control.

- The CNS relies on information from three sensory systems: proprioceptive, visual, and vestibular. Each system contributes a unique role in maintaining balance. The ability of the CNS to select, suppress, and combine these inputs is called sensory organization. Proprioceptive inputs are dominant when the surface is firm and fixed. Visual cues are particularly important when somatosensory inputs are unreliable (changing surfaces). The vestibular system, on the other hand, is dominant when a conflict exists between somatosensory and visual cues and plays a major role in ambulation.
- Technological advances in the examination of appropriate sensory organization provide valuable information of both sensory organization and motor control.

PEDIATRIC *Perspectives*

- Control of balance and coordination progresses throughout childhood. The concepts of balance, coordination, and postural control are closely interrelated (see also "Pediatric Perspectives" in Chapter 12). Much continued research is needed to understand the development and refinement of postural control in children as they acquire adult postural and movement skills.[1]
- Children begin to learn anticipatory postural strategies to coordinate posture and locomotion with the onset of voluntary sitting and crawling.[2] During perturbations of stance, 4- to 6-year-old children have greater and more variable responses than do younger children. It has been suggested that the difference may be the result of a period of transition, as visual sensory input becomes less important and other somatosensory information becomes more important in postural control and balance.[3] Children do not demonstrate adult values for muscle onset latencies for postural responses and control of movement until 10 to 15 years of age.[2]
- Childhood deficits in balance and postural stability may be related to deficits in the proprioceptive system, owing to incomplete development or injury. Balance and coordination in sports may be adversely affected by attention deficit hyperactivity disorder (ADHD).[4] Chronic otitis media and effusion in the inner ear significantly affect balance and coordination skills in 4- to 6-year-old children. These skills improve after tympanostomy tube insertion.[5]
- Children with neurologic and musculoskeletal diagnoses may have impaired balance and coordination, which may be related to multiple factors, such as sensory system deficits, impaired ROM and strength, and abnormal muscle tone. Patients must be treated at developmentally correct stages of balance and control. For example, children with cerebral palsy show deficits in sensorimotor organization and muscular coordination. These deficits affect their anticipatory activities.[6]

1. Horak FB. Assumptions underlying motor control for neurologic rehabilitation. In: MJ Lister, ed. Contemporary management of motor control problems, Proceedings of the II Step conference. Alexandria, VA: Foundation for Physical Therapy, 1991:11–28.
2. Haas G, Diener HC, Rupp H, Dichgan J. Development of feedback and feedforward control of upright stance. Develop Med Child Neurol 1989;31:481–488.
3. Shumway-Cook A, Woollacott M. The growth of stability: postural control from a developmental perspective. J Motor Behav 1985;17:131–147.
4. Hickey G, Frider P. ADHD: CNS function and sports. Sports Med 1999;27:11–21.
5. Hart MC, Nichols DS, Butler EM, Burin K. Childhood imbalance and chronic otitis media with effusion: effect of tympanostomy tube insertion on standardized tests of balance and locomotion. Laryngoscope 1998;108:665–670.
6. Nashner LM, Shumway-Cook A, Marin O. Stance posture control in select groups of children with cerebral palsy: deficits in sensory organization and muscular coordination. Exper Brain Res 1983;49: 393–409.

- The major muscle groups that control the center of gravity over the base of support include the paraspinals, abdominals, hamstrings, quadriceps, gastrocnemius, and tibialis anterior. Coordinated actions among muscles result in joint-specific movements and indirect, inertial forces on the neighboring joints. Therefore, the anatomic classification of a muscle may differ from its functional classification.
- The primary movement patterns for controlling balance include an ankle strategy, hip strategy, and stepping strategy. The strategies vary in muscle recruitment, body movements, and joint axes. Inadequate ROM, decreased strength, pain, swelling, and joint instability can decrease the normal limits of stability. Dysfunction in any of these factors creates an offset center of gravity, compromising movement patterns.
- Treatment of musculoskeletal problems include strengthening and range of motion, techniques to effect abnormal tone, and several coordination activities to improve the timing of postural reactions.

REFERENCES

1. Shumway-Cook A, McCollum G. Assessment and treatment of balance disorders. In: PC Montgomery, BH Connolly, eds. Motor control and physical therapy. Hixson, TN: Chattanooga Group, Inc., 1993:123–138.
2. Kauffman TL, Nashner LM, Allison LK. Balance is a critical parameter in orthopedic rehabilitation. New Technol Phys Ther 1997;6:43–78.
3. Nashner LM. Sensory, neuromuscular, and biomechanical contributions to human balance. In: PW Duncan, ed. Balance: proceedings of APTA Forum. Alexandria: APTA, 1990:33–38.

4. Nashner LM. Evaluation of postural stability, movement and control. In: S Hasson, ed. Clinical exercise physiology. St. Louis: Mosby, 1994:199–234.
5. McCollum G, Leen T. Form and exploration of mechanical stability limits in erect stance. J Motor Behav 1989;21:225–238.
6. Hobeika CP. Equilibrium and balance in the elderly. ENT 1999; 78:558–566.
7. Horak FB, Shupert CL. Role of the vestibular system in postural control. In: SJ Herdman, ed. Vestibular rehabilitation. Philadelphia: Davis, 1994:22–46.
8. Dietz V, Horstmann GA, Berger W. Significance of proprioceptive mechanisms in the regulation of stance. Prog Brain Res 1989;80:419–423.
9. Dorman J, Fernie GR, Holliday PJ. Visual input: its importance in the control of postural sway. Arch Phys Med Rehabil 1978;59: 586–591.
10. Horak FB. Clinical measurement of postural control in adults. Phys Ther 1987;67:1881–1885.
11. Hain TC, Hillman MA. Anatomy and physiology of the normal vestibular system. In: SJ Herdma, ed. Vestibular rehabilitation. Philadelphia: Davis, 1994:3–21.
12. Shumway-Cook A, Horak FB. Assessing the influence of sensory interaction on balance. Phys Ther 1986;66:1548–1550.
13. Horak FB, Nashner LM. Central programming of posture control: adaptation to altered support surface configurations. J Neurophysiol 1986;55:1369–1381.
14. Diener HC, Horak FB, Nashner LM. Influence of stimulus parameters on human postural responses. J Neurophysiol 1988;59: 1888–1905.
15. DiFabio RP, Badke MB. Relationships of sensory organization to balance function in patients with hemiplegia. Phys Ther 1990;70: 543–548.
16. Horak FB, Diener HC, Nashner LM. Postural strategies associated with somatosensory and vestibular limits of stability. Exp Brain Res 1992;82:167–171.
17. Badke MB, DiFabio RP. Balance deficits in patients with hemiplegia: considerations for assessment and treatment. In: PW Duncan, ed. Balance: proceedings of the APTA Forum. Alexandria, VA:. APTA, 1990:130–137.
18. Shumway-Cook A, Horak FB. Rehabilitation strategies for patients with peripheral vestibular disorders. Neurology clinics. Philadelphia: Saunders, 1990.
19. American Physical Therapy Association. Guide to physical therapist practice, second edition. Phys Ther 2001;81:1–768.
20. National Athletic Trainers' Association. Athletic training educational competencies. 3rd ed. Dallas: NATA, 1999.

CHAPTER 12

Posture, Body Mechanics, and Spinal Stabilization

Ginny Keely, MS, PT

Treating the spine can be an ominous task for the novice practitioner. The spine, with its intricacies, might intimidate one who is looking for a black-and-white picture that dictates specific intervention. It has been estimated that 5.6% of the U.S. population, or approximately 10 million people, have back pain at any one point in time.[1] It is, therefore, important for all practitioners to gain a reasonable arsenal of intervention skills aimed at getting the client back to work or play. This chapter gives the clinician a framework in which to treat individuals with spinal injuries, with the intended outcome of returning the client to premorbid level of function.

■ *Scientific Basis*

BIOMECHANICAL CONSIDERATIONS

Although the spine is actually just a series of joints, the intimate relationships between the joints give the spine a variety of special qualities. The anterior-posterior curves enable the spine to sustain compressive loads 10 times greater than if the column were straight.[2] The hydraulic nature of the disks permits controlled movement while transferring forces vertically to the trabecular system of the adjacent vertebral bodies.[2] The synovial facet joints guide motion in multiple planes, permitting the human body to move freely in three dimensions. Together, the vertebral bodies, disks, facet joints, supportive ligaments, and muscles coalesce to create an extremely dynamic structural system.[2]

POSTURE

To function in a world with strong gravitational forces, the body has adapted by integrating delicate architectural and dynamic supportive designs, allowing for relatively effortless upright positioning. This design, however, is combated by twenty-first century lifestyle. Most people, regardless of age, have lived a life full of sitting, flexed postures, and restricted activity and movement. Good posture "is a state of musculoskeletal balance that protects the supporting structures of the body against injury or progressive deformity."[3] This musculoskeletal balance is important not only at rest but also with the dynamic activity of the body in motion.

To achieve balance, one must consider both dynamic and inert structures responsible for postural equilibrium. Muscles provide dynamic counterforces to moments of extension and flexion caused by gravitational torque at joints and require an intact nervous system to provide sensorimotor feedback.[4] The inert osseous and ligamentous structures provide passive tension at joints and support for weight bearing in the upright posture. At equilibrium, the line of gravity falls near or through the axes of rotation of the joints and compression forces are optimally distributed over weight-bearing surfaces.[5] Gravitational forces are then balanced by countertorque generated either by inert structures or by minimal muscle activity.[5] When the center of mass moves, the line of gravity falls a distance away from the joint axes, often approaching the limits of the base of support. A need exists for increased countertorque to balance gravitational forces and maintain upright posture.[5]

When considering spinal alignment and the interplay of inert and dynamic structures, the clinician should note the influence of the lower biomechanical chain. Structural or functional faults may contribute to a less-than-optimal foundation on which the spine must function. Structural alignment issues include limb length difference and bony alignment of the femur, and functional problems include postural and muscle imbalances about the hip, knee, or foot.

Structural Malalignment

Limb length differences may lead to spinal asymmetry by effectively lowering the pelvis on one side and elevating the other. For example, if a patient has a short left extremity, the pelvis will drop on the left, carrying the spine with it. Hence, the spine will be leaning to the left. As the individual seeks optical righting, a compensatory curve of the lumbar spine may occur back to the right. If an overcorrection is achieved, yet another compensatory curve back to the left may be noted in the thoracic spine. This positioning asymmetry leads to unnatural forces through the spine. The concave side of the curve has increased facet weight bearing and narrowing of the intervertebral foramen, and the hydraulic disk is at risk for injury on the convex side. In addition, the muscles on the convex side tend to lengthen and become weaker, whereas the muscles on the concave side tend to shorten.

Femoral structure may also influence spinal mechanics. If a patient has coxa vara, the pelvis tends to be brought into a position of anterior tilt, or anterior inclination. The opposite is true with coxa valga, in which the pelvis tends toward a posterior tilt, or posterior inclination. If the pelvis is positioned in an anterior tilt, the lumbar spine is brought into a greater lordosis. An accentuated anterior tilt increases forces on the posterior elements of the spine, such as the facet joints, putting these structures at risk for injury. Conversely, if the pelvis is tilted posteriorly, the lumbar spine may lose normal lordosis. This position of relative kyphosis may put the anterior structures at risk for injury, especially the disk. With the loss of lordosis, the annular structure of the disk is stressed posteriorly and may lead to annular incompetence and possibly an inability for the annulus to adequately control the nucleus.[6,7]

Knee posture may also effect stress in the spine. A genu valgum, or "knock-kneed," posture tends to guide the pelvis into either an anterior or a posterior tilt because of compensatory femoral rotation. With faulty knee alignment in the frontal plane, the hip tends to compensate in the transverse plane with either a medial or a lateral rotation. The pelvis then responds with sagittal plane compensation, leading to excessive anterior or posterior tilt. Again, these postures direct forces through the spine in an anterior or posterior manner, as discussed previously. Owing to effects on pelvic position, genu recurvatum (knee hyperextension) may also promote a shearing compensation in the upper lumbar spine. The spine transitions from an excessive lordosis caused by an excessive anterior pelvic tilt and adopts a position of flexion (kyphosis) to bring the body into anterior-posterior balance.[6]

Functional (Muscle) Imbalance

Functional imbalance is a dysfunction in the musculoskeletal system, potentially leading to a less-than-optimal spinal foundation. The musculoskeletal system can be likened to a balanced system of guy wires or springs attached to a structural foundation (Fig. 12-1). The over-

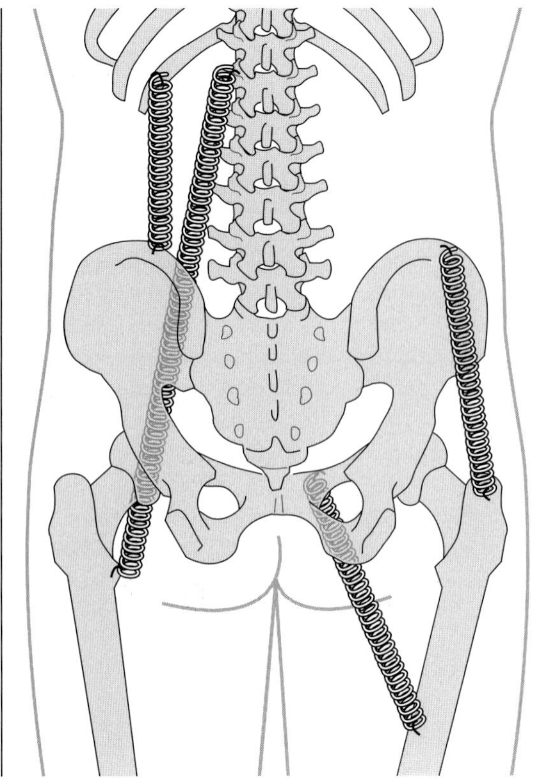

FIGURE 12-1 Springs demonstrate a mechanical model of lumbopelvic stability.

all length of the supportive guy wires affects the balance of the structural foundation. In addition, the extensibility, or quality of overall length of the supportive guy wire, affects the balance within the system.

Janda and Jull[8] suggested that the pelvic crossed syndrome may affect the balance of the muscles surrounding the joints of the lower extremity. For example, if the pelvis is in a position of anterior tilt, the muscular system may develop compensatory qualities. The hip flexors, placed in a relaxed position, may shorten along with the lumbar extensors. Conversely, the gluteals and abdominals are in a lengthened position, subjecting them to stretch weakness. Given that it weakens the passive components of the muscles, chronic stretch may neurologically inhibit the active components, making the muscle less stiff.[9,10] Similarly, the chronically shortened muscles may lose passive elasticity and be actively facilitated toward a higher state of contractility, becoming increasingly stiff.[9,10] Because of these factors, it is a difficult task to overcome the postural tendency promoted by the crossed pelvic syndrome.[8]

Balance of the musculature around the pelvis is important not only for postural reasons but also because the iliopsoas, tensor fascia lata, quadriceps, hamstrings, gluteus maximus, hip rotators, abductors, and adductors play a crucial role in the ability of the pelvis to appropriately transmit ground reaction forces.[4] Table 12-1 lists the primary muscles involved in postural assessment.

BODY MECHANICS

Proper body mechanics are considered crucial both for control of symptoms and for prevention of future episodes of back pain. However, no one definition of proper body mechanics is accepted, which can lead to confusion in patient management. Floyd and Silver[11] advocated full posterior pelvic tilt with lumbar flexion for lifting, which employs the neurologic protective mechanism of extensor muscle relaxation in the full end of range position. This end range relaxation suggests that a posterior pelvic tilt may protect the spinal musculature from injury.

McGill[12] supported the idea of extreme anterior pelvic tilt to protect the spine during lifting, but this may compromise the posterior structures that are not designed for such weight-bearing capabilities. McGill countered with the idea of pelvic and lumbar "neutral" for lifting and for most functional tasks. As described later, this neutral position varies among individuals.

The appropriate (proper) body mechanics can greatly influence the musculoskeletal environment in which functional tasks are performed, leading to improper stresses in the spine.[12] Consider the potential effect of shortened or stiff hamstring muscles. While performing a task such as squatting, short or stiff hamstrings will limit the ability of the pelvis to maintain its relatively neutral alignment because of the effect the muscles at their attachments on the ischial tuberosities. As the hamstrings become taught

TABLE 12-1 Postural Muscles Prone to Loss of Flexibility or Weakness

Muscles Prone to Tightness	Muscles Prone to Weakness
Erector spinae	Rectus abdominus
Quadratus lumborum	Serratus anterior
Iliopsoas	Gluteus maximus, medius, and minimus
Tensor fascia lata	Lower trapezius
Piriformis	Vastus medialis and lateralis
Rectus femoris	Short cervical flexors
Hamstrings	Extensors of upper limb
Gastroc-soleus	Tibialis anterior
Pectoralis major	
Upper trapezius	
Levator scapula	
Sternocleidomastoid	
Scalenes	

Adapted from Janda V, Jull G. Muscles and motor control. In: LT Twomey, JT Taylor, eds. Physical therapy of the low back. Clinics in physical therapy series. New York: Churchill Livingstone, 1987:253–278.

throughout hip flexion, the muscles will eventually pull on the ischial tuberosities, causing the pelvis to tilt posteriorly. A similar phenomenon occurs in the upper extremity with overhead reaching. A stiff or short latissimus dorsi muscle (extending from the posterior aspect of the pelvis to the intertubercular groove of the humerus) can limit the ability of the humerus to move upward, causing the pelvis to tilt anteriorly to allow for a greater range of overhead reach.

As noted earlier, the body functions most efficiently when in a state of postural equilibrium. When the center of mass moves, the line of gravity falls away from joint axes, often toward the perimeter of the base of support. In this situation, the muscles act to balance gravitational forces and maintain postural balance.[13] If a joint remains in a locked (or close-packed) position, the gravitational forces are attenuated and the inert support structures are at risk.[5] Therefore, the basic idea of proper body mechanics is the safe maintenance of a loose-packed joint position while external gravitational forces are imposed, often near the limits of the base of support and while supporting external loads. To achieve this balance, the client needs both the knowledge of safe joint position and the necessary muscular strength to maintain musculoskeletal balance.

SPINAL STABILIZATION

The idea of spinal stabilization evolved because of the belief that to recover and maintain health, patients with low back pain must exercise.[14] Such functional exercise techniques emphasize movement re-education and apply a combination of principles derived from neurodevelopmental techniques, proprioceptive neuromuscular facilitation (Chapter 8), and basic body mechanics. The goal of this type of training is not only to improve the patient's physical condition and symptoms but also to facilitate efficient movement.[14,15]

The basic philosophy behind stabilization training is that spinal pain is a movement or postural disorder that has either resulted in or perpetuated spinal dysfunction.[14] The actual pathoanatomy of spinal pain is poorly understood. Multiple potential pain generators exist in spinal pain syndromes, and often the anatomic structure at fault does not matter.[4] The crucial matter is to determine the activities and postures in which the patient is unable to tolerate stresses. The concept of stability of the spine actually considers a combination of the osseoligamentous system, muscle system, and neural control system.[16] The clinician should avoid getting caught up in the guessing game of pathoanatomic diagnosis and focus on improvement of function and, hence, stability. Therefore, the basis of functional stabilization training is to provide the patient with movement awareness, knowledge of safe postures, and functional strength and coordination that promotes management of spinal dysfunction. Freedom of movement while maintaining a stable foundation is the goal. Table 12-2 presents the expectations and goals that should be considered when developing an individualized stabilization program.[15]

Many practitioners use exercise in the treatment of low back problems. However, the type of exercise and the emphasis in training are not standardized. What is known from research investigations is that exercise programs facilitate management of spinal symptoms.[17–23] O'Sullivan et al.[24] demonstrated a significant decrease in pain and disability immediately, 3 months, 6 months, and 30 months after initiating an exercise intervention. In a retrospective study, Saal and Saal[21] found that a high percentage of patients with objective radiculopathy had successful outcomes with stabilization training, even when surgery had previously been recommended. Nelson et al.[20] demonstrated that a large number of patients for whom surgery was recommended had successful outcomes in the short term by performing aggressive strengthening exercises. Thus, although it has been shown that exercise is beneficial, a variety of training programs have been used.

The exercise format for stabilization emphasizes both strength and endurance, as well as addresses proprioception. If a client is aware of the safe-functioning neutral position of the spine, then the ability to maintain safe posture is the key. This ability has a basic strength requirement; but, because postural muscles must have endurance, the strengthening exercises should progress toward endurance.[12,25] Consider the evidence that shows patients with back pain have selective wasting of the type 1 (slow-oxidative) muscle fibers.[26] The loss of type 1 fibers renders the muscles less equipped for endurance

TABLE 12-2 Expectation and Goals of a Spinal Stabilization Program

Patients complain less and become more functional with exercise intervention.
The neurologic influences of muscles and joints are inseparable; thus the clinician must be concerned with the neuromotor system and not treat muscles and joints in isolation.
Regardless of anatomic involvement or stage of recovery, all patients with low back pain can engage in a training program.
Patients are trained to improve physical capacity; to facilitate more functional movement; and to prevent, control, or eliminate symptoms.
Training should include increasing flexibility, strength, endurance, and coordination.

Reprinted with permission from Biondi, B. Lumbar functional stabilization program. In: Goldstein TS, ed. Functional rehabilitation in orthopedics. Gaithersburg, MD: Aspen, 1995:133–142.

activities.[4] This information provides further incentive to address endurance as much as strength.

Therefore, the practitioner needs to identify the muscles on which to focus when initiating any type of therapeutic exercise regime. Research suggests that the core stabilizers are not the larger, external muscles—such as the rectus abdominus and external oblique muscles—but rather the inner, deep muscles—such as the lumbar multifidus (segmentally), the transversus abdominus, and (to some extent) the internal oblique muscles. The multifidus muscles are important for reducing shear forces in the lumbar spine;[21,22] and recent evidence supports the ability of the lumbar extensor muscles, even at low levels of activity, to increase lumbar posteroanterior stiffness.[12,27,28]

Through ultrasonographic imaging, Hides et al.[29] identified selective ipsilateral multifidus wasting at the level of spinal injury. Although they identified selective wasting of the type 2 (fast-twitch) fibers, they also found an internal structural change of the type 1 fibers, described as "moth eaten" in appearance.[30] This selective wasting of muscle appears to have long-lasting implications for recovery.[30] Again, emphasis in training of the type 1 fibers is warranted. The multifidus atrophy develops acutely and continues for at least 10 weeks, even when pain-free status has been achieved, with or without exercise intervention.[31] However, in the experimental group that received exercise therapy, multifidus size was restored. On follow-up, individuals in the exercise group had a significantly lower recurrence rate of pain than those in the control group.[16]

Indahl et al.[32] demonstrated in porcine experiments that, although the multifidus muscles increased in electrical activity when subjected to annular stimulation, they underwent reflex inhibition when saline was injected into the associated facet joint, demonstrating a complex pattern of neurologically mediated events. It has been postulated that the loss of muscle size of the multifidus after injury is not related to the presence of electrical activity. In fact, it may be possible that because of high electrical activity, the muscle undergoes wasting as a result of the increased metabolic demands.[29]

The transversus abdominus muscle has been confirmed as a primary stabilizer of the lumbar spine. In fact, support by the transversus abdominus is considered to be the most important of the abdominal muscles. Its action seems to be independent of the other abdominal muscles and is most closely tied to the function of the diaphragm and pelvic floor muscles and intimately relates to the thoracolumbar fascia. The transversus abdominus, with some contribution from the internal oblique muscle, assists in increased intra-abdominal pressure. Its normal action, along with the action of deep fibers of the lumbar multifidus muscles, may function to form a deep internal corset. This pattern of motor control is disrupted in patients with low back pain.[16]

Given that stabilization as an exercise intervention is meant to both condition the muscles and address motor programming, the obvious question is whether motor programs can really be changed. One concept to emphasize is that stabilization training in general works the core stabilizers in their natural fashion—not as prime movers but as primary stabilizers. The limbs are providing the resistance, and the core muscles respond to the postural challenge. In healthy individuals, the stabilizers act in a feedforward manner; the trunk muscles precede the limb muscles in order of motor recruitment.[33] In other words, the trunk muscles "turn on" in preparation for the limb movement. Conversely, in the patient population, the firing of the abdominal muscles is delayed, often occurring after the limb movement.[34]

Recent findings support the idea that skill training can indeed change the motor firing pattern of abdominal muscle activity in response to limb movement.[16,35] In addition, some researchers have demonstrated that it is possible to alter movement patterns and muscle recruitment patterns by training individuals in spinal stabilization techniques.[36,37]

Finally, in addition to working the core stabilizers, conditioning of the major postural muscles is encouraged. These muscles include the gluteals, erector spinae, latissimus dorsi, and lower-extremity muscles. Clinicians should include upper-extremity exercises as an adjunct, because spinal stresses increase as upper-extremity loads are maneuvered.

■ *Clinical Guidelines*

POSTURE

Addressing posture is probably the single most important aspect of treating spinal injuries. By examining an individual's posture using the vertical compression test, the implications of postural faults are easily demonstrated.[38] During the test, forces of gravity in the vertical plane are exaggerated and stress points are manifested. The patient usually is able to feel the gravitational stresses, and postural correction then becomes a powerful tool.

To examine the ability of an individual to attenuate loads through the body in relaxed stance, provide a smooth, direct downward pressure through the trunk, accentuating gravitational load. This action essentially provides the clinician with a visual representation of the potential effects of increased gravitational load on a patient in the standing position. The results of the test can be used to project the possible shearing forces exerted on the body when required to maintain an upright position for an extended period of time (Fig. 12-2).

After postural correction, employ the vertical com-

FIGURE 12-2 The vertical compression test.

PURPOSE: Examine vertical loading responses throughout the system.

POSTION: Client standing relaxed. Clinician on stool behind.

PROCEDURE: Clinician applies gravitational overpressure directly down through client's shoulders.

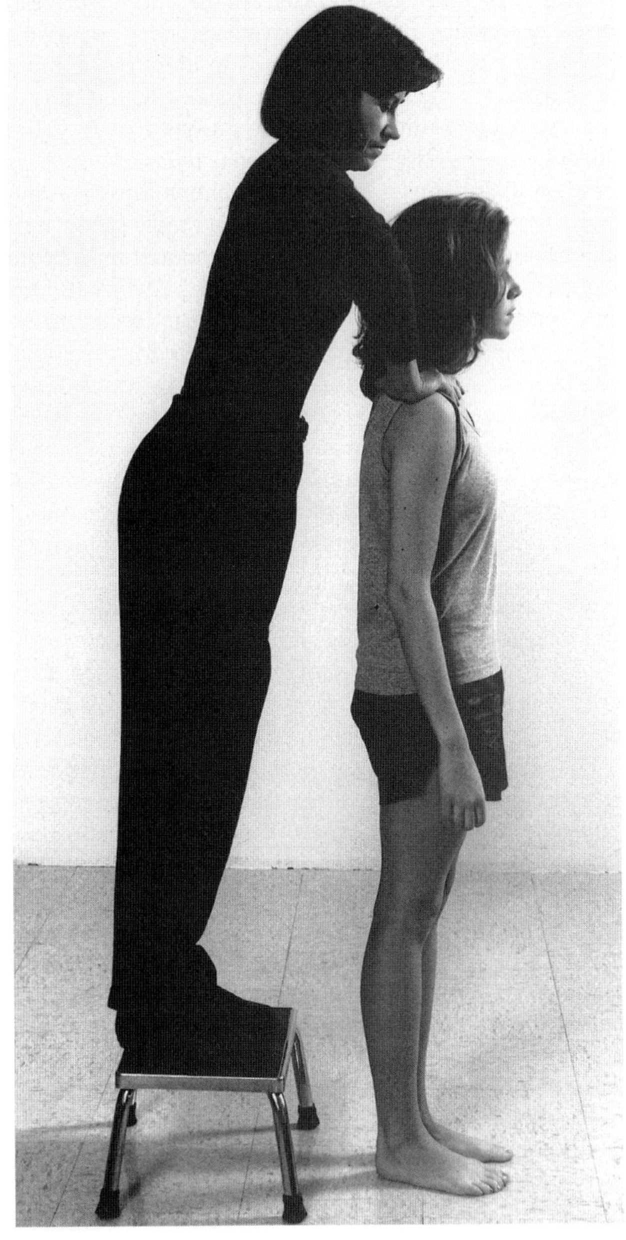

pression test again. A firm resistance to gravity that is balanced through the load-bearing joints will diffuse the forces, enabling the client to feel the difference in an immediate and applicable way. Regardless of diagnosis, the patient must be educated regarding posture if any noticeable postural inefficiencies are present, as most individuals demonstrate.

BODY MECHANICS

Although body mechanics are dynamic while posture appears static, each is truly an extension of the other. When the body moves through space, gravitational forces impart moments of force that vary in direction and intensity. The body must constantly adapt to these forces, but the uninformed individual is not aware of potentially efficient and safe positions in which to best handle the external forces. Therefore, it is imperative to observe the client in functional movements, scrutinizing the mechanics of the movement to identify inefficient and potentially unsafe maneuvers.

Functional testing need not be complicated. Simple observation of normal activities can be quite valuable. This examination can begin as soon as the client stands from the seated position. Notice the position of the body over the legs. Observe whether the individual uses momentum or pushes from the upper extremities to attain the standing position. Is the pelvis in an extreme position as it moves forward over the lower extremities? Is there unnecessary internal rotation torque of the femurs, with accompanying pronation of the subtalar or midtarsal joints? Is the thoracic spine in a compromised position of end-range kyphosis during the movement to standing? Any of these compensatory movements indicates decreased ability to withstand the forces of gravity for that particular maneuver. Look for similar compensatory behaviors in all functional tests, including partial squatting, unilateral balance, lifting an item from the floor, reaching forward or overhead, pushing or pulling, and the prone leg lift for multifidus stability.

Frequently, body mechanics are compromised not only by the patient's lack of understanding of safe functional performance but by a physical limitation that makes proper performance impossible. Recall the example of stiff hamstrings and the influence on squatting. Loss of mobility in the hamstrings will limit the ability of the pelvis to maintain neutral alignment, because the hamstrings may mechanically influence the pelvis into a posterior tilt. The clinician with a trained eye should watch for such compensations and seek to address the physical as well as the functional limitations.

SPINAL STABILIZATION

If the goal is to improve the protective stabilizing ability of the spinal muscles, it is imperative that the exercise load not overtax the muscles. If the muscles are fatigued, this may create compensation and, potentially, inhibition of the targeted muscles. Initially, the spinal stabilization program begins with the learning of an isolated contraction of the targeted muscle, which enhances the client's proprioceptive abilities needed for the progression of exercise. Light resistance with isolated contraction follows, with gradual progression to functional and weight-bearing activities. Although limb movement alone imposes the initial challenge to the muscle, resistance to the limbs follows as the client progresses. In the early phases, it is important for the client to perform slow movements, because the proximal stabilizing muscles may weaken or become inhibited when exposed to ballistic limb movement.[39]

Stabilization exercise is encouraged not only for young adults but for all ages. Adolescents have been successfully treated with these techniques, and it is well established that exercise in the aging population has numerous health benefits.[40] Remember to monitor risk factors in older adults when teaching them an exercise program.

Neutral Position

The neutral position, also called the "functional range of motion," is the position in which the spine is asymptomatic or least symptomatic, and corresponds to the optimal position within which the spine functions most efficiently.[14] This position, or range of motion (ROM), varies among individuals and pathologies. Exercising at the end of ROM in either direction is not recommended.[12]

When given the opportunity to identify the least painful position, most people will indicate a relatively neutral position. This position is roughly achieved when the spine is resting and the patient is in the hook-lying position. With the hips flexed to approximately 60°, as naturally occurs in hook lying, the lumbar spine tends to adopt a position that is closest to the mid-range. Therefore, the hook-lying position is a good one for initiating the patient's discovery of the neutral position.

The client's least painful position may be one of relative flexion of the lumbar spine, corresponding to a posterior pelvic tilt (called a flexion bias).[15] Some clients are most comfortable toward the extension ROM of the lumbar spine, with an anteriorly tilted pelvis, which indicates an extension bias.[15] Although these biases may change as the pathology changes, the clinician should always be aware of patient's bias when designing an exercise prescription.

Training Progression

The clinician should consider the following basic principles when beginning a training progression: (1) monitor the effects of weight bearing, (2) use stable before unstable postures, (3) use simple motions before combined movements, and (4) integrate gross motions before isolated, fine motor patterns. The patient's tolerance to weight bearing or load bearing should be kept in mind when prescribing exercise, because some movements inherently involve more gravitational forces than others. An exercise in supine naturally decreases the gravitational stresses, whereas a loaded upright activity could exacerbate a condition in a patient with load sensitivities. The supine position also naturally provides more external stability than does the quadruped, kneeling, or upright position. Simple movements should be mastered before progressing to motions that require stability in diagonal planes, which challenge the body in three planes of motion. Last, the patient should be competent in mass body movements before the clinician superimposes isolated movements. For example, the action of rising from the seated position is less challenging than rising from the seated position and simultaneously reaching for the phone.

To teach a client stabilization concepts, begin by helping the client produce and explore lumbopelvic movement in the sagittal plane (anterior-posterior direction), which is best done in the supine position. Then ask the client to identify the position in which symptoms are reduced or absent. This position constitutes the neutral position. If the client is asymptomatic within a range of movement, then he or she is free to move within the neutral ROM rather than maintain a strict neutral position.

After the client accomplishes muscle control to maintain the neutral position (or ROM), teach the client to perform simple movements, gradually progressing to advanced, functional actions.

Individuals progress at different rates. The easiest way to help the client maintain the neutral ROM is to assist him or her with the use of external support, referred to as passive prepositioning. For example, the neutral position for a patient with a flexion bias is to be adequately supported in a supine position with the hips and knees in the 90/90 position, which encourages lumbar flexion. In contrast, the neutral position for a patient with an extension bias may be achieved with passive support to the spine in extension. The clinician may place a towel roll under the lumbar spine for support or simply ask the patient to allow the lower extremities to lie flat, which tilts the pelvis anteriorly and extends the lumbar spine. Exercising in this supported position assists the patient in maintaining a safe position for the spine.

Active prepositioning refers to the next level of stabilization in which the client uses muscular contraction to maintain a safe, stable posture for exercise. After exploring lumbopelvic motion and identifying the neutral position, the patient actively contracts the deep stabilizers to maintain the neutral position. When the patient can achieve adequate active contraction, the clinician can begin to focus on challenging the stabilizing musculature. The patient should begin with slow, controlled limb movement, while the clinician looks for any sign of subtle compensation. One common error is for the patient and clinician to get stuck in this phase of active co-contraction in preparation for movement. When time does not permit the clinician to help the patient move to a more advanced phase of intervention, the patient's concept of stabilization is of rigid holding to protect the spine. It is important that the patient does not move while the spine is locked in with isometric holding but rather progresses to the next phase, dynamic stabilization.

In the dynamic stabilization phase, the muscles (via proprioceptive properties) protect the spine from unwanted motions. Muscles are not precontracted to protect the spine from undesired movement, but the muscles are on call, so to speak, and are recruited as needed to control spinal movements within the safe range. This phase also requires that the individual has the ability to freely transition from use of agonist and antagonist stabilizing musculature.

Functional Loss Characteristics

Of particular importance in the development of a stabilization program are the patient's functional loss characteristics: position sensitivity, weight-bearing sensitivity, stasis sensitivity, and pressure sensitivity. Although they may be found in isolation or may occur in combination, they will be discussed individually.[12,15]

Position Sensitivity

The patient who is position sensitive is usually the easiest to treat. Such a patient can easily identify the position of comfort when searching for the neutral position and, when given the tools to manage the spine in or about that position, can learn to satisfactorily control symptoms. In addition to stabilization training, these individuals need to have a good understanding of which postures in daily living tend to place them in a precarious position. For example, patients with a flexion bias should be taught to avoid the relaxed standing posture, because it creates an anterior pelvic tilt and lumbar extension.

Weight-Bearing Sensitivity

A common finding, weight-bearing sensitivity is manifest quickly in an examination. A person who is weight-bearing sensitive frequently employs load-reducing maneuvers. For example, if the clinician notices the patient is slouched in a chair with the buttocks forward and the trunk leaning back on the upper thoracic spine, the patient may be seeking the most supine position available at the moment. It is tempting to interpret this behavior as poor posture, but the position may be used as a load-reducing maneuver. Individuals with weight-bearing sensitivity will do anything possible to decrease the influences of gravity. In the examination room, such patients tend to lean on the upper extremities for support, often shifting position to vary the weight distribution.

To progress to an exercise program for patients with this functional loss characteristic, the clinician needs to be creative in developing exercises that keep the spine unloaded or that actually provide distraction through exercise. Examples include the basic principles of unloading via non-weight-bearing positions. Another consideration is the use of traction harness supports for both gravity-eliminated and antigravity positions. Eventual progression might include upright unweighting exercises, such as pull-ups and dips, while paying attention to basic stabilization principles.

Stasis Sensitivity

Stasis sensitivity is commonly found in individuals with hypermobile or unstable conditions. This sensitivity is evidenced by the tendency for the patient to prefer moving to staying still and to feel worse in any sustained posture. The position, unless close to anatomic neutral, is irrelevant; if the posture is sustained, pain occurs. Nights are often difficult, because the body remains still during sleep. The patient may need to get up in the night and walk around to decrease symptoms. Treatment considerations for these patients should include adherence to a relatively anatomic neutral posture, with controlled flexion/extension movement permitted during functional activities. Aerobic exercise, because of its oscillatory effects, often helps reduce symptoms. However, the emphasis should be on control of spinal movement during activity.

Pressure Sensitivity

Patients with pressure sensitivity on the posterior aspect of the spine will need modifications to any supine exercise and will best tolerate any activity in which there is no external pressure applied to the spinous processes or sacrum. For supine positioning, place two mats side by side with a slight gap to suspend the pressure-sensitive areas between the supportive surfaces.

Examination

A thorough examination is always an important aspect of stabilization training and exercise prescription. As indicated, muscle imbalances may limit appropriate performance of certain exercises, and these imbalances must be dealt with before advancing the program. Compensatory movements during exercise may indicate a physiologic condition that warrants further investigation. Always pay close attention to pain response and to compensatory movements that may occur with activity. Pain during safe exercise is often different from the symptoms for which the patient sought treatment. Often, the muscle action will trigger different, but benign, symptoms related to muscle activity and not to pathology.

When embarking on a stability program for a patient with a hypermobile segment, it is important to have some objective measures regarding the stabilizing function of the multifidus muscles. The recommended testing procedure for segmental multifidus testing is shown in Figure 12-3. The lumbar spine is flexed up to the level of the involved segment; an attempted lateral displacement of the femurs will be poorly resisted in the presence of weak multifidi. This pressure should be light.

The multifidi primarily function as contralateral rotators; but because the forces are applied through the pelvis, the side on which the pressure is applied is the side providing the resistance. In other words, if the pressure is applied to the femur on the left side (with the force directed toward the right), the left multifidus is being tested (Fig. 12-3). Because the multifidus muscles are inhibited at the

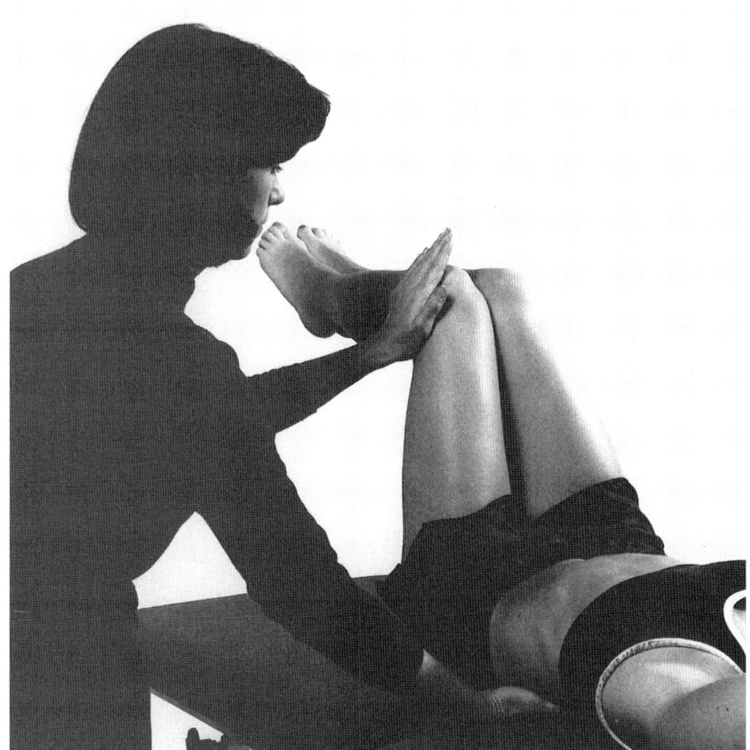

FIGURE 12-3 Segmental multifidus muscle testing.

PURPOSE: Examine core stability of the segmental lumbar muscles.

POSTION: Client lying supine. Clinician palpating intersegmentally to flex the lower trunk up, isolating to the desired level.

PROCEDURE: Clinician gives gentle, gradual lateral pressure to distal femurs, creating a rotational force through the lumbar spine. Clinician compare side to side and to segments above and below, observing for weakness, as demonstrated by lack of resistance to the rotational force.

level of spinal injury,[29] it is helpful to track the function of the multifidus using this testing procedure.

An alternate method of multifidus testing is a screening procedure recommended by Richardson et al.[16] This test relies on palpation and comparison of the contractions on each side. With the patient in the prone position, the clinician palpates adjacent to the spinous process and asks the patient, "Gently swell out your muscles under my fingers without moving your spine or pelvis." The clinician assesses the ability for the muscles to perform this action. This technique can also be used as a training tool for isolated multifidus contraction.[16]

Another objective measurement that helps document recovery is the assessment of weight-bearing symmetry. Using two scales side by side, observe the load distribution on examination and on re-examination. As the spine gains stability, weight distribution should be increasingly symmetrical, providing that no other biomechanical factors are interfering with the balance of load.

Summary: Spinal Stabilization

Movement with stability is the ultimate goal of stabilization training. The client should develop freedom of movement, without rigid spinal-holding patterns, and should function more efficiently during all activities. This improved movement is accomplished through enhanced proprioceptive abilities, strength, postural endurance, and balanced, efficient motor programming.

■ *Techniques*

POSTURE

Making changes in posture is often difficult and frustrating for both the client and the clinician. It seems that even if the client's posture can be corrected, he or she drifts back into the old dysfunctional position as soon as appropriate posture is no longer the focus of concentration. Therefore, in addition to educating the patient on posture in a proprioceptive manner, adjuncts should be used to help reinforce proper posture throughout the day. The objective is to offer some useful postural correction and education techniques and then to suggest adjuncts to assist the patient in maintaining the postural changes.

The use of the vertical compression test, as indicated earlier, is recommended on initial examination and after postural correction, to evaluate the patient's static alignment (Fig. 12-2). After correction procedures, the vertical compression test checks the correction both for examination purposes and to illustrate the difference to the patient. Often the patient will feel off balance and must be convinced of the benefits of the change. Usually, a mirror or photograph will help demonstrate the value of the correction.

To correct faulty posture, the use of verbal and physical cues is recommended. Begin from the foundation and move superiorly. Use of a plumb line helps when the client is initially learning to look for postural deviations.[5] If the knees are locked into hyperextension, ask the patient to soften them. If the pelvis is anteriorly tilted, provide manual cues while asking the client to tuck the tail under. For example, to encourage inferior movement of the sacrum, the clinician places a finger of one hand on the sacrum and taps or presses lightly in an inferior direction while a finger on the hand is placed on the midline of the abdomen inferior to the umbilicus and skin-drags the anterior abdomen in a superior direction. If pelvis is posteriorly tilted, the clinician can reverse the same manual cues and ask the client to tip the pelvis forward as though it were a bucket and he or she were trying to pour water out of the front of it.

For a patient with a rounded, forward shoulder posture, addressing the upper trunk will alter the faulty posture inferiorly. Place a finger on the upper sternum, and tap it gently, asking the patient to breathe while lifting the sternum up and forward slightly, then to exhale without allowing the chest to drop (Fig. 12-4). Besides offering the cervical spine relief from the often-associated forward head posture, this technique has the added benefit of promoting abdominal breathing.

Although a temporary solution, simple taping is a powerful tool for postural education. Both in the lumbar and thoracic spine, posterior taping offers a primitive, but effective, form of biofeedback: The tape pulls when the patient moves into a flexed posture. To tape the lumbar spine, begin in the standing or prone position. Ask the patient to produce and explore lumbopelvic movement, coming to rest in the neutral position. Then apply (1) horizontal anchor strips at the thoracolumbar junction and the sacrum, (2) diagonal strips to form an X across the low back (Fig. 12-5), (3) a few longitudinal strips from anchor to anchor, and (4) a couple of horizontal closing strips. Thoracic taping can be applied in a similar manner, emphasizing the direction of desired support. Athletic tape usually works well for these techniques but usually quickly loosens. Fortunately, taping does not take long to make an impact. As soon as the client sits in the car, the learning is intensified. Other, more adhesive types of tape are available, and they may be used to maintain postural feedback over a longer period of time. However, the clinician must be aware of any potential skin allergies that may preclude leaving the tape on for more than a few hours.

Additional methods for promoting maintenance of corrected posture include techniques that periodically remind the client to self-correct. Setting a watch to beep every 30 min or so is an easy method. Clients who work at a computer may use an alarm program that sounds every 30 min; besides serving as a reminder of postural correction, it may encourage the client to stand up and perform 1 min of stretching exercises.

FIGURE 12-4 Technique for correcting faulty posture.

PURPOSE: To correct a rounded, forward-shoulder posture.

POSTION: Client standing. Clinician standing to side.

PROCEDURE: Clinician places a finger on client's upper sternum and taps it gently, asking client to breathe while lifting the sternum up and forward slightly and then to exhale without allowing chest to drop.

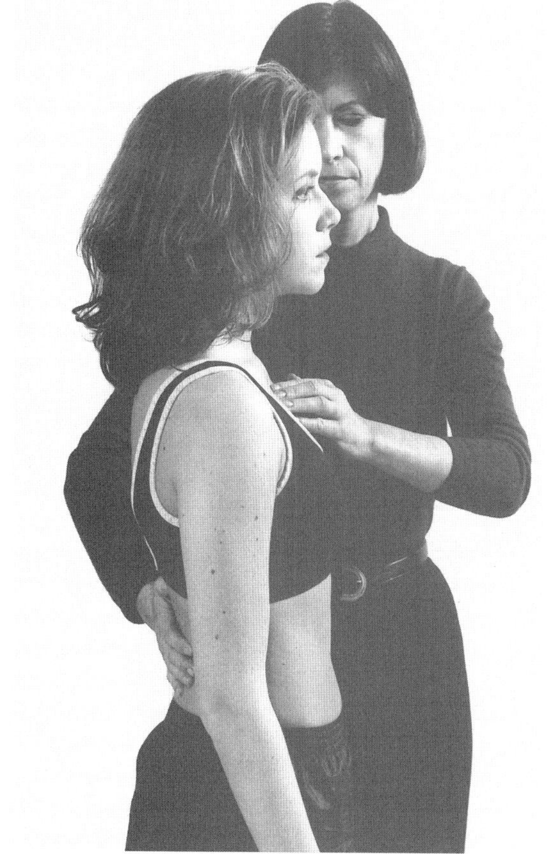

FIGURE 12-5 Lumbar spine taping to provide feedback.

PURPOSE: To provide primitive postural feedback.

POSTION: Client standing in a neutral lumbopelvic position.

PROCEDURE: Clinician applies horizontal anchor strips at the thoracolumbar junction and sacrum, diagonal strips in an X across the low back, a few longitudinal strips from anchor to anchor, and a couple of horizontal closing strips.

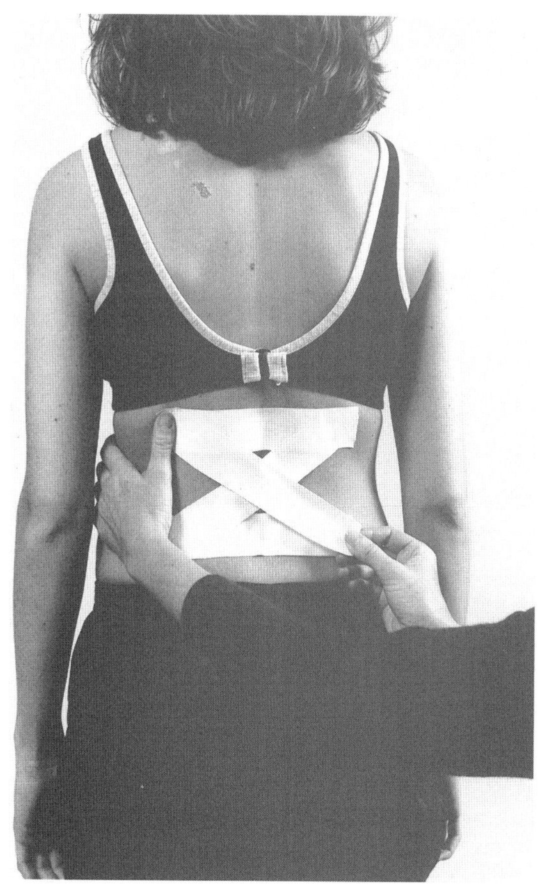

BODY MECHANICS

Before moving on to techniques of body mechanics education, the importance of the lower extremities must be discussed. One of the most frustrating aspects of training body mechanics is the fact that lower extremity strength can be the limiting factor in one's ability to move efficiently and safely through daily activities. The most basic of body mechanics education is use of proper lifting techniques. When lifting from the floor, the individual must achieve a position that is close to the floor, which requires strong lower extremities that can safely lower and raise the body. Therefore, lower extremity strength is as fundamental to spinal care as is spinal strength.

By following a few basic ergonomic principles, workers can protect themselves on the job (Table 12-3). Patient education in these basic concepts will provide guidance for a lifetime of active prevention of workplace injury or exacerbation of symptoms.

When possible, videotape the client performing on the job or videotape simulated job or sports activities. Review the tape in slow motion, looking for subtle movement faults of which the patient may be unaware. When dealing with a work or sports environment, it is important for the clinician to understand the necessary activities. The clinician can seek out educational videos on the sport or job or can obtain the assistance of a reputable teaching professional, work manager, or coach to gain knowledge in basic techniques. This information, combined with professional knowledge on biomechanics and rehabilitation, provides a wealth of intervention potential for the client in question and for future clients.

Obstacle course training is a powerful way to assist the patient in problem solving while focusing on maintaining a functional, neutral posture. Varying the environment in which an individual is performing a task is known to improve overall learning. Therefore, setting up a simple obstacle course in the clinic is an inexpensive and valuable tool for effective training and can provide objective measures in the form of time to completion. Examples of tasks that can be used are pushing a weighted cart, pulling a vacuum cleaner, lifting cuff weights from the floor to an overhead shelf, placing a child seat into the back of a car, bending over to scrub the bathtub, leaning over the sink to simulate brushing the teeth, moving wet clothes from a washer to dryer, and sitting in an office chair and reaching to answer the phone or use the computer.

TABLE 12-3 Summary of Basic Ergonomic Principles

Summary of Basic Ergonomic Principles
Keep frequently used materials close to avoid reaching.
Work should be positioned at elbow height for sitting and standing.
Heavier objects should be placed lower and lighter objects, higher.
Keep loads close to the body
Push loads instead of pulling, whenever possible.
Maintain neutral posture.
Eliminate excessive repetition.
Minimize fatigue by avoiding static loads and grips, taking breaks, and rotating stressful jobs.
Use adjustable workstations and chairs; change postures frequently.
Provide clearance and access so that proper movements are possible.
Create a comfortable environment with adequate lighting and temperature.
Eliminate vibration.

SPINAL STABILIZATION

Initiation of Training

Before beginning an exercise routine, the tissue should be prepared and the clinician should try to optimize the healing environment.[4] For the patient with lumbar pathology, the exercise preparation technique of choice is aerobic activity. In fact, aerobic exercise itself has been shown to have positive effects on low back pain.[41] This activity may be performed in numerous postures, and the clinician should consider the patient's specific characteristics and positional bias when choosing an aerobic modality. Giving consideration to the client's specific concerns, the clinician may recommend walking, bicycling, using a ski machine, or supine bicycling (Chapter 10). Occasionally, the client is not ready for aerobic exercise; in this case therapeutic modalities may be used to prepare the tissue for intervention.

The aerobic activity in the initial phases of stabilization training should be specifically for warm-up purposes and should not be overly aggressive. Fast, or ballistic, movements of the extremities can be detrimental to the training of the core stabilizers and should be reserved for those individuals who have demonstrated proper stabilization techniques in early phase activities.

The individual's flexibility and mobility must be considered so that all stabilization exercises are safe and appropriate. Simply stated, specific flexibility or mobility limitations may interfere with the physical performance of an activity. For example, if the hip is unable to flex beyond 100° before recruiting the pelvis into a posterior tilt, any exercise requiring more than 100° of hip flexion is unsafe. Be careful to watch for compensation that may originate from such a physical limitation. The clinician should use other therapeutic interventions to correct the limitation to allow for progression of the stabilization program.

The clinician begins stabilization training by providing the patient a relatively easy position in which to produce and explore lumbopelvic motion (this is usually the hooklying position). One good method of instruction is for the clinician to ask the patient to envision the face of a clock on his or her abdomen, with 12:00 at the belly button and 6:00 at the pubic bone. The clinician then asks the patient to alternately tilt the pelvis so that 12:00 rocks toward the floor and then 6:00 rocks toward the floor. The clinician then instructs the patient to move back and forth from the 12:00 to 6:00 positions gently, slowly, and with awareness 10 times each direction. The patient then identifies the point within that range that is most comfortable. Because this point is the most comfortable spot, training is focused on teaching the patient how to stay near that point during daily life. As noted, this position is referred to as the neutral or functional position of the spine and should be emphasized and maintained for all movements performed during spinal stabilization activities.

When progressing a patient to a new exercise, the clinician should always ensure proprioceptive accuracy before embarking. Again, the initial phase of stabilization training should include isolated stabilizing muscle contractions (passive preconditioning), followed by challenge to the stabilizing musculature via limb movement (active preconditioning), with eventual progression to functional activities for neuromotor retraining (dynamic stabilization). Each new exercise should be initiated with the patient exploring the lumbopelvic motion, safely and accurately identifying the neutral position. Remember that the neutral position may change as the pathology changes; therefore, the patient should re-explore each movement with each new activity. The pelvic rocking has the added benefit of providing input to the type 2 mechanoreceptors[42] and thus reducing pain.

As the patient demonstrates awareness of the neutral, or functional position, the clinician begins to train the isolated transversus abdominus contraction. The clinician asks the client to place a finger or two just medial to the anterior superior iliac spine (ASIS) and lightly press into the tissue. Then the patient is told to draw the abdominal muscles inward and upward, without altering the spinal position, and to feel a simultaneous tensing in the pelvic floor muscles. An alternate position for transversus contraction is in quadruped next to a mirror.[16] As the transversus contraction is achieved, the abdomen draws upward, narrowing the waist. With either technique, the idea is to isolate contraction and avoid overexertion, which tends to recruit all of the abdominal muscles.

A great tool for assisting the patient in awareness of abdominal contraction is a biofeedback instrument. Simple, single channel electromyographic devices can give the patient auditory and visual feedback regarding electrical activity in the targeted muscles. If choosing this adjunct, the clinician should remember to document the parameters during each session in which the device is used to obtain additional objective information. Usually, if needed at all, the use of electromyography will be necessary for only a few visits. Recommended placement for electrodes is just inferior and medial to the ASIS.[43]

Phase I: Basic

If the patient understands the concepts of selective muscle contraction and the neutral spine position, the next aspect of training is to challenge the muscle's ability to maintain postural control while subject to perturbation. This challenge is accomplished via subtle movement of the upper and lower extremities. Again, emphasize slow, controlled movement with awareness. Parameters used during phase I are presented in Table 12-4.

The main thing to remember during phase I is that protocols are not used; instead the clinician is encouraged to use his or her imagination to best facilitate the patient's learning. The usual approach is to follow a developmental sequence path, beginning with supine exercises (including bridging) and progressing to prone, quadruped, kneeling, and standing exercises. This framework may be adapted to specific patient situations, and some postures may need to be avoided according to patient tolerance and abilities. For example, if a patient has particularly tight rectus femoris muscles but the positional bias for intervention is flexion, the bridging posture may be too difficult, owing to the anatomic limitations. These important data are obtained from physical examination and through careful observation of the patient while he or she is performing the exercises.

In addition, it must be emphasized that the neutral (functional) position of the spine should be maintained during all activities. If the patient performs an activity and the neutral position cannot be maintained, pain will

TABLE 12-4 Phase I (Basic) Stabilization Training

Goals
Improve proprioceptive awareness
Increase strength, flexibility, and coordination
Become proficient in basic body mechanics
Promote independence in exercise
Decrease symptoms
Exercises
Short lever arms
Minimal, if any, weights
Stable, supported postures

occur, which indicates that the program is being progressed too aggressively.

Supine Activities

Supine exercises typically begin with simple, supported, upper extremity movement. This movement may be performed bilaterally for balanced abdominal recruitment or unilaterally for asymmetrical recruitment that challenges the spine in the transverse plane (rotation). The patient should be asked to lift the arms overhead first without abdominal contraction, because the lumbar spine will usually extend slightly and the patient will become aware that movement of the upper extremities can influence the spine (Fig. 12-6).

To progress from upper extremity movement, have the client attempt to lift one lower extremity slightly and then lower it before attempting to lift the other. The tendency is for the patient to get a rotational shift in the pelvis and lumbar spine during the transition from one side to the other. If this rotation occurs, the clinician should emphasize that maintaining a level pelvis during the transition will promote depth in the contraction of the core stabilizers (Fig. 12-7).

One method used to facilitate deep stabilizer recruitment is to ask the patient to imagine that gum is stuck on the bottom of one shoe. As the patient tries to lift the foot, he or she imagines the gum pulling strongly back down. After the foot has been lifted just a few inches, the patient imagines that the foot is being pulled back down, and the patient should permit the foot to slowly return to the support surface. Supine exercises can be progressed by having the patient lift one leg and the contralateral arm simultaneously. This activity is sometimes referred to as the dying bug exercise (Fig. 12-8).

Another technique to facilitate deep stabilizer recruitment is manual resistance. The clinician applies gentle

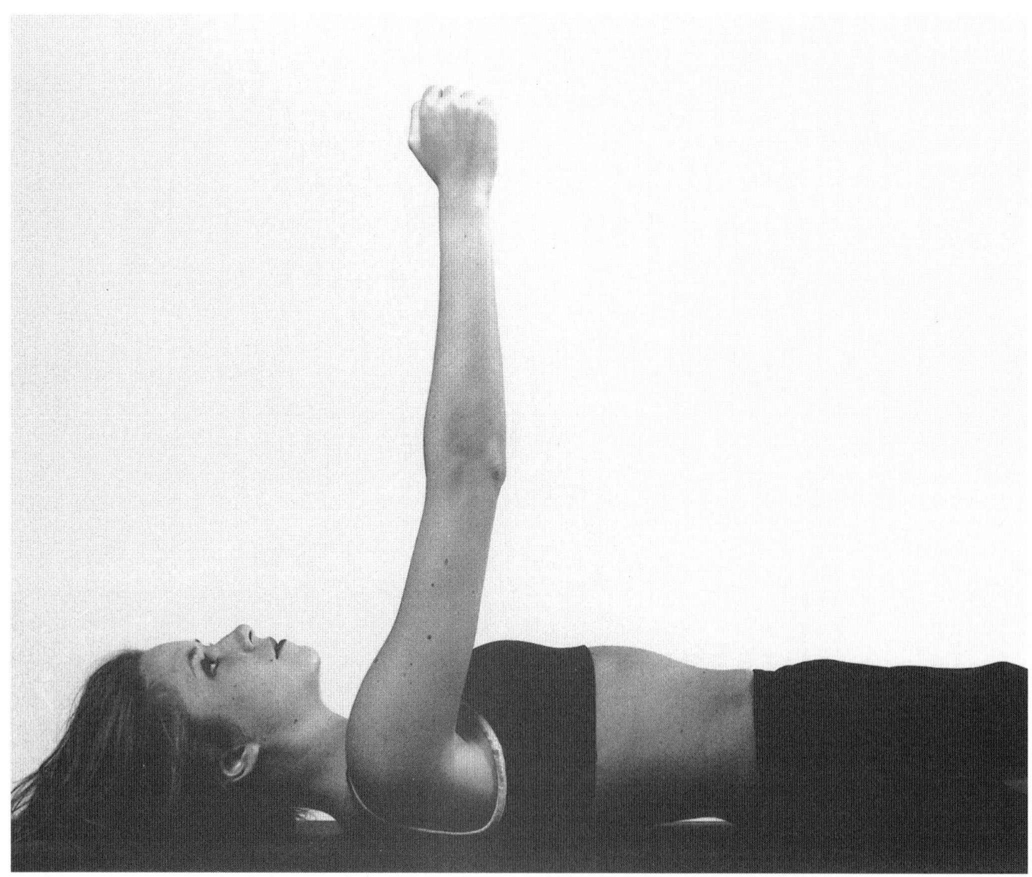

FIGURE 12-6 **Unilateral upper extremity lift in supine.**

PURPOSE: Facilitate proprioceptive awareness of abdominal contractions associated with upper extremity movement.

POSTION: Client lying supine in neutral lumbopelvic position.

PROCEDURE: Client lifts one arm overhead, noting forces that occur in lumbar spine. Client counteracts forces with abdominal contraction, maintaining a still lumbopelvic spine.

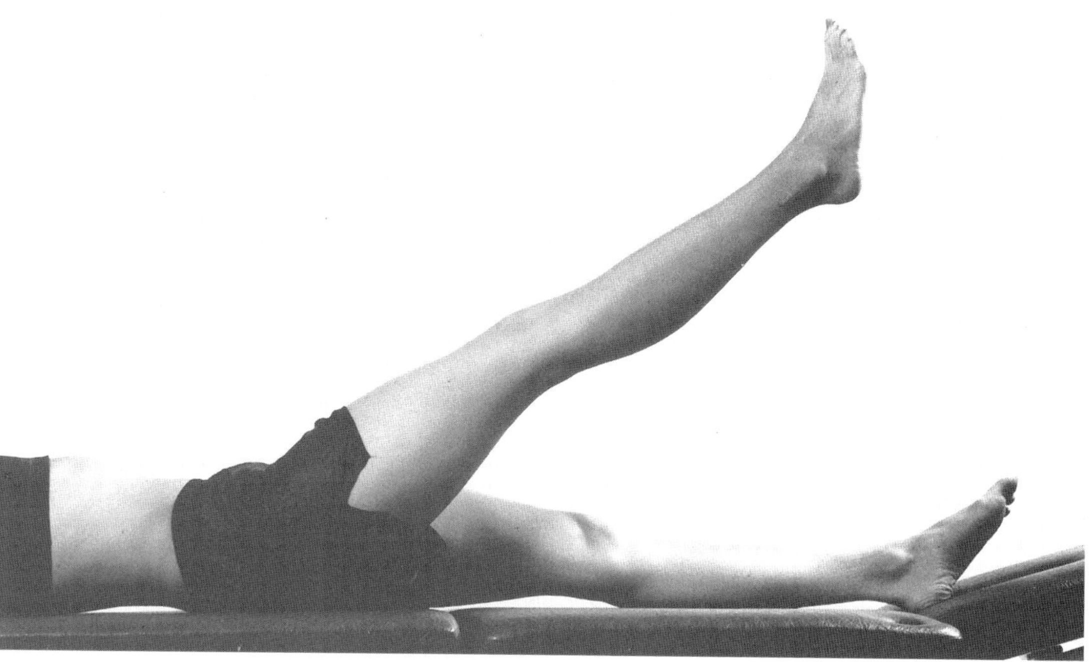

FIGURE 12-7 **Unilateral lower extremity lift in supine.**

PURPOSE: Facilitate proprioceptive awareness of abdominal contractions associated with lower extremity movement.

POSTION: Client lying supine in neutral lumbopelvic position.

PROCEDURE: Client lifts one limb slightly and then lowers it, while counteracting forces with abdominal contraction and maintaining a still lumbopelvic spine.

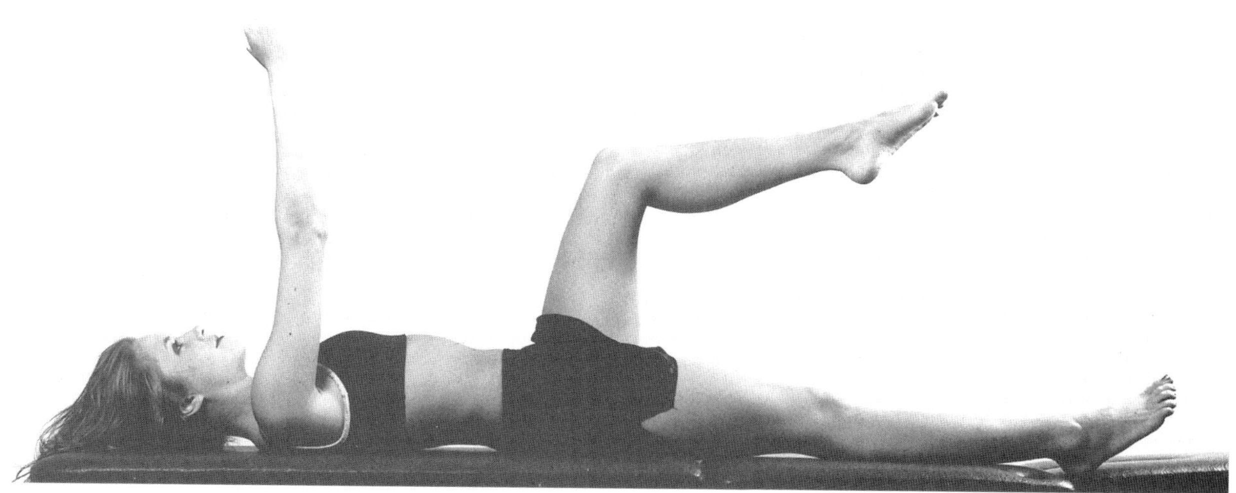

FIGURE 12-8 **Dying bug exercise in supine.**

PURPOSE: Facilitate proprioceptive awareness of spinal stress with limb movement and to strengthen the abdominal stabilizers.

POSTION: Client lying supine in neutral lumbopelvic position.

PROCEDURE: Client raises right arm and left leg and then left arm and right leg (similar to a supine running motion).

NOTE: Emphasis should be placed on control, before speed. Resistance is optional. Neutral position of spine should be maintained.

resistance to the limbs, either supported or unsupported, to facilitate irradiation of contraction from the stronger muscles to the targeted, deeper muscles.[44]

The initial stabilization experience for the patient is more of a learning session than an exercise session. The clinician should remember this when providing directions for the home exercise program. The patient should be instructed to take time to practice the movements instead of being told to do specific sets of repetitions. The patient should also be advised to practice in a quiet environment that is conducive to concentration. This initial training is probably the most important aspect to the overall success of the stabilization program. If the patient becomes sloppy with movements early on, neither pain reduction nor improvement in functional performance will occur.

To increase the challenge to the stabilizing muscles in supine, exercises can be advanced so that the limbs are no longer providing support. Advancement of exercise should include the addition of ankle and hand weights or exercise tubing for further challenge. As the patient improves in the ability to maintain a stable trunk with these exercises, both the duration and the speed of the activity should increase.

Exercising supine can include bridging activities, which can be challenging, especially when progressing to single lower extremity support. Bridging exercises not only challenge the core stabilizers but also require strong gluteal contraction. All motions should be performed slowly at first, with speed increasing as the patient's abilities increase. As with all exercises, it is possible to add weights, tubing, or manual resistance to increase the level of difficulty (Figs. 12-9 and 12-10).

Prone Activities

Prone exercises are excellent for strengthening the lumbar extensors and gluteal muscles and provide a direct challenge to the anterior stabilizing muscles to hold the pelvis from posterior tilting. The clinician should watch for sequence of contraction, emphasizing the stabilizing muscle contraction before any gluteal activity. If gluteals are recruited first, prevention of extension moment through the low back is impossible. If the patient has a flexion bias or has difficulty with prone positioning, use of pillows for abdominal support is recommended. Again, to progress the exercises, use upper and lower extremity lifts to challenge the core stabilizers (Figs. 12-11 and 12-12).

Quadruped exercises offer less external support than supine and prone exercises (Figs. 12-13 and 12-14). Therefore, these activities are usually begun after the more supported postures. The patient's hands should be placed directly below the shoulders and the knees below the hips. Have the patient gripping a towel or hand weight if he or she has difficulty with the wrist extension position in

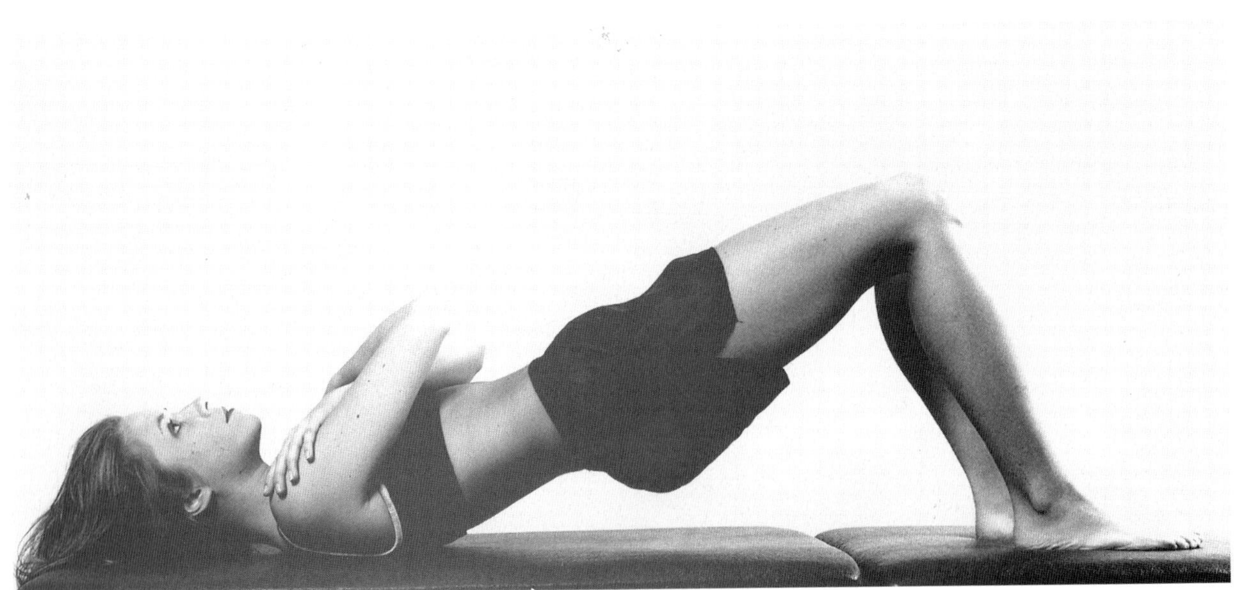

FIGURE 12-9 **Bridge position.**

PURPOSE: Facilitate proprioception and isolate stabilizing muscles and hip extensors.

POSTION: Client hook lying.

PROCEDURE: Client elevates hips while maintaining lumbopelvic neutral position.

NOTE: Client raises hips only as high as proper form can be maintained. Resistance is optional.

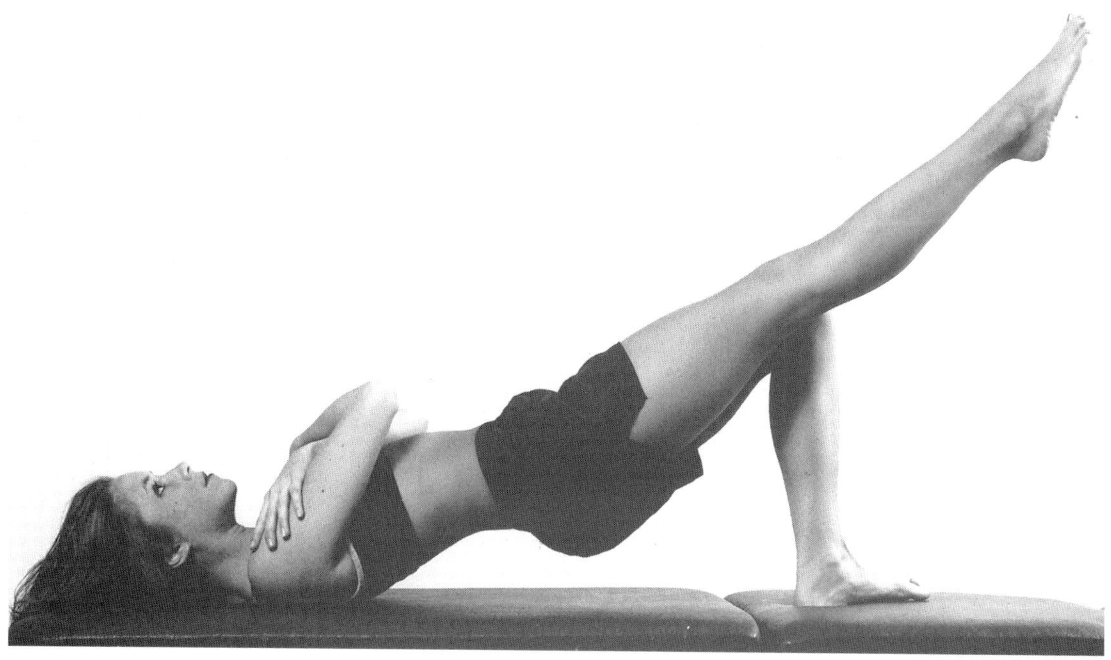

FIGURE 12-10 **Unilateral lower-extremity lift in bridge position.**

PURPOSE: Progress the bridging exercise to emphasize rotational stability and balance.

POSTION: Client lying in bridge position in lumbopelvic neutral position.

PROCEDURE: Client extends one leg while maintaining neutral pelvis.

NOTE: Requires solid contraction of the gluteals. Resistance is optional.

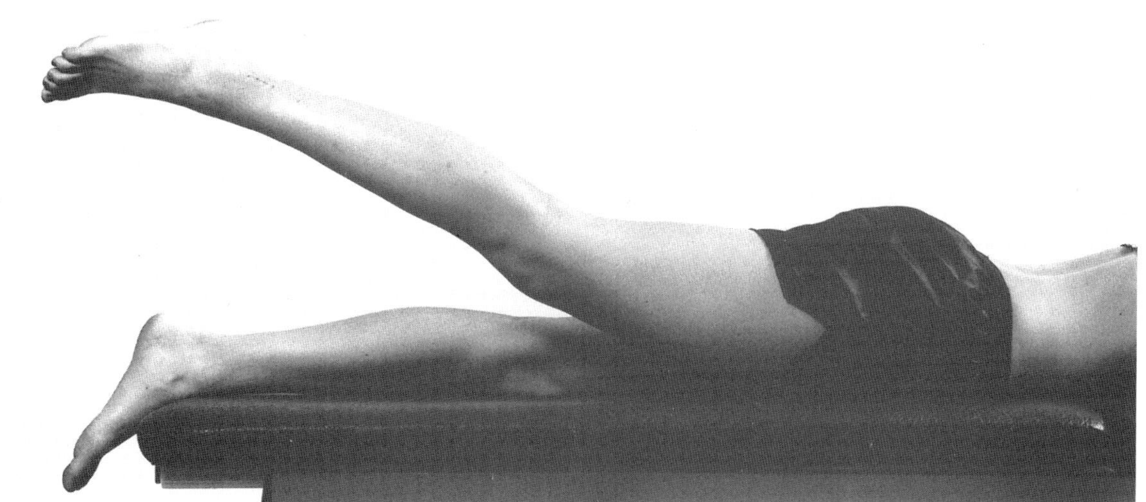

FIGURE 12-11 **Unilateral hip extension in prone.**

PURPOSE: Facilitate proprioception while attempting limb movement in a new position.

POSTION: Client lying prone with arms overhead or by side.

PROCEDURE: Client barely lifts leg, focusing on gluteal contraction and avoiding lumbar rotation.

NOTE: Clinician may palpate ASIS to observe for excessive anterior pelvic tilting or rotation through pelvis. Resistance is optional.

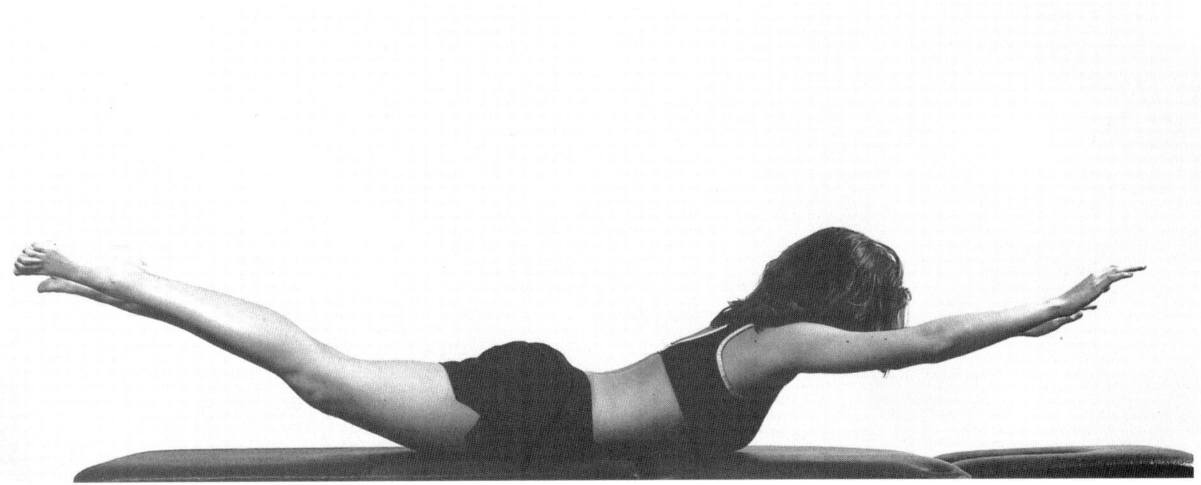

FIGURE 12-12 Bilateral upper and lower extremity lift in prone.

PURPOSE: Provide endurance strengthening of stabilizing muscles of trunk while facilitating proprioceptive awareness.

POSTION: Client lying prone in the Superman position.

PROCEDURE: Client barely lifts all four extremities off the support surface.

NOTE: May be performed with static holds or limbs can be moved various patterns. Resistance is optional.

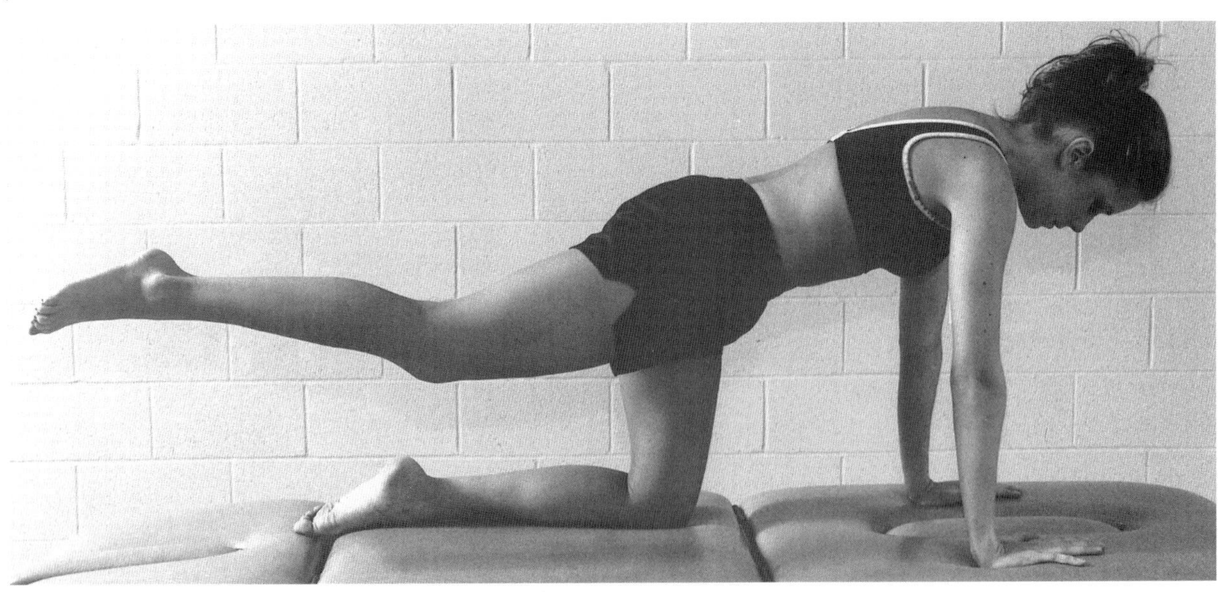

FIGURE 12-13 Unilateral lower extremity lift in quadruped.

PURPOSE: Facilitate proprioception while attempting limb movement in a new position.

POSTION: Client kneeling in quadruped, with hands directly beneath shoulders and knees directly below the hips.

PROCEDURE: Client produces and explores lumbopelvic motion and locks in neutral position. The client extends one hip so foot just clears support surface (to avoid unnecessary lumbar extension).

NOTE: Resistance is optional.

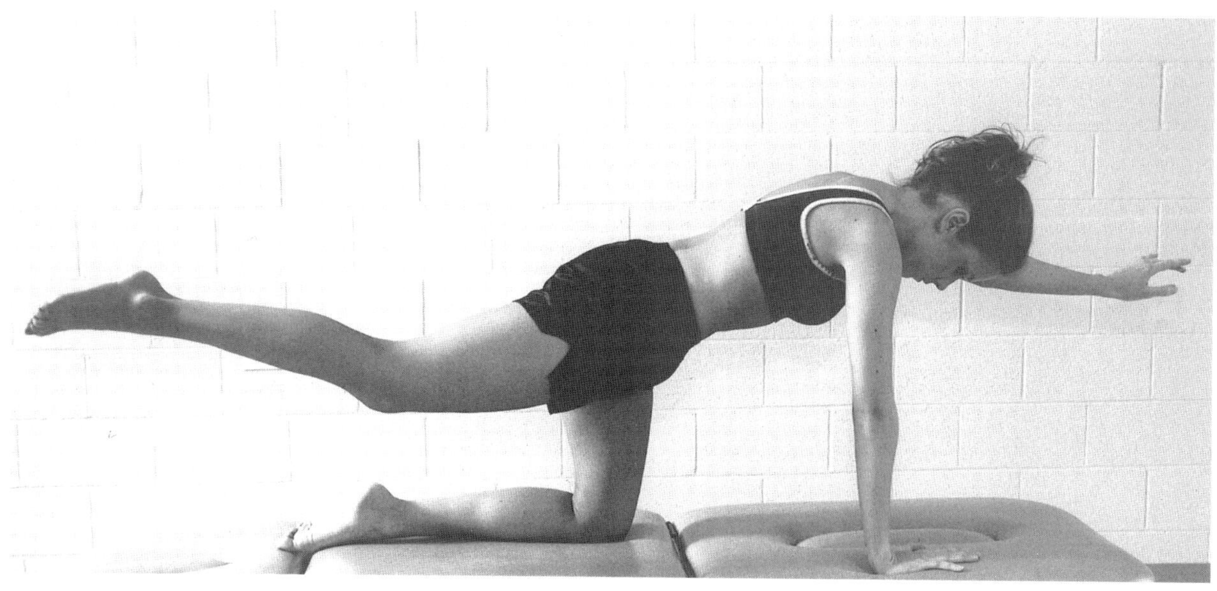

FIGURE 12-14 **Opposite upper and lower extremity lift in quadruped.**

PURPOSE: Provide endurance and strengthening of stabilizing muscles of trunk while facilitating proprioceptive awareness.

POSTION: Client kneeling in quadruped with hands directly beneath the shoulders and knees directly below the hips.

PROCEDURE: Client starts in neutral position, extends one hip and flexes opposite shoulder while maintaining neutral cervical positioning.

NOTE: Resistance is optional.

quadruped. Care should be given to the thoracic spine, making sure that the scapulae are stable and that thoracic kyphosis is relatively neutral. The tendency is for the thoracic spine to arch into flexion. Patients often attempt to lift the leg high during lower extremity extension, resulting in lumbar extension. Keeping the foot low along the support surface will usually eliminate lumbar extension and may improve contraction of the stabilizing multifidus. Another common error is excessive lateral weight shift toward the supporting lower extremity. To reduce this tendency, the clinician can position the patient next to a wall, effectively blocking a weight shift.

Kneeling and Standing Activities

To continue the developmental progression, the client is advanced to kneeling, a position of less stability and potentially greater challenge then the quadruped position. Simple alternate shoulder flexion, with or without weights, can be a great exercise to begin functional stabilization of the spine (Fig. 12-15).

Although it is a more challenging position for stability, standing should be addressed early. As soon as the client understands the neutral position, the clinician should begin to teach basic body mechanics. Include supine to sit, sit to stand, forward bending, and basic lifting as soon as possible. Lunges while maintaining the neutral position of the spine are excellent. Such activities can be used as a part of a home exercise program. The clinician should continue to refine functional activities as the patient is progressed to more advanced training.

Phase II: Advanced

Table 12-5 summarizes the goals and exercises of phase II, the advanced program. In addition to adding weights and increasing the lever arm for any of the aforementioned exercises, training a patient for return to dynamic activity requires dynamic exercises. Use of unstable surfaces is recommended to add challenge and reality to the dynamic spinal stabilization training program. An unstable surface can range from a foam floor mat to single leg support on a foam roll. Clinicians can also use therapeutic balls, ankle platforms, balance boards, and slider boards (Figs. 12-16 to 12-20).

To address true learning and endurance, any one exercise may be performed for 2 to 5 min. Although thousands of repetitions are required to create a new habit, learning retention can be promoted by varying the environment of an activity and changing the order in which activities are performed.[39] Therefore, it is recommended that activities be rotated in and out of an exercise routine. Feedback to the patient should be monitored. Initial training requires quite a bit of immediate verbal and manual cuing, but the clinician's assistance should quickly diminish so that the patient concentrates on

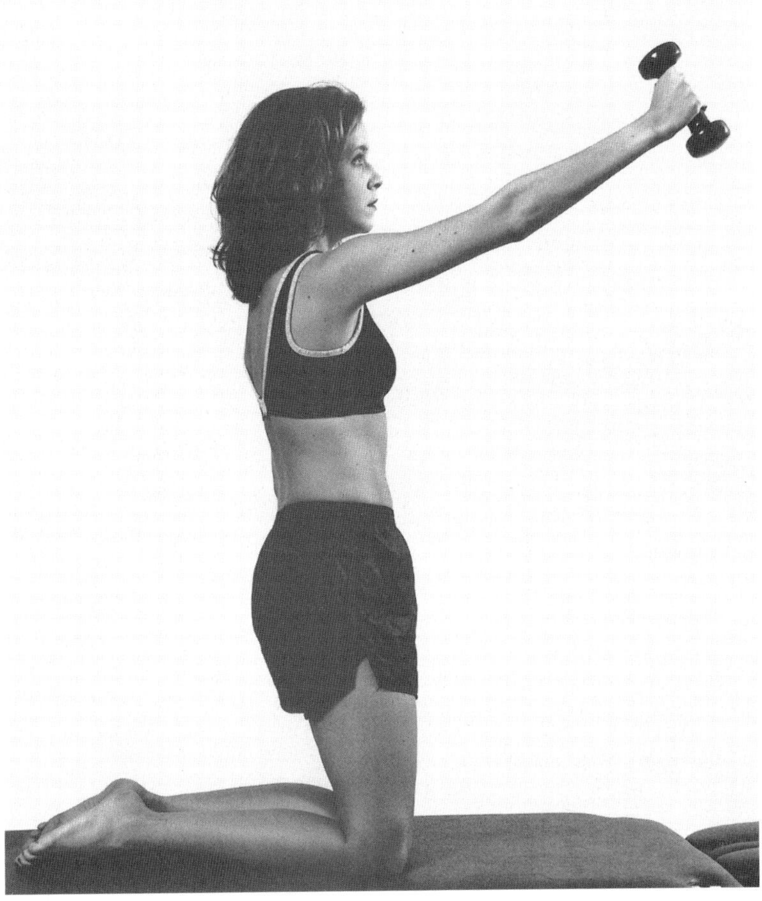

FIGURE 12-15 Kneeling upper extremity lift.

PURPOSE: Facilitate proprioception while attempting limb movement in a new position. Strengthening shoulder girdle and trunk-stabilizing muscles.

POSTION: Client kneeling tall in neutral lumbopelvic position.

PROCEDURE: Client lifts one arm overhead, only as high as possible without losing form. Client alternates arms.

NOTE: Resistance is optional.

TABLE 12-5 Phase II (Advanced) Stabilization Training

Goals
Train for endurance
Focus on specific coordination training
Achieve controlled and safe functioning in combined axes
Exercises
Longer lever arms
Less stable surfaces
Transitional and functional movement patterns and postures
Move around combined axes
Increased speed, repetition, and weights for functional endurance training

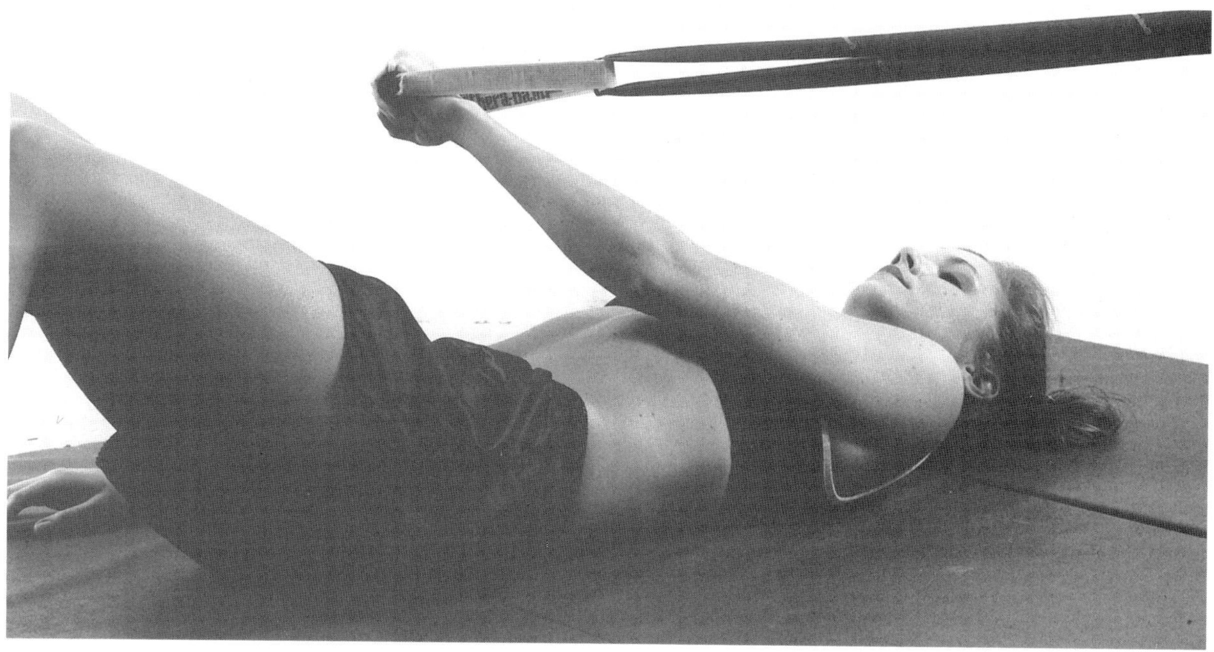

FIGURE 12-16 **Upper extremity exercise in supine with weights (PNF pattern).**

PURPOSE: Strengthen stabilizing musculature in a stable, functional pattern.

POSTION: Client hook lying in neutral lumbopelvic position.

PROCEDURE: Client performs upper extremity diagonal patterns against resistance. Client maintains neutral spine position.

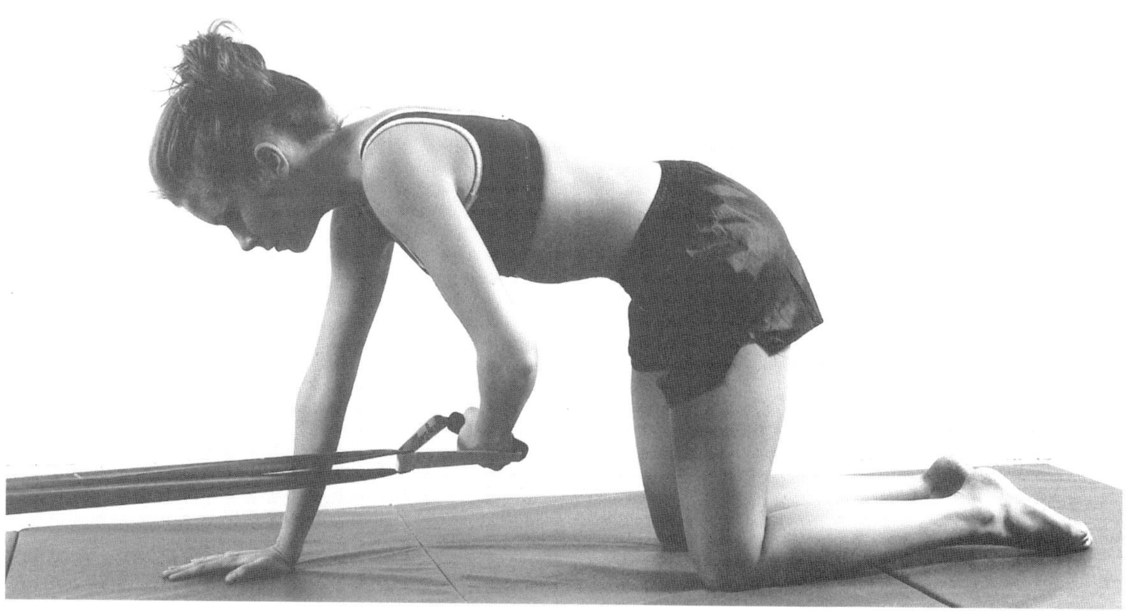

FIGURE 12-17 **Upper extremity exercise in quadruped with weights (PNF pattern).**

PURPOSE: Strengthen stabilizing musculature in a stable, functional pattern.

POSTION: Client kneeling in quadruped in neutral lumbopelvic position.

PROCEDURE: Client performs upper extremity diagonal patterns against resistance. Client maintains neutral spine position.

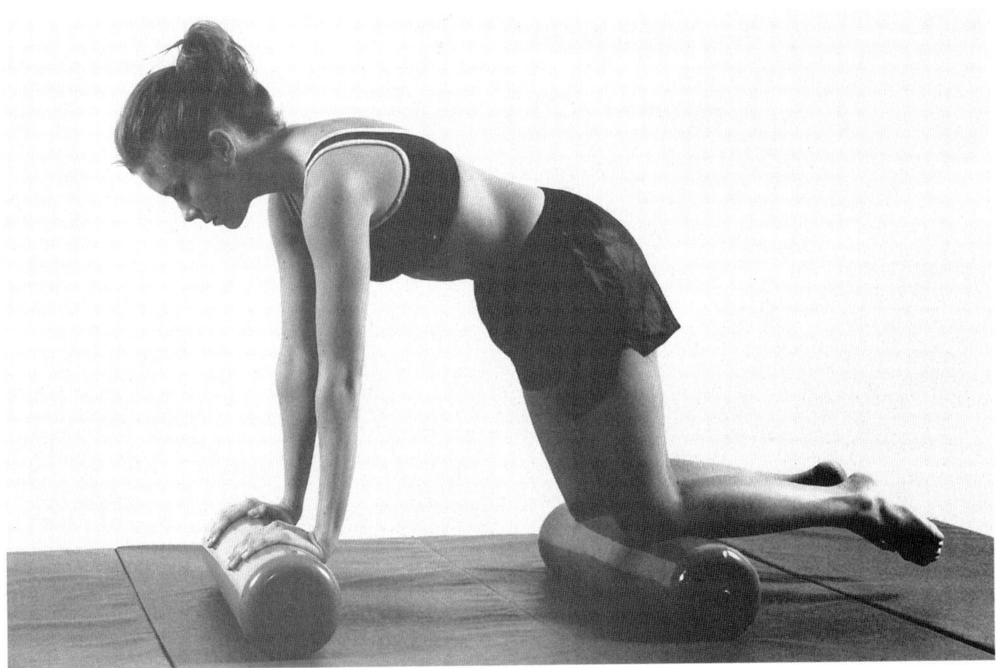

FIGURE 12-18 **Use of foam roller in quadruped.**

PURPOSE: Challenge trunk stability on unstable surfaces.

POSTION: Client kneeling in quadruped with hands and knees on foam rollers.

PROCEDURE: Client maintains lumbopelvic control.

NOTE: To increase the muscular and proprioceptive challenge, client flexes arms or extends hips and knees

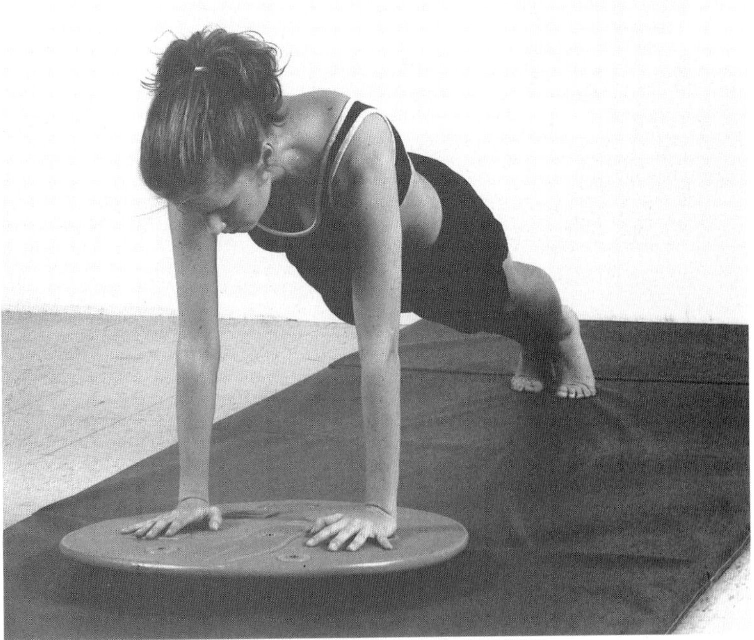

FIGURE 12-19 **Use of balance board in prone.**

PURPOSE: Challenge trunk stability on unstable surfaces.

POSTION: Client lying in pushup position in neutral lumbopelvic position with hands on balance board.

PROCEDURE: Client weight shifts side to side, front to back, or in diagonals or may perform pushup activity. Client maintains neutral spine position.

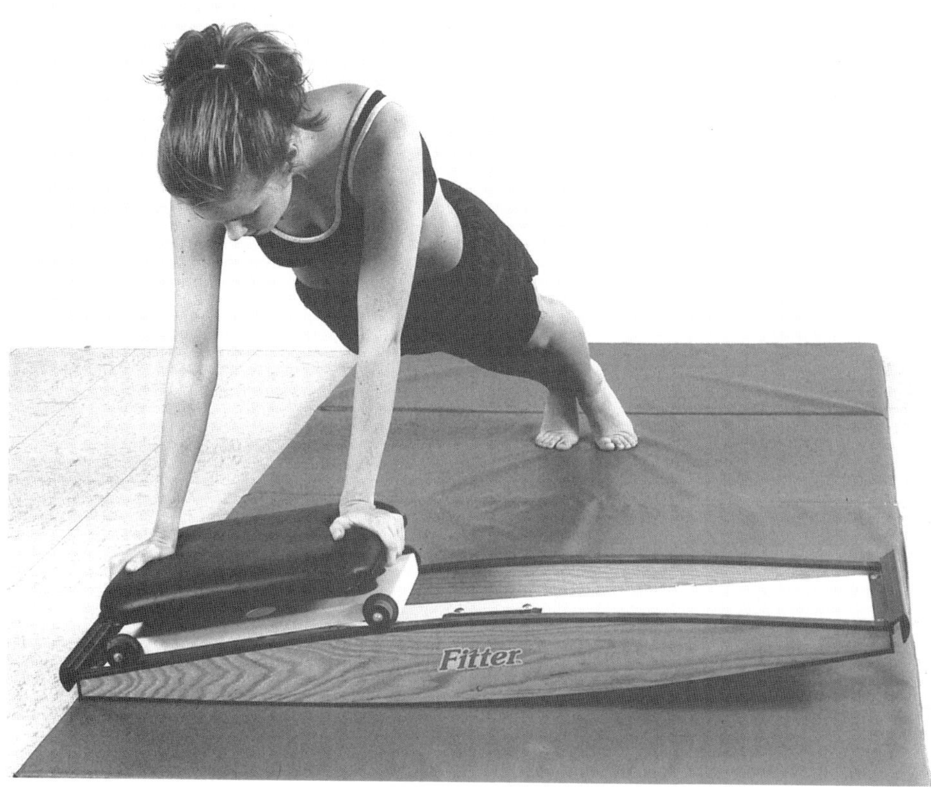

FIGURE 12-20 **Use of sliding board in prone.**

PURPOSE: Challenge trunk stability on unstable surfaces.

POSTION: Client lying in pushup position in neutral lumbopelvic position with hands on sliding board.

PROCEDURE: Client weight shifts side to side or performs pushup activity. Client maintains neutral spine position.

providing self-feedback. The clinician should then provide feedback after the patient completes a particular bout of activity.[45]

The use of a patient journal or flow sheet is recommended to track and encourage compliance. The more the patient feels responsibility for the rehabilitation plan, the more successful the outcome. Again, the goal is for the patient to learn new motor skills; practice, practice, practice is necessary for new movement patterns to become second nature.

Spinal Consideration: Therapeutic Ball

Among the wide variety of activities and props that can be used to add challenge to a dynamic spinal stabilization program, the therapeutic ball has become popular. Thus this section reviews a spinal stabilization program that uses the therapeutic ball to treat individuals with spinal dysfunction. Such a program promotes activity patterns that use appropriate muscles working in a coordinated fashion; the goal is returning the individual to pain-free movement.

As for other techniques of spinal stabilization, two points must be emphasized. First, it is important that the therapeutic ball activities do not cause or increase spinal pain. Second, the clinician must carefully monitor the quality of the patient's movement to ensure that the neutral position is maintained during all activities. Finding and maintaining the neutral (functional) position of the spine enables the patient to perform the exercises without pain and allows the patient to move the arms and legs with less fatigue.

Therapeutic ball exercises can be performed in the supine and prone positions. From the supine position, bridging (and modifications of bridging) are emphasized (Figs. 12-21 and 12-22). Prone exercises include activities in which the upper extremity, lower extremity, and both extremities can be used to challenge the muscles required to stabilize the spine in the neutral position (Figs. 12-23 to 12-27).

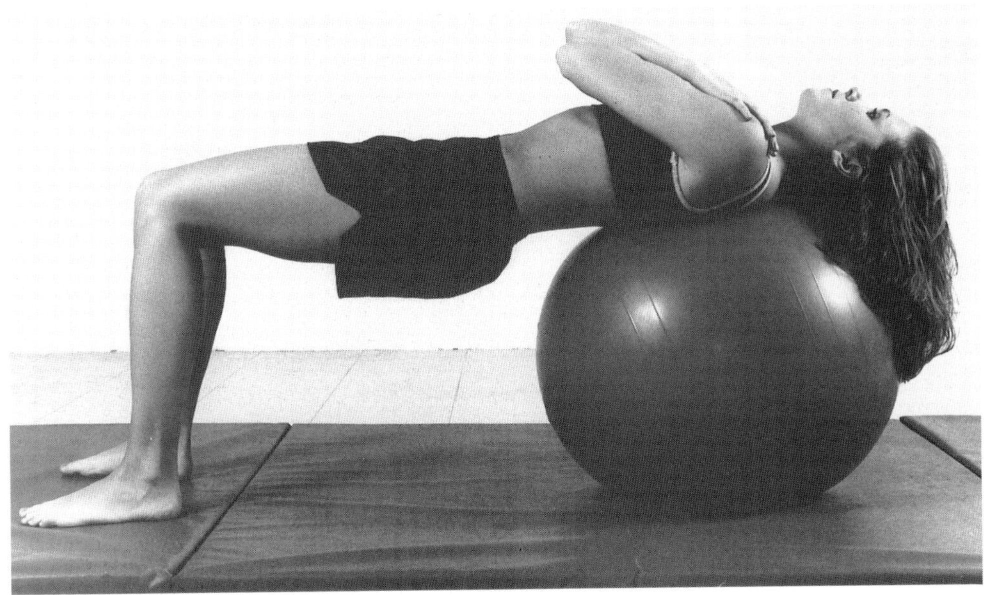

FIGURE 12-21 Use of therapeutic ball in bridging.

PURPOSE: Challenge stabilizing musculature on an unstable surface and in a position that requires endurance and strength of the gluteals.

POSTION: Client lying supine with the head, neck, and upper thoracic spine supported on therapeutic ball.

PROCEDURE: Client elevates hips to maintain upper thoracic position on ball. Client elevates hips while maintaining lumbopelvic neutral position.

NOTE: Client raises hips only as form can be maintained.

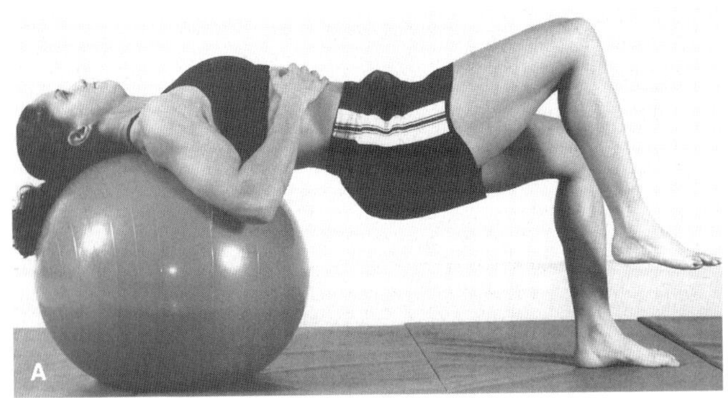

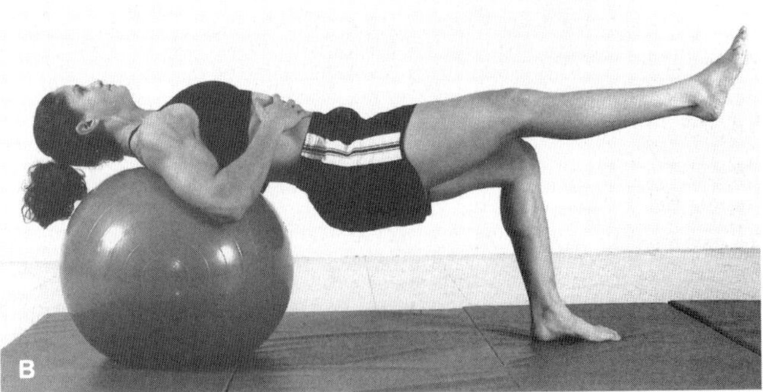

FIGURE 12-22 Unilateral lower extremity lift on therapeutic ball in bridge position.

PURPOSE: Challenge stabilizing musculature on an unstable surface and in a position that requires endurance and strength of the gluteals.

POSTION: Client lying in bridge position in lumbopelvic neutral with hips elevated.

PROCEDURE: Client lifts one foot off support surface while maintaining lumbopelvic neutral and solidly contracting gluteals (panel A).

NOTE: To increase difficulty, client extends one leg while maintaining lumbopelvic neutral (panel B).

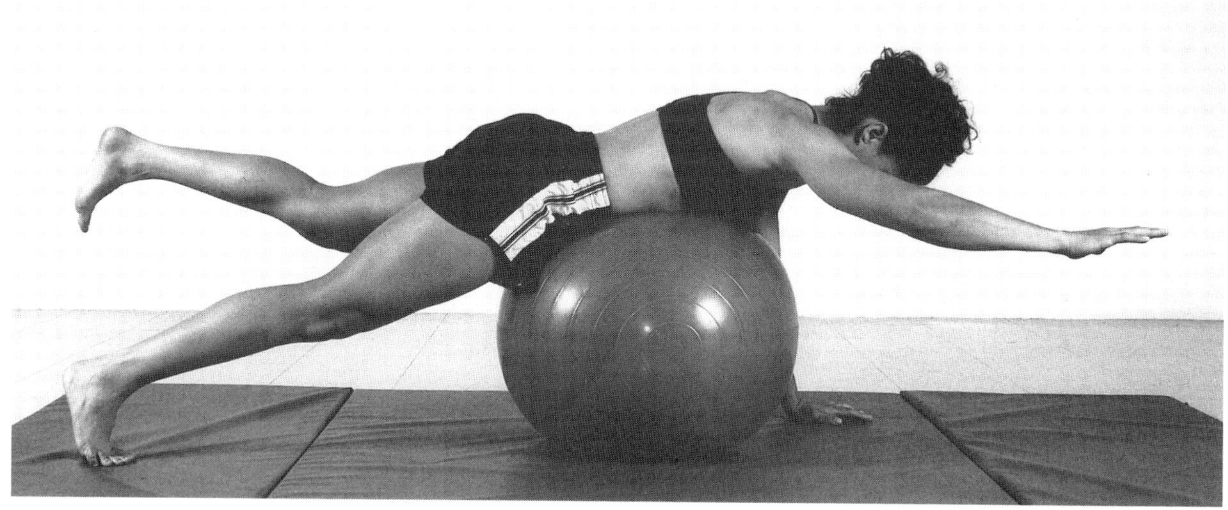

FIGURE 12-23 Upper and lower extremity lift over therapeutic ball.

PURPOSE: Challenge spinal stability, emphasizing spinal extensor muscles.

POSTION: Client lying in prone over therapeutic ball with body horizontal or shoulders higher than hips. Client in neutral lumbopelvic and cervical spine position.

PROCEDURE: Client lifts arms, legs, or opposite arm and leg.

NOTE: Resistance is optional. More hip flexion encourages lumbar flexion; more hip extension encourages lumbar extension.

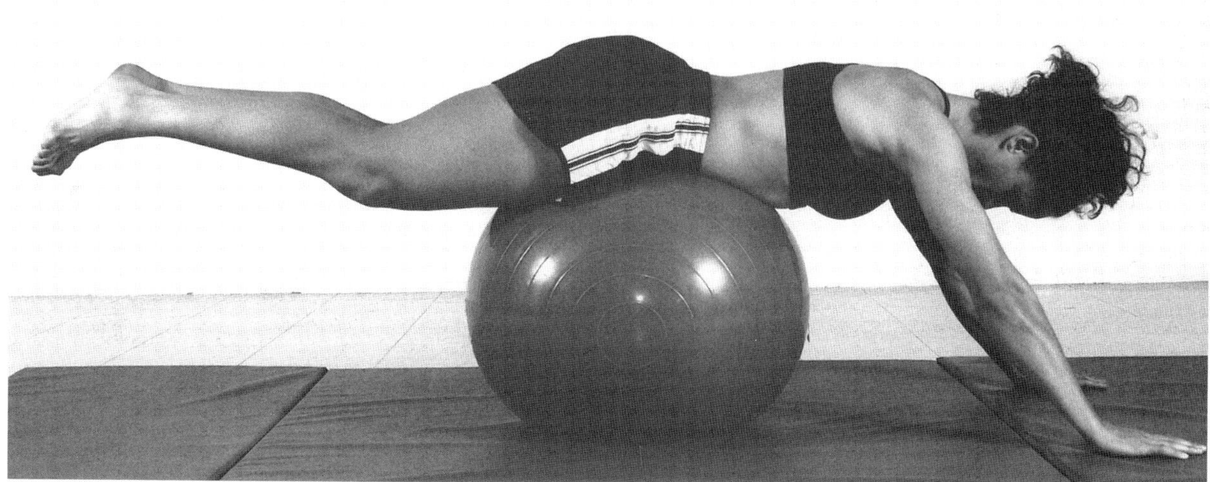

FIGURE 12-24 Bilateral lower extremity lift over therapeutic ball.

PURPOSE: Challenge spinal stability, emphasizing spinal extensor muscles.

POSTION: Client lying in pushup position with therapeutic ball under hips. Client in neutral lumbopelvic and cervical spine position.

PROCEDURE: Client maintains neutral spine position.

NOTE: Clinician may provide manual resistance at trunk or legs to increase challenge.

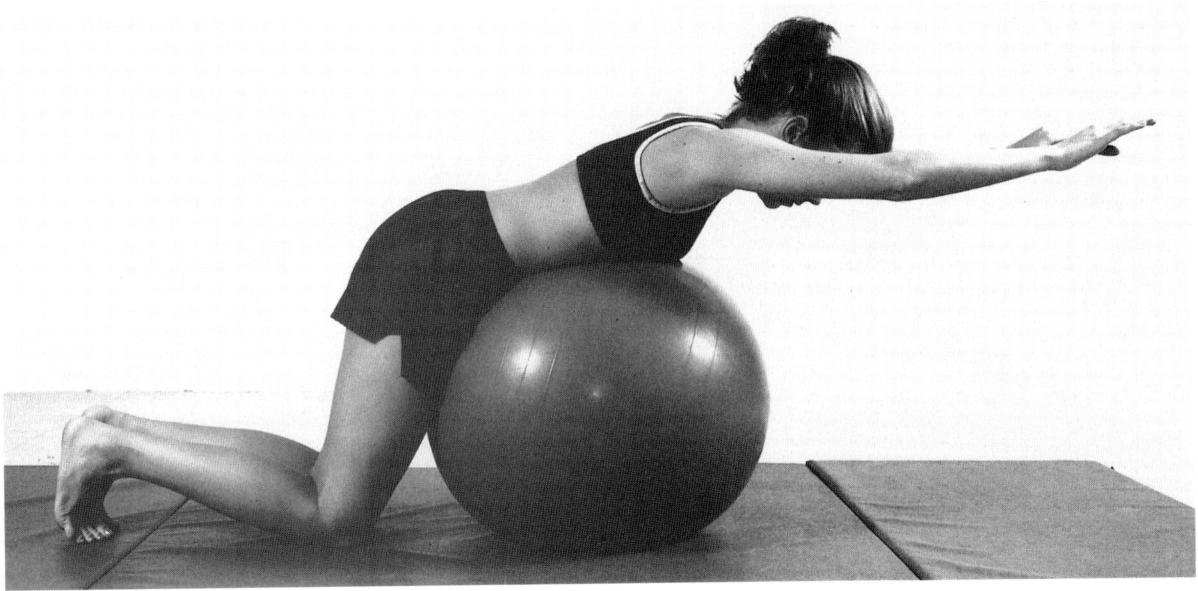

FIGURE 12-25 **Scapular retraction with knees flexed on therapeutic ball.**

PURPOSE: Strengthen upper back and shoulder girdle muscles.

POSTION: Client kneeling in quadruped with therapeutic ball under hips and knees on floor.

PROCEDURE: Client flexes shoulders overhead in Superman position and holds position.

NOTE: To increase challenge, client performs upper extremity movements (swimming, reciprocal flexion/extension). Resistance is optional.

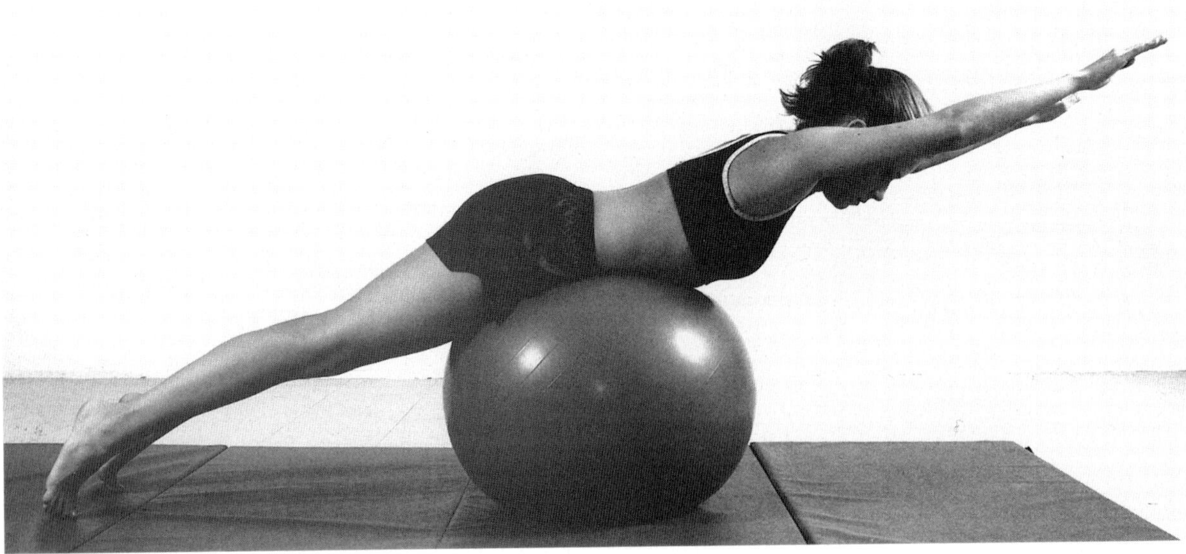

FIGURE 12-26 **Scapular retraction with knees extended on therapeutic ball.**

PURPOSE: Strengthen upper back and shoulder girdle muscles.

POSTION: Client kneeling in quadruped with therapeutic ball under hips and knees on floor.

PROCEDURE: Client extends hips and knees, keeping ball under hips. Client flexes shoulders overhead in Superman position and holds position.

NOTE: To increase challenge, client performs upper extremity movements (swimming, reciprocal flexion/extension). Resistance is optional.

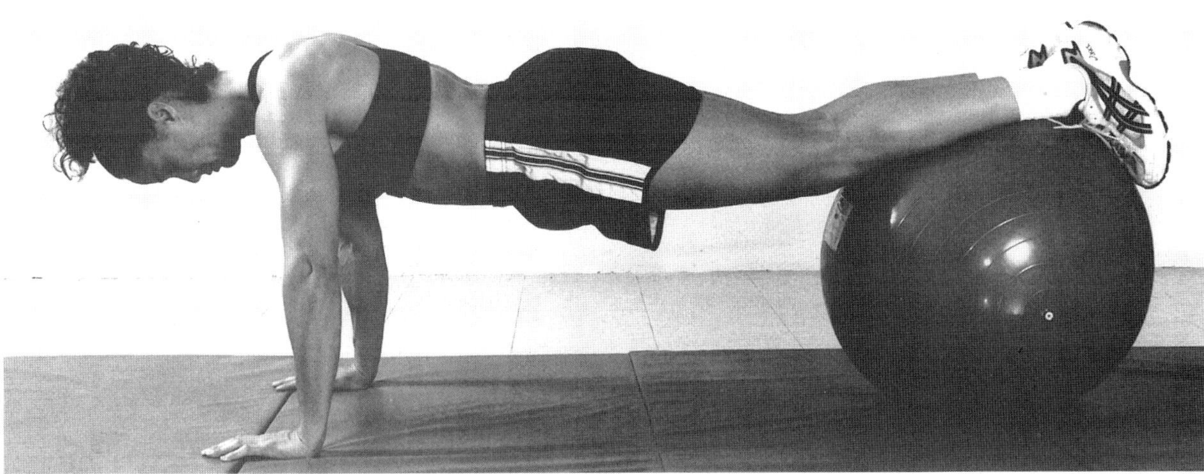

FIGURE 12-27 **Gluteal-abdominal hold with therapeutic ball.**

PURPOSE: Strengthen upper back and shoulder girdle muscles.

POSTION: Client in quadruped with therapeutic ball under shin or ankles (depending on desired level of challenge).

PROCEDURE: Client holds position or shifts weight bearing forward and backward and side to side. Client maintains neutral spine position.

CASE STUDY

PATIENT INFORMATION

A 22-year-old female college student presented to the clinic with the diagnosis of L4-L5 disk injury. She reported right low back and right lower extremity pain with duration of 2 weeks. The patient described the pain as dull and achy, with numbness in the right calf. She rated her pain as 3/10, with the worst being 5/10. The patient believed her pain was the result of an increase in frequency and duration of sitting over the previous 4 months. Her medical history was significant for microscopic diskectomy at L5-S1 4 years earlier. She reported that her calf numbness had been present since the surgery. Her symptoms were worse with sitting, bending, and hamstring stretching and better with distraction. The patient's goals were to lift weights, jog, and swing a golf club without pain.

Examination revealed positive neural tension signs in the right lower extremity and decrease in both active and passive segmental stability at L4-L5. Repeated movement testing revealed centralization with standing extension and peripheralization with standing flexion. The use of a vertical compression test caused an increase in pain (4/10); performance of the test after a postural correction did not change the pain response. The piriformis and gluteus medius muscles on the right demonstrated moderate soft tissue restriction. The right Achilles reflex was absent, and decreased sensation was present in the distribution of S1. The patient reported that these findings were related to the previous injury and surgery. She had decreased flexibility of the hamstrings bilaterally, and a positive straight-leg-raising (SLR) test at 50° on the right. Lower abdominals and L4-L5 multifidus stability tests demonstrated 3+/5 strength. Findings indicated sciatic nerve inflammation and annular incompetency at the level of L4-L5.

LINKS TO

Guide to Physical Therapist Practice and *Athletic Training Educational Competencies*

Pattern 4F of the *Guide*[3] relates to the diagnosis of this patient. This pattern is described as: "impaired joint mobility, motor function, muscle performance, range of motion, or reflex integrity secondary to spinal disorders." Included in the patient diagnostic group of this pattern are nerve root disorders. Anticipated goals include an increase in the "ability to perform physical tasks," using verbal instruction and demonstration and modeling for teaching, and an increase in the ability to "perform physical tasks related to work and leisure activities," using aerobic endurance activities, balance and coordination training, posture awareness training, strengthening, and stretching.

The *Competencies*[46] refers to treatment of athletes using a variety of techniques. The teaching objectives listed under the competencies of this domain indicate that the athletic trainer, upon graduation from an accredited program, will be able to "describe indications, contraindications, theory and principles for the incorporation and application of various contemporary therapeutic exercises including exercises to improve dynamic joint stability, neuromuscular coordination, postural stability, and proprioception." Demonstration of "segmental stabilization techniques" is also emphasized, "including trunk and cervical stabilization."

INTERVENTION

Initial goals of intervention were to educate the patient on the neutral spine and appropriate body mechanics and improve neural tension signs. Patient was treated with pain-free stretching of the hamstrings (see Fig. 3-7) and piriformis. The patient was taught the proprioceptive neutral posture in the unloaded supine position and was taught the body mechanics of supine to sit and straight-back bending (as bending forward to brush teeth).

PROGRESSION

One Week After Initial Examination

At the 1-week follow-up, the patient was able to control her leg symptoms with an extension-biased posture. Her SLR had improved to 75° bilaterally, and a faint Achilles reflex was present on the right. The vertical compression test resulted in pain rated as 2/10; performance of the test after postural correction resulted in no pain. Abdominal and multifidus strength were graded as 4/5.

Given this improvement, the goals of intervention were revised to address active segmental stability. Intervention consisted of the following:

1. Use of lumbar taping for biofeedback for extension-biased posturing (Fig. 12-5).
2. Stretches: hamstrings, piriformis.
3. Initiation of supine and prone active prepositioning stabilization activities (Figs. 12-6, 12-7, and 12-11).

Two Weeks After Initial Examination

After 2 weeks of intervention, the patient presented with normal abdominal and multifidus strength, a negative vertical compression test, a negative SLR test, and positive neural tension signs. She continued to avoid sitting because it aggravated the symptoms. The goals of intervention were to improve neural tension signs and increase sitting tolerance. Intervention consisted of the following:

1. Treadmill walking focused on maintaining stability of lumbopelvic spine (see Fig. 10-8).
2. Continued stretching.
3. Increase stabilization activities: supine activities using weights for upper (Fig. 12-16) and lower extremities; dying bug exercise (Fig. 12-8).

Three Weeks After Initial Examination

After 3 weeks of intervention, the patient presented with negative neural signs. She continued to avoid sitting because it aggravated the symptoms. The goals of intervention were to improve sitting tolerance and begin dynamic stabilization activities. Intervention consisted of the following:

1. Treadmill jogging focused on maintaining stability of lumbopelvic spine.
2. Continued stretching.
3. Increase stabilization activities: upright lunge and push/pull weighted cart.

Four Weeks After Initial Examination

At the 4-week follow-up, the patient presented with no positive objective findings. The goals of intervention were to progress dynamic stabilization activities, including running 2 miles without onset of lower-extremity pain and to initiate a gym weightlifting program. Intervention consisted of the following:

1. Recumbant bicycling focused on maintaining stability of lumbopelvic spine and continued treadmill work: combined total up to 60 min (see Fig. 10-4).
2. Increase stabilization activities: resisted baseball swing using elastic band and throwing a ball.
3. Gym weightlifting program: leg press, hamstring curls, lunges (Fig. 9-12), pull-ups, dips, and proprioceptive neuromuscular facilitation (PNF) with elastic band (see Fig. 8-20).

OUTCOMES

After 5 weeks of intervention, the patient was able to control her leg and back symptoms and had resumed prior activities. She had met all goals and was discharged to a home stabilization program to be completed three times per week. All exercises were to be performed to fatigue, and a gym program was to be completed two or three times per week.

SUMMARY

- Intervention for the individual with low back pain can be challenging. If a painful problem is caused or perpetuated by a movement disorder, the clinician needs

GERIATRIC *Perspectives*

- The ability to maintain an erect posture during static and dynamic movement requires a complex coordination of systems: central nervous, motor, somatosensory, and biomechanical. In healthy old age, the ability to maintain an upright posture and alignment remains intact. The classic flexed posture depicted by the media is largely the result of a combination of age-related changes and neurologic and musculoskeletal disorders.[1]
- Spinal flexibility does change with aging and may decrease as much as 50% compared to younger adults.[2] Spinal flexibility is an essential component of typical movement and, therefore, may affect biomechanical performance of functional tasks.[3] With advancing age, altered neuromuscular control, decreased muscle strength, and degenerative joint changes will result in a tendency to stand with slightly flexed hips and knees, rounded shoulders, forward head, increased kyphosis, and decreased lumbar lordosis. These postural changes affect flexibility in extension and axial rotation and may limit the ability to take a deep breath.[4]
- Postural re-education, flexibility, and spinal stabilization exercises may result in tremendous functional gains for most older adults. In sedentary older adults, the trunk flexors are more prone to weakness and tightness whereas trunk extensors are more prone to stretch weakness. Iliopsoas, tensor fascia lata, and hip adductor muscles are usually tight as well. Caution should be exercised when designing programs for spinal stabilization for older adults, especially if using prone positioning and a balance board. Overall health, strength, and presence of co-morbid conditions (e.g., osteoporosis) should be examined closely.
- Activities using the therapeutic ball may be problematic and may require adaptations for safety. Use of a foam roll or square of foam on the floor may be a better choice. To further improve safety, the training may take place within parallel bars or within reach of a stabilizing surface or person.

1. Pathy MSJ. Neurologic signs of old age. In: RC Tallis, HM Fillit, JC Brocklehurst, eds. Brocklehurst's textbook of geriatric medicine and gerontology. 5th ed. London: Churchill Livingstone, 1998.
2. Schenkman M, Shipp KM, Chandler JM, et al. Relationships between mobility of axial structures and physical performance. Phys Ther 1996;76:276–285.
3. Bergstrom G, Anainsson A, Bjelle A, et al. Functional consequences of joint impairment. Scand J Rehabil Med 1985;17:183–190.
4. Goldstein TS. Geriatric orthopaedics. Gaithersburg, MD: Aspen, 1999.

to focus on correcting the faulty movement pattern. A thorough examination will assist the clinician in choosing appropriate intervention strategies that can facilitate more efficient, comfortable function. The clinician should remember to:

- Observe the patient in functional tasks.
- Examine how the patient is responding to gravitational forces.
- Evaluate the lower biomechanical chain for deficits that may lead to increased spinal stresses.
- Educate the patient in static posture before progressing to dynamic activities.
- Emphasize proprioceptive awareness before progressing the patient to higher-level exercises.
- Train the patient in supported positions before progressing to more challenging, unsupported conditions.
- Use tactile and verbal cues to facilitate the desired movements and muscle contractions.
- Notice that the neutral position varies among individuals and may change as the pathology changes.
- Focus on the core stabilizers: the multifidus, transversus abdominus, and internal obliques.
- Include the whole body in the training regimen.
- Exercise postural muscles with endurance-training principles.
- Monitor the patient's responses to weight bearing, movement, and static postures; modify exercises as needed.
- Watch for subtle compensatory movements during training.
- Incorporate functional tasks in training, either mimicking an activity in the clinic or conducting treatment sessions in the actual environment in question.
- Include flexibility, strength, endurance, functional movement re-education, and coordination in the complete training package

- The clinician should understand that the ultimate goal is to facilitate function. Thus, the clinician should help the patient focus on active participation in the recovery process, because this form of intervention is geared

PEDIATRIC Perspectives

- Age affects posture and movement throughout the lifespan. Children are not expected to conform to adult standards for posture and movement, primarily because the developing child has much greater flexibility and mobility than the adult.[1] The child is developing muscular, vestibular, visual, and other systems during growth and maturation. Children, therefore, cannot be expected to have the same motor programs as an adult.
- The literature fails to describe the exact sequence of postural response development in children. Variations in descriptions are likely owing to children using multiple postural control strategies as their sensory and motor systems develop.[2] Very young children commonly have immature and unsteady control of posture and gait. Postural abilities needed to control balance and lower extremity musculature are not attained until 5 or 6 years of age.[3] By 7 to 10 years of age, children demonstrate similar eyes-closed postural sway to adults.[2]
- Most postural deviations in the growing child are developmental and related to age. Such deviations usually improve without treatment as a part of neuromuscular development. Examples include protruding abdomen posture, varus/valgus lower extremity alignment, and flat feet.[1] A young child is not likely to have habitual postural faults and could be harmed by corrective measures that are not needed. Rather, development and maturation will correct most minor childhood postural faults. Postural faults may develop in response to intense childhood participation in some sports such as gymnastics, swimming, and dance. Severe postural deviations should be treated regardless of age.[1]
- Scheuermann's kyphosis can occur in the adolescent,[4] which can mistakenly be attributed to poor posture; caution is required. Radiologic studies confirm this diagnosis.
- In infants, the posterior (extensor) muscle group of the trunk develops first, making an imbalance between trunk extensors and flexors. The abdominals are relatively much stronger in adults than in children.[1] Therefore, although trunk stabilization exercises are appropriate for all age groups, young children may have difficulty with mastery of stabilization exercises owing to incomplete strength development of the abdominals.

1. Kendall FP, McCreary EK, Provance PG. Muscles: testing and function. 4th ed. Baltimore: Williams & Wilkins, 1993.
2. Campbell SK. Pediatric physical therapy. Philadelphia, : Saunders, 1995.
3. Breniere Y, Bril B. Development of postural control of gravity forces in children during the first 5 years of walking. Exper Brain Res 1998;121:255–262.
4. Salter, RB. Textbook or disorders and injuries of the musculoskeletal system. 3rd ed. Baltimore: Williams & Wilkins, 1999.

toward, not only reduction of symptoms, but prevention of reinjury. It is not a quick fix but a lifelong learning process.

- The current level of quality research in this area gives the clinician scientific evidence to support a program of developing motor control and muscle function for rehabilitation of low back injuries. In this process, the client should develop freedom of movement, without rigid spinal holding patterns. Efficiency in functional movements should be enhanced through improved proprioceptive abilities, strength, postural endurance, and balanced and efficient motor programming.

REFERENCES

1. Loney PL, Stratford PW. The prevalence of low back pain in adults: a methodological review of the literature. Phys Ther 1999;79:384–396.
2. Kapandji IA. The physiology of the joints. Vol. 3 Edinburgh, UK: Churchill Livingstone, 1982.
3. American Physical Therapy Association. Guide to Physical Therapist Practice, second edition. Phys Ther 2001;81:1–768.
4. Porterfield J, DeRosa C. Mechanical low back pain: perspectives in functional anatomy. Philadelphia: Saunders, 1991.
5. Kendall FP, McCreary EK, Provance PG. Muscle testing and function. 4th ed. Baltimore: Williams & Wilkins, 1993.
6. Riegger-Krug C, Keysor JJ. Skeletal malalignments of lower quarter: correlated and compensatory motions and postures. J Orthop Sports Phys Ther 1996;23:164–170.
7. Levine D, Whittle MW. The effects of pelvic movement on lumbar lordosis in the standing position. J Orthop Sports Phys Ther 1996;24:130–135.
8. Janda V, Jull G. Muscles and motor control. In: LT Twomey, JT Taylor, eds. Physical therapy of the low back. Clinics in physical therapy series. New York: Churchill Livingstone, 1987: 253–278.
9. Cholewicki J, McGill SM. Mechanical stability of the in vivo lumbar spine: implications for injury and low back pain. Clin Biomech 1996;11:1–15.
10. Johansson H, Sjolander P, Sojka P. A sensory role for the cruciate ligaments. Clin Orthop Rel Res 1991;268:161–178.
11. Floyd WF, Silver PHS. The function of the erector spinae muscles in certain movements and postures in man. J Physio 1955; 129:184–190.
12. McGill SM. Low back exercises: evidence for improving exercise regimes. Phys Ther 1998;78:754–765.

13. Norkin CC, Levangie PK. Joint structure and function: a comprehensive analysis. 2nd ed. Philadelphia: Davis, 1992.
14. Morgan, D. Concepts in functional training and postural stabilization for the low back injured. Top Acute Care Trauma Rehab 1988;2:8–17.
15. Biondi, B. Lumbar functional stabilization program. In: Goldstein TS, ed. Functional rehabilitation in orthopedics. Gaithersburg, MD: Aspen, 1995:133–142.
16. Richardson C, Jull G, Hodges P, Hides J. Therapeutic exercise for spinal segmental stabilization in low back pain. London: Churchill Livingstone, 1999.
17. DiFabio RP. Efficacy of comprehensive rehabilitation programs and back school for patients with low back pain: a meta-analysis. Phys Ther 1995;75:865–878.
18. Frost H, Klaber J, Moffett JA, et al. Randomized controlled trial for evaluation of a fitness program for patients with chronic low back pain. Br Med J 1995;310:151–154.
19. Frost H, Lamb SE, Klaber J, et al. A fitness program for patient with chronic low back pain: 2-year follow-up of a randomized controlled trial. Pain 1998;75:273–279.
20. Nelson BW, Carpenter DM, Dreisinger TE, et al. Can spinal surgery be prevented by aggressive strengthening exercises? A prospective study of cervical and lumbar patients. Arch Phys Med Rehab 1999;80:20–25.
21. Saal JA, Saal JS. Nonoperative treatment of herniated lumbar intervertebral disc with radiculopathy. Spine 1989;14:431–437.
22. Saal JA. Dynamic muscular stabilization in the nonoperative treatment of lumbar pain syndromes. Orthop Rev 1990;19:691–700.
23. Weber D, Woodall WR. Spondylogenic disorders in gymnasts. J Orthop Sports Phys Ther 1991;14:6–13.
24. O'Sullivan PB, Twomey LT, Allison GT. Evaluation of specific stabilizing exercise in the treatment of chronic low back pain with radiologic diagnosis of spondylolysis or spondylolisthesis. Spine 1997;22:2959–2967.
25. Lee HWM. Progressive muscles synergy and synchronization in movement patterns: an approach to the treatment of dynamic lumbar instability. J Manual Manipulative Ther 1994;2:133–142.
26. Mannion AF, Weber BR, Dvorak J, et al. Fiber type characteristics of the lumbar paraspinal muscles in normal healthy subjects and in patients with low back pain. J Orthop Res 1997;15:881–887.
27. Cholewicki J, Panjabi MN, Khachatryan A. Stabilizing function of trunk flexor-extensor muscles around a neutral spine posture. Spine 1997;22:2207–2212.
28. Shirley D, Lee M, Ellis E. The relationship between submaximal activity of the lumbar extensor muscles and lumbar posteroanterior stiffness. Phys Ther 1999;79:278–285.
29. Hides JA, Stokes MJ, Saide M, et al. Evidence of lumbar multifidus muscle wasting ipsilateral to symptoms in patients with acute/subacute low back pain. Spine 1994;19:165–172.
30. Rantanen J, Hurme M, Falck B, et al. The lumbar multifidus muscle five years after surgery for a lumbar intervertebral disc herniation. Spine 1993;18:568–574.
31. Hides JA, Richardson CA, Jull GA. Multifidus muscle recovery is not automatic after resolution of acute, first-episode low back pain. Spine 1996;21:2763–2769.
32. Indahl A, Kaigle AM, Reikeras O, Holm SH. Interaction between the porcine lumbar intervertebral disc, zygapophyseal joints, and paraspinal muscles. Spine 1997;22:2834–2840.
33. Hodges PW, Richardson CA. Contraction of the abdominal muscles associated with movement of the lower limb. Phys Ther 1997;77:132–142.
34. Hodges PW, Richardson CA. Inefficient muscular stabilization of the lumbar spine associated with low back pain: a motor control evaluation of transversus abdominus. Spine 1996;21:2640–2650.
35. O'Sullivan PB, Twomey LT, Allison GT, Taylor J. Specific stabilizing exercise in the treatment of chronic low back pain with a clinical and radiological diagnosis of lumbar segmental instability. Paper presented at the 10th biennial conference of the Manipulative Physiotherapists Association of Australia. St Kilda, Melbourne, 1997. [Cited in Richardson C, Jull G, Hodges P, Hides J. Therapeutic exercise for spinal segmental stabilization in low back pain. London: Churchill Livingstone. 1999.]
36. Elia DS, Bohannon RW, Cameron D, Albro RC. Dynamic pelvic stabilization during hip flexion: a comparison study. J Orthop Sports Phys Ther 1996;24:30–36.
37. O'Sullivan PB, Twomey LT, Allison GT. Altered abdominal muscle recruitment in patients with chronic back pain following a specific exercise intervention. J Orthop Sports Phys Ther 1998;27:114–124.
38. Saliba VL, Johnson GS. Lumbar protective mechanism. Functional orthopedics I. Course outline. San Antonio, TX: The Institute of Physical Art, 1999.
39. Umphred, D. Neurological rehabilitation. 3rd ed. St. Louis: Mosby, 1995.
40. Menard D, Stanish WD. The aging athlete. Am J Sports Med 1991;17:187–196.
41. Nutter P. Aerobic exercise in the treatment and prevention of low back pain. Occup Med 1988;3:137–145.
42. Wyke BD. Neurological aspects of low back pain. In: MIV Jayson, ed. The lumbar spine and back pain. London: Sector, 1976:189–256.
43. Barnett J, Zaharoff A. Surface EMJ in dynamic lumbar stabilization training. Unpublished manuscript. Feb 2000.
44. Voss DE, Ionta MK, Myers BJ. Proprioceptive neuromuscular facilitation: patterns and techniques. 3rd ed. Philadelphia: Harper & Row, 1985.
45. Frank JS, Earl M. Coordination of posture and movement. Phys Ther 1990;70:855–863.
46. National Athletic Trainers' Association. Athletic training educational competencies. 3rd ed. Dallas: NATA, 1999.

CHAPTER 13

Aquatic Therapy

Jean M. Irion, EdD, PT, SCS, ATC

Historical documentation of the use of water as a healing medium can be traced as far back as 2400 B.C.E. in the Proto-Indian culture. The original use of water as a healing medium solely by immersion in water does not coincide with the current use and perception of aquatic therapy. Not until the latter part of the 1890s did aquatic rehabilitation move from passive immersion to a treatment technique that involved active patient participation.[1] The purpose of this chapter is to provide an overview of the use of aquatic therapy for treatment of clients with musculoskeletal dysfunction of the spine or extremities. A discussion of the physical properties and fluid dynamics of water provides the scientific basis that substantiates the use of a water medium for rehabilitation. Clinical guidelines and specific therapeutic techniques, including the appropriate use of therapeutic aquatic equipment are discussed next. The chapter concludes with a case study, demonstrating the physical properties, fluid dynamics, and therapeutic techniques presented in this chapter.

■ *Scientific Basis of Aquatic Therapy*

PHYSICAL PROPERTIES OF WATER

Several physical properties of water are introduced in this section. The effect of these properties should be considered first when determining whether a client is an appropriate candidate for aquatic therapy. The inclusion of aquatic therapy in a plan of care needs to be substantiated by one or more of these properties of water.

Relative Density (Specific Gravity)

The relative density, or specific gravity, of a substance is the ratio of the density of a given substance to the density of water.[2] The "substance" referred to in the definition of specific gravity is a human body or the extremity of a human body. Pure water has a specific gravity of 1. Generally, the human body, with air in the lungs, has a specific gravity of 0.974, slightly less than the specific gravity of water.[3–5] If a person's body or extremity has a specific gravity < 1, it has a tendency to float; whereas if a person's body has a specific gravity > 1, it has a tendency to sink. The average male body has a greater density than a female body. The differences in specific gravity between the sexes can be accounted for by the differences in the percentage of lean body mass to fat content.

Lean body mass is made up of bone, muscle, connective tissue, and organs with a relative density close to 1.1.[6] Fat mass includes both essential body fat plus any excess fat and has a relative density of about 0.9.[6] Therefore, an individual who is highly fit and muscular and has a relatively high proportion of lean body mass will have a density that exceeds 1 and thus will have a tendency to sink. In contrast, a person who has a greater overall fat mass, particularly excess fat, will have a body density < 1 and have a tendency to float.

The specific gravity of the client needs to be taken into consideration when placing him or her in an aquatic medium. The clinician must determine whether the client is a "sinker" or a "floater" when making safety decisions about where and in what position to place the client. The specific gravity must also be taken into consideration when choosing which flotation devices are needed to optimize therapeutic treatment in the water. Safety may be compromised if the clinician places a client who has minimal swimming skills and who has a tendency to sink in the deep end of a pool to perform an exercise without the assistance of an appropriate flotation device. Furthermore, such a client will expend excess energy just to stay afloat and maintain the body in the required position instead of maximizing the use of the water for therapeutic purposes.

Likewise, placing a flotation device on a client who already has a tendency to float may cause the client to work hard simply to gain control over the level of buoyancy when attempting to maintain the required position in the water. If the client is unable to maintain an extremity in the optimal position for exercise in the water, the clinician may add a buoyancy device to that extremity to allow it to be positioned properly.

Buoyancy

It is important for any clinician using a water environment for a therapeutic intervention to understand the concept of buoyancy. The Archimedes principle states that when a body is fully or partially immersed in a fluid at rest, the body experiences an upward thrust equal to the weight of the fluid displaced.[3,6] Buoyancy is defined as the upward thrust acting in the opposite direction of gravity and is related to the specific gravity of an immersed object.[2] As mentioned, a person or extremity with a specific gravity < 1.0 will have a tendency to float. In this instance, the upward thrust exerted by the water on the person is greater than the weight of the fluid displaced by the person. Therefore, the individual has a tendency to float.

Buoyancy must also be considered as a force that can assist, resist, or support movement of a person or an extremity in the water. Figure 13-1 illustrates the concept of buoyancy as a force on a lever arm (the extremity) at various angles of movement of the hip into abduction in the water. The following definitions clarify the concept of buoyancy as a force on an extremity moving in the water:[3,6]

Moment of force: the turning effect of the force about a point.

Moment of buoyancy (*F*): $F \times d$, where *F* is the force of buoyancy, and *d* is the perpendicular distance from a vertical line through *P* to the center of buoyancy(P is the point about which the turning effect buoyancy is exerted).

Center of buoyancy (*CB*): center of gravity of the displaced liquid

As the leg moves further into hip abduction toward the surface of the water (shown in Figure 13-1 as L_1, L_2, and L_3,) the distance between *P* and *CB* (shown in the figure as d_1, d_2, and d_3) becomes greater. The longer the distance, the greater the turning effect, or moment of force, on the limb. Thus as the limb moves closer to the surface of the water toward a horizontal position, the effect of buoyancy becomes greater.

The effect of buoyancy on the movement of an extremity is also affected by the length of the extremity and the presence of a buoyancy device at the end of the extremity. The effect of buoyancy by changing the length of the lever arm is shown in Figure 13-2 by the movement of the hip into abduction with the knee flexed to 90°. In this example, shortening the length of the lever arm by shortening the limb length brings the *CB* closer to *P*, which in turn shortens the distance between *CB* and *P*. Therefore, the force of buoyancy is less.

The effect of adding a buoyancy device to the end of an extremity being moved in the water is demonstrated in Figure 13-3. If a buoyancy device is placed on the ankle while the client performs hip abduction, the CB moves distally, thereby increasing the distance from *P*. Thus the effect of buoyancy on the movement of that limb is increased.

Buoyancy Assist Movements

The examples of hip abduction exercises described in Figures 13-1 to 13-3 are buoyancy assist movements; the extremity is moving from a vertical position in the water to a

FIGURE 13-1 Effect of buoyancy increasing with increased hip abduction

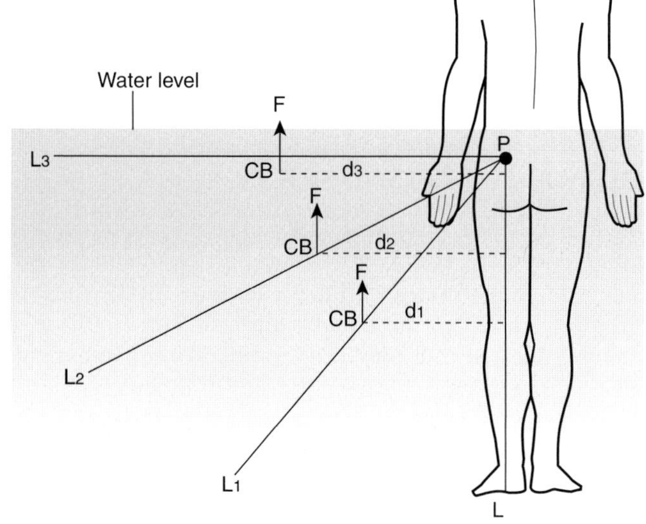

FIGURE 13-2 The effect of lever arm length on buoyancy, using hip abduction in a 90° flexed position as an example.

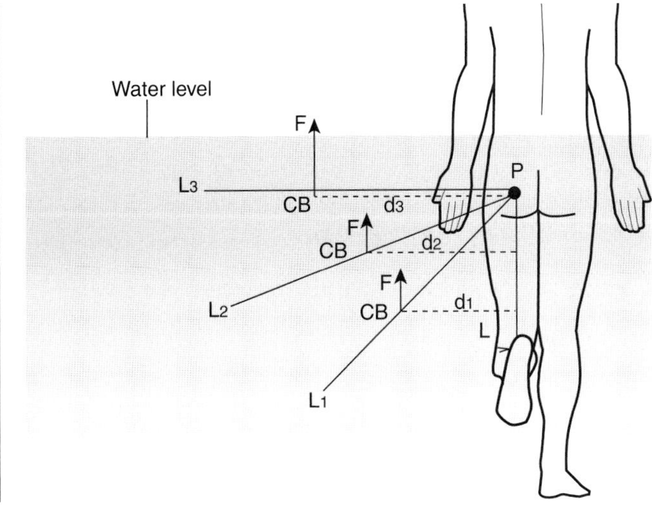

horizontal position, parallel with the water's surface (Fig. 13-4). For exercises that use buoyancy to assist movement, the clinician should use great caution when altering the length of the lever arm of an extremity or when adding a flotation device to the end of an extremity. If the patient does not have the volitional control to stop or slow the movement, any prescribed restriction in range of motion (ROM) could be exceeded. A shorter lever arm might be initially called for when using a buoyancy assist activity for a patient with restricted ROM. However, an added device that assists the effect of buoyancy on the extremity's movement might cause the patient to exceed his or her safe range, and thus caution is called for.

Buoyancy assist movement can be used for isometric muscle contractions at various angles through an arc of movement of a joint or limb. For the patient to perform a buoyancy assist movement in which he or she is actively contracting, the patient must control the movement by both eccentric and concentric muscle contractions. For example, if the patient is concentrically performing shoulder abduction while standing vertical in a pool, the shoulder adductors are acting eccentrically to control the speed of the shoulder movement into abduction.

Buoyancy Resist and Support Movements

Buoyancy can provide resistance and support to movements in the water. Buoyancy resist is defined as the movement of an extremity from a starting horizontal position (parallel to the water's surface) deeper into the water (to a vertical position). This movement is directly opposite of a buoyancy assist movement. An example of a buoyancy resist movement is shoulder adduction performed from a starting position of 90° abduction moving toward shoulder adduction (a vertical position in the water) (Fig. 13-5). The

FIGURE 13-3 The effect of buoyancy is altered by the addition of a flotation device (*closed ovals*) at the end of the extremity.

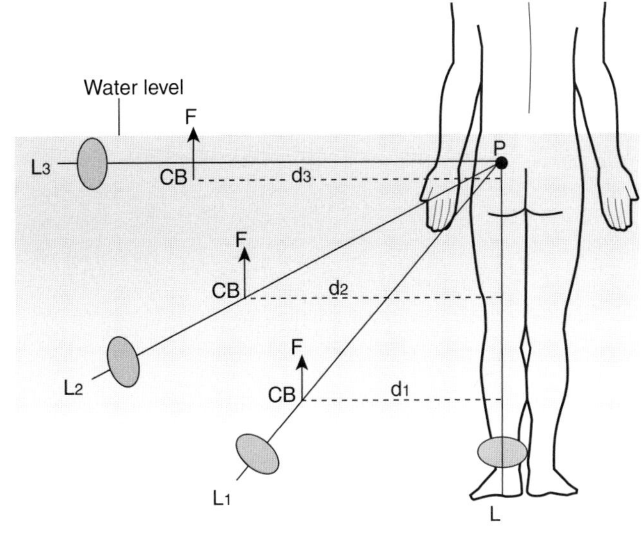

FIGURE 13-4 **Buoyancy assist hip abduction.**

PURPOSE: To improve hip abduction ROM or initiate active-assistive strengthening of hip abductors.

POSITION: Client standing in waist-deep or deeper water with lower extremity adducted beside contralateral limb. Contralateral limb firmly planted on bottom of pool.

PROCEDURE: Client actively initiates hip abduction movement, allowing buoyancy to passively or actively assist movement of hip to a fully abducted position.

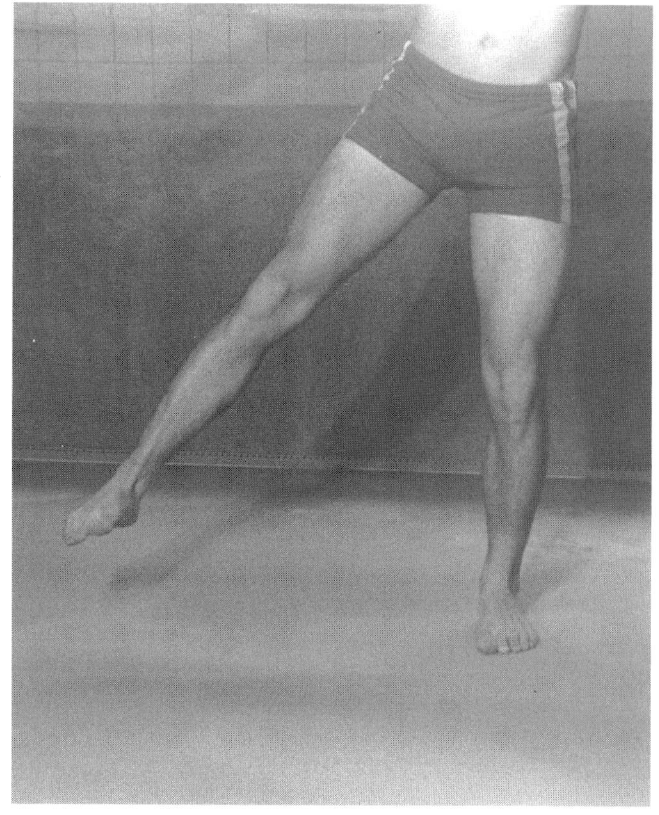

FIGURE 13-5 **Buoyancy resist shoulder adduction.**

PURPOSE: To improve strength of shoulder adductor muscles.

POSITION: Client standing in shoulder-deep water with both lower extremities firmly planted on bottom of pool. One upper extremity starts in approximately 90° of shoulder abduction.

PROCEDURE: Client actively moves abducted extremity away from water's surface to shoulder adducted position, stopping when extremity contacts side of body.

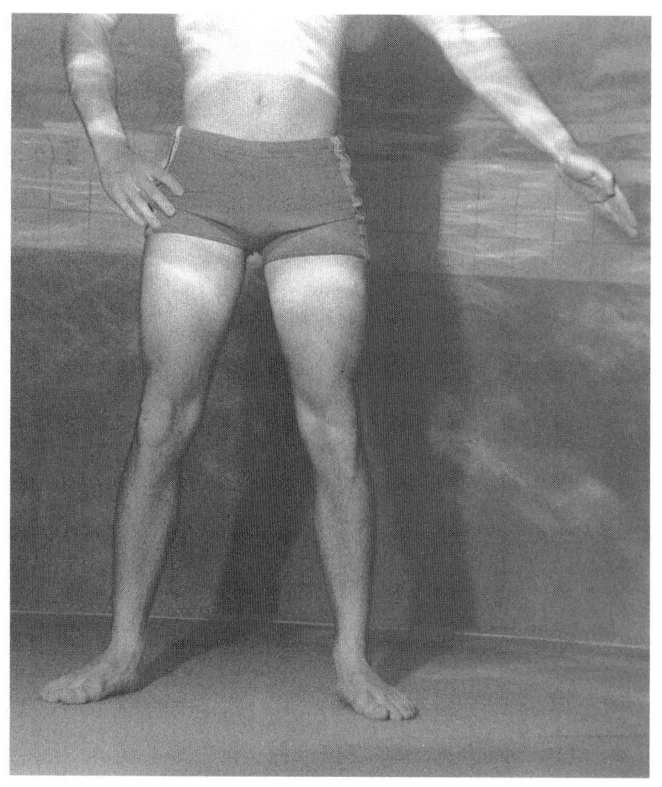

force of buoyancy in these resist movements is greater when the limb is closer to the surface of the water, decreasing as the movement approaches a more vertical position.

Buoyancy support movements are performed when an extremity is lying on the water's surface (or just below it) and is moved parallel to the surface. For example, the patient positions the shoulder in 90° of abduction and then performs horizontal abduction and adduction movements. Buoyancy support can be equated to a gravity-eliminated movement performed on land. Progression of the intensity of an exercise in the water can be achieved merely by altering a movement from buoyancy assist to buoyancy support to buoyancy resist.

Joint Loading

Buoyancy also plays a significant role in the progression of weight-bearing status in the water. Such progression performed in water is not only more comfortable and safer but also more easily quantifiable than any technique used for clinically determining weight-bearing status on land. Suspended vertical activities in the deep end of the pool allow exercises to be performed with no weight bearing and with minimal effects of gravity on the body. These movements, however, mimic functional movements on land, thus allowing rehabilitation to start much sooner and more safely. Harrison et al.[7,8] investigated quantification of the percentage of weight bearing for immersion levels at C7, the xiphoid process, and the anterior superior iliac spine (ASIS) for standing and during ambulation. The subjects were able-bodied males and females with no abnormalities in gait. The weight-bearing status for males was consistently slightly higher at a given water level than for the female counterparts.

The results of the studies of Harrison and colleagues[7,8] provide a safe range of weight-bearing status for the three water levels. Standing activities in water to C7 is 8 to 10% weight bearing for females and males, to the xiphoid process is 28% for females and 35% for males, and to the ASIS is 47% for females and 54% for males. Ambulation at a slow pace revealed the following ranges of safe weight bearing for males and females: in water to C7, up to 25% weight bearing status; to the xiphoid process, 25 to 50%, and to the ASIS, 50 to 75%.

Clinically, the use of the decreased joint-loading environment of the water allows for earlier, safer, and more comfortable rehabilitation. Clients who have pathologies that are exacerbated by gravitational forces in a vertical position of the body on land are prime candidates for early initiation of aquatic intervention. Such conditions include degenerative disk disease; facet joint pathologies; partial discectomies; spinal fusions; compression fractures of the spine from trauma or osteoporosis; degenerative joint disease of the spine or extremities such as osteoarthritis, stress fractures, and joint replacements; iliosacral and sacroiliac dysfunction; and early open or closed reduction of fractures of the pelvis and lower extremity for which significant and lengthy weight-bearing restrictions have been imposed.

Hydrostatic Pressure (Pascal's Law)

Pascal's law states that, at any given depth, the pressure from a liquid is exerted equally on all surfaces of the immersed object.[2] Hydrostatic pressure is also directly proportional to the depth of immersion of the body part below surface level. Water exerts a pressure of 22.4 mm Hg/foot of water depth.[4,9] If an individual is immersed vertically in water at a depth of 4 feet, the hydrostatic pressure at his or her feet is 88.9 mm Hg, roughly four times greater than the hydrostatic pressure at the surface of the water.

Hydrostatic pressure can be used for many purposes in rehabilitation. Pressure exerted at the feet of a patient who is standing vertically in water is slightly higher than the diastolic blood pressure, aiding in the resolution of edema in an injured part.[4,9] In addition, the hydrostatic pressure at a 4-foot depth more than doubles the pressure of the standard elastic bandage.[10] Peripheral edema in the foot and ankle, which may occur in many lower extremity injuries, can be decreased through the use of hydrostatic pressure.

Several studies comparing cardiovascular responses to vertical aerobic exercise on land to an equivalent level of vertical exercise in water have identified hydrostatic pressure as one of the primary contributing factors for the differences noted.[11–15] The cardiovascular system appears to work more efficiently in water and, therefore, has a significant effect on the exercise parameters used in aerobic water exercise compared to land. This modification in parameters is discussed later in this chapter.

Because hydrostatic pressure exerts an equal force at a given level of water depth, the water provides a safe, supportive, and forgiving environment in which to start early balance and proprioceptive training. Compression on all submerged surfaces of the body by the hydrostatic pressure of the water also activates peripheral sensory nerve endings for early proprioceptive input to the trunk and extremities.

Viscosity, Cohesion, Adhesion, and Surface Tension

The combined properties of viscosity, cohesion, adhesion, and surface tension serve as a source of resistance for movement in water. All liquids share a property known as viscosity, which refers to the magnitude of internal friction among individual molecules in a liquid.[9] Viscosity affects an individual or object moving in a fluid, acting as a form of resistance when the water molecules stick to the surface of the object attempting to move through the water. Likewise, viscosity is a time-dependent property of a liquid and is described as distance over time. The faster an object moves through a liquid, the greater the viscosity and, therefore, the greater the resistance to movement.[9]

Cohesion is the force of attraction among molecules within the same substance, such as the attraction of one water molecule to another adjacent water molecule. Adhesion is the force of attraction among molecules of two different types of matter such as air and water at the air–water interface or water and glass molecules at the water–glass container interface. Surface tension is a force created by the cohesive and adhesive properties of the water molecules at the air–water interface. Surface tension acts as a resistance for movement in the water (e.g., when an extremity moves from the water to the air and vice versa).[7]

All four of these properties can provide a graded progression of resistive exercise. Modifications such as speed of movement, size of the surface area of the body moving in the water, and breaking of surface tension allow for a gradual progression or regression in the intensity of an exercise. Documentation of the increased tolerance to the viscosity and cohesive and adhesive properties is readily done by indicating the speed of movement, length of time the activity is performed, and extent of the body's surface area involved in the exercise. In addition, these four properties have a tendency to slow down movements normally performed on land; thus water enables a client to practice a movement in a more controlled environment. These slower movements also allow the clinician to observe and examine movement patterns and provide feedback to the client for modification, as needed, particularly in the presence of poor movement patterns.

Refraction

Refraction causes the bending of light rays as they pass from a more dense to a less dense medium and vice versa.[4,6] In aquatic therapy, refraction occurs when light rays pass from air to water. Consideration of this property is important when the clinician is viewing the position of a body part from above the water level. The position of the trunk or extremities appears distorted and in the wrong position. Careful consideration of the true body position needs to occur before correction of the client is undertaken. An experienced aquatic therapist begins to compensate for the property of refraction and is able to correct the perception of body position before correcting the actual position of the client.

FLUID DYNAMIC PROPERTIES OF WATER

Several fluid dynamic properties must be taken into consideration before initiating an aquatic intervention: streamline versus turbulent water flow; formation of wakes, eddies, and drag force; and movement of a streamlined versus an unstreamlined object through water. The effects of these properties, in conjunction with the physical properties of water, need to be considered each time a plan of care is developed for a client.

Streamlined Versus Turbulent Water Flow

Streamlined, or laminar, flow of water is defined as a steady, continuous flow of water molecules in one direction in which the molecules are all traveling parallel to each other.[6] Once the flow of water reaches a critical velocity level, the water molecules begin to move in an irregular fashion, causing rotary movements of the molecules (known as eddies) and creating a turbulent water flow.[6] The frictional resistance to movement of an object or body provided by both a streamlined and a turbulent water flow increases with increasing velocity of flow. The resistance to movement into a turbulent flow of water is considerably greater than that of streamlined flow. In a streamline flow, resistance is directly proportional to velocity, whereas, in turbulent flow, resistance is proportional to the square of the velocity.[6]

When using a therapeutic pool in which turbulent flow can be created to offer resistance to an exercise or movement, progression of the velocity of the turbulent flow of water must be performed with caution. A small increase in the velocity of a turbulent flow of water significantly increases the intensity of the exercise being requested of the client.

One advantage to using a therapeutic pool in which turbulent flow can be regulated is the decreased need for various types of exercise equipment to provide increased resistance to movement. Performing exercises against or into a turbulent flow of water is an excellent means of incorporating balance and coordination activities into the plan of care.

Eddies, Wakes, and Drag Force

Movement of a body or object in water causes turbulent flow of water around and behind the object or body. These irregular patterns of water movement, known as eddy currents, occur around and behind a body or object when it moves in the water.[6] In addition, a pressure gradient is formed by moving a body or object through water. Pressure is increased in front of the object and decreased behind the object. The wake is an area of reduced pressure created behind a person or object moving in the water. Within the wake, eddy currents begin to form as the turbulent flow of water going around the body or object begins to flow into the lower pressure area. Flow of water into the wake also creates a drag force on the body. Drag force is the tendency for a person or object to be pulled back into the wake. As the velocity of the body or object increases, the drag force increases, creating a greater resistance to movement.[6]

Several clinical implications need to be considered when applying the concepts of eddies, wakes, and drag force to the rehabilitation process. Because the wake is an area of reduced pressure in the water, the clinician should maximize its use in gait training. To lower the resistant for the patient, allow the client to walk behind the clinician in his or her wake.[6] Gradual progression in gait training to increase the water resistance for the client during ambulation can be achieved by changing his or her position in relation to the clinician.

Many clients have a tendency to lean forward from the trunk to overcome drag force. Verbal and visual cues need to be provided to help the client overcome this and perform movement in the water in a safer neutral spine position. In addition, caution must be taken when directing a client to change direction of movement when in the water. The client will be working against a turbulent flow and the water movement when starting in the opposite direction. A great deal of balance and coordination is needed to maintain an upright position against these obstacles.

Streamlined Versus Unstreamlined Movement

Turbulent flow can be created by movement of an object through water. An object can be either streamlined or unstreamlined. A streamlined object has a narrow surface area that moves through the water, demonstrated by the water paddle shown in Figure 13-6. A streamlined object disturbs the water less than an unstreamlined object. In contrast, an unstreamlined object has a broad surface area that moves through the water, demonstrated by a hydrotone bell (aquatic exercise equipment) shown in Figure 13-7. Movement of an unstreamlined object in the

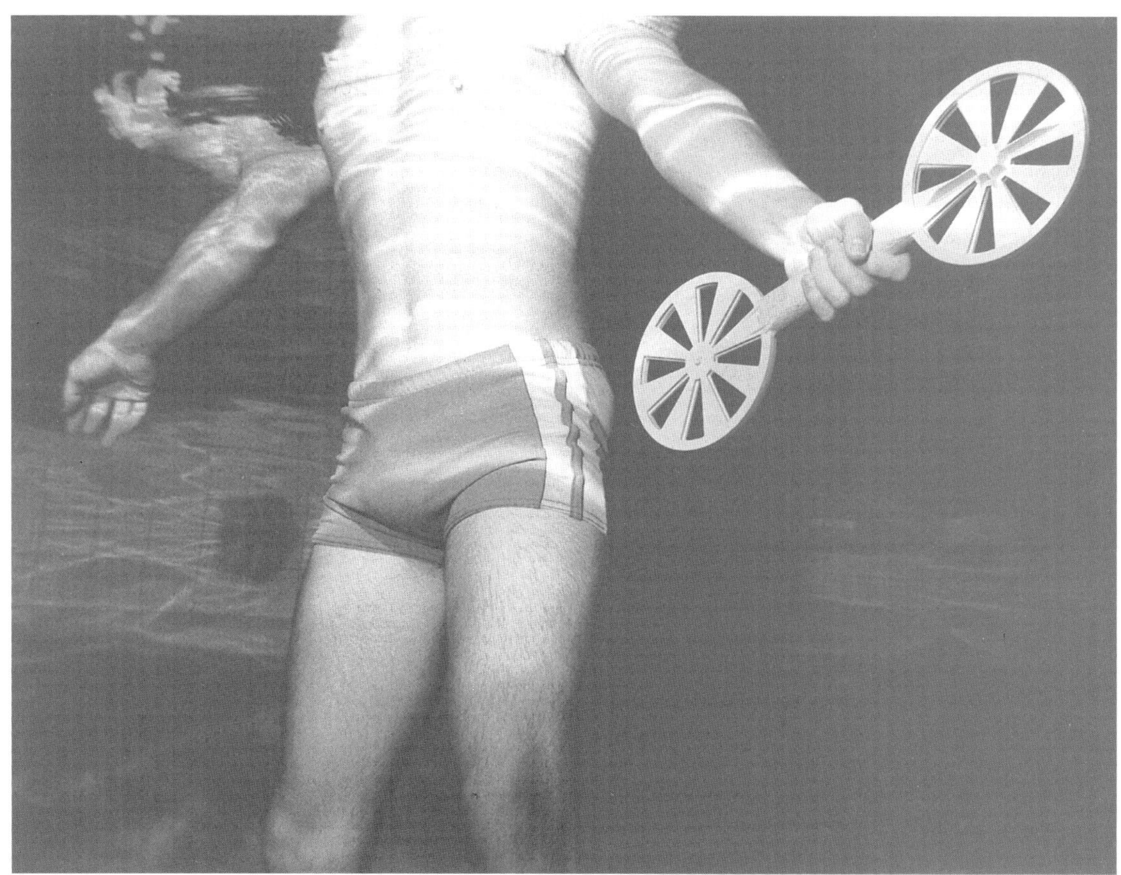

FIGURE 13-6 Movement of streamlined exercise paddle.

PURPOSE: To increase resistance to movement of an extremity through water by using a piece of equipment.

POSITION: Client standing in shoulder-deep water with both feet planted firmly on bottom of pool. Client holding onto a water paddle with one upper extremity, which is in a fully adducted, elbow extended, forearm supinated position. Paddle oriented so narrowest surface (streamlined) will be moved through water.

PROCEDURE: Client performs shoulder abduction to 90°, maintaining arm position while moving streamlined water paddle through water.

FIGURE 13-7 Movement of unstreamlined exercise bell.

PURPOSE: To increase resistance to movement of an extremity through water by using a piece of equipment.

POSITION: Client standing in shoulder-deep water with both feet planted firmly on bottom of pool. Client holding onto a bell with one upper extremity, which is in a fully adducted, elbow extended, forearm supinated position. Bell oriented so broadest surface (unstreamlined) will be moved through water.

PROCEDURE: Client performs shoulder abduction to 90°, maintaining arm position while moving unstreamlined bell through water.

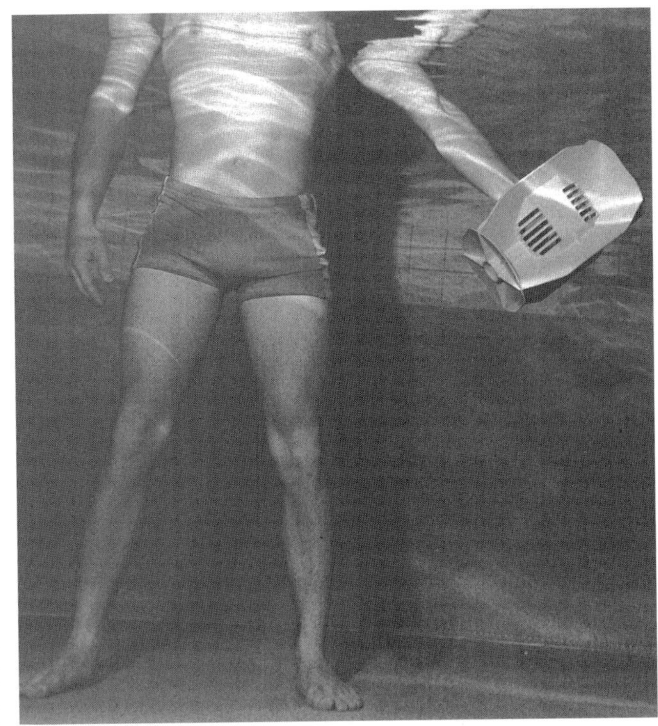

water causes greater water disturbance and thus greater resistance. Going from a streamlined to a more unstreamlined piece of equipment is one means of progressing the level of resistance for exercise in a water environment. This progression is also easily documented by indicating the change in the streamlined nature the equipment being used.

A patient can alter the streamlined nature of the body by altering his or her position or the position of a body part, thus changing the resistance provided by the water. When a patient walks sideways, a narrower, streamlined surface of the body is in contact with the water. When a patient walks forward, a broader, unstreamlined surface of the body is in contact with the water. To create even more resistance, the clinician can have the patient hold a piece of unstreamlined equipment, such as a kickboard, in front of the body while walking forward in the water (Fig 13-8).

Altering the position of an extremity as it moves through the water to alter the resistance provided is another means of changing the intensity of an exercise. When the shoulder is in abduction with the forearm supinated, it is more streamlined than when the shoulder is in abduction with the forearm in a neutral position. Adding a pair of aqua gloves can create a more unstreamlined surface, increasing the intensity of the exercise (Fig. 13-9). Caution must be taken when adding a piece of equipment to an exercise or changing the body position from streamlined to unstreamlined. A relatively small change in the streamline nature of an exercise can significantly change the overall resistance level of an exercise and stress a joint or other structure beyond the patient's safe parameters.

A thorough knowledge and understanding of the fluid dynamic properties of water is vital if a clinician chooses to incorporate aquatic intervention into a client's plan of care. Simply applying the principles of therapeutic intervention on land, well known to the clinician, to the aquatic environment will not maximize the use of the water medium. A lack of knowledge of the properties of water may sometimes not only be an ineffective form of therapeutic intervention but also compromise the safety of the client.

■ *Clinical Guidelines*

INDICATIONS

The previous section emphasized the need for the clinician to fully understand and apply the physical and fluid dynamic properties of water when developing an aquatic intervention plan that best benefits the client. A knowledgeable clinician can make decisions about the appropriateness of aquatic intervention for a given client. Table 13-1 lists impairments and functional limitations that indicate the use of aquatic intervention before or in conjunction with land-based therapy. Justification for reim-

FIGURE 13-8 **Forward walking with kickboard.**

PURPOSE: To increase resistance to forward movement provided by water, increasing intensity of walking program.

POSITION: Client standing in chest- to shoulder-deep water holding kickboard parallel to front of trunk, between waist and chest height.

PROCEDURE: Keeping kickboard under water, client walks forward at a pace that allows client to feel water resistance while safely maintaining an upright position.

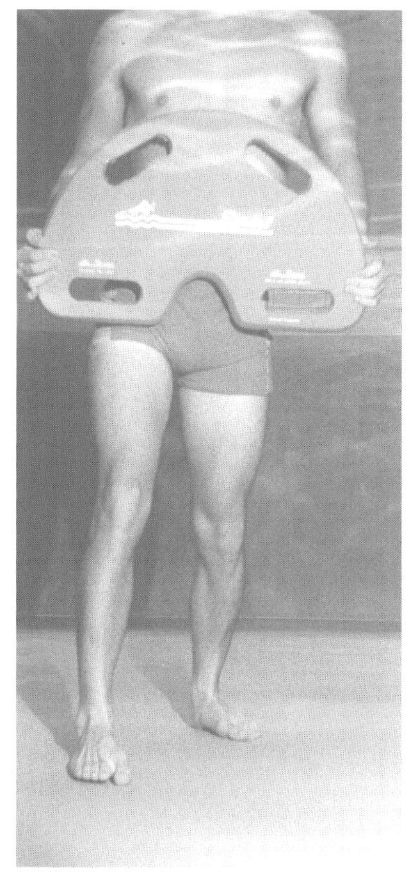

FIGURE 13-9 **Shoulder abduction with aqua glove.**

PURPOSE: To increase resistance to movement of an extremity through water by maintaining an unstreamlined body position and using a piece of unstreamlined equipment.

POSITION: Client standing in shoulder-deep water with both feet planted firmly on bottom of pool. Client wearing one or two aqua gloves with upper extremity in a fully adducted, elbow extended, forearm neutral, fingers abducted position.

PROCEDURE: Client performs shoulder abduction to 90°, maintaining arm and hand position while moving unstreamlined gloved hand through water.

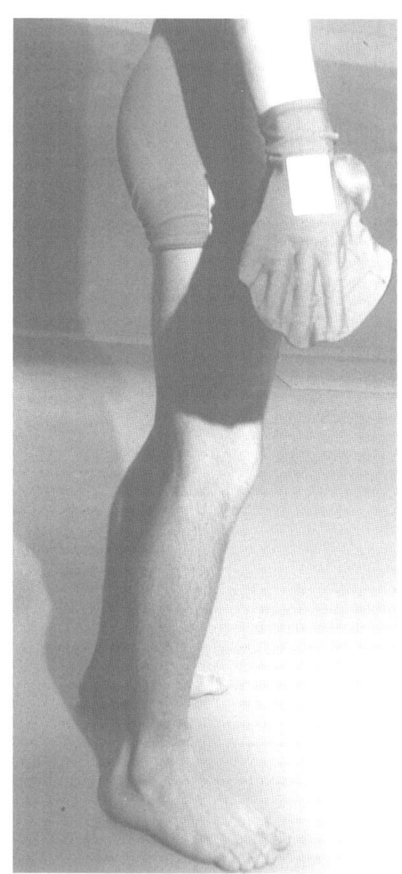

TABLE 13-1 Indications for Aquatic Intervention: Impairments and Functional Limitations

Decreased range of motion
Pain with movement or functional activity on land
Balance, proprioception, and/or coordination deficits
Decreased strength
Cardiovascular compromise or deconditioned status
Weight-bearing restrictions on land
Peripheral edema in extremity
Gait deviations not easily corrected on land
Lack of progress with traditional land-based program
Difficulty with heat dissipation during exercise on land
Exacerbation of symptoms with land exercise
Poor movement patterns not easily correctable on land

bursement of aquatic intervention to third-party payers is enhanced when the clinician is able to indicate specific impairments and functional limitations that would be more positively influenced by an aquatic medium than a land-based gravity-influenced environment. Benefits of aquatic intervention as part of a rehabilitation program are listed in Table 13-2.

TABLE 13-2 Benefits of Aquatic Intervention

Initiation of rehabilitation sooner than on land in many instances
Positive psychological benefit of being able to do more in water than on land
Assist in edema control
Relaxed environment owing to warm water
Initiation of controlled active movements earlier than on land
Less pain with movement than on land
Initiation of dynamic functional movement patterns earlier than on land
Good carryover to movement patterns on land
Good environment for proprioceptive and sensory input
Forgiving environment for balance and coordination training
Options available for gradual increase of exercise intensity
Gait deviations and poor movement patterns more easily detected than on land
Easier progression of weight-bearing status than on land
Ability to completely de-weight the spine and extremity joints
Better heat dissipation and heat tolerance in below thermoneutral water temperature than on land
Enhanced cardiovascular function in below thermoneutral water temperature than on land

HISTORY

Aquatic therapy, more than land-based therapy, requires a thorough history taking. The clinician must always review background information on a client before initiating any therapeutic intervention. The aquatic environment presents a greater risk management environment than a comparable land-based environment. Gathering important background information assists the clinician in providing a more risk-free environment for both the client and the clinician. The background information provides specific data that can assist the clinician in developing a plan of care for a client, including safe entry and exit techniques from the pool, avoiding unsafe movement patterns, determining of safe exercise parameters, and appropriately supervising the client. Table 13-3 provides a list of important information the clinician should gather during history taking and before initiating an aquatic intervention.

CONTRAINDICATIONS AND PRECAUTIONS

Several authors have composed lists of contraindications and precautions for aquatic therapy for various patient populations.[3,6,16,17] The contraindications and precautions most applicable to a client base with musculoskeletal and neuromuscular dysfunction are given in Tables 13-4 and 13-5. Each facility, however, must develop and modify such contraindications and precautions based on the types of patients it serves. Knowledge and expertise of the professional and support staff affect a facility's choices in determining appropriate and safe candidates for aquatic intervention. For example, a client who has a thoracic compression fracture secondary to osteoporosis and requires the use of an oxygen tank for chronic obstructive pulmonary disease may not be accepted at all aquatic therapy facilities. One institution may not feel comfortable managing this client safely in a pool environment, whereas another facility may be able to modify an aquatic program for this client while staying within safe exercise parameters.

SAFE EXERCISE PARAMETERS

Water temperature, in conjunction with depth of water, body composition, and intensity of exercise, must be con-

TABLE 13-3 History on Client

History on Client
Contraindications to aquatic intervention
Safety needs and precautions of the patient
Medical status and medical history
Current medications
Prior involvement in land or aquatic therapy intervention
Transfer ability on land
Use of assistive device on land
Weight-bearing status on land
Work, leisure, and exercise activity status before injury
Need for use of protective brace or splint during aquatic intervention
Comfort level in water
Ability to swim
Joints or structures affected
Precautions for allowable ROM
Pain level baseline
Psychological status
Available active and passive ROM at affected joints
Functional limitations
Other important objective impairment information
Level of healing of surgical incision
Static and dynamic balance capabilities
Sensory status
Impairments and functional limitations determined from land-based program
Goals of aquatic intervention

sidered when recommending the level of exercise for an aquatic treatment program. Water temperature above and below thermoneutral temperature (31 to 33°C; 88 to 90.5°F) significantly changes cardiovascular responses to exercise compared to an equal intensity and type of exercise on land. Heart rate during head-out of water, light to moderate intensity cycling or walking/jogging in thermoneutral temperature water is not significantly different from that for the same intensity exercise performed on land. In contrast, heart rate is usually 10 beats per minute (bpm) lower for moderately heavy, strenuous, and maximal exercise in water below thermoneutral temperature.[18]

As water temperature increases above the thermoneutral level, heart rate, overall cardiovascular demands, and core body temperature all increase to potentially unsafe levels.[18,19] Evaporation of sweat is the primary means of cooling the body temperature in air, whereas conduction and convection are the primary means of heat gain or loss by the body in water. Heat exchange in water is greater than in air because heat conductance in water and the specific heat of water are approximately 25 to 1000 times greater, respectively.[18] When water temperature is greater than skin temperature, heat gain by an immersed body is greater than heat loss. Clients should avoid exercising at moderate to high intensities in a warm water pool to lessen or eliminate the chances of heat illness, particularly when immersed to chest level and above.

When water temperature is < 31°C (88°F), heart rate decreases by as much as 17 to 20 bpm and stroke volume increases during moderate- to high-intensity, vertical, deep water exercise.[11–15,18] It is speculated that immersion in cool water causes peripheral vasoconstriction so the body can maintain core body temperature. This vasoconstriction augments central blood volume, which, in turn, increases

TABLE 13-4 Contraindications to Aquatic Intervention

Contraindications to Aquatic Intervention
Excessive fear of water
Fever or high temperature
Untreated infectious disease
Open wound
Contagious skin disease
Surgical incision with sutures or staples in place
Partial opening of a surgical incision
Serious cardiac conditions that cause cardiac compromise
Uncontrolled seizure disorder

cardiac preload. The increase in cardiac preload thus increases stroke volume, which provides a strong stimulus via the baroreceptors to decrease heart rate.[11–15,18] The cardiovascular changes seen during deep water vertical exercise are attributed to hydrostatic pressure and a more efficient cardiovascular system during exercise in cooler water. These changes are also attributed to the decreased demand on the cardiovascular system to dissipate the heat produced from exercise. Generally, higher intensity aerobic exercise is recommended at water temperatures between 26 and 28°C (78.8 and 82.4°F).[20]

The rating of perceived exertion (RPE) scoring system for intensity of exercise, originally developed by Borg, has been used successfully by many practitioners to accurately determine level of exercise intensity in water.[20]

TABLE 13-5 Precautions to Aquatic Intervention

Precautions to Aquatic Intervention
Seizure disorder controlled well with medications
Recently healed surgical incision
Absent or impaired peripheral sensation
Diabetes
Postural hypotension
Significant balance or vestibular disorder
Respiratory dysfunction
Colostomy
Difficulty with bowel or bladder control
Tracheostomy tube
Fear of water
Compromised vision without corrective lenses
Compromised cardiac or respiratory system (poor endurance or asthma)

Wilder and Brennan[15] modified the Borg scale for water-running exercise programs. The specifics of the five-point Brennan scale are discussed later in this chapter.

Water depth affects heart rate. Heart rate is generally 8 to 11 bpm lower in chest-deep water during an aerobic shallow-water vertical exercise session compared to an equal intensity of exercise on land.[18] In addition, body composition affects a person's exercise response while immersed in water at different temperatures. Sheldahl et al.[21] investigated the effect of water-immersed cycling on obese and lean women at 20, 24, and 28°C (68, 75.2, and 82.4°F). Lean women exhibited a fall in rectal core temperature during cycling at 20 and 24°C, whereas obese women had no change. In addition, energy expenditure was greater in the lean women at the two lower water temperatures because of shivering. Shivering is a mechanism used in cool water temperatures to maintain body temperature.[21]

In summary, several factors about the client, water, and intended exercise need to be taken into consideration when determining exercise intensity levels. Water temperatures at or above the thermoneutral level are used primarily for lower-intensity exercises such as ROM; flexibility; relaxation and pain control; low-level balance, coordination, and proprioceptive training; gait training; specific low-intensity functional training; and beginning level core- and trunk-strengthening exercises. In contrast, water temperatures below thermoneutral should be used for cardiovascular endurance training, higher intensity local muscle endurance and strengthening, plyometrics training, cross-training, interval training, and some sport- or work-specific functional training. In addition, the target heart rate for land exercise should not be used to determine the target heart rate for more strenuous aerobic water exercise. The target heart rate should be modified to 10 to 20 bpm less than the desired target heart rate on land for a desired level of exercise intensity and depth of water.

ORGANIZATION OF A TREATMENT SESSION

Generally, an aquatic treatment session for a client with musculoskeletal dysfunction lasts 30 to 60 min. Depending on the conditioning level of the client and any comorbid conditions or precautions, the initial aquatic session may last only 10 to 15 min. An increase in the total time of immersion can be increased gradually over 1 or 2 weeks, as the client tolerates. Each treatment session usually consists of the following seven components, listed with the time allotted for each:

Warm-up: 5 to 15 min.
ROM and flexibility: 5 to 15 min.
Strengthening and stabilization: 13 to 15 min.
Endurance training: 15 to 20 min.
Coordination, balance, and proprioception: 5 to 15 min.
Functional activities: 5 to 15 min.
Cool-down: 5 to 15 min.

The general organization of a treatment program can be modified to emphasize work in one or more aspects of an aquatic program based on the patient's impairments, functional limitations, and goals. For example, during the early phases of an aquatic therapy intervention for a patient with adhesive capsulitis of the shoulder, more emphasis may be placed on manual therapy techniques to the glenohumeral joint and the scapulothoracic articulation, in addition to ROM and flexibility exercises; and less emphasis may be placed on strengthening at the shoulder. The extra time spent on ROM and flexibility alters the organization and time spent on the various components of a treatment session.

INTEGRATION WITH LAND ACTIVITIES AND RETURN TO FUNCTIONAL LAND REHABILITATION

Emphasis in today's health-care environment is on justification of the need for a particular intervention. This is especially true for aquatic therapy, particularly when the patient's primary functional activities are not conducted in a water environment. A definite link needs to be made between aquatic intervention and improvement in functional activities or skills on land. The plan of care chosen by the clinician—whether that intervention is performed solely in water, solely on land, or land and water in combination—needs to relate directly to the achievement of functional land goals.

The decision to include aquatic intervention in a plan of care for a client begins at the time of initial examination, during which impairments or functional limitations are determined. Then the clinician must begin to justify the need for aquatic intervention, which can be achieved by showing that a treatment program using specific physical and hydrodynamic properties of water is more effective and will achieve the patient's goals more quickly than a similar land-based program. Documentation of the reasons for aquatic intervention instead of or in conjunction with land intervention is begun at the same time the clinician develops the plan and rationale for the specific regimen. The clinician should emphasize how the properties of water can be used to achieve land skills.

When treating patients with musculoskeletal dysfunction, the clinician will generally choose one of the following three options when deciding if it is appropriate to include aquatic therapy as part of the program: wet to dry transition, dry to wet transition, and wet only.[22]

Wet to dry transition is defined as a treatment intervention that begins in an aquatic environment and eventually transfers to a land-based intervention. This option is recommended for clients who are not able to tolerate axial and compressive forces on joint structures in a land-based program and for whom these forces are contraindicated because of the specific injury, illness, or a surgical intervention.[22]

Dry to wet transition is indicated for clients for whom a land-based program exacerbates the condition.[22] Such a client is transferred to an aquatic intervention after having begun a land-based program. Gradual progression back to a land-based program is indicated once the client is ready and relatively pain free.

A *wet-only program* is recommended for clients who have a complete inability to tolerate a land-based treatment program or who prefer aquatic therapy. Clients with pathologies such as rheumatoid arthritis, osteoarthritis, fibromyalgia, spinal stenosis, significant degenerative disk disease, and chronic pain syndromes fit well into the wet-only option. Upon discharge from intervention services, a maintenance program of wet-only exercise is often the only option these clients have for continued, regular exercise.

A fourth option is a combined wet and dry program (discussed in more detail later in this chapter). Clients who need to function on land but, because of their pathology, cannot tolerate the rigors of a land-only intervention program prefer this option. Clients who are not progressing as quickly as anticipated in a land-only program benefit from a combined intervention, which allows the clinician to capitalize on the water's physical properties to enhance the therapy and to decrease the daily stresses on the client's affected structures. By altering between land and water therapeutic interventions, the clinician is able to combine the best of both aquatic and land environments and to provide the client with several options for a continued home program after discharge.

In addition, clients who require variety and stimulation to adhere to an intervention program may benefit from the combined wet and dry option. Clients with long-term musculoskeletal or neuromusculoskeletal dysfunction who require years of intervention to increase function, maintain function, or prevent deterioration of function do well with this option. Understandably, these clients can become bored with a land-only program, and the clinician is challenged at every treatment session to keep these clients motivated so that functional goals in the school and home environments can be achieved in a timely manner. Clinicians treating clients with chronic dysfunctions report better results when using a combined land and water intervention.

The clinician must re-examine the patient on a regular basis to justify the continued use of aquatic therapy beyond the initial treatment session(s). The use of aquatic intervention cannot be stagnant in nature, and its effectiveness in achieving desired functional land goals must be documented for each patient.

■ *Techniques*

Aquatic therapeutic techniques that are used to address common physical impairments and functional deficits are presented in this section. Some techniques use aquatic exercise equipment to support the trunk in a vertical or horizontal position, support an extremity in an appropriate position, add resistance to increase the intensity of an exercise, or add turbulence to increase the intensity of an exercise.

FLEXIBILITY AND RANGE OF MOTION

Chapters 2 to 4 present information on ROM and mobilization. Aquatic intervention is a great supplement to those techniques. Warm water, with its buoyancy property, provides an excellent medium for enhancing and improving flexibility and range of motion in the spine and extremities.[23] Immersion in warm water promotes relaxation and increases tissue temperature, enhancing the extensibility of the musculotendinous and soft tissues surrounding the joint and allowing the stretch to be more efficient.

Floating in supine is a buoyancy support position for shoulder abduction used early in an exercise program designed for improving ROM. This position is especially useful when a buoyancy assist position is too difficult for the client to control. After the client has developed the motor control needed for working within safe parameters, buoyancy assist positions for increasing ROM can be added to the program. Buoyancy devices can also be used to improve ROM (Figs. 13-10 and 13-11).

Manual spine and extremity mobilization techniques

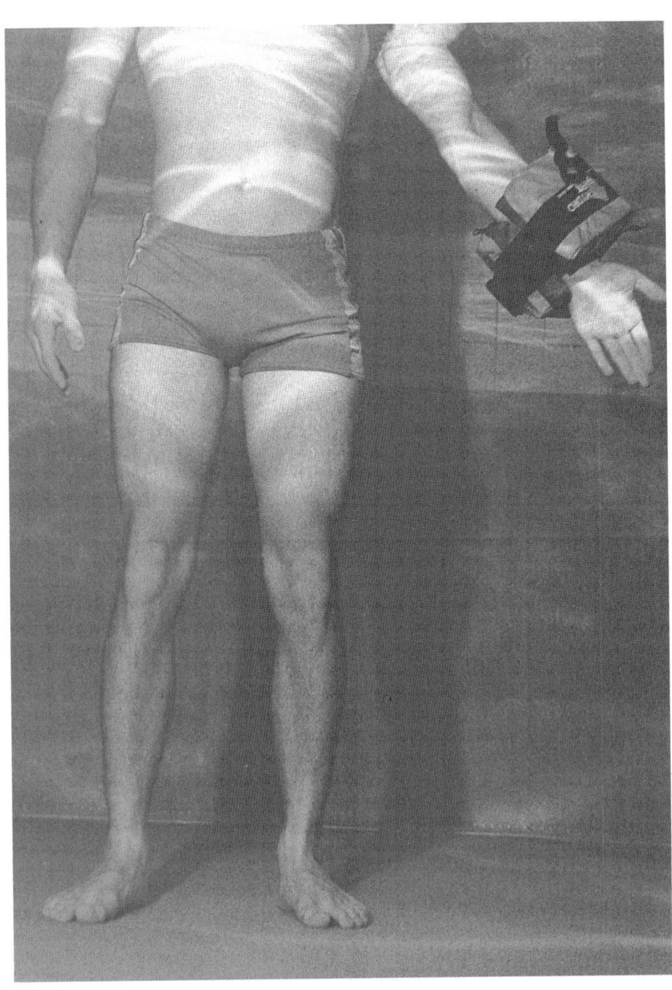

FIGURE 13-10 **Standing shoulder abduction with buoyancy cuff.**

PURPOSE: To enhance effect of buoyancy for improving ROM at shoulder joint.

POSITION: Client standing in shoulder-deep water with both feet planted firmly on bottom of pool. Client wearing buoyancy cuff on forearm just above wrist with upper extremity in a fully adducted, elbow extended, forearm supinated position.

PROCEDURE: Client initiates shoulder abduction, while maintaining arm position and allowing buoyancy to perform or assist movement of upper extremity to a 90° abducted position.

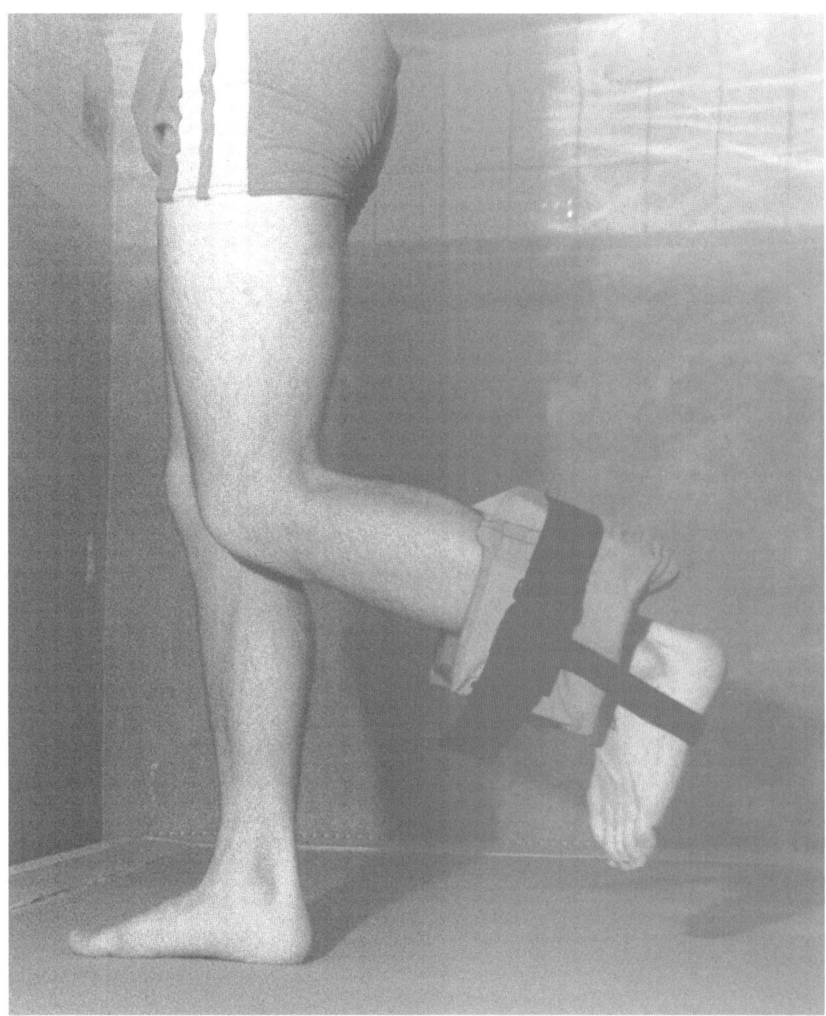

FIGURE 13-11 Standing knee flexion with buoyancy cuff.

PURPOSE: To enhance effect of buoyancy for improving ROM at knee joint.

POSITION: Client standing in waist-deep water with one foot planted firmly on bottom of pool. Client wearing buoyancy cuff just above ankle on one lower extremity, which is in a knee extended position.

PROCEDURE: Client initiates knee flexion, allowing buoyancy to perform or assist movement of lower extremity to allowable end point of flexion.

have been adapted for use in an aquatic treatment program (Figs. 13-12 to 13-14).[24–27] The use of a buoyancy assist position with or without a buoyancy device can also be used to increase the extensibility of muscles, such as the hamstrings, or for adherent nerve root stretch,[26] as shown in Figure 13-15. Optimum muscle stretch on land for improving extensibility is generally thought to be 30 sec of low-load stretching without pain for uninjured musculotendinous tissue.[28] Stretches of shorter duration and repeated several times may be more tolerable during the tissue-healing phase of rehabilitation.

GAIT TRAINING

An aquatic environment is ideal for reintroducing a gait pattern to clients whose gait has been compromised by pain or other restrictions or has been minimized by injury or surgery. Early weight-bearing can be initiated in the supine position in the water by use of closed-kinetic-chain weight-bearing activity (Fig. 13-16). The clinician offers unilateral weight bearing on the plantar surface of one foot. At the same time, resistance is offered to dorsiflexion of the ankle and flexion of the hip and knee on the contralateral extremity at the dorsum of the foot,

FIGURE 13-12 **Posterior and anterior mobilization glide at the talocrural joint.**

PURPOSE: To increase ankle dorsi and plantarflexion ROM.

POSITION: Client floating supine, supported with flotation devices about the cervical spine and pelvis and with affected ankle in a relaxed, slightly plantarflexed position. Contralateral ankle may be supported with a floatation device, if necessary. Clinician standing at client's feet, facing client.

PROCEDURE: Clinician places stabilizing hand over posterior distal end of tibia and mobilizing hand on plantar surface of foot just distal to talocrural joint, over talus. Mobilizing hand pushes talus toward bottom of pool.

NOTE: Posterior mobilization technique shown. For anterior mobilization, clinician places stabilizing hand over anterior distal end of tibia and mobilizing hand cups calcaneous. Mobilizing hand pushes calcaneous toward surface of water.

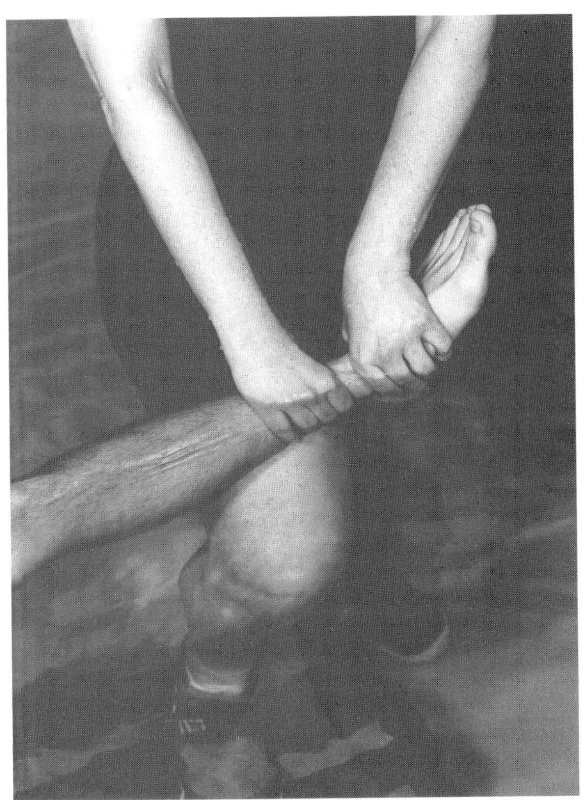

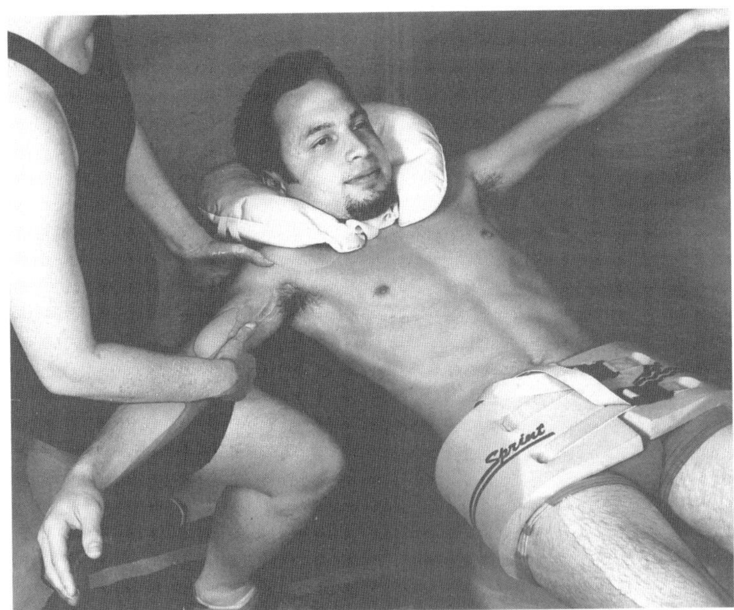

FIGURE 13-13 **Inferior mobilization glide at glenohumeral joint.**

PURPOSE: To increase shoulder abduction ROM.

POSITION: Client floating supine supported with flotation devices about the cervical spine and pelvis and with the affected upper extremity floating at the surface of water in a comfortable level of shoulder abduction. Ankles may be supported with flotation devices, if necessary. Clinician standing just above the affected shoulder, facing client's shoulder.

PROCEDURE: Clinician places forearm under humerus and grasps its proximal-medial aspect with supporting hand. Clinician places web of mobilizing hand over superior surface of head of humerus just distal to glenohumeral joint. Mobilizing hand pushes head of humerus inferior toward client's feet.

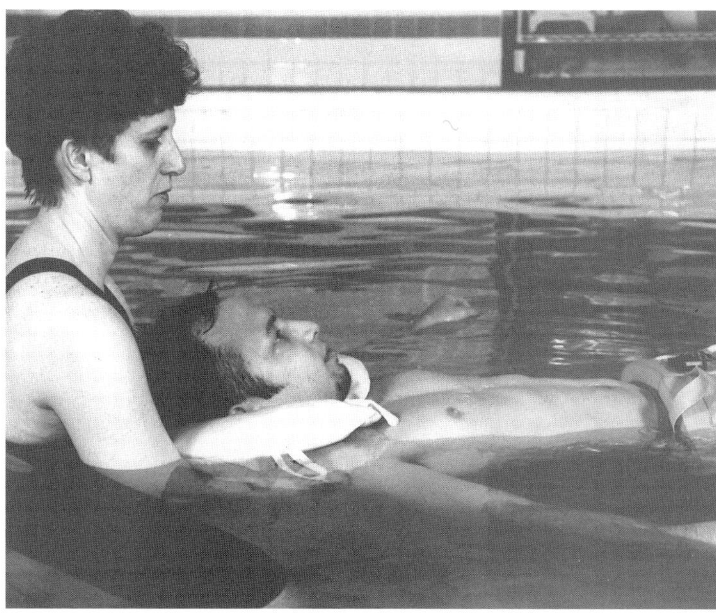

FIGURE 13-14 **Thoracic extension mobilization.**

PURPOSE: Passively improve segmental extension of thoracic spine.

POSITION: Client floating supine supported with flotation devices about the cervical spine and pelvis. Ankles and wrists may be supported with floatation devices, if necessary. Clinician standing above the client's head facing client.

PROCEDURE: Clinician overlaps index fingers under thoracic segment to be mobilized. Overlapped fingers move toward water's surface, performing anterior to posterior oscillations.

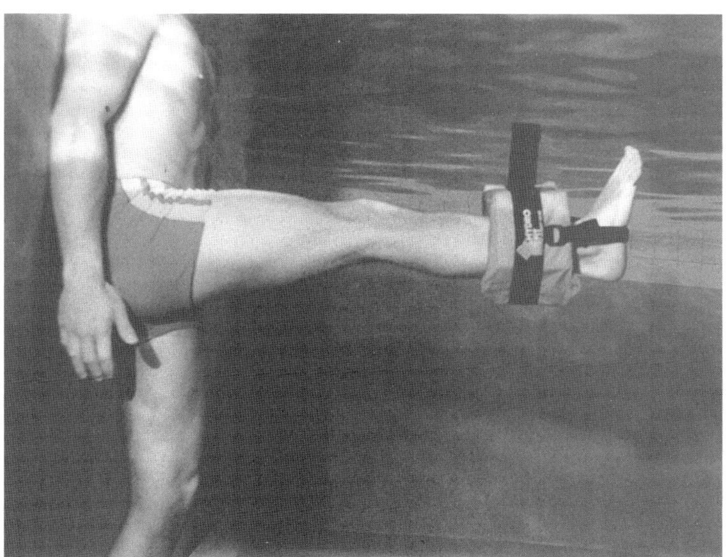

FIGURE 13-15 **Adherent nerve root or hamstring stretch with buoyancy cuff.**

PURPOSE: To passively mobilize and stretch an adherent nerve root or stretch hamstring muscle.

POSITION: Client standing in waist- to chest-deep water with back against side of pool and one foot planted firmly on bottom of pool. Client wearing buoyancy cuff just above ankle on one lower extremity, which is in a 90° hip flexed position.

PROCEDURE: Client allows buoyancy cuff to extend knee to limits of toleration (without causing significant discomfort).

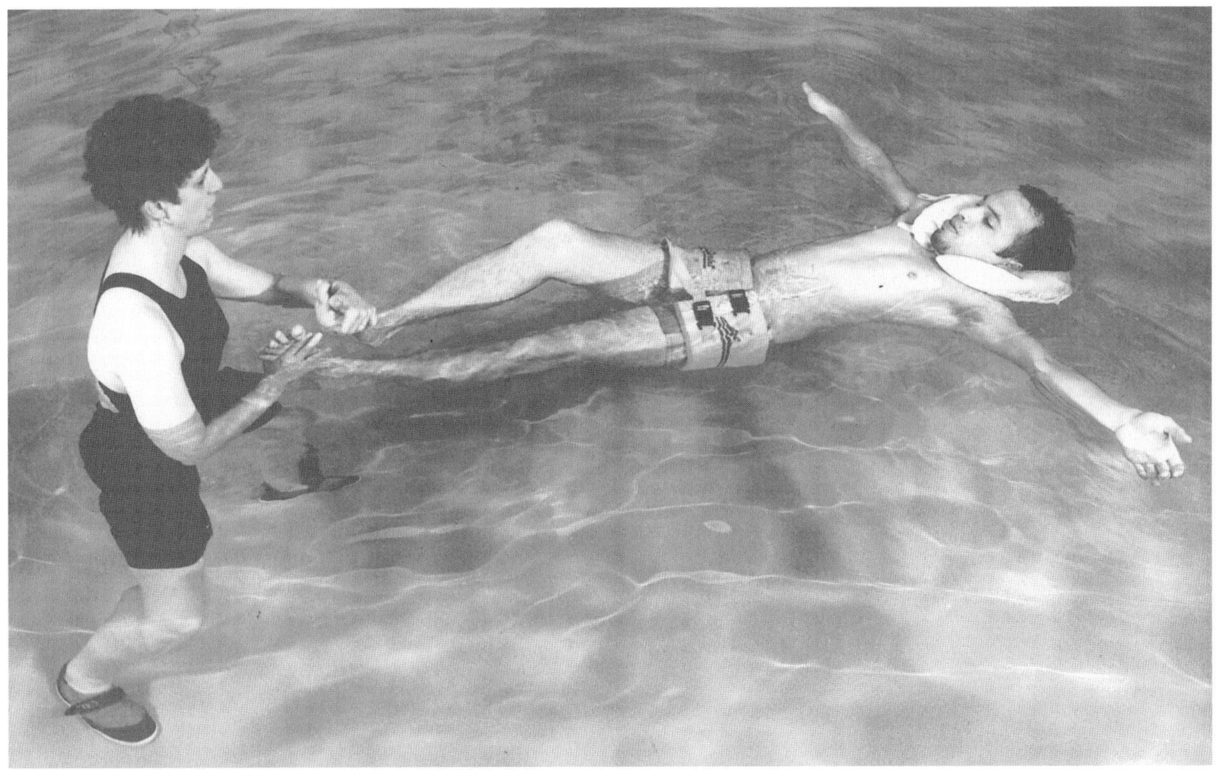

FIGURE 13-16 **Pregait activity in supine with tactile input.**

PURPOSE: To introduce early weight bearing and sequencing of the gait pattern.

POSITION: Client floating in supine supported with flotation devices about the cervical spine and pelvis. Wrists may be supported with flotation devices, if necessary. Clinician facing client's feet.

PROCEDURE: Clinician places hands on dorsum of client's feet while client flexes slightly at one knee and hip and simultaneously dorsiflexes foot of same extremity. Clinician allows client to actively flex hip and knee to about 20° and dorsiflex ankle as far as tolerated. Client isometrically holds position for 5 to 10 sec and repeats as tolerated.

mimicking the beginning of the swing phase against gravity on land.

The client can be progressed to vertical gait activities initiated with deep-water walking (a reduced weight-bearing state). If appropriate, the client can be advanced to walking in shoulder-deep water and then to shallower water to increase the weight bearing.

Water's viscosity and cohesion offer several benefits to gait training. They add resistance to, and thus help strengthen, the muscles used during gait activities. Viscosity and cohesion also have a tendency to slow cadence, which allows the clinician to carefully examine the client's gait, assess for deviations, and offer corrections via manual or verbal cuing. Furthermore, along with hydrostatic pressure, viscosity and cohesion make water much more forgiving than land for clients who have difficulty with balance. Recovery from a fall is much easier in water than on land for both the client and the clinician.

Gait training can be performed on stairs in a water environment by using an aquatic step bench (Fig. 13-17) or the pool's steps. The step bench can be placed in different depths of water, depending on the weight bearing desired by the clinician. Aquatic step benches and removable (portable) stairs are available in a variety of heights. The patient may use a kickboard or water noodle for balance and support during early gait training; as the patient gains control, the floatation device can be removed (Fig. 13-18).

STRENGTHENING

Chapters 5 and 6 discuss enhancing muscle strength. Strengthening can also be part of an aquatic program. Progression of strength exercises can be done safely by exploring the physical and hydrodynamic properties of water. These properties in conjunction with the physiologic properties of muscle fibers allow the clinician to address muscle strengthening versus local muscle endurance. Methods for increasing the intensity of aquatic exercises are presented in Table 13-6.

FIGURE 13-17 **Step bench with forward step up.**

PURPOSE: To initiate gait training for stair climbing.

POSITION: Client standing in waist-high or deeper water in front of a step bench.

PROCEDURE: Client initiates a step-up motion, leading with limb requested by clinician. Once both lower extremities are on bench, client steps off bench.

NOTE: Clinician determines the leading limb and whether client steps backward or forward.

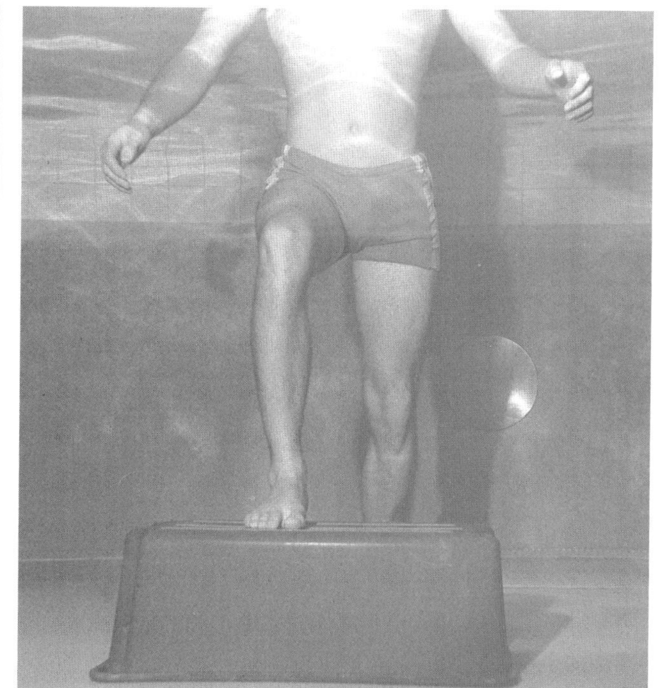

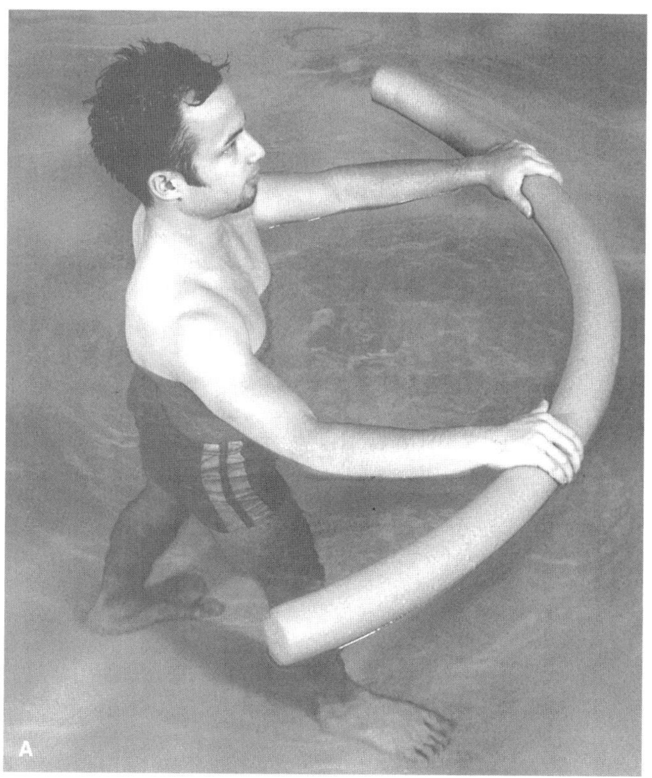

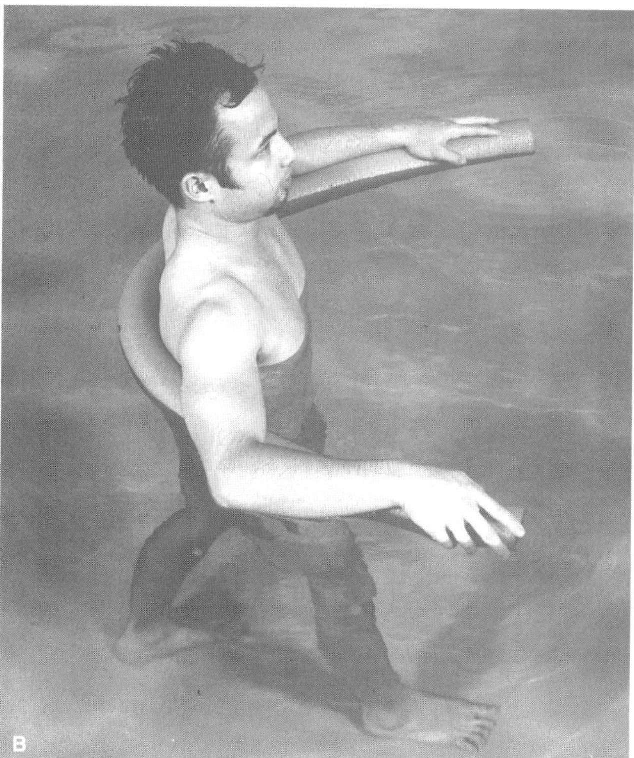

FIGURE 13-18 **Forward ambulation with water noodle.**

PURPOSE: To initiate gait training with some assistance for balance.

POSITION: Client standing in slightly above waist- to chest-deep water, holding on to a water noodle with both hands. Noodle is placed in front of client (panel A) or is wrapped under client's arms (panel B).

PROCEDURE: Client walks forward while holding on to water noodle.

NOTE: As balance improves, clients can hold on to noodle more loosely.

TABLE 13-6 Methods for Increasing the Difficulty of Aquatic Strengthening Activities

Move from buoyancy assist to buoyancy support to buoyancy resist
Increase speed of movement
Decrease length of lever arm for active movements with buoyancy assist
Increase length of lever arm with buoyancy resist
Add a buoyancy device to the end of the extremity for buoyancy resist activities
Increase size and irregularity of buoyancy device used for resistive activities
Increase size and irregularity of resistive device
Add turbulence to the direction of movement
Increase the number of repetitions of an exercise
Increase in overall time for performance of an exercise
Decrease rest time between exercises

Emphasis on muscle strength or endurance can be achieved by manipulating the number of repetitions of an exercise, the work:rest ratio in a given cycle, and the total duration of a particular exercise. Both closed- and open-chain exercises for the extremities can be performed in an aquatic environment. Some examples of extremity strengthening exercises are given in Figures 13-19 to 13-21. Trunk and multiple joint strengthening techniques are discussed in the next section.

CORE AND TRUNK STRENGTHENING

Chapter 12 provides background on spinal stabilization. Several clinicians have modified those concepts for use in an aquatic environment.[22,26,29–31] A spinal stabilization rehabilitation program incorporates the client's pain-free position of the neutral spine.[32] Neutral spine is defined as being approximately at the mid-range between the extremes of lumbopelvic spinal flexion and extension and is the position in which the patient is most comfortable.[30]

It is common for patients with spinal dysfunction to use movement patterns that take the spine out of the neutral position, especially when the extremities and spine are moved simultaneously. Patients seem to use these inappropriate patterns to compensate for pain that occurs during functional movement on land.[30] Unfortunately, these poor compensatory patterns can become habitual, perpetuating the pain and spinal dysfunction. Thus, the primary goals of spinal stabilization exercises are to facilitate and teach efficient and effective movement patterns from a sound neutral spine.[32]

The aquatic environment is an ideal medium for spinal stabilization exercises. Training the client to achieve total spinal alignment, proper posture, and neutral positioning should be the initial goal of an aquatic spinal stabilization program.[29] Once spinal alignment and proper postural awareness are obtained, the clinician uses the aquatic environment to help the client gain dynamic control over spinal movement. This control allows the client to develop better synergistic functional movement patterns and increase ROM, flexibility, and strength.

The aquatic environment enhances awareness of proper posture and body mechanics and eliminates the potentially harmful and painful compressive and shear forces that gravity places on spinal structures such as the disks and facet joints.[22,29,30] Any movement of the body in the water forces the client to stabilize at the spine and trunk to overcome the forces of the water. An aquatic-based spinal stabilization program can benefit patients with discogenic pain, nerve root impingement or irritation, postural syndrome, facet joint syndrome, chronic pain, and sacroiliac or iliosacral dysfunction. A water-based program is also recommended for patients recovering from surgical procedures such as laminectomy, diskectomy, and spinal fusion.

Stabilization exercises can be performed in deep or shallow water for the cervical, thoracic, and lumbar levels of the spine. The advantage of doing these exercises in deep water, particularly for patients with lumbar spine dysfunction, is to decrease the compressive forces on bony and soft tissue structures by suspending the client in the water with a flotation device about the trunk. The disadvantage of using deep water in the initial stages of a spinal stabilization program is the lack of position sense provided by weight bearing through the lower extremities or contact of the spine and posterior trunk against a surface, such as the pool wall. For most clients, deep-water spinal stabilization techniques are more difficult because the client must rely almost completely on coordinated contractions of the muscles of the pelvis and trunk to allow pain-free movement.[30]

In contrast, for clients who are weight-bearing sensitive on land, deep water may be more comfortable and is a good choice for initial spinal stabilization activities. Strengthening the scapular stabilizers is the primary emphasis of a stabilization program for cervical and thoracic pathologies and for shoulder dysfunctions, such as rotator cuff tendonitis. All exercises are performed within the client's pain-free ROM in a slowed and controlled manner.[30]

Progression is achieved in a spinal stabilization program by moving the client from small-excursion movement at one joint to large-excursion dynamic movements at multiple joints, while maintaining a safe, balanced, and neutral spine position. Dynamic control of these movements is achieved through stabilization of the pelvis and lumbar spine through the co-contraction of agonist and antagonist

FIGURE 13-19 **Knee flexion and extension strengthening with buoyancy device.**

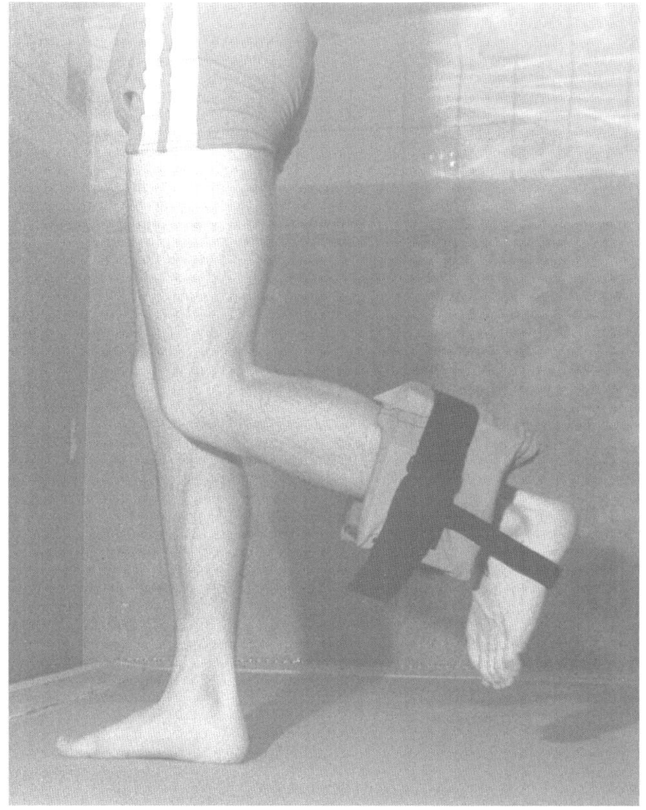

PURPOSE: To increase strength in the quadriceps and hamstring muscle groups.

POSITION: Client standing in waist-deep water with one foot planted firmly on bottom of pool. Client wearing buoyancy device near ankle on one lower extremity with hip in neutral position and knee fully extended. Client holding on to side of the pool for balance and support, as needed.

PROCEDURE: Client actively flexes and extends at the knee joint while maintaining hip and spine in neutral and upright position.

NOTE: There should be no flexion or extension at hip or trunk.

FIGURE 13-20 **Shoulder flexion and extension strengthening with aqua glove.**

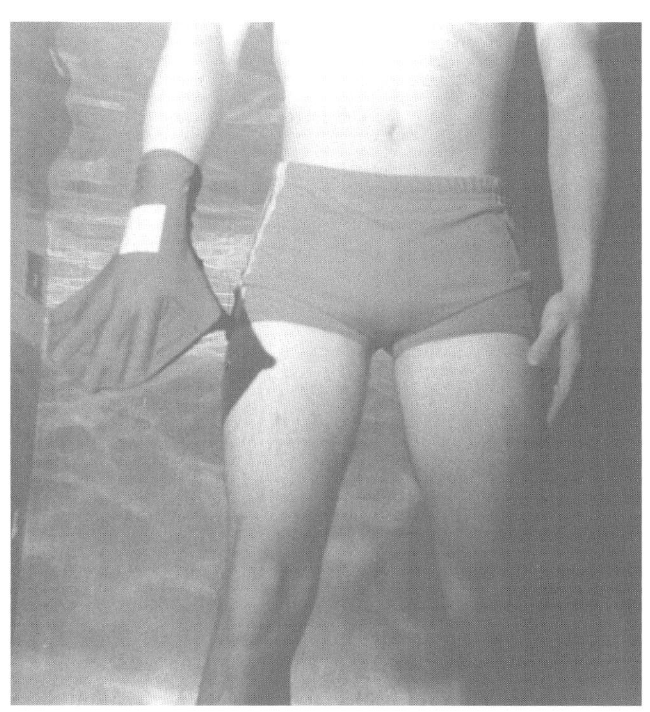

PURPOSE: To increase strength in shoulder flexors and extensors.

POSITION: Client standing in shoulder-deep water with arms at sides, elbows extended, forearms in full pronation, and fingers abducted. Client wearing aqua gloves.

PROCEDURE: Client simultaneously, or alternately, moves upper extremities to 90° shoulder flexion, back through neutral, to full shoulder extension while maintaining arm position.

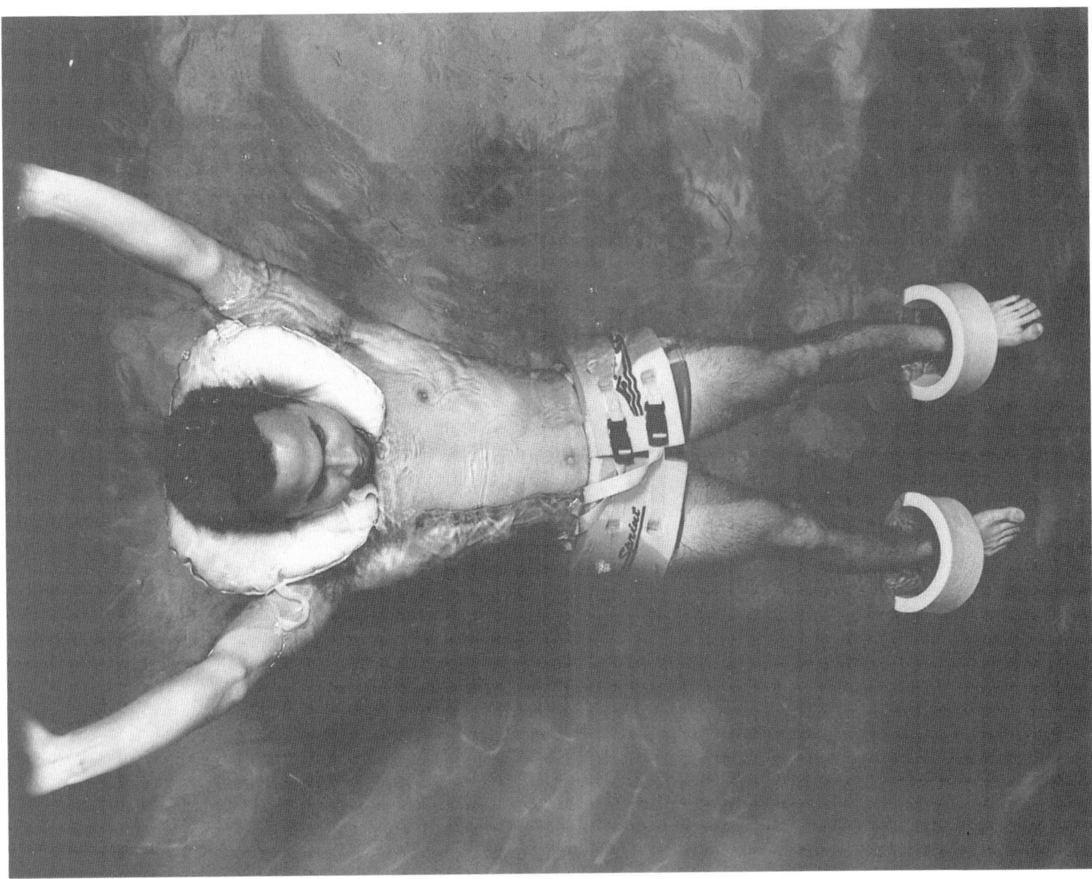

FIGURE 13-21 Closed-chained upper-extremity push-pull.

PURPOSE: To strengthen muscle groups in a closed-chain format.

POSITION: Client floating supine with shoulders fully flexed overhead and elbows maintained in almost full extension.

PROCEDURE: With hands pressed flat on side of pool or grasping railing or handles, client pushes upper extremities into the pool side or railings.

NOTE: If handles or railings are available, client may alternate between pushing body away from and pulling it back into side of pool.

trunk muscles (e.g., abdominals, gluteus maximus, and latissimus dorsi) in a synergistic pattern that enhances maintenance of the neutral spine position. Examples of spinal stabilization exercises for patients with lumbopelvic dysfunction are given in Figures 13-22 to 13-24. Examples of deep-water spinal stabilization exercises and their normal progression are given in Table 13-7. An example of a scapular and spinal stabilization exercise for cervical, thoracic, and shoulder dysfunction is given in Figure 13-25.

BALANCE, PROPRIOCEPTION, AND COORDINATION

Balance, proprioception, and coordination activities can be initiated in the water for the trunk and extremities. For the purposes of this chapter, balance is defined as the ability to maintain the center of gravity over the base of support, as in standing balance.[33] Proprioception is defined as the awareness of posture, movement, and changes in equilibrium and the knowledge of position, weight, and resistance of objects in relation to the body.[33] Coordination can be defined as the ability of different components of the neuromusculoskeletal system to work together to produce smooth controlled, and accurate movements.[33] Coordination deficits occur when muscles fail to fire in sequence or when the central nervous system (CNS) is unable to direct movement activities accurately. These three components are part of the entire motor control concept (see Chapter 11).

Several of the exercises used to improve balance and proprioception not only challenge these systems but also serve as dynamic stabilization activities. Proximal stability is required of the trunk and proximal joints of the extremities to successfully and safely perform these activities, thus challenging the entire neuromusculoskeletal system.

FIGURE 13-22 **Mini-squats with back to side of pool.**

PURPOSE: To experience and practice neutral spine position while superimposing functional squatting.

POSITION: Client standing in chest-deep water with back against side of pool and feet about shoulder-width apart. Client standing with hips and knees flexed to 20 to 30° and hands on hips.

PROCEDURE: Client finds and holds neutral spine position. Client then performs isometric co-contraction of the abdominal and gluteal muscles while maintaining neutral position and performing mini-squats to 50 to 70° of hip and knee flexion, as tolerated.

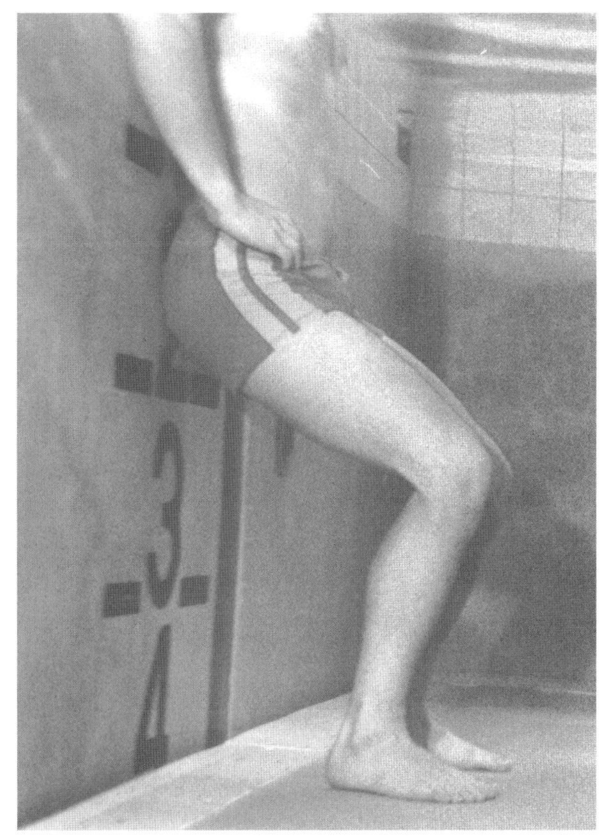

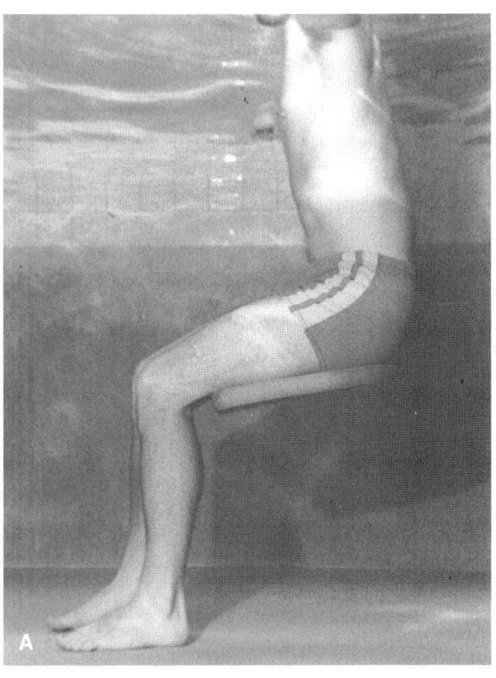

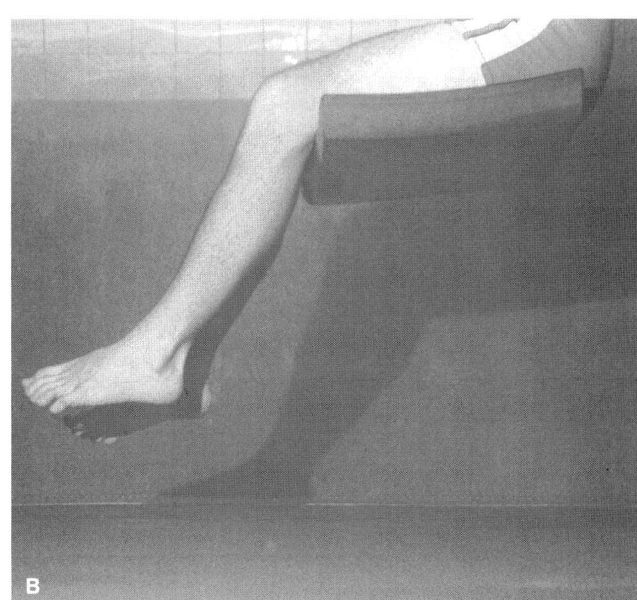

FIGURE 13-23 **Breastroke with wonder board.**

PURPOSE: To practice maintenance of neutral spine position in sitting while moving upper extremities.

POSITION: Client sitting on wonder board in approximately 4 ft. of water with spine in neutral position and upper extremities floating in front (Panel A).

PROCEDURE: Client maintains neutral position while performing isometric co-contractions of the abdominal and gluteal muscles. Then client superimposes breaststroke movements of upper extremity (Panel B).

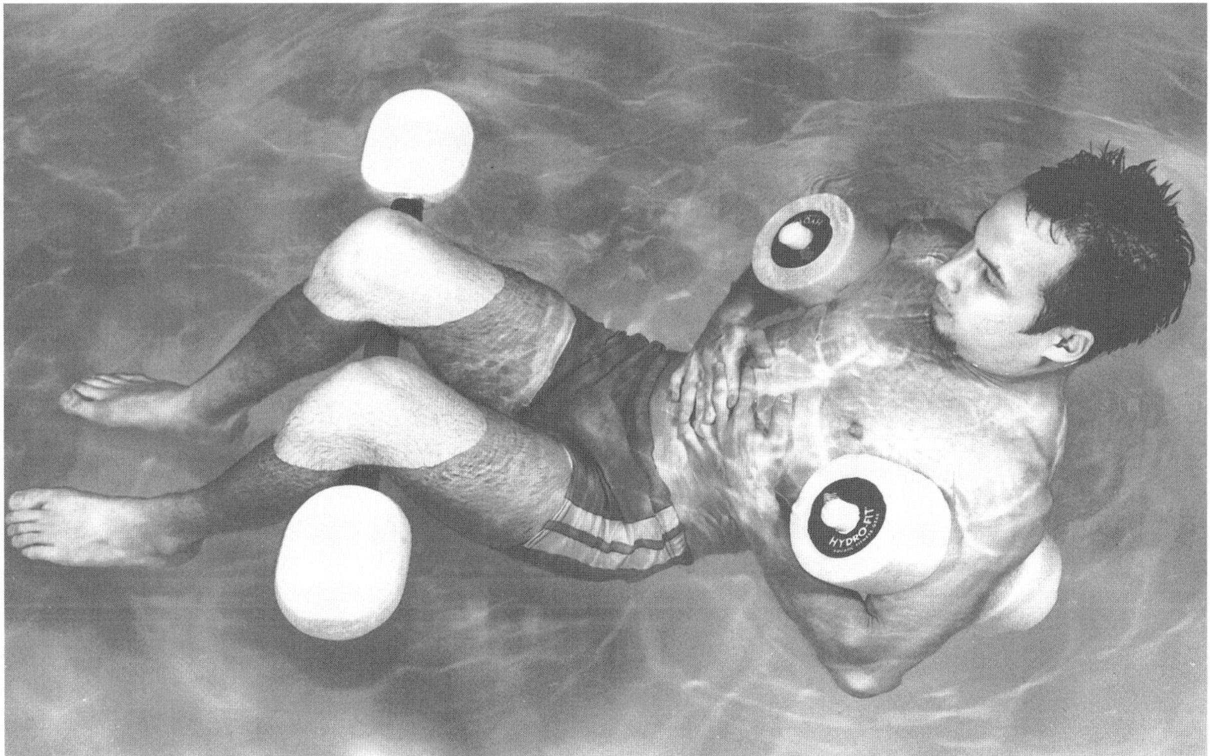

FIGURE 13-24 Abdominal strengthening in neutral lumbar spine position.

PURPOSE: To increase abdominal strength while protecting spine in a neutral position.

POSITION: Client floating supine in 3 to 4 ft of water supported by floatation devices under knees and on upper extremities. Cervical spine may be supported with floatation device, if necessary. Client floating with knees flexed over barbell and hips in neutral or slightly flexed position.

POSITION: Client tucks chin and flexes slightly at hip, performing an abdominal crunch while maintaining a neutral spine position.

A desired intensity of a balance, proprioceptive, and coordination activity can be achieved in several ways. One way is to simply have the client perform the skill at a faster, yet safe, speed. Decreasing the level of support provided by the clinician, piece of equipment, or side of pool also progresses the intensity of the exercise. Increased difficulty can also be achieved by adding turbulence, which is accomplished by increasing the speed of the water's movement, if possible.

Some exercises used in the water for balance, proprioception, and coordination are listed in Table 13-8 and shown in Figures 13-26 and 13-27. Furthermore, several more advanced plyometric activities (discussed next) can be used as well.

PLYOMETRICS

The concept of plyometrics has its roots in Europe, where it was first known as "jump training."[34] The term was coined in 1975 by Fred Wilt, an American track-and-field coach; and following its Latin derivation, it can be interpreted to mean "measurable increases." Plyometrics are most commonly used by athletes to incorporate sports-specific jumping, hopping, bounding, and leaping skills in the rehabilitation process. Plyometric exercises enable a muscle to reach maximum strength in as short a time as possible.[34]

Plyometric exercise requires activities in which eccentric muscle contractions are rapidly followed by a movement completed by concentric contractions. It is postulated that eccentric–concentric muscle contraction not only stimulates the proprioceptors sensitive to rapid stretch but also loads the serial elastic components with a tension force from which the individual can rebound[34] (see Chapter 9).

Plyometric activities can be progressed from low to high intensity within six categories: jumping in place, standing jumps, multiples hops and jumps, bounding, box drills, and depth jumps.[34] The aquatic environment is an

TABLE 13-7 Deep-Water Spinal Stabilization Exercises[a]

Single knee to chest
Bilateral knee to chest
Side sit-ups
Hip abduction–adduction
Lower-extremity bicycling propulsion
Lower-extremity walking or reciprocal arm swing while sitting on barbell or kickboard
Squats while standing on barbell
Squats with quarter and half turns
Upper-extremity breaststroke forward and backward while standing on barbell
Forward steppage gait with lower extremity crossing midline

[a]All activities performed while maintaining a neutral spine via co-contraction of abdominals and gluteal muscles.

ideal medium for beginning plyometric training before progressing the client to training on land. Furthermore, aquatic plyometrics can be done with specificity to the requirements of sport, work, or leisure activity. Plyometric training in the water can be performed with equipment, such as aquatic step benches, elevated platforms, and balls of different sizes and weights (Figs. 13-28 and 13-29).

CARDIOVASCULAR ENDURANCE TRAINING

Intervention for musculoskeletal disorders usually emphasizes regaining strength, ROM, and functional capabilities. Unfortunately, cardiovascular rehabilitation to improve the client's endurance level is seldom mentioned. Yet most clients whose physical activity level has been significantly reduced during the time of injury recovery have suffered a decline in overall cardiovascular performance. Studies have confirmed that a significant decline in cardiovascular function occurs during a period of decreased physical activity.[35,36] Thus, it is important to include some form of cardiovascular endurance training to ensure full recovery of the client with a musculoskeletal dysfunction.

Chapter 10 presents a detailed description of land-based cardiovascular programs. Cardiovascular training can also be performed in an aquatic environment. Deep- or shallow-water running, walking, and cross-country skiing are excellent choices.

Before including a cardiovascular endurance component to a treatment program, the clinician must be familiar with the client's cardiovascular and cardiopulmonary history and current medications. Some prescribed medications alter the heart rate response to a given intensity level

FIGURE 13-25 Simultaneous alternating push-downs with buoyant dumbbells.

PURPOSE: To provide strengthening for scapular and posterior shoulder muscles for proximal stabilization in cervical and thoracic areas.

POSITION: Client standing in shoulder-deep water with shoulders and forearms in neutral position and elbows slightly flexed while holding a buoyant dumbbell in each hand. Client holding spine in neutral position with co-contraction of abdominal and gluteal muscles.

PROCEDURE: Client pushes one dumbbell down toward pool floor and allows the contralateral dumbbell to float toward water surface by extending shoulder and flexing elbow in a controlled manner.

NOTE: Dumbbell remains submerged below water surface when client achieves full shoulder extension and elbow flexion.

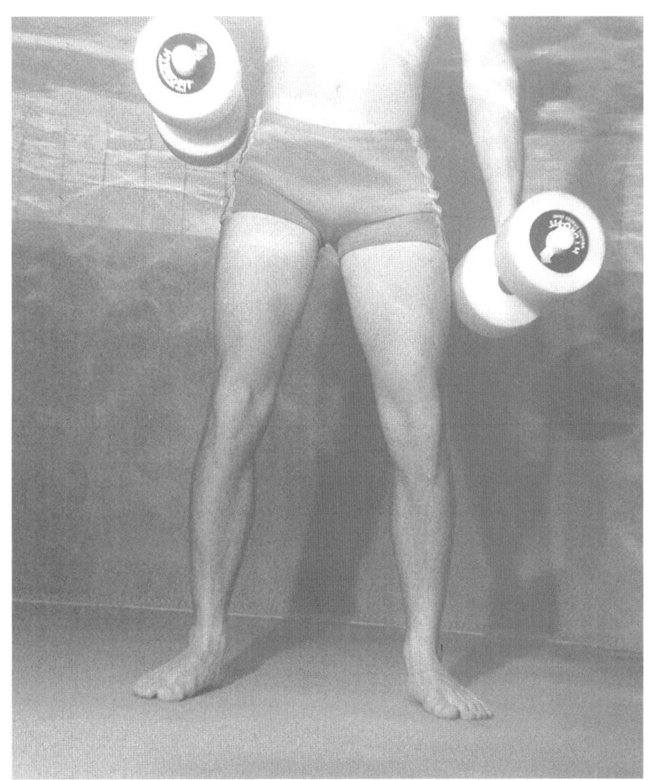

TABLE 13-8 Balance, Proprioceptive, and Coordination Activities in an Aquatic Environment

Balance
Stork standing on injured and uninjured limbs while arms create turbulence (e.g., by breaststroking)
Stork standing while performing a variety of levels of squats with arms held in a variety of positions (e.g., mini squats with both arms over head)
Sitting on kickboard while clinician creates turbulence
Single- or double-leg squatting while standing on buoyant dumbbell
Proprioception
Stork-standing on injured and uninjured limbs while moving contralateral lower extremity into different positions of hip flexion, abduction, extension, and external rotation, with and without the knee flexed
Deep-water running for three to five strides followed by a pirouette; repeat
Coordination
Braiding gait sideways in different depths of water with and without arm movement
Backward and forward heel-toe walking holding onto side of pool and progressing to middle of pool
Side stepping while crossing arms in front and back of trunk
Stork-standing while performing squats and asymmetrical arm movement patterns
Sitting on buoyant barbell while performing the vertical breaststroke
Rocking horse while crossing arms in front and back of trunk

of exercise. Clinicians must also understand the cardiovascular response to immersion and exercise in the aquatic environment, as discussed earlier.

Deep-water running gained popularity as a form of cardiovascular training in the 1980s when Gold Medal–marathoner Joan Benoit Samuelson began running in a pool during recovery from a sport-related injury. Several studies investigated the effect of cardiovascular vertical training in deep- and shallow-water running and underwater cycling. These studies showed improvement in cardiovascular function comparable to a land-based regimen of similar intensity. The studies noted that aquatic training prevented the decline in cardiovascular fitness level normally seen during an episode of decreased physical capabilities.[14,37–40] Research has also shown the importance of instruction in, and maintenance of, proper deep-water running form for optimal outcome in cardiovascular fitness training.[11,41,42]

Deep-water running is described as simulated running in the deep end of a swimming pool, avoiding contact with the bottom of the pool. Buoyancy in the water eliminates the impact with the ground experienced when running on land.[43,44] Proper form and body position are important and are described in Table 13-9. Patients may run in place by using a tether strap or may chose to run over a given distance in the pool. It is recommended the patient wear a commercially available flotation device or vest to assist in maintaining proper form (Fig. 13-30). The motions of cross-country skiing can also be used for cardiovascular training (Table 13-10). The intensity of the cardiovascular endurance program can be increased by adding equipment (e.g., aqua gloves or fins) to increase the resistance to movement in the water by increasing the surface area of the body part.

Monitoring the intensity of an aerobic endurance exercise in the water is performed in one of three ways: target heart rate (THR), RPE, and cadence. Target heart rate should fall in the range of 60 to 90% of maximal heart rate using the following formula:

$$\text{Maximal heart rate} = 220 - \text{age (years)} - 15 \text{ bpm}$$

For the deconditioned client, it may be best to use a THR in the 40 to 60% range. For more detailed information on monitoring aerobic activities, see chapter 10.

The Brennan scale is useful when using RPE to determine intensity of exercise in the water (Table 13-11).[43,44]

FIGURE 13-26 **Braiding sideways walking.**

PURPOSE: To improve dynamic balance, coordination, and proprioception.

POSITION: Client standing in waist- to neck-deep water.

PROCEDURE: Client steps out sideways with leading leg then steps with trailing leg, placing it alternately in front and behind leading leg with each step.

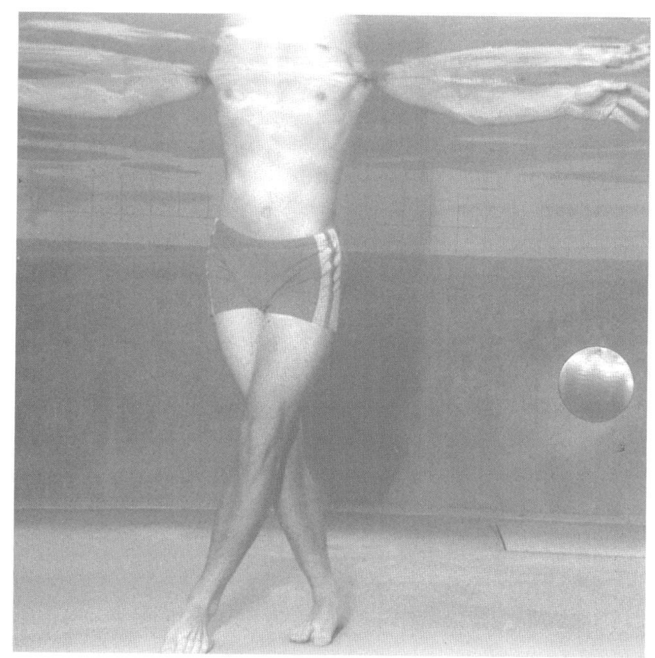

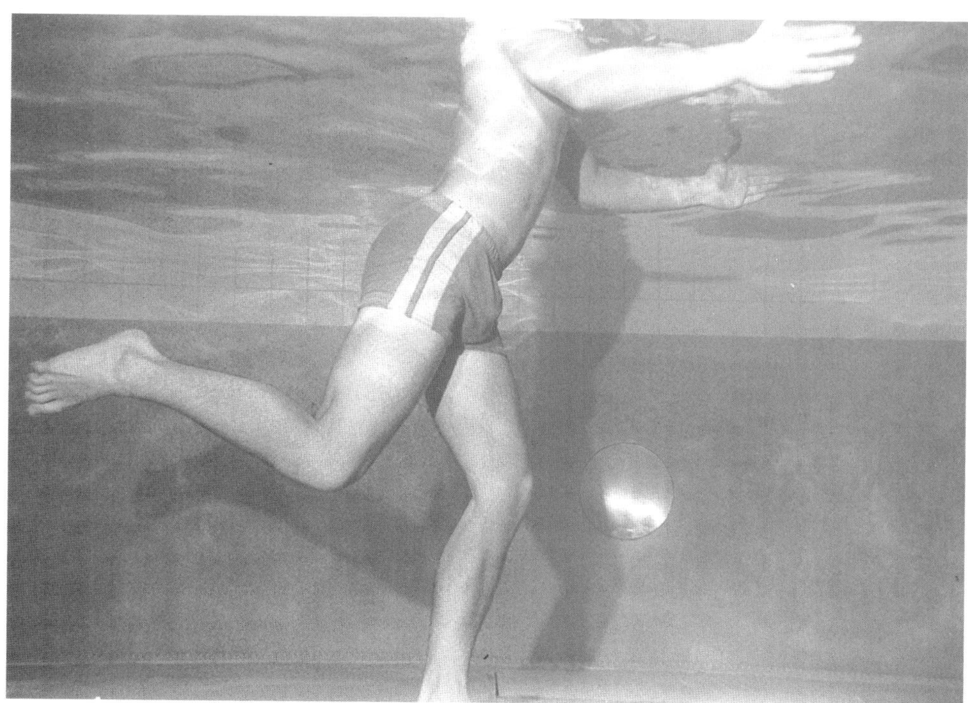

FIGURE 13-27 **Rocking horse.**

PURPOSE: To challenge and enhance balance, coordination, and proprioception.

POSITION: Client standing in waist- to shoulder-deep water with arms resting at side and forearms in a neutral position.

PROCEDURE: Client leaps forward, shifting all weight to leading leg with hip and knee flexed, while crossing one arm over the other in horizontal adduction across front midline; then client kicks trailing leg behind, with hip extended, knee flexed, and ankle plantarflexed. Next, client steps back onto trailing leg (keeping the hip extended, knee flexed, and ankle plantarflexed) and takes weight fully off leading leg (keeping hip and knee flexed), while crossing one arm over the other beyond the back midline. Client repeats movement.

NOTE: Trailing and leading legs and arm crossed on top can be switched or alternated.

FIGURE 13-28 **Directional plyometric jumping.**

PURPOSE: To improve power jumping skills.

POSITION: Client standing in waist- to shoulder-deep water with hips and knees slightly flexed.

PROCEDURE: Client jumps forward, backward, right, and left (north, south, east, and west).

NOTE: Clinician can determine a direction pattern beforehand or randomly select and cue direction as client jumps.

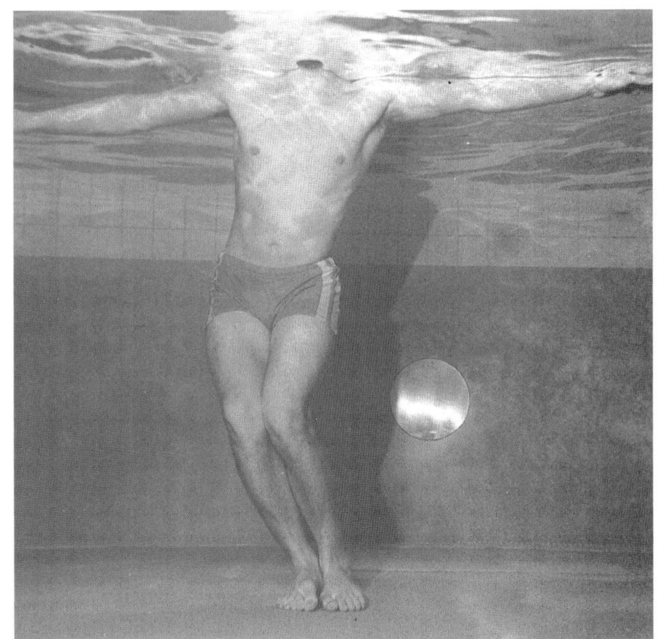

FIGURE 13-29 **Lateral box jumps.**

PURPOSE: To improve lateral power jumping skills.

POSITION: Client standing in mid-trunk- to shoulder-deep water, with hips and knees slightly flexed, beside aquatic step bench.

PROCEDURE: Client jumps up and to side, placing both feet simultaneously onto step bench, and then jumps off to side, placing both feet simultaneously on pool floor.

NOTE: Client performs exercise from both sides of bench.

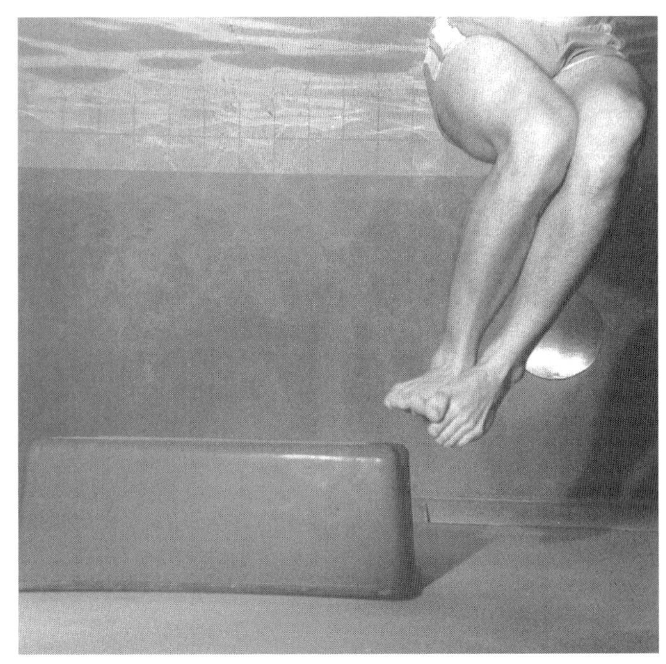

TABLE 13-9 Deep-Water Running Form
Water line at shoulder level
Head looking straight forward
Trunk slightly forward of vertical
Spine in neutral position
Upper-extremity motion identical to that used on land
Primary arm motions from shoulder
Shoulder flexion brings hands to just below water line 8 to 12 in. from chest
Extension brings hands just below hips
Hands slightly clinched with thumbs on top
Elbows primarily flexed but undergo a slight degree of extension and flexion
Lower-extremity motion requires attention to detail
Maximum hip flexion of 60–80°
As hip flexes, knee extends
When maximum hip flexion is reached, leg should be perpendicular to the horizontal
Hip and knee extend together
Knee reaches full extension when hip is in neutral
As hip extends beyond neutral, knee begins to flex
Ankle in dorsiflexion when hip is in neutral
Ankle in plantarflexion when hip is extended beyond neutral
Dorsiflexion re-assumed when hip is flexed and leg extends
Inversion and eversion accompany dorsiflexion and plantarflexion, as seen on land

The Brennan scale, an adaptation of the Borg RPE scale, and is a five-point scale with increments of 0.5 that uses verbal descriptors ranging from very light to very hard. Descriptors of on-land running activities for each point on the scale are included, which makes it easy for athletes and coaches to correlate aquatic activity to an established land-based training session.[43,44]

Cadence is the third means of establishing exercise intensity for cardiovascular training in the water. Cadence is defined as the number of times the right leg moves through a complete gait cycle each minute.[43,45] Wilder et al.[45] found a significant correlation (0.98) between cadence and heart rate during graded exercise testing in the pool. Cadence is most useful as a guide for exercise intensity when interval training is incorporated into a treatment program. See Table 13-11 for cadence rates appropriate for clinicians or coaches setting up interval-type training session for distance runners and sprinters.[43] Deep-water running interval training can closely mimic a land-based interval training session. This form of interval training has become popular not only with athletes who are recovering from injury but also with athletes who are including water running as a regular component of a cross-training program.

CROSS-TRAINING AND MAINTENANCE PROGRAMS

Many clinicians who develop rehabilitation programs for their clients incorporate a cross-training regimen when integrating water-based with land-based exercise. Some facilities are beginning to incorporate both land- and water-based exercises into work conditioning and functional restoration programs designed for injured workers. This combination maximizes the benefits of both environments, adds fun, and prevents boredom.[46]

Once a client returns to maximum improvement and is ready for discharge from services, there is no reason why the clinician cannot recommend continued individual participation in aquatic exercise in conjunction with land exercise. The clinician should recommend continuation of water exercise if the physical properties of water can be

FIGURE 13-30 Deep-water running with floatation device.

PURPOSE: To improve or maintain cardiovascular endurance.

POSITION: Client standing suspended in deep water by floatation device.

PROCEDURE: Client runs in place for a designated period of time at a designated pace.

NOTE: Client may wear floatation device around waist or may wear wet vest. Client must be taught proper water-running technique.

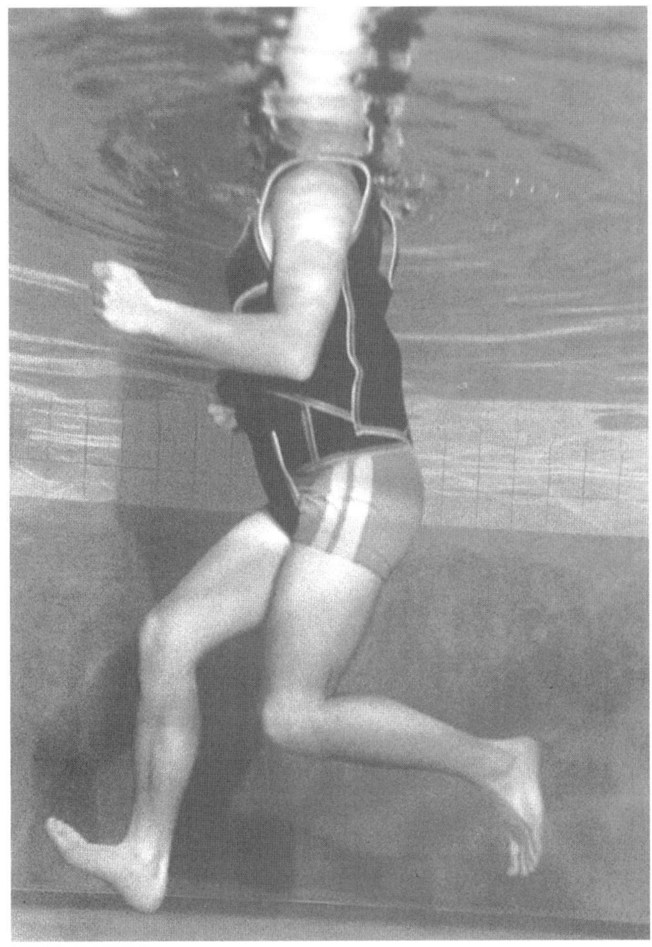

used to the benefit of the client. For clients who cannot tolerate land-based exercise (e.g., those with rheumatoid arthritis and osteoarthritis), water exercise may be the sole means of a maintenance program. For other clients, water can serve as a viable medium for cross-training. A training program of aerobic exercise such as running, walking, or cross-country skiing can be performed on both land and in water on alternating days. Even for the highly trained athlete, little to no loss in performance has been observed when water running is substituted for or performed in conjunction with land running.[11,37–39] Land and water aerobic programs can be alternated quite easily for most clients.

Strength training can be alternated between a land program (using free weights, elastic bands, circuit training, or exercise machines) and a comparable water program (using assistive and resistive buoyancy and unstreamlined equipment). Trunk stabilization exercises can continue in the water environment. Facilities around the country are beginning to offer non-therapeutic aquatic exercise classes for prevention of spine pain and for continued progress of clients who have been discharged from therapeutic services.

For many clients, aquatic exercise serves as a welcome change of pace, improving overall well-being and creating a positive attitude to exercise. Anecdotal reports indicate improved long-term adherence to exercise when incorporating a cross-training regimen that includes both land and water. The aquatic environment may also help prevent or

TABLE 13-10 Cross-Country Skiing Form

Use flotation belt or vest
Maintain vertical position
Reciprocal flexion and extension of upper and lower extremities
Very slight flexion maintained in bilateral elbows and knees
Movement occurs primarily at hips and shoulders through a tolerated ROM
May add aqua gloves or paddles to upper extremities to increase resistance
May add fins to lower extremities to increase resistance

TABLE 13-11 Brennan RPE Scale Correlated to Cadences and Land Equivalents for Distance Runners and Sprinters

	Distance Runners		Sprinters	
Brennan Score	**Cadence**	**Land Equivalent**	**Cadence**	**Land Equivalent**
1.0 very light	< 60	Brisk walk	< 74	> 800 m
1.5	60–64		75–59	
2.0 light	60–64	Easy jog	80–84	600–800 m
2.5	65–69		85–90	
3.0 somewhat hard	70–74	Brisk run	90–94	400–600 m
3.5	75–80		95–99	
4.0 hard	80–84	5-K or 10-K race	130–134	200–400 m
4.5	85–90		135–139	
5.0 very hard	> 90	Short track intervals	> 113	50–200 m

FIGURE 13-31 Lifting plastic crates.

PURPOSE: To practice a functional lifting technique.

POSITION: Client standing in waist-deep water in diagonal squat lifting position (one foot slightly in front, wide base of support, and neutral spine) while holding a plastic crate close to body between thighs, with elbows flexed at 20 to 30°.

PROCEDURE: While maintaining neutral spine by co-contracting abdominal and gluteal muscles, client squat lifts to 50 to 70° of hip and knee flexion, keeping elbows slightly flexed.

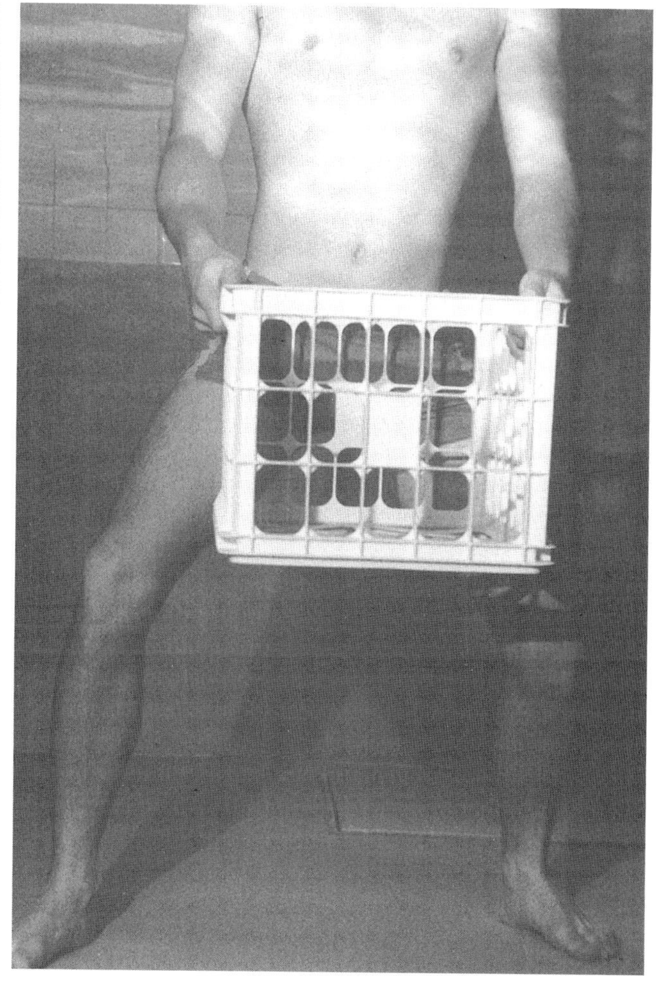

alleviate the exacerbation of symptoms, allowing the former patient to stay pain-free and functional for leisure and work activities on a long-term basis.

FUNCTIONAL TRAINING

Incorporation of functional training into an aquatic rehabilitation program is vital to transition a client to the land environment in which function will be performed on a regular basis. Functional activities performed in the water serve as initial training for carryover to safe performance on land. The type of functional training incorporated depends on the tasks and skills required by, and goals of, the client. Some activities used in an aquatic program are as simple as transfer skills from vertical (standing) to sitting and vice versa. Bed mobility training can be achieved by teaching transitions from supine, through side lying to prone and back to supine on the long-body-axis in a horizontal position on the surface of the water.

FIGURE 13-32 Tennis swing with paddle.

PURPOSE: To practice a sport-specific technique.

POSITION: Client standing in mid-trunk-deep water in forehand tennis stroke position while holding on to a water paddle (panel A) or table tennis paddle (panel B).

PROCEDURE: Client repetitively swings paddle through water, mimicking a forehand tennis stroke with appropriate technique.

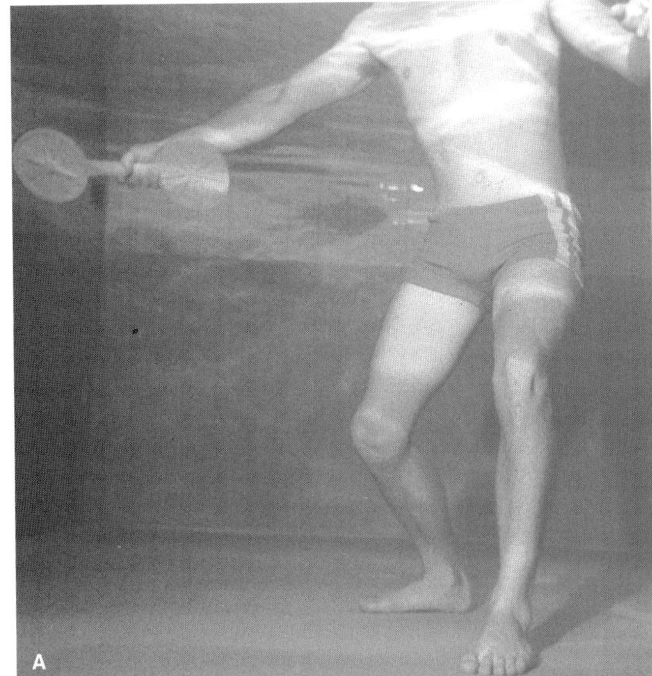

A

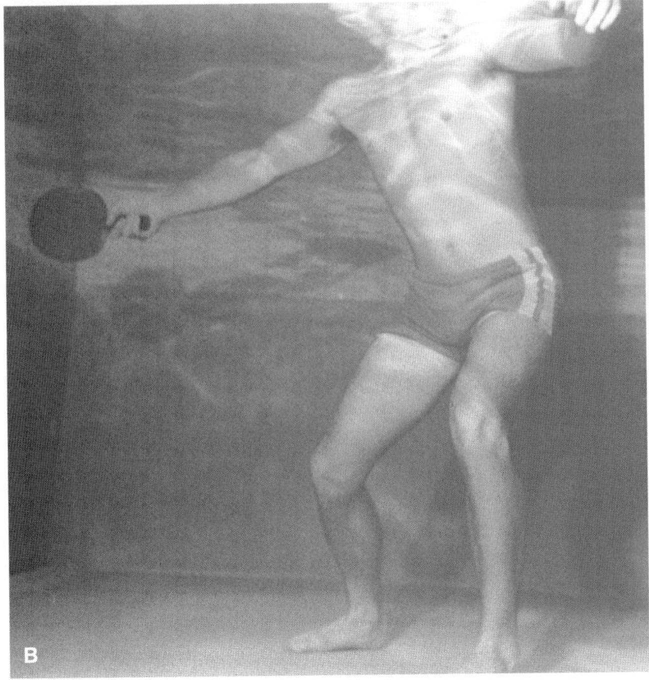

B

More complex, multitask, sport-specific, or functional work activities can also be initiated in the water. An example of functional skill training is lifting plastic crates with different numbers of holes in them to alter resistance (Fig. 13-31). Sport-specific skills include mimicking a tennis swing while holding a water paddle (Fig. 13-32).

CASE STUDY

PATIENT INFORMATION

A 19-year-old defensive back football player presented to the clinic with a long-term history of low back pain (LBP) of insidious onset and aggravated by any sports participation. The current bout of LBP began 2 months earlier, when the patient was dead lifting as part of his weight-training program. At the time of the lifting incident, the athlete stated his trunk was stuck in a forward-flexed position. An MRI study, ordered by an orthopedic surgeon within days of the onset of pain, revealed a two-level disk herniation at the L4-5 and L5-S1 interspaces. Radiographs revealed moderate degenerative joint disease for the patient's age throughout the lumbar spine. The physician recommended redshirting the athlete for his freshman year and referred him to the clinic to prepare him for college football training and conditioning for the following spring's off-season training.

The patient's chief complaint was pain (7 out of 10) in the low back from the level of L1 to S1 centrally and bilaterally into the erector spinae musculature with radiation of pain into the right buttock and posterior thigh. The patient also reported pain in the lumbar spine and right buttock after sitting for a prolonged period of time during classes and while traveling in a car; inability to do household chores such as vacuuming and sweeping; and pain with lower-extremity weight training, jogging on land, and recreational sports activities such as basketball.

The initial examination revealed an altered standing posture with a forward head position and decreased lumbar lordosis on the sagittal view. Active ROM of the lumbar spine revealed decreased lumbar flexion secondary to pain in the spine and right buttock. Repeated lumbar flexion active ROM increased lumbar pain and peripheralized the radiation of pain into the right posterior thigh and calf. Myotome assessment revealed bilateral weakness and pain in the lumbar spine with resistive hip flexion, knee extension, and ankle dorsiflexion (right side more than left). Passive posterior-anterior segmental mobility testing of the lumbar spine revealed hypomobility, but no pain, from levels T12 through L3 with hypermobility and pain noted at levels L4 and L5. Manual muscle testing revealed weakness in the rectus abdominis and bilateral tightness in the hip flexors and hamstring musculature (right greater than left). All other examination procedures were within normal limits.

Based on the mechanism of injury, the examination findings, and the results of the diagnostic testing, the patient was diagnosed with lumbar disk disease at the L4-L5 and L5-S1 levels with associated radiculopathy into the right lower extremity.

LINKS TO

Guide to Physical Therapist Practice* and *Athletic Training Educational Competencies

Musculoskeletal pattern 4F of the *Guide*[47] relates to the diagnosis of this patient. This pattern is described as "impaired joint mobility, motor function, muscle performance, range of motion, or reflex integrity secondary to spinal disorders." Included in the diagnostic group of this pattern is intervertebral disk disorder and the anticipated goal is "ability to perform physical tasks related to self-care, home management, community and work (job/ school/play) integration or reintegration and leisure activities using aquatic exercises."

The therapeutic exercise domain in the *Competencies*[48] refers to treatment of athletes using a variety of techniques. The teaching objectives listed under the competencies of this domain indicate that the athletic trainer, upon graduation from an accredited program, will be able to "describe indications, contraindications, theory and principles for the incorporation and application of various contemporary therapeutic exercises including aquatic therapy." Later, demonstration of aquatic therapy is emphasized.

INTERVENTION

The goals of intervention were as follows:

- Decrease pain by at least three levels on a visual analog scale at rest and with light activities of daily living (e.g., sweeping and vacuuming).
- Maintain a neutral spine position via better core strength of abdominal and gluteals during sitting and housecleaning activities.
- Adhere to recommended energy conservation techniques and posture and body mechanics during functional activities.
- Increase strength in the trunk and lower extremities.
- Eliminate pain during lower-extremity resistive testing.
- Obtain full pain-free repeated trunk flexion ROM.
- Return to safe and pain-free participation in off-season foot-

ball training, including weight training, cardiovascular conditioning, and agility drills of running and cutting.

Football contact practice was delayed until the following fall training session. Treatment was initiated on land for the first month and consisted of the following:

1. Central posterior to anterior glides from T12 through L3, progressing from grades 1 through 4 as tolerated to increase segmental mobility (see Fig. 4-8).
2. Prone on elbow positioning and prone press-ups, emphasizing extension at the upper lumbar levels by stabilizing the lower lumber levels with a mobilization belt (see Fig. 2-8).
3. Instruction in proper posture, body mechanics, and energy conservation techniques for prolonged sitting, light house cleaning, and proper lifting.
4. No lifting during activities of daily living.
5. Use of a lumbar support cushion for sitting in class and driving and instruction on the need for frequent, short standing breaks with active trunk extension.
6. Early spinal stabilization techniques, emphasizing abdominal and gluteal sets in supine and sitting and maintenance of the neutral spine position during activities of daily living.
7. Bridging activities superimposed on a neutral spine (see Fig. 12-9).
8. Gym ball activities to address spinal stabilization and core strengthening (see Figs. 12-21 to 12-23).
9. Use of ice after exercise and for pain control, as needed.

PROGRESSION

Four Weeks After Initial Examination

Toward the end of the first month, the patient's pain and weakness symptoms began to subside. However the athlete was unable to tolerate progression to more aggressive standing, strengthening, and weight-bearing activities (e.g., jogging) because of increased symptoms. Thus, a 2-week program of aquatic therapy was initiated:

1. Deep-water suspended vertical hanging with a flotation device under each axilla and 2.5-lb weights on each ankle.
2. Deep-water vertical suspended exercises with a flotation device under each axilla with the spine held in neutral with co-contraction of abdominals and gluteals, unilateral and bilateral knee to chest hip ROM exercises and hip abduction and adduction with knees extended.
3. Deep-water walking forward and backward.
4. Deep-water jogging or running forward and backward (Fig. 13-30).
5. Side lying running forward and backward.
6. Shallow-water (shoulder to chest deep) exercises with the spine held in neutral position by co-contraction of abdominals and gluteals: walking forward and backward, sidestepping while wearing aqua gloves, hamstring stretching with back against the wall (Fig. 13-15).

All of these exercises were performed under clinician supervision two times per week in the minimal pain range for the spine and lower extremities. There was no increase in peripheral symptoms. The patient also performed the exercises in an independent home exercise program an additional one to two times per week.

Six Weeks After Initial Examination

After 2 weeks of aquatic intervention, the patient reported an increase in length of time spent in sitting without pain, an increased ability to perform abdominal and gluteal co-contraction, no pain when standing in active forward flexion, and no complaints of pain into the right buttock.

Aquatic intervention was thus continued for 4 weeks more, progressing duration, repetitions, and speed of movement in the water, placing greater emphasis on abdominal and gluteal control in the neutral spine position, and increasing the excursion of movement of the trunk and lower extremities. The athlete was seen once a week by the clinician and continued with his independent exercise program an additional one or two times per week. The following exercises were added to the aquatic program:

1. Deep-water suspended vertical exercises: side sit-ups; squats (Fig. 13-22); upper-extremity breaststroke forward and backward while standing on a barbell; upper-extremity breaststroke or reciprocal arm swing (as during walking) forward and backward while sitting on a barbell or kickboard (Fig. 13-23).
2. Shallow-water exercises: forward and backward jogging interval training; running progression; plyometric directional drills with and without a step bench and superimposing a variety of arm positions and movements (Fig. 13-28); replication of running patterns and catching a football.

OUTCOMES

During the final 2 weeks of the aquatic intervention, the clinician prescribed and supervised a gradual return to lower-extremity and trunk weight training and a progression of jogging and running drills on land. At the end of the aquatic intervention, the patient had met all long-term goals and was discharged from the clinician's care. He was given guidelines for continued progression of exercises in the water to be used for cross-training with the prescribed land exercises. Parameters for safe progression of a land weight training and running drills were also provided by the clinician.

GERIATRIC Perspectives

- Exercising in water results in reduction of stresses on weight-bearing joints and is an ideal medium for rehabilitation of older adults with precautions and contraindications.[1–3] Before initiating a water program for older individuals, the clinician should recommend a medical checkup for blood pressure and other medical problems. In addition, a listing of current prescribed and over-the-counter medications (including vitamin and herbal supplements) should be obtained using the "brown bag" technique (the patient is told to place all frequently taken medications in a bag and to bring them in). Medications of particular concern are the antihypertensives and cardiac drugs that may limit the body's cardiovascular responses.
- With aging, the body's thermoregulating capacity is reduced and may limit the older individual's ability to adapt to central heat gain or loss. Furthermore, the patient's comfort, safety, and skill in the water should be evaluated. The clinician should determine the need for a life jacket or lift.[4]
- Most accidents in older adults involved in aquatic therapy and exercise occur when entering and exiting the pool and are caused by poor balance, slow recovery time after loss of balance, dizziness, and tripping over objects left at the side of the pool. Special consideration should be given to the entry ramp in regard to hand railings, nonslip surfaces, and organization of the pool side and changing areas.
- If possible, older individuals with vision problems should wear corrective lenses during the sessions. Hearing aids, however, should not be worn in the water. Thus instructions should be discussed with the patient before he or she removes the aid to enter the water.
- Older adults benefit from the socialization of group aquatic rehabilitative sessions; however, individualized therapy with qualified staff is more appropriate for frail older adults. Owing to the age-related increase in central processing time and response time, exercise instruction should be slow paced and clearly demonstrated.
- An emergency procedure should be carefully devised, discussed, and practiced with all staff involved in the pool area. In addition, the plan should be clearly outlined and posted near the designated telephone.

1. Heyneman CA, Premo DE. A "water-walkers" exercise program for the elderly. Pub Health Rep 1992;107:213–216.
2. Stevenson J, Tacia S, Thompson J, Crane C. A comparison of land and water exercise programs for older individuals. Med Sci Sports Exerc 1988;22(Suppl 20):537–540.
3. Selby-Silverstein L, Pricket N, Dougherty M, et al. Effect of aquatic therapy on temporal spatial parameters of gait in the frail elderly. Phys Ther 1999;79:S47–S51.
4. Kimble D. A case study in adaptive aquatics for the geriatric population Clin Manage 1986;6:8–11.

SUMMARY

- This chapter provided an overview of the use of aquatic therapy intervention for a client with musculoskeletal dysfunction of the spine and extremities. Several aspects of the water environment and the client must be taken into consideration before implementing aquatic techniques in a plan of care. The clinician must consider the physical properties of water each time a clinical decision is made to use an aquatic intervention for a particular patient.
- Justification for the use of the aquatic medium in a plan of care either by itself, or in conjunction with land intervention, depends on the individual needs of the client. Proper use of the physical properties of water enhances the plan of care and may speed recovery. There are many treatment options and parameters for aquatic intervention, and a careful review of the client's impairments, functional limitations, and precautions or contraindications must be undertaken before introducing specific aquatic techniques in a plan of care.
- Several types of aquatic equipment are available. Addition of any piece of aquatic equipment should have a purpose that fills a treatment need. The clinician must carefully evaluate the client's ability to safely use and tolerate a piece of equipment before adding it to the aquatic intervention program.
- The information presented in this chapter provides the clinician with guidelines, treatment options, and a knowledge base when deciding to use an aquatic environment as a component of patient's treatment plan.

PEDIATRIC *Perspectives*

- Water can be an excellent and fun exercise medium for all ages of children. To increase success with children, the clinician should focus on play with therapeutic purposes.
- The principles of specific gravity and buoyancy are excellent reasons to use aquatic therapy for support during exercise interventions used with children. Water can be used for assistance or resistance, depending on the exercise prescription. Specific benefits include weight relief, ease of movement, and success with activities. These benefits allow the child to explore movement more freely, strengthen muscles, and practice functional activities. Working in water may allow children to learn to perform movements and activities too difficult to accomplish on land.[1,2]
- Aquatic therapy offers children opportunities for social interaction and may help promote development of independence and a positive body image.[3] Some children (sinkers and nonswimmers) may need floatation assistance for safety and stability during aquatic exercise, depending on their height and the depth of the water. Be careful when using water wings, because the buoyancy is lost if the child's shoulder musculature fatigues.[2]
- If the pool is too deep for a child to touch the bottom, a submerged table or step can be used to adjust water depth for appropriate levels for exercise. Alternatively, the child could stand on the thighs of the clinician, who stands in a partially squatted position.[2]
- Aquatic therapy can be used for both rehabilitation and general exercise for pediatric patients who have a variety of diagnoses, including cerebral palsy, spina bifida, traumatic brain injury, Waardenburg syndrome,[1] and orthopedic dysfunction.[3] It is an excellent choice for children with juvenile rheumatoid arthritis for treatment of both strength and flexibility impairments.[4,5] Water is also an excellent medium for general exercise in this same population because joints are supported, compressed, and protected. Aquatic exercise has been described as an appropriate and safe intervention for children with osteogenesis imperfecta.
- Be sure to monitor water temperature when children are participating in aquatic exercise. Extremes of temperature may be difficult for children to manage owing to their less efficient thermoregulatory systems.
- All children participating in aquatic exercise must be carefully supervised by a qualified individual. Most aquatic therapy for children is one on one rather than in groups. Pool-side charts and pictures help children remember the motions of the exercises.[2] Aquatic exercise may begin as early as 6 months of age to facilitate weight bearing and supported and assisted active exercise.[4]

1. Duval R, Roberts P. Aquatic exercise therapy: the effects on an adolescent with Waardenburg's syndrome. Phys Ther Case Rep 1999;2:77–82.
2. Styer-Acevedo JL. Aquatic rehabilitation of the pediatric client. In: R Ruoti, P Morris, A Cole, eds. Aquatic rehabilitation. Philadelphia: Lippincott, 1997:151–172.
3. Campion M. Hydrotherapy in pediatrics. Gaithersburg, MD: Aspen Systems, 1985.
4. Campbell SK. Pediatric physical therapy. Philadelphia: Saunders, 1995.
5. Wright FV, Smith E. Physical therapy management of the child and adolescent with juvenile rheumatoid arthritis. In: JM Walker, A Helewa, eds. Physical therapy in arthritis. Philadelphia: Saunders, 1996:211–244.

REFERENCES

1. Irion JM. Historical overview of aquatic rehabilitation. In: R Ruoti, P Morris, A Cole, eds. Aquatic rehabilitation. Philadelphia: Lippincott, 1997:3–14.
2. Wilson JD, Buffa AJ, eds. College physics. 3rd ed. Englewood Cliffs , NJ: Prentice Hall, 1997.
3. Haralson K. Therapeutic pool programs. Clin Manage 1986;5: 10–17.
4. Becker BE. Aquatic physics. In: R Ruoti, P Morris, A Cole, eds. Aquatic rehabilitation. Philadelphia: Lippincott, 1997:15–23.
5. Bloomfield J, Fricker P, Fitch K. Textbook of science and medicine in sport. Champaign, IL: Human Kinetics, 1992.
6. Skinner AR, Thomson AM. Duffield's exercise in water. 3rd ed. Philadelphia: Bailliere Tindall, 1989:4–46.
7. Harrison R, Bulstrode S. Percentage weight bearing during partial immersion in the hydrotherapy pool. Physiother Practice 1987;3:60–63.
8. Harrison RA, Hillman M, Bulstrode S. Loading of the lower limb when walking partially immersed: implications for clinical practice. Physiotherapy 1992;78:164–166.
9. Becker BE. Biophysiologic aspects of hydrotherapy. In: BE Becker, AJ Cole, eds. Comprehensive aquatic therapy. Boston: Butterworth-Heinemann, 1997:17–48.
10. Genuario SE, Vegso J. The use of a swimming pool in the rehabilitation and reconditioning of athletic injuries. Contemp Orthop 1990;20:81–397.
11. Butts NK, Tucker M, Smith R. Maximal responses to treadmill and deep water running in high school female cross country runners. Res Q Exer Sport 1990;62:236–239.
12. Christie JL, Sheldahl LM, Tristani FE, et al. Cardiovascular reg-

ulation during head-out water immersion exercise. J Appl Physiol 1990;69:657–664.
13. Frangolias DD, Rhodes EC. Metabolic responses and mechanisms during water immersion running and exercise. Sports Med 1996;1:38–53.
14. Ritchie SE, Hopkins WG. The intensity of exercise in deep water running. Int J Sports Med 1991;27–29.
15. Wilder RP, Brennan DK. Physiological responses to deep water running in athletes. Sports Med 1993;16:374–380.
16. Cole AJ, Moschetti M, Eagleston TA, Stratton SA. Spine pain: aquatic rehabilitation strategies. In: BE Becker, AJ Cole, eds. Comprehensive aquatic therapy. Boston: Butterworth-Heinemann, 1997:73–101.
17. Cirullo, JA. Considerations for pool programming and implementation. In: JA Cirullo, ed. Orthopaedic physical therapy clinics of North America. Philadelphia: Saunders, 1994:95–110.
18. Cureton KJ. Physiologic responses to water exercise. In: R Ruoti, P Morris, A Cole, eds. Aquatic rehabilitation. Philadelphia: Lippincott, 1997:39–56.
19. Choukroun ML, Varene P. Adjustments in oxygen transport during head-out immersion in water at different temperatures. J Appl Physiol 1990;68:1475–1480.
20. Thein JM, Brody LT. Aquatic-based rehabilitation and training for the elite athlete. J Orthop Sports Phys Ther 1998;27:32–41.
21. Sheldahl EM, Buskirk ER, Loomis JL, et al. Effects of exercise in cool water on body weight loss. Int J Obesity. 1982;6:2942.
22. Cole AJ, Eagleston RE, Moschetti M, et al. Spine pain: aquatic rehabilitation strategies. J Back Musculoskel Rehab 1994;4:273–286.
23. Thein L, McNamara C. Aquatic rehabilitation of patients with musculoskeletal conditions of the extremities. In: R Ruoti, P Morris, A Cole, eds. J Aquatic rehabilitation. Philadelphia: Lippincott, 1997:59–83.
24. Babb R, Simelson-Warr A. Manual techniques of the lower extremities in aquatic physical therapy. J Aquatic Phys Ther 1996;4:9–15.
25. Schrepfer RW, Babb RW. Manual techniques of the shoulder in aquatic physical therapy. J Aquatic Phys Ther 1998;6:11–15.
26. Cirullo JA. Aquatic physical therapy approaches for the spine. In: JA Cirullo, ed. Orthopaedic physical therapy clinics of North America. Philadelphia: Saunders, 1994:179–208.
27. Mickel C, Shepherd J. Towards the localization of the lumbar postero-antero mobilization technique in water in the treatment of low back pain: a clinical note. Manual Ther 1998:162–163.
28. Bandy WD, Irion JM. The effect of time on static stretch on the flexibility of the hamstring muscles. Phys Ther 1994;74:845–849.
29. McNamara CA. Aquatic spinal stabilization exercises. J Aquatic Phys Ther 1997;5:11–17.
30. Cercone K. Dynamic aquatic therapy for the low back. Aquatic Phys Ther Rep 1995;4:6–10.
31. Konlian C. Aquatic therapy: making a wave in the treatment of low back injuries. Orthop Nurs 1999;18(1):11–20.
32. Saal J. Nonoperative treatment of herniated lumbar intervertebral disc with radiculopathy. Spine 1989;14:431–437.
33. Thomas CL ed. Taber's cyclopedic medical dictionary. 18th ed. Philadelphia: Davis, 1993.
34. Chu D. Jumping into plyometrics. Champaign, IL: Leisure, 1992.
35. Coyle EF, Hemmert Mk, Coggan AR. Effects of detraining on cardiovascular responses to exercise: role of blood volume. J Appl Physiol 1986;60;95–99.
36. Coyle EF, Martin WH, Simacore DR, et al. Time course of loss of adaptations after stopping prolonged intense endurance training. J Appl Physiol 1984;57:1857–1864.
37. Eyestone ED, Fellingham G, George J, et al. Effect of water running and cycling on maximum oxygen consumption and 2 mile run performance. Am J Sports Med 1993;21:41–44.
38. Bushman BA, Flynn MG, Andres FF, et al. Effect of four week deep water run training on running performance. Med Sci Sports Exer 1997;29:694–699.
39. Wilber RL, Moffatt RJ, Scott BE, et al. Influence of water run training on the maintenance of aerobic performance. Med Sci Sports Exer 1996;28:1056–1062.
40. Quinn TJ, Sedory DR, Fisher BS. Physiological effects of deep water running following a land based training program. Res Q Exer Sports 1994;65:386–389.
41. Frangolias DD, Rhodes EC. Maximum and ventilatory threshold responses to treadmill and water immersion running. Med Sci Sports Exer 1995;27:1007–1013.
42. Michaud TJ, Brennan DK, Wilder RP. Aquarunning and gains in cardiorespiratory fitness. Strength Condition Res 1995;9:78–84.
43. Bushman B. Athletes propel deep water running to prominence. Biomechanics. 1999;32:43–49.
44. Wilder RP, Brennan DK. Techniques of water running. In: BE Becker, AJ Cole, eds. Comprehensive aquatic therapy. Boston: Butterworth-Heinemann, 1997:123–134.
45. Wilder RP, Brennan DK, Schotte DE. A standard measure for exercise prescription for aqua running. Am J Sports Med 1993;21: 45–48.
46. Stephens-Bogard K. A dip in the pool. Adv Directors Rehab 1999;8:37–40.
47. American Physical Therapy Association. Guide to physical therapist practice, second edition. Phys Ther 2001;81:1–768.
48. National Athletic Trainers' Association. Athletic training educational competencies. 3rd ed. Dallas: NATA, 1999.

CHAPTER 14

Functional Progression: Lower Extremity

Steven R. Tippett, PhD, MS, PT, SCS, ATC
Michael L. Voight, DHSc, PT, OCS, SCS, ATC

Barbara Hoogenboom, PT, SCS, ATC (Case Study 3)
Reta Zabel, PhD, PT, GCS (Case Study 4)

Rehabilitating injured individuals so they can resume preinjury activity levels is both a science and an art. Intervention to regain preinjury function must begin promptly after injury and proceed until the patient is once again performing at the highest possible level. Therapeutic measures must be incorporated that sufficiently prepare the healing tissue for the inherent demands of a given activity; but just as important, these interventions must take place at the appropriate time during the healing process. A rehabilitation program that does not adequately address the function of the injured tissue will result in inadequate physiologic loading, minimizing the readiness of the tissue to return to activity. Therapeutic intervention too late or too early in the rehabilitation program may predispose the patient to reinjury.

Functional progression is a series of graduated activities that maximize the individual's readiness to return to activities. The science of functional progression entails functional tissue loading. The art of functional progression involves tissue loading in an activity-specific fashion. This chapter presents the scientific basis of functional progression and offers guidelines for progression and examples of program implementation after macrotraumatic and microtraumatic injuries.

The clinician routinely establishes treatment goals, which are addressed during the formal rehabilitation program. The goals are directed at pain, swelling, loss of muscle strength, and loss of joint range of motion (ROM). Simply satisfying these clinical goals does not ensure that the patient is ready to return to work or athletic competition. Reducing pain and swelling and increasing strength and ROM must be accompanied by specific activities that are interjected in the treatment program in a safe and timely manner.[1] After satisfying the clinical goals and before being released from the formal treatment program, the patient must be challenged in specific activities to help ensure his or her readiness for work or competition. This challenge is where the functional progression program comes into play.

Functional progression is defined as a series of specific, basic movement patterns that are graduated according to difficulty of the skill and the patient's tolerance.[2] The concept of functional progression was first introduced as a formal strengthening and agility program for West Point cadets who had undergone knee injury.[3] As functional progression was embraced by rehabilitation team members, the typical program became more activity-specific and took into consideration the psychological ramifications of the injured patient undergoing rehabilitation.[4,5]

■ *Scientific Basis*

RATIONALE

Just like any component of the rehabilitation program, functional progression must be based on sound scientific rationale. Whether the patient has sustained a fracture, sprain, or strain, the functional progression program imparts needed stress to the healing tissue. According to Wolf's law, after a bone injury, the bone remodels and adapts its material properties to the mechanical demands placed on it.[6] The same principles apply to soft tissue healing. In the animal model, scar tissue is fragile for the first 4 to 5 days after injury owing to a relative lack of significant extracellular matrix. Scar tissue rapidly increases in bulk from day 5 to day 21 via fibroplasia. The fibroplasia phase of wound healing is characterized by increased collagen deposition, which peaks approximately 14 days after injury. Most of the newly synthesized collagen is type III, which is thought to be responsible for early stabilization of the developing collagen meshwork. Small, closely packed, randomly assigned collagen fibers are present before 21 days after injury. Loose fascicle formation is present at day 14, and interlacing fascicles are seen by day 21. At this time, the predominant collagen is type I, which is important to the long-term properties of the extracellular matrix.[7]

Stress to the randomly assigned collagen fibers results in fiber orientation along these specific lines of stress. For example, stress applied to healing medial collateral ligaments (MCLs) in rats has been shown to result in increased tensile strength and decreased joint laxity compared to nonexercised animals.[8] Stress designed to increase tension within healing MCLs in rabbits results in increased total collagen and more longitudinal orientation of collagen fibers than in a control group.[9] Prolonged immobilization, on the other hand, has been shown to decrease ultimate load and energy-absorbing capacity of the bone–ligament interface of the MCL in rabbits.[10]

Applying this basic scientific rationale in the clinical setting, a series of college football players with complete tears of the MCL of the knee treated with early protected motion and physical therapy were able to return to full-contact activities in an average of 9 weeks. Average follow-up at 46 months revealed 85% of the athletes with good or excellent results. Approximately 40% of the knees revealed no side-to-side valgus laxity, and the remaining 60% of the knees demonstrated less than 5 mm of valgus laxity.[11] Mobilization and other forms of short-term stress to healing tissue are effective in localizing stress to target tissues.[9]

SPECIFIC ADAPTATIONS TO IMPOSED DEMAND

Stress to healing tissue must be activity-specific and must be applied in a timely manner. This is the point at which the art of functional progression enters the picture. The specific adaptations to imposed demands (SAID) principle governs the type of stress that must be applied to the healing injury.[4] To maximize the efficacy of the functional progression program, activities must mirror the demands that will be placed on the patient once he or she returns to work or competition. An intimate knowledge of the activity and, more important, the specific duties required of the patient in a given environment are necessary prerequisites for a successful program.

Obviously, a football player has different physical demands than a baseball player, an ice skater has different demands than a hockey player, and a soccer player has different demands than a wrestler. When prescribing and administering a functional progression program for any of these patients, a good working knowledge of the specific activity is an absolute prerequisite. The same can be said for prescribing and advancing the functional progression program for any athlete involved in any sporting activity. It is the duty of the rehabilitation professional to understand the specifics of a sport well enough to confidently prescribe the functional progression program. If the clinician does not possess this knowledge, it is incumbent on him or her to identify and secure the resources that will provide this information. Often, the athlete or coach is a valuable resources when formulating the functional progression program.

Taking this notion one step further, the rehabilitation professional must also possess a thorough understanding of the athlete's specific roles in a given sport. For example, in football the demands on an offensive lineman are different from those on a defensive back; thus the functional progression program for each of these football players must address the individual demands. The lineman must be able to assume a down position and is involved with run blocking, pass blocking, and double-team blocking on the line of scrimmage. On the other hand, the defensive back generally engages in action away from the line of scrimmage and is involved with back pedaling, cutting, jumping, and sprinting. It is clear why the clinician must seek a depth of knowledge regarding the sport-specific responsibilities of the patient.

According to the SAID principle, for the functional progression program to be complete, stress on the healing tissue must reflect the demands of a given activity. The physical demands on the patient must be analyzed globally and then broken down by level of difficulty and then progressed according to the patient's tolerance. Physical demands consist of the gross fundamental movements required for a given task as well as specific tissue function. Examples of fundamental movements include stationary positions, such as standing, squatting, and kneeling. Stationary efforts may entail open-chain or closed-chain activities and may take place with both feet on the ground (bilateral support activities) or with only one weight-bearing lower extremity (unilateral support activities). Functional requirements also include dynamic body segment movements, such as jumping (bilateral nonsupport) and hopping (unilateral nonsupport), and may involve straight-plane or mulitplane activities.

Examples of tissue function are the role of the ligament as a primary or secondary stabilizer; the role of the muscle in providing dynamic restraint to the injured joint as a prime mover, synergist, or antagonist; and the role of the injured muscle as primarily generating concentric, eccentric, or isometric contractions. Activity-specific static and dynamic ROM along with flexibility demands must also be taken into consideration when designing the functional progression program. Finally, for activities to be functional in terms of energy requirements (anaerobic or aerobic), the duration of the drills must be sport-specific.

NEUROMUSCULAR CONTROL

Observing the coordinated and integrated movements of the triple jump, a dismount from the parallel bars, or dribbling a basketball around a screen for a jump shot, it is obvious that there must be something more to functional progression than breaking down skills step by step and hoping for skill integration. Sporting activities are complex movements requiring not only a variety of movements and positions but a smooth transition from one position or movement to another. In the competitive environment, the athlete does not routinely think about each of the basic movement patterns required to perform complex sport skills. As the athlete becomes more proficient in a given sport, the basic skills became second nature. In other words, the athlete is able to perform these activities at a subconscious level. Therefore, progression through a functional program means that primitive skills in the program are integrated from the conscious to the subconscious level.

A patient's ability to function at the subconscious level involves integration of incoming information from the environment, which involves neuromuscular control. To reestablish neuromuscular control after injury, the functional progression program must incorporate activities that entail balance, proprioception, coordination, power, speed, and agility.[12–16] Neuromuscular control is the motor response to sensory information from the environment and is under the influence of four crucial elements: proprioception and kinesthetic awareness, functional motor patterns, dynamic joint stability, and reactive neuromuscular control.[17] Lower-extremity functional progression activities in the closed-kinetic chain facilitate proprioceptive and kinesthetic re-education of the weight-bearing joints. Functional motor patterns are the heart and soul of functional progression, beginning at the conscious level and progressing to the subconscious.

Reactive neuromuscular training is an example of a program designed to restore dynamic stability and enhance cognitive appreciation of the joint's position and movement of the joint after it is injured. The design and implementation of this type of training program are critical for restoring the synergy and synchrony of muscle-firing patterns required for dynamic stability and fine motor control, thereby restoring both functional stability about the joint and enhanced motor-control skills.[18]

Dynamic stability is initially stressed via bilateral support activities in a single plane as the patient produces self-generated oscillations that create a shift in the body's center of gravity. Shifting of the center of gravity results in the upper body being pulled in a given direction over the fixed lower extremities. The patient is required to generate lower-extremity isometric contractions to offset this weight shift and thus remain in a stable position. These oscillating techniques for isometric stabilization aid in the integration of visual, mechanoreceptor, and equilibrium reaction by using isometric contractions of target musculature offsetting the shift in the center of gravity in a single plane or in multiple planes.

The reactive neuromuscular training program can be progressed from slow- to fast-speed activities, from low- to high-force activities, and from controlled to uncontrolled activities. Initially, these exercises should evoke a balance reaction or weight shift in the lower extremities and ultimately progress to a movement pattern.[18] Examples of specific reactive neuromuscular-training techniques are presented later in this chapter.

BENEFITS OF FUNCTIONAL PROGRESSION

The functional progression program provides benefits to many individuals involved in the rehabilitation program. Of course, the program provides discernible physical benefits for the patient, but it also provides less tangible psychological benefits for the injured individual. A well-devised and efficiently implemented program is also rewarding for the rehabilitation professional and those interested in the care of the patient (coach, parent, employer, etc).

Physical Benefits for the Patient

The physical benefits of a functional progression program can be inferred from the earlier discussion of the underlying scientific principles. Specifically, the program promotes optimal healing of the injured tissue and maximum postinjury performance, which occur only when the program is exactly as its name implies, functional. Loading tissue in a controlled fashion promotes tissue healing. Applying loads in a graduated fashion according to the specific demands of the healing tissue promotes organization of collagen.

For example, after a first-degree proximal hamstring strain in a softball player, active-assisted hip flexion and knee extension to regain ROM and isometric, isotonic, or isokinetic hip extension and knee flexion to regain strength are certainly appropriate interventions for addressing the athlete's impairment. Without focusing on deceleration activities of the hip and knee via eccentric muscle contraction in the closed-kinetic-chain, however, specific tissue function will not be dealt with. Without stressing a return to running in the functional progression, the athlete risks reinjury the first time he or she is required to run in a competitive situation. Stressing the healing hamstring muscles according to functional demands in the sporting activity facilitates optimal healing. Functional demands in this case means two joint eccentric muscle contractions for lower extremity deceleration.

Functional progression also assists in maximizing postinjury performance. By progressing through functional skills during the rehabilitation program, the athlete should be fully prepared to resume sports participation. An ideal functional progression program is one in which the athlete has had the opportunity to complete all activities required for competition before actually returning to the competitive environment. For a softball player with a hamstring strain, the return to a running program should entail not only straight ahead sprinting but also base running and positional running requirements. After progressing through the sport-specific running sequence, the athlete should be ready to resume all competitive softball running requirements.

Psychological Benefits for the Patient

Benefits of a sound functional progression program for the patient are not just physical in nature. The program also provides psychological benefits to the recuperating patient. After injury, the athlete frequently undergoes a period of anxiety as a result of changes in daily routine, many of which the individual is not able to control. Before the injury, the athlete was accustomed to daily practice and competition schedules. The athlete was used to daily interactions with teammates, coaches, and other personnel. After injury, these routines are altered, which may result in mood disturbances. Such mood changes have been observed to occur within 24 hr after injury and have been noted to dissipate as successful recovery progresses.[19]

Functional progression can also assist in minimizing the stress of being injured. The rehabilitation professional depends on information from the patient when designing an effective program, making the client an active participant in his or her own rehabilitation program. During the functional progression program, the patient is given physical tasks to accomplish. By becoming an active, involved participant and realizing genuine progress at each step, the client regains some of the control that was lost a result of being injured. Functional progression also enhances the patient's self-confidence. As progress is achieved through the functional progression program, the patient is provided with a sense of accomplishment. As these accomplishments build on one another, the patient becomes more confident in specific physical abilities, which in turn provide a foundation for more difficult activities in the functional progression program.

During the rehabilitation process, patients who demonstrate positive psychological factors such as positive self-talk, goal setting, and mental imagery, attained desired rehabilitation goals more quickly than patients who do not demonstrate those factors.[20] Adherence to a rehabilitation program has been linked not only with the effectiveness of the program but also with social support, goal and task mastery orientation, self-motivation, high pain tolerance, and the ability to adapt to scheduling and environmental conditions.[21] Goal setting and goal accomplishment are common themes to successful programs. A functional progression program is made up of a series of physical tasks for the patient to conquer, and each step in the program is a goal for the patient to attain. The rehabilitation professional should work with the client to set realistic goals and prescribe a functional progression program to satisfy these goals. As the patient meets each goal, his or her self-confidence is advanced. As final functional progression activities take place in a group setting, a sense of once again belonging is a positive psychological benefit for the patient.

Benefits for the Rehabilitation Professional

Almost immediately after an injury, the patient and everyone involved with the patient (coach, spouse, parent, employer) want to know the answer to one important question: When will the patient be able to work or play again? Functional progression can provide all of these individuals, as well as the rehabilitation professional, a gauge of progress. With an idea of preinjury functional demands, the clinician is able to design a functional progression program that provides an indirect assessment of where the patient is at in the rehabilitation program and where the patient needs to go. The patient and concerned individuals should be able to visualize the functional progression program on a continuum, be able to see where the patient is along that continuum, and thus have an effective estimate of the patient's progress in his or her rehabilitation efforts.

■ Clinical Guidelines

Before initiating weight-bearing activities in the lower-extremity functional progression program, certain prerequisites must be met, including control of swelling and pain, adequate ROM and flexibility to perform the desired activities, adequate strength to perform the desired activities, and sufficiently healed tissue that can tolerate the stress of the desired activities. Care should also be taken to ensure sufficient proximal (spine and pelvis) strength, ROM, and flexibility. Soft tissue healing time constraints depend on the severity of injury. The rehabilitation professional should have a thorough knowledge of the status of the injury and how healing is progressing. Indications that activities may be overzealous and exceeding healing time constraints include increases swelling, pain, abnormal gait, substitution in movement, loss or plateau in ROM or strength, and documented increase in laxity of a healing ligament.

The challenge of returning an athlete safely to competition in the shortest time possible is made inherently more difficult because of the very nature of therapeutic exercise. As indicated, inadequate stress to healing tissue results in poor preparation for the return to competition. On the other hand, too much stress is also counterproductive. Dye's [22] "envelope of function" is an excellent way to conceptualize the advancement of the functional progression program. He described the envelope of function as the "range of load that can be applied across an individual joint in a given period of time without supraphysiologic overload or structural failure." Activity can be described in terms of applied loads and frequency of loading. High-loading activities can be performed for only a short amount of time before exceeding the envelope of function. Low-loading activities can be performed for a longer time; however, a finite frequency for lighter loading also exists before exceeding the envelope.

A practical example of the envelope of function is the progression from bilateral nonsupport activities (jumping) to unilateral nonsupport activities (hopping) for a patient with an anterior cruciate ligament injury. As the patient progresses from jumping to hopping, the load increases; thus to avoid exceeding the envelope, the total duration of exercise should be decreased appropriately. Overuse injuries can be prevented by scheduling periods of reduced activity during a buildup in activities.[7] As noted, the signs of excessive loading are an increase in swelling or pain, a loss in ROM or strength, and an increase in laxity of the healing ligament. One problem is that the health-care professional does not know that the therapeutic activities are too aggressive until after the signs of excessive loading are seen. So how does the rehabilitation professional progress the program? When does the program need to be slowed down? Perhaps the best answer to these critical questions lies in the staging of overuse injury.

Healthy tissue is in dynamic balance: Bone is constantly being deposited and reabsorbed, collagen is synthesized and undergoes catabolism, and injured soft tissue undergoes degeneration and regeneration. When these processes are in equilibrium, all is well. When bone resorption exceeds deposition or when soft tissue degeneration exceeds regeneration, normal equilibrium is disrupted. One of the symptoms of musculoskeletal disequilibrium is pain. Several authors have classified overuse injuries into stages based on pain before, during, and after activity.[23,24] In these staging systems, pain gradually increases to the point at which performance is negatively affected. As a general guideline, activities that do not cause pain during exertion and activities that cause pain for less than 2 hr after exertion are allowed. Pain during activity that negatively affects performance, pain that persists for more than 2 hr after activity, pain that affects activities of daily living, and pain at night indicate that activity restriction is required (Table 14-1).

For example, consider a grade 1 hamstring strain in a softball player. Three-quarter-speed sprinting from a stationary start was noted to cause minimal discomfort after the workout that subsided in less than 30 min after termination of activity. Full-speed sprinting from a stationary start caused no pain during the activity but did cause localized pain in the proximal posterior thigh for 6 hr after the workout. Based on the athlete's response to full-speed sprinting, the clinician determined that the activities were too aggressive and that the speeds needed to be decreased.

The clinician should now have a good understanding of the basics of the functional progression process. Each program must be individualized based on the injury and the demands placed on the patient. The following sequences and case studies will provide a better understanding of the depth that the clinician must consider when prescribing a functional progression program. The case studies also introduce the concept of specific tissue loading. These studies are intended to provide a template for clinician reference and are not intended to be prescriptive or all inclusive. The ideal functional program is one developed by the clinician in conjunction with the individual athlete in a specific setting.

TABLE 14-1 Classification System for the Effect of Pain on Athletic Performance[a]

Level	Description of Pain	Sports Activity
1	No pain	Normal
2	Pain only with extreme exertion	Normal
3	Pain with extreme exertion 1–2 hr after activity	Normal or slightly decreased
4	Pain during and after any vigorous activity	Somewhat decreased
5	Pain during activity that forces termination	Markedly decreased
6	Pain during daily activities	Unable to perform

[a]Reprinted with permission from Fyfe I, Stanish WD. The use of eccentric training and stretching in the treatment and prevention of tendon injuries. Clin Sports Med 1992;11:601–624.

Techniques

This section presents some of the more common functional progression activities used to train patients. As indicated, the key to an efficient and successful functional progression program is in the careful progression of easier tasks followed by more difficult tasks. Therefore, this section emphasizes suggestions for the progression of a number of activities referred to as "sequences." Note that the patient does not necessarily perform each sequence independently of other sequences. Several types of sequences may overlap. For example, in one exercise session, the athlete may be sprinting full speed forward in a straight plane but performing cutting activities at only half speed. Furthermore, not every sequence presented is used for all athletes. The extent to which each sequence is emphasized depends on the sport and the specific position the client plays within the sport.

REACTIVE NEUROMUSCULAR TRAINING SEQUENCE

Reactive neuromuscular training can be as simple as static control with little or no visible movement or as complex as a dynamic plyometric response (chapter 9) requiring explosive acceleration, deceleration, or change in direction. Early activities include single-leg stance, uniplaner activities in which the patient pulls on exercise tubing while maintaining balance, and isometric activities that include minimal joint motion. The patient can be progressed from isometric activities to exercises that used controlled concentric and eccentric contractions through a full ROM, such as the squat and lunge. Finally, ballistic and impact activities, such as resisted walking, running, and bounding, can be introduced in the advanced stages of rehabilitation.[18]

Single-Leg Stance

The client should stand bearing full weight with equal distribution on the affected and unaffected lower extremity. Placing a 6- to 8-in. step stool under the unaffected lower extremity will cause a weight shift to the affected lower extremity, placing greater emphasis on the affected side. At the same time, the unaffected extremity can still assist with balance reactions (Fig. 14-1).

The exercise can be made more difficult by using an unstable surface, which will also increase the demands on the mechanoreceptor system. Single or multidirec-

FIGURE 14-1 **Single leg stance on step stool.**

PURPOSE: Reflex stabilization, using static compression of the articular surfaces to facilitate isometric contraction of muscles of the lower extremity.

POSITION: Standing, feet shoulder's width apart (assume left side is involved extremity).

PROCEDURE: Place uninvolved extremity on step stool, forcing greater weight shift to the involved side.

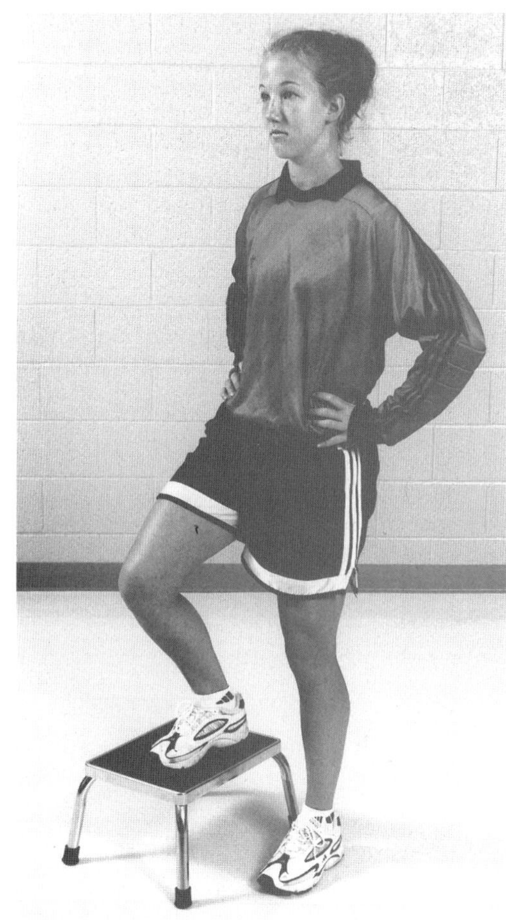

tional rocker devices or bolsters assist the progression to the next phase (Fig. 14-2).

Uniplaner Exercise

Exercise tubing can be used for uniplaner exercise, by pulling two pieces of tubing toward the body and returning the tubing to the start position in a smooth, rhythmical fashion with increasing speed. Changes in direction (anterior, posterior, medial, or lateral weight shifting) create specific planar demands. Each technique is given a name that is related to the weight shift produced by the applied tension. The body reacts to the weight shift with an equal and opposite stabilization response. *Therefore, the exercise is named for the cause and not the effect.*

During performance of these exercises, the athlete should make little or no movement the lower extremity. If movement is noted, resistance should be decreased to achieve the desired stability. Uniplaner activities are described in Figures 14-3 to 14-6.

Multiplanar Exercises

The basic exercise program can be progressed to multiplaner activity by combining the proprioceptive neuromuscular facilitation (PNF) diagonal patterns and chop and lift patterns of the upper extremities (Fig. 14-7). The patterns from the unaffected and affected sides cause a multiplaner stress that requires isometric stabilization. The client is forced to automatically integrate the isometric responses that were developed in the previous uniplaner exercises.

Squat

The squat is used because it employs symmetrical movement of the lower extremities, which allows the affected lower extremity to benefit from the visual and proprioceptive feedback from the unaffected lower extremity. A chair or bench can be used as a ROM block (range-limiting device) if necessary. The block may minimize fear and increase safety (Figs. 14-8 to 14-10).

FIGURE 14-2 **Single leg stance on unstable surface.**

PURPOSE: Reflex stabilization, using static compression of the articular surfaces to facilitate isometric contraction of muscles of the lower extremity.

POSITION: Standing on involved extremity (left) on bolster.

PROCEDURE: Patient maintains balance while standing on bolster.

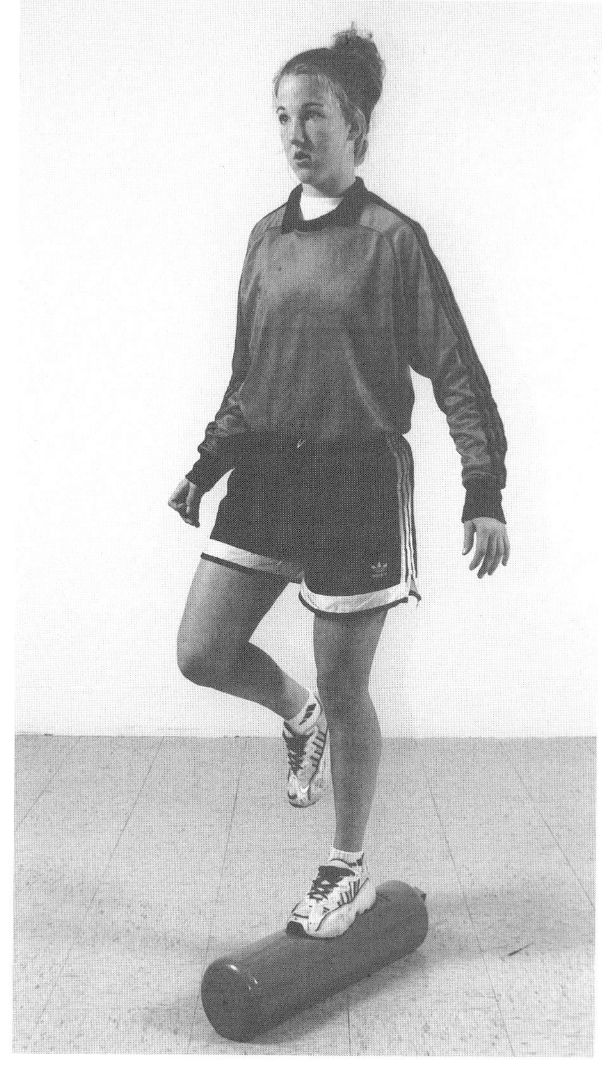

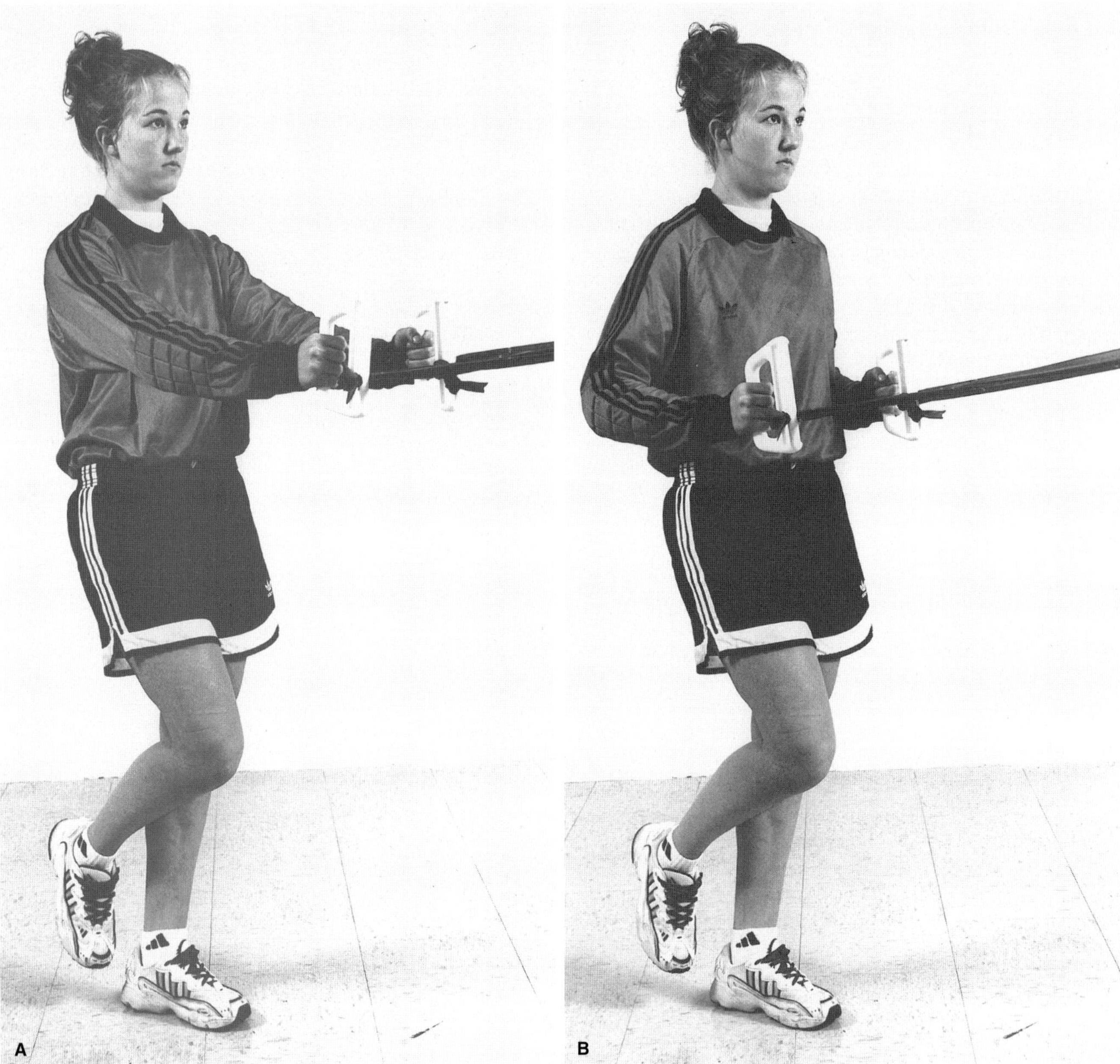

FIGURE 14-3 Uniplanar anterior weight shift.

PURPOSE: Static stabilization, demonstrating stability required to achieve motor learning and control in a single plane of motion.

POSITION: Standing on involved extremity (left) facing the tubing.

PROCEDURE: Patient holds tubing in both hands (panel A). Maintaining balance on involved extremity, patient pulls the tubing toward body in a smooth motion (panel B). This positioning causes a forward weight shift, which is stabilized with an isometric counterforce consisting of hip extension, knee extension, and ankle plantar flexion.

FIGURE 14-4 **Uniplanar posterior weight shift.**

PURPOSE: Static stabilization, demonstrating stability required to achieve motor learning and control in a single plane of motion.

POSITION: Standing on involved extremity (left) with back to the tubing.

PROCEDURE: Maintaining balance on involved extremity, patient moves tubing away from body in a smooth motion. This positioning causes a posterior weight shift, which is stabilized by an isometric counter force consisting of hip flexion, knee flexion, and ankle dorsiflexion.

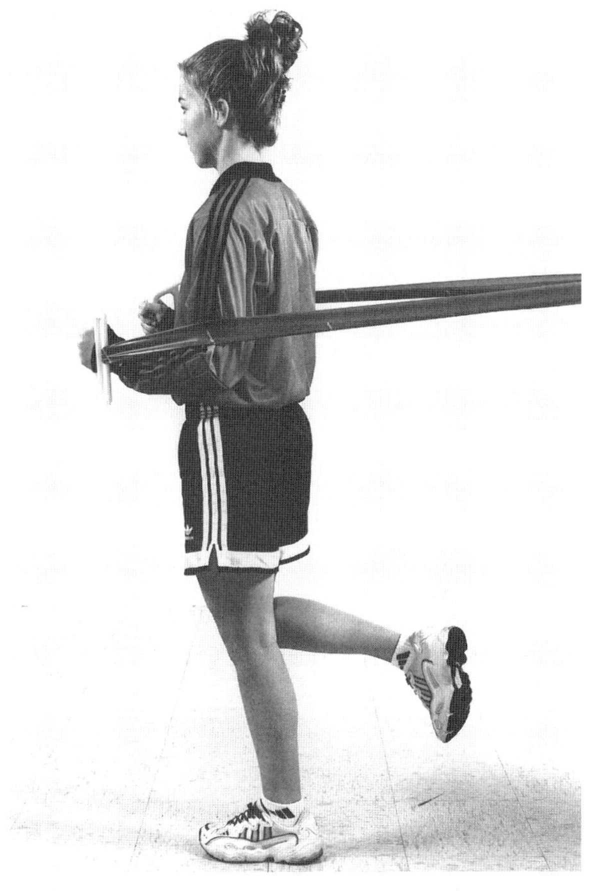

FIGURE 14-5 **Uniplanar medial weight shift.**

PURPOSE: Static stabilization, demonstrating stability required to achieve motor learning and control in a single plane of motion.

POSITION: Standing on involved extremity (left) with uninvolved extremity closest to the tubing.

PROCEDURE: Maintaining balance on involved extremity, patient pulls tubing with one hand in front of body and other hand behind body in a smooth motion. This positioning causes a medial weight shift, which is stabilized with an isometric counter-force consisting of hip adduction, knee co-contraction, and ankle inversion.

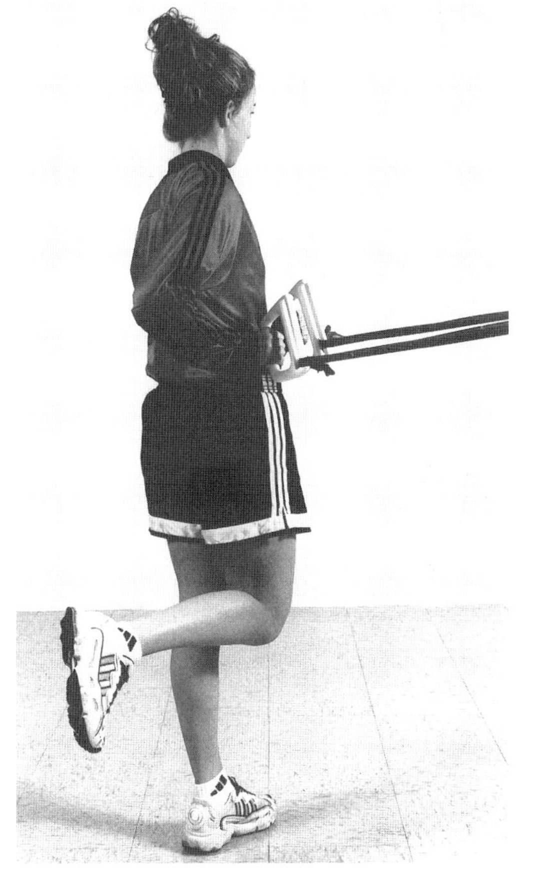

FIGURE 14-6 **Uniplanar lateral weight shift.**

PURPOSE: Static stabilization, demonstrating stability required to achieve motor learning and control in a single plane of motion.

POSITION: Standing on involved extremity (left) with involved extremity closest to tubing.

PROCEDURE: Maintaining balance on involved extremity, patient pulls tubing with one hand in front of body and other hand behind body in a smooth motion. The lateral shift is stabilized with an isometric counter-force consisting of hip abduction, knee co-contraction, and ankle eversion.

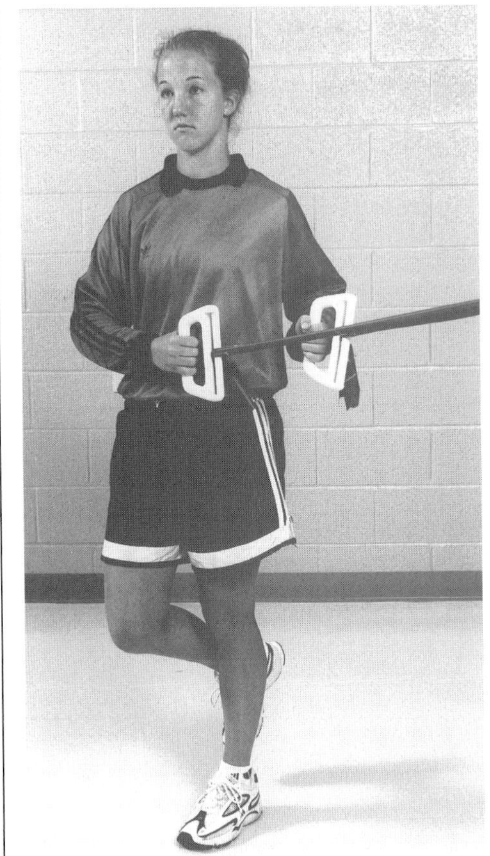

FIGURE 14-7 **Multiplanar PNF lift technique.**

PURPOSE: Static stabilization, demonstrating stability required to achieve motor learning and control in multiple planes of motion.

POSITION: Standing on involved extremity (left).

PROCEDURE: Maintaining balance on involved extremity, patient performs PNF lift technique.

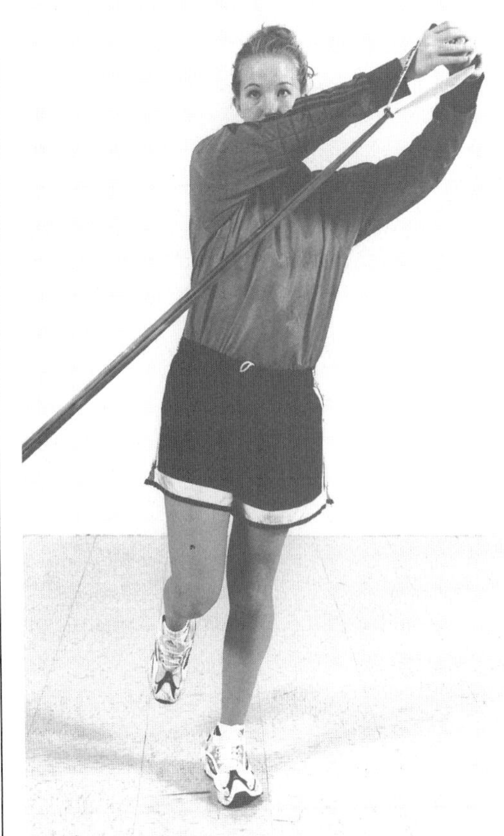

FIGURE 14-8 **Squat: anterior weight shift (assisted).**

PURPOSE: Stimulation of dynamic postural response, facilitating concentric and eccentric contractions.

POSITION: Standing, facing tubing, with belt around waist and feet shoulder's width apart (assume involved side is left lower extremity).

PROCEDURE: Patient squats to the height of the chair in a smooth, controlled motion, and then returns to standing. The anterior weight shift facilitates the descent phase of the squat; the hip flexors, knee flexors, and ankle dorsiflexors are load dynamically with eccentric contractions during the return to standing. This activity is great for retraining shock absorption activities that occur during landing.

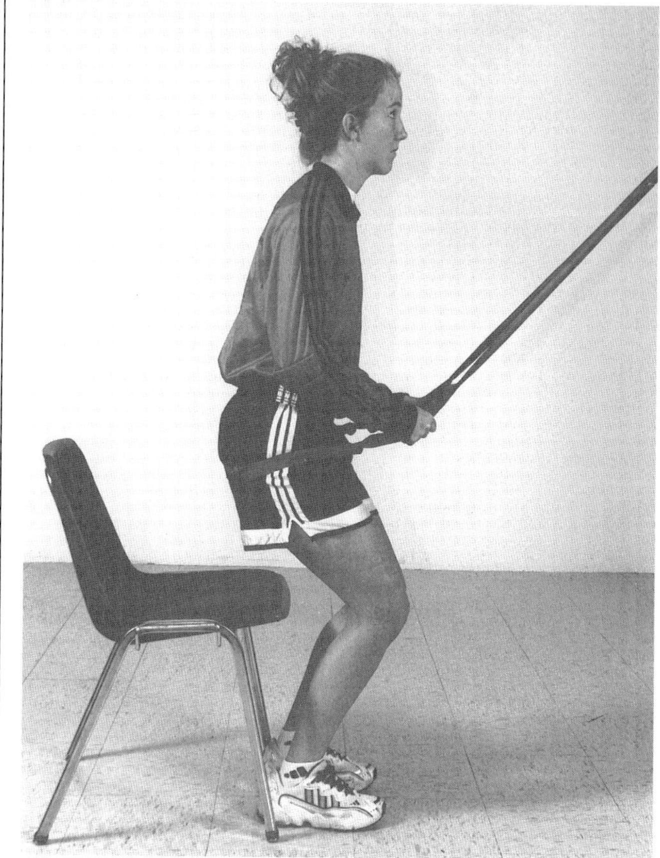

FIGURE 14-9 **Squat: posterior weight shift.**

PURPOSE: Stimulation of dynamic postural response, facilitating concentric and eccentric contractions.

POSITION: Standing on involved extremity (left), facing away from tubing, with belt around waist and feet shoulder's width apart.

PROCEDURE: Patient squats to the height of the chair in a smooth, cortrolled motion, and then returns to standing. This technique facilitates the accent phase of the squat; the hip extensors, knee extensors, and ankle plantar flexors are loaded dynamically with eccentric contractions during the return to sitting. The posterior weight shift is a great activity for learning the take-off position for sprinting and jumping.

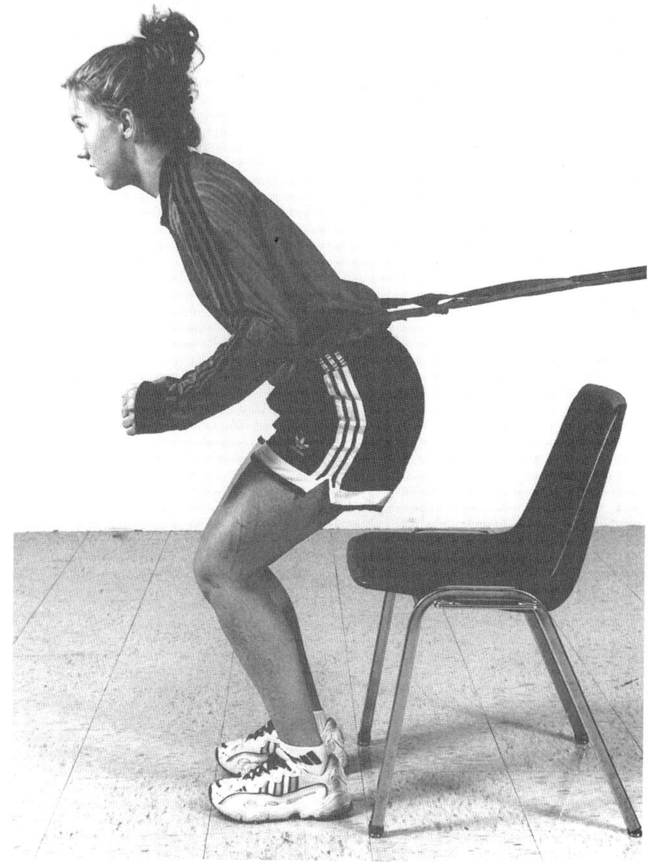

FIGURE 14-10 Squat: medial weight shift.

PURPOSE: Stimulation of dynamic postural response, facilitating concentric and eccentric contractions.

POSITION: Standing with uninvolved extremity closest to tubing, belt around waist, with feet shoulder's width apart (assume involved extremity is left lower extremity).

PROCEDURE: Patient squats to the height of the chair in a smooth, controlled motion, and then returns to standing. This technique places less stress on the affected lower extremity and allows the patient to lean onto the unaffected lower extremity without incurring excessive stress or loading.

NOTE: The lateral weight shift technique is not illustrated, but it is the same as shown in Fig. 14.10 except with the tubing pulling lateral (to the patient's left) instead of pulling medial (to patient's right as is shown in Fig. 14.10). This lateral weight shift exercise will place a greater stress on the affected lower extremity, thereby demanding increased balance and control. The exercise simulates a single leg squat but adds balance and safety by allowing the unaffected extremity to remain on the ground.

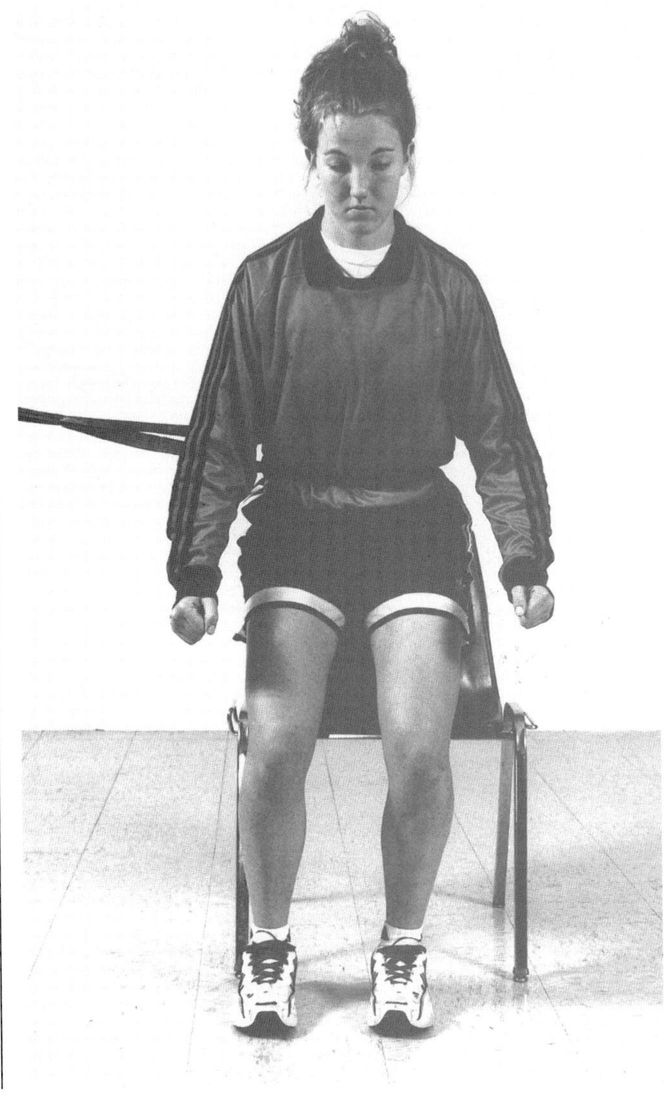

Lunge

The lunge is more specific than the squat in that it simulates sports and normal activity. The exercise decreases the base of support while producing the need for independent disassociation. The ROM can be stressed to a slightly higher degree. If the client is asked to alternate the lunge from the right to the left leg, the clinician can easily compare the quality of the movement between the limbs (Fig. 14-11 to 14-13).

Resisted Walking

Resisted walking uses the same primary components used in gait training. The applied resistance of the tubing, however, allows a reactive response unavailable in nonresisted activities. The addition of resistance permits increased loading and brings about the need for improved balance and weight shift.

Resisted Running

Resisted running simply involves jogging or running in place with tubing attached to a belt around the waist. The clinician can analyze the jogging or running activity, because this is a stationary drill. The tubing resistance is applied in four different directions, which provides simulation of the different forces that the client will experience on return to full activity (Figs. 14-14 to 14-16).

Resisted Bounding

Bounding is an exercise in which the client jumps off one foot and lands on the opposite foot, essentially jumping from one foot to the other. Bounding places greater emphasis on the lateral movements, and its progression follows the same weight-shifting sequence as the resisted running exercise. Side-to-side bounding in a lateral-resisted exercise promotes symmetrical balance and

FIGURE 14-11 **Lunge: anterior weight shift.**

PURPOSE: Stimulation of dynamic postural response, facilitating concentric and eccentric contractions.

POSITION: Standing, facing tubing, with feet shoulder's width apart (assume involved side is left lower extremity).

PROCEDURE: Leading with involved extremity, patient lowers into lunge position in a smooth, controlled motion, and then returns to standing. This positioning will increase the eccentric loading on the quadriceps with deceleration on the downward movement. For the upward movement, the patient is asked to focus on hip extension, not knee extension.

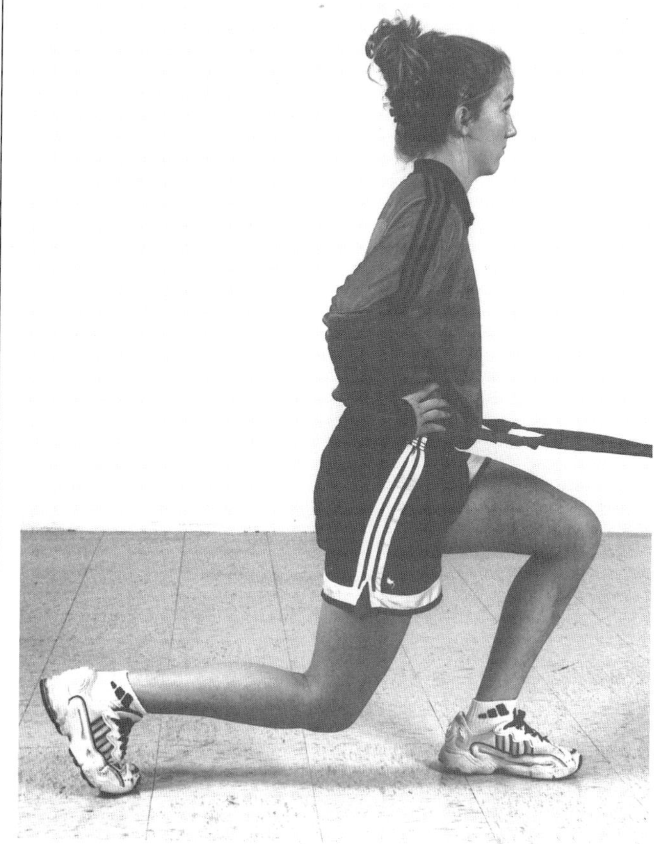

FIGURE 14-12 **Lunge: posterior weight shift.**

PURPOSE: Stimulation of dynamic postural response, facilitating concentric and eccentric contractions.

POSITION: Standing, facing away from tubing, with feet shoulder's width apart (assume involved extremity is left lower extremity).

PROCEDURE: Leading with involved extremity, patient lowers into lunge position in a smooth, controlled motion, and then returns to standing. When lowering self into lunge, patient must work against resistance because the tubing is stretched; when at the low point of lunge position, the patient is assisted back up by the tubing.

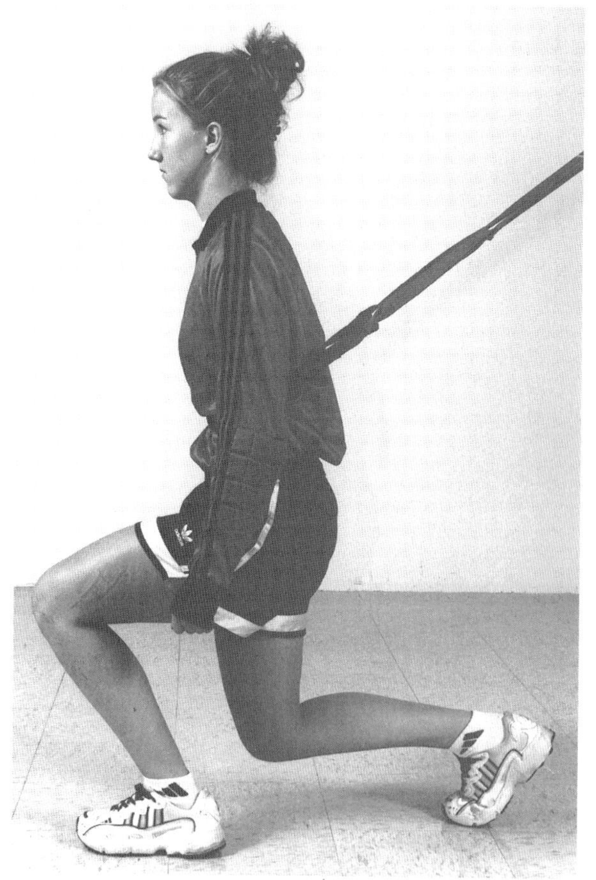

FIGURE 14-13 **Lunge: medial weight shift.**

PURPOSE: Stimulation of dynamic postural response, facilitating concentric and eccentric contractions.

POSITION: Standing with uninvolved extremity closest to tubing, with feet shoulder's width apart (assume involved extremity is left lower extremity).

PROCEDURE: Leading with involved extremity, patient lowers into lunge position in a smooth, controlled motion, and then returns to standing. Medial weight shift causes the ankle inverters to fire in order to maintain the position, which may facilitate ankle stability.

NOTE: The lateral weight shift is not illustrated, but is the same as shown in Fig. 14.13 except with the tubing pulling lateral (to patient's left) instead of pulling medial (to patient's right as is shown in Fig. 14.13). The lunge with lateral weight shift is performed by positioning the patient with the affected lower extremity closest to the resistance. This lateral weight shift causes firing of the ankle everters, which may be great for ankle stability.

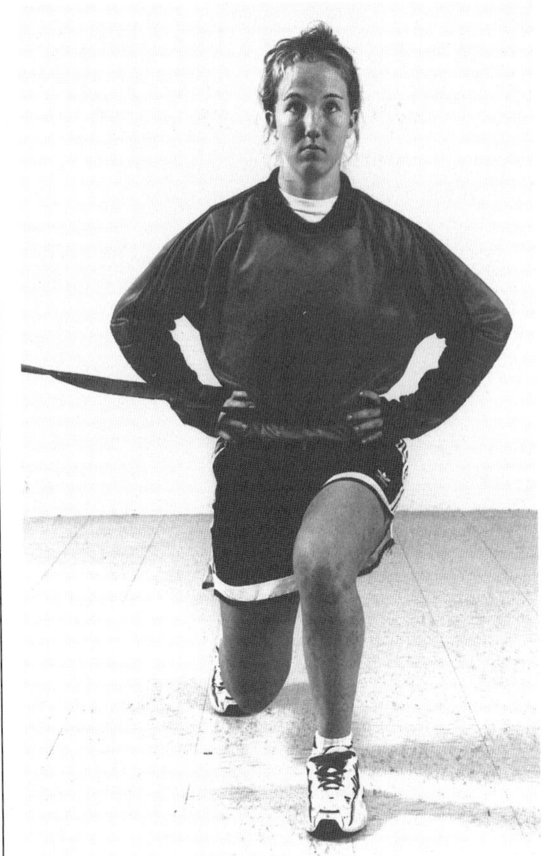

FIGURE 14-14 **Stationary run: anterior weight shift.**

PURPOSE: Stimulation of dynamic postural response, introducing impact and ballistic exercise and improving balance and weight shift.

POSITION: Standing, facing tubing, with feet shoulder's width apart (assume involved side is left lower extremity).

PROCEDURE: Patient starts with light jogging in place and can progress to "butt kicks"; same distance from origin of tubing should be maintained. The anterior weight shift run is probably the most difficult technique to perform correctly and is, therefore, taught last. This technique simulates deceleration and eccentric loading of the knee extensors.

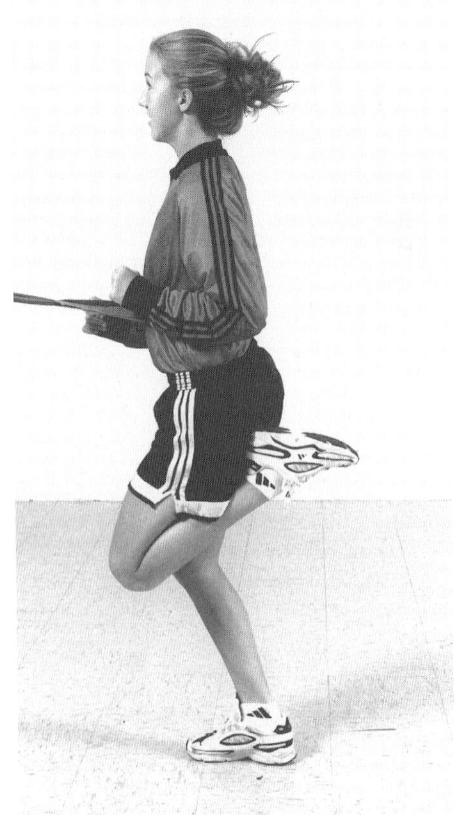

FIGURE 14-15 **Stationary run: posterior weight shift.**

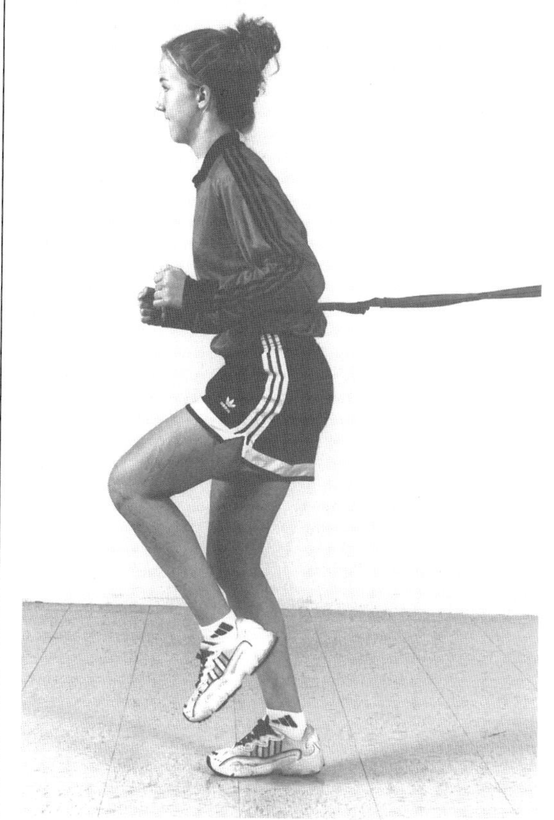

PURPOSE: Stimulation of dynamic postural response, introducing impact and ballistic exercise and improving balance and weight shift.

POSITION: Standing, facing away from tubing, with feet shoulder's width apart (assume involved extremity is left lower extremity).

PROCEDURE: Patient starts with light jogging in place and can progress to running in place; same distance from origin of tubing should be maintained. The most advanced form of the posterior weight shift run involves the exaggeration of the hip flexion called "high knees." This technique simulates the acceleration phase of jogging or running.

FIGURE 14-16 **Stationary run: medial weight shift.**

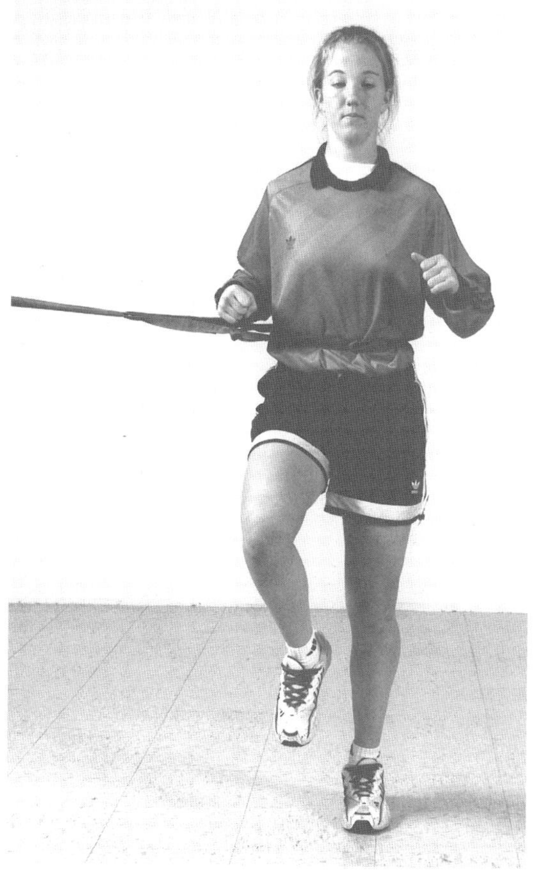

PURPOSE: Stimulation of dynamic postural response, introducing impact and ballistic exercise and improving balance and weight shift.

POSITION: Standing with uninvolved extremity closest to tubing, with feet shoulder's width apart (assume involved extremity is left lower extremity).

PROCEDURE: Patient starts with light jogging in place and can progress to running in place; same distance from origin of tubing should be maintained. This technique simulates the forces that the patient will experience when cutting or turning quickly away from the affected side. (For example, the exercise will facilitate cutting left in a patient with a left lower extremity problem.)

NOTE: The lateral weight shift technique is not illustrated, but it is the same as shown in Fig. 14.10 except with the tubing pulling lateral (to the patient's left) instead of pulling medial (to patient's right as is shown in Fig. 14.16). This technique simulates the forces that the patient will experience when cutting or turning quickly towards the affected side. (For example, this exercise will facilitate cutting right in a patient with a left lower extremity problem.)

endurance required for progression to higher levels of strength and power applications. Before using the tubing, the client should learn the bounding activity by jumping over cones or other obstacles. The tubing can then be added to provide the secondary forces that cause anterior, posterior, medial, or lateral weight shifting (Figs. 14-17 to 14-19).

AEROBIC SEQUENCE

It is valuable for a sufficient aerobic base (chapter 10) to be established initially in the functional progression program to allow the client to demonstrate his or her ability to tolerate the additional stress of running, before the program is progressed to short duration, sprinting, and jumping activities.

Jogging 20 steps and walking 20 steps for a total of 20 min at a very slow pace is the initial stage for returning the client to aerobic activity. The client can then be progressed to jogging 4 to 5 min and walking 2 to 3 min for a total treatment time of 20 to 40 min at a slow pace or at the client's tolerance. Caution should be used if running around any curves or corners. Suggested frequency of the initial program is three times per week.

The jogging program can be progressed as shown in Table 14-2, which outlines a jogging program for an individual who wants to develop an aerobic base. If the client is a distance runner, he or she can be further progressed to a program similar to that presented in Tables 14-3 and 14-4. The programs in these tables are examples only, each program must be individualized according to the client's response to treatment.

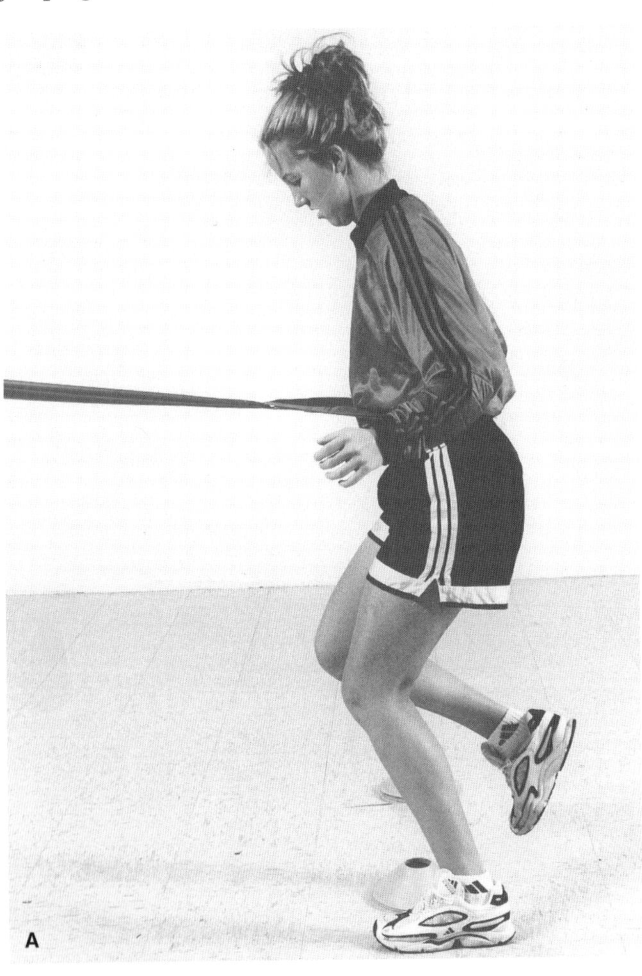

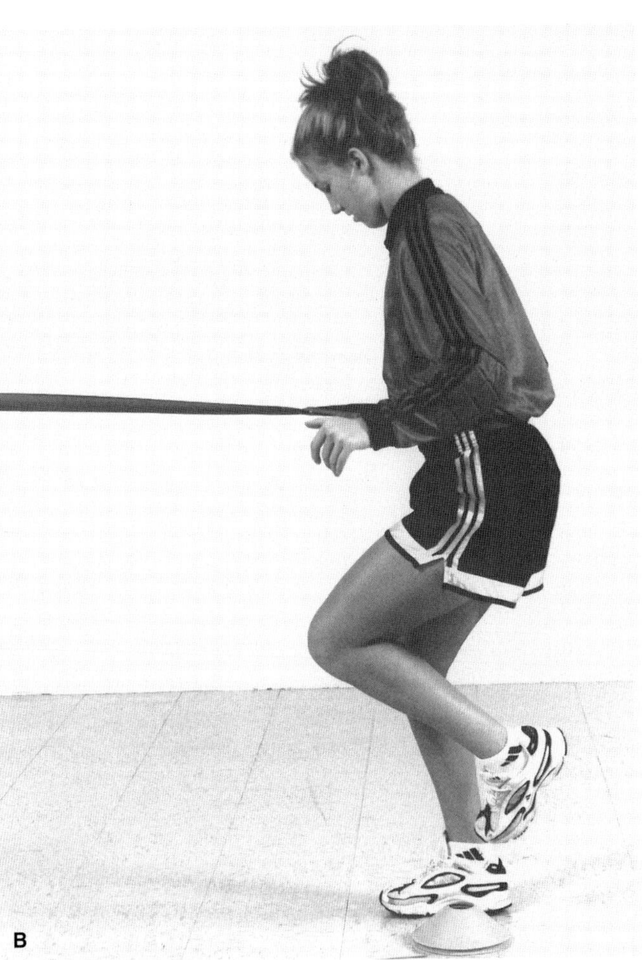

FIGURE 14-17 Bounding: anterior weight shift.

PURPOSE: Stimulation of dynamic postural response, promoting balance and endurance in preparation for progression to higher level lower extremity exercise.

POSITION: Standing, facing tubing, with feet shoulders width apart (assume involved extremity is left lower extremity).

PROCEDURE: Patient takes off of one foot, jumps over cones that are set at a prescribed distance, and lands on the opposite foot. The technique is then repeated in the opposite direction. This exercise will assist in teaching deceleration and lateral cutting movements.

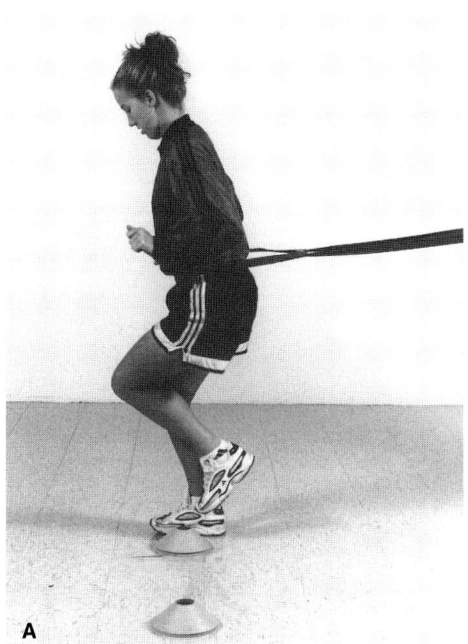

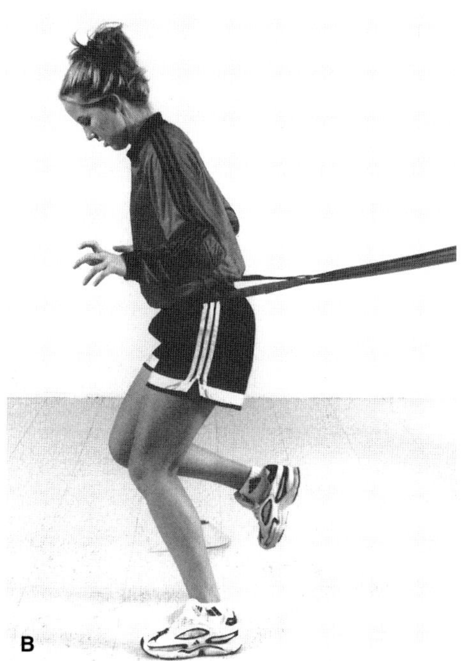

FIGURE 14-18 **Bounding: posterior weight shift.**

PURPOSE: Stimulation of dynamic postural response, promoting balance and endurance in preparation for progression to higher level lower extremity exercise.

POSITION: Standing, facing away from tubing, with feet shoulder's width apart (assume involved extremity is left lower extremity).

PROCEDURE: Patient takes off of one foot, jumps over cones that are set at a prescribed distance, and lands on the opposite foot. The technique is then repeated in the opposite direction. This exercise will assist in teaching acceleration and lateral cutting movements.

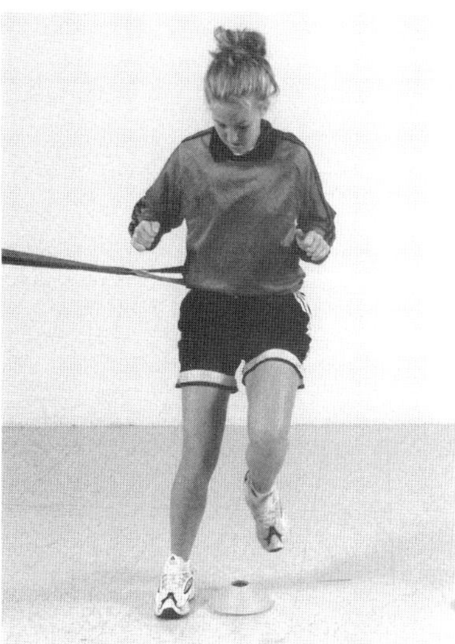

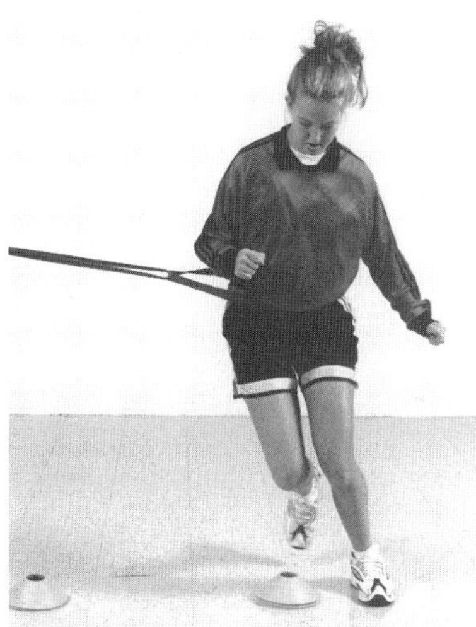

FIGURE 14-19 **Bounding: medial weight shift.**

PURPOSE: Stimulation of dynamic postural response, promoting balance and endurance in preparation for progression to higher level lower extremity exercise.

POSITION: Standing, with uninvolved extremity closest to tubing, with feet shoulder's width apart (assume involved side is left lower extremity).

PROCEDURE: Patient takes off of one foot, jumps over cones that are set at a prescribed distance, and lands on the opposite foot. The technique is then repeated in the opposite direction. The medial weight shift bound is used as an assisted plyometric exercise because the impact on the involved extremity (left) is greatly lowered owing to the pull of the tubing.

NOTE: The lateral weight shift technique is not illustrated, but is the same as shown in Fig. 14.19 except with the tubing pulling lateral (to the patient's left) instead of pulling medial (to patient's right as is shown in Fig. 14.19). This exercise is the most strenuous of the bounding activities since it actually accelerates the body weight onto the affected lower extremity. This shift to the affected extremity is, however, necessary so that the clinician can observe the ability of the affected limb to perform a quick direction change and controlled acceleration/deceleration.

TABLE 14-2 Jogging Program

Day 1	Day 2	Day 3	Day 4	Day 5	Day 6	Day 7
0.5-mile jog on track; jog straights and walk curves	0.5-mile jog on track; jog straights and walk curves	0.5-mile jog on track; jog straights and walk curves	0.5-mile jog on track; jog straights and walk curves	0.5-mile jog on track; jog straights and walk curves	Off	0.5-mile jog on track; jog straights and walk curves
Day 8	**Day 9**	**Day 10**	**Day 11**	**Day 12**	**Day 13**	**Day 14**
1.5-mile jog on track	1.5-mile jog on track	2-mile jog on track	2-mile jog on track	Off	2-mile jog on track	3-mile jog on track
Day 15	**Day 16**	**Day 17**	**Day 18**	**Day 19**	**Day 20**	**Day 21**
3-mile jog on track	3-mile jog on track	2-mile jog on track	4-mile jog on track	4-mile jog on track	Off	Regular team conditioning

SPRINT SEQUENCE: STRAIGHT-PLANE ACTIVITY

Once jogging and running are painless and gait deviations absent, the sprint sequence should be initiated. The client may continue the aerobic program when the sprint sequence is added to the functional progression program. Straight-ahead sprinting is progressed from half speed to three-quarter speed, and finally to full speed. Once the client is able to tolerate straight-ahead sprints at three-quarter speed, half-speed backward sprints are added. The client is eventually progressed to full-speed backward sprints (Table 14-5).

When the client is able to tolerate three-quarter-speed backward sprinting, half-speed lateral sprints (also called carioca, braiding, or cross-overs) are added. When the client can perform the three sprints (forward, backward, and lateral) at full speed, then other activities can be added such as high stepping or, for a basketball player, dribbling a ball while sprinting. These drills are limited only by the ingenuity of the clinician.

JUMP–HOP SEQUENCE

Functional progression activities for the lower extremity progress from simple to complex, from bilateral activities (jumps) to unilateral activities (hops), from activities with the feet on the ground (support) to activities in which the feet leave the ground (nonsupport), from slow speeds to faster speeds, and from straight-plane activities to mulitplane activities. Specific activities and a suggested order of progression are found in Table 14-6.

CUTTING SEQUENCE: MULTIPLE-PLANE ACTIVITY

Of primary importance to the functional progression of most athletes is the cutting sequence. The cutting sequence begins with figure-eight running and progresses to actual cutting activities in which the athlete plants the foot and accelerates in a different direction. Gentle figure-eight running can be initiated using a distance of about 40 yd and running at half speed. For example, initially the full length of a basketball court could be used, and the athlete could change directions by running long, easy curves (Fig. 14-20). The speed of running at this distance is then increased to three-quarter and finally to full speed. Once full-speed figure-eights can be performed at this distance, the distance is decreased to about 20 yd, so the figure-eights are smaller and the maneuvering area is tighter; the athlete begins at half speed. For example, the

TABLE 14-3 Running Progression for Distance Runner (Every Other Day)

Day 1	Day 2	Day 3	Day 4	Day 5	Day 6	Day 7
2 miles	Off	2.5 miles	Off	3.0 miles	Off	3.5 miles
Day 8	**Day 9**	**Day 10**	**Day 11**	**Day 12**	**Day 13**	**Day 14**
Off	4.0 miles	Off	4.5 miles	Off	5.0 miles	Off

TABLE 14-4 Running Progression (Daily)

Day 1	Day 2	Day 3	Day 4	Day 5	Day 6	Day 7
5 miles	2 miles	5 miles	2.5 miles	5 miles	3 miles	Off
Day 8	**Day 9**	**Day 10**	**Day 11**	**Day 12**	**Day 13**	**Day 14**
5 miles	3.5 miles	5 miles	4 miles	5 miles	4.5 miles	Off
Day 15	**Day 16**	**Day 17**	**Day 18**	**Day 19**	**Day 20**	**Day 21**
5 miles	5 miles	5 miles	Off	5 miles	6 miles	5 miles
Day 22	**Day 23**	**Day 24**	**Day 25**	**Day 26**	**Day 27**	**Day 28**
6 miles	5 miles	6 miles	5 miles	5 miles	6 miles	7 miles

figure-eight would now be performed on only half of a basketball court (Fig. 14-20). The athlete is again progressed to three-quarter and then to full speed. The sequence is repeated at about 10 yd. For example, the figure-eight would now be performed between the baseline and the free throw line (Fig. 14-20). Of course, this progression could be performed in other settings besides a basketball court.

Running figure-eights can then be replaced by cutting drills in which the athlete is first asked to jog to a given spot, plant the involved extremity, and cut toward the uninvolved side. If required, the athlete may need to perform cuts at 45°, 60°, and finally 90° (Fig. 14-21). The speeds at which the athlete approaches the spot at which the extremity is planted is progressively increased.

After full-speed 90° cutting is achieved without difficulty, speeds are again decreased and the athlete begins the same cutting sequence on verbal or visual command, which more closely simulates the environment to which the individual is attempting to return. Running to a predetermined point before cutting allows the athlete to plan the movement in advance; this preparation is not available in actual practice or game conditions. Table 14-7 presents an example of a figure-eight and cutting sequence. This sample functional progression program must be individualized to the client, based on his or her response the activity.

Case Studies

Several case studies are given in this chapter to integrate information from all the previous chapters and to present information across the lifespan.

CASE STUDY 1

PATIENT INFORMATION

A 15-year-old high school female soccer player was injured during an intrasquad game 2 days before the examination. The athlete engaged in contact just after completing a crossing pass and developed a valgus stress to the knee. She felt immediate medial knee pain and was unable to continue participation. She was able to bear minimal weight on the leg after

TABLE 14-5 Sprint Sequence Using Straight-Plane Activities

Sprint at half speed
Sprint at three-quarter speed; backward sprint at half speed
Sprint at full speed; backward sprint at three-quarter speed; lateral sprint at half speed
Backward sprint at full speed; Lateral sprint at three-quarter speed
Lateral sprint at full speed

TABLE 14-6 Jump–Hop Sequence

Loading	Activity	Intensity/Frequency
Bilateral support	Leg press	3 sets for 3 sec; increase by 30 sec until 2-min duration is reached
	Mini-squat	
Unilateral support	One-leg press	3 set for 30 sec; increase by 15 sec until 1-min duration is reached
	One-leg mini-squat	
Straight plane, bilateral, nonsupport	Front-to-back jumps	Multiple sets at sport-specific duration of at least 30 sec
	Side-to-side jumps	
	Vertical jumps	
	Horizontal jumps	
Straight plane, unilateral, nonsupport	Front-to-back hops	Multiple sets at sport-specific duration of at least 30 sec
	Side-to-side hops	
	Lateral stepping	
	Lunges	
	Vertical hops	
	Horizontal hops	
Multiple plane, bilateral, nonsupport	Diagonal jumps	Multiple sets at sport-specific duration of at least 30 sec
	V jumps	
	5-dot drill	
Multiple plane, unilateral, nonsupport	Diagonal hops	Multiple sets at sport-specific duration of at least 30 sec
	V hops	
	5-dot drill	

the injury. No immediate swelling was noted, no pop was felt or heard, and no episodes of the knee locking or catching were experienced. She was seen in the emergency department the same day of the injury and was placed in a 30° immobilizer and issued crutches.

At the initial visit, the athlete was able to bear partial weight with the assistance of axillary crutches. Active ROM of the knee was 18 to 99° of flexion, which was limited by medial knee pain. Passive ROM of the knee was 5 to 105° of flexion, which was limited by hamstring spasm and medial knee pain. Volitional quadriceps recruitment with an isometric contraction was less via palpation than the opposite side. The knee demonstrated no intra-articular effusion, and less than 1 cm of peri-articular swelling was noted when measured at the joint line and compared to the other knee.

Tenderness to palpation was noted at the middle third of the medial joint line. The distal femoral epiphysis in skeletally immature athletes can be damaged via this same mechanism of injury.[25] However, palpation of the epiphysis did not reveal any tenderness. Ligamentous examination for lateral, anterior, and posterior straight-plane instability and for anteromedial, anterolateral, and posterolateral instability revealed no asymmetrical problems. Approximately 5 mm of instability was noted with valgus stress at 30° of flexion; an end point was present that was accompanied by pain (6 on a 0 to 10 scale). The minimal instability was present at the joint line and not at the distal femoral epiphysis. Based on the examination and evaluation, the patient was diagnosed with a second-degree medial collateral ligament sprain.

LINKS TO

Guide to Physical Therapist Practice and *Athletic Training Educational Competencies*

Using the *Guide*,[26] the clinician found that this patient was grouped in musculoskeletal practice pattern 4D. This pattern is

FIGURE 14-20 **Running figure-eights in a progressively smaller maneuvering area.**

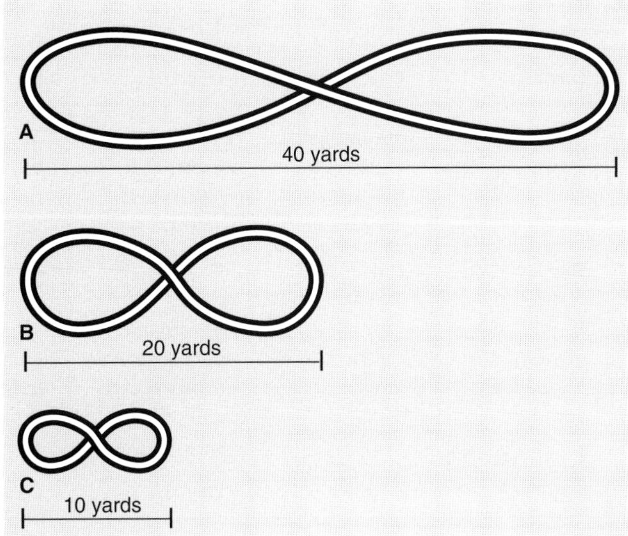

definded as "impaired joint mobility, motor function, muscle performance, and range of motion associated with connective tissue dysfunction." Anticipated goals for this patient as they relate to functional progression include increasing motor function; improving joint mobility, weight-bearing status, strength, power, and endurance; protecting the injured body part; and minimizing the risk of recurrent injury.

The *Competencies*[27] refers to the ability to "revise goals and objectives and develop criteria for progression and return to competition based on level of function and patient outcomes." In addition, teaching objectives include "functional rehabilitation and reconditioning."

INTERVENTION

Goals for the early stage of intervention focused on minimizing the inflammatory process that accompanies healing. The patient was instructed to use the crutches with toe-touch weight bearing. She was also told to apply ice to the medial knee after exercise and for 20 to 30 min every 4 hr when awake. The athlete was instructed in quadriceps isometrics—10-sec contractions for 10 repetitions 10 times a day (see Fig. 6-9)—and bent-knee leg raises—three sets of 20 repetitions twice a day while in the immobilizer (see Fig. 6-14). The immobilizer was to be removed four to five times a day and the athlete was to perform 90 to 40° open-chain, gravity-resisted knee extensions—three sets of 20 repetitions. The patient be-

FIGURE 14-21

Progression for cutting activities in which the cuts become sharper and thus more difficult. 1, 45° cut; 2, 60° cut; 3, 90° cut.

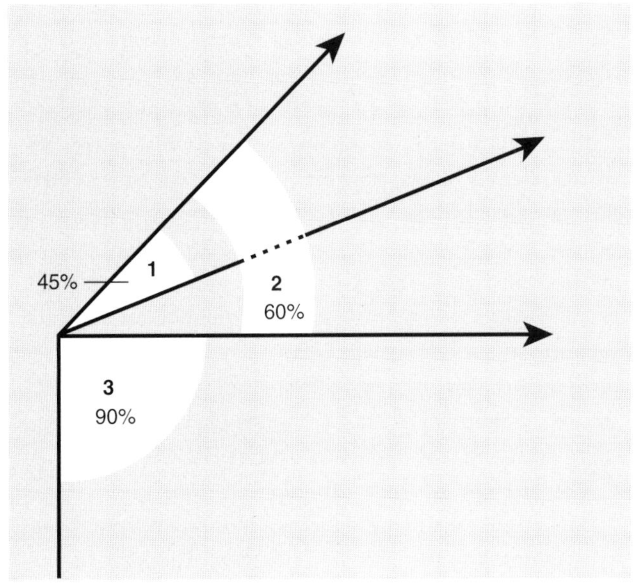

TABLE 14-7 Figure-Eight and Cutting Sequence[a]

Day 1	Day 2	Day 3	Day 4	Day 5	Day 6	Day 7
40-yd figure-eights at a jog	40-yd figure-eights at a half-speed sprint	40-yd figure-eights at a half-speed sprint.	40-yd figure-eights at a full-speed sprint	20-yd figure-eights at a half-speed sprint	20-yd figure-eights at a full-speed sprint	10-yd figure-eights at a half-speed sprint
Day 8	**Day 9**	**Day 10**	**Day 11**	**Day 12**	**Day 13**	**Day 14**
10-yd figure-eights at a full-speed sprint	Off	45° straight cuts at set location at a half-speed sprint	45° straight cuts at set location at a full-speed sprint	45° straight cuts on command at a full-speed sprint	Off	60° straight cuts at set location at a half-speed sprint
Day 15	**Day 16**	**Day 17**	**Day 18**	**Day 19**	**Day 20**	**Day 21**
60° straight cuts at set location at a full-speed sprint	60° straight cuts on command at a full-speed sprint	Off	90° straight cuts at a set location at a half-speed sprint	90° straight cuts at a set location at a full-speed sprint	90° straight cuts on command at a full-speed sprint	Off

[a]Perform 2 sets of 10 repetitions.

longed to a health club with access to an upper-extremity ergometer (see Fig. 10-10), so she was taught how to monitor her pulse, given a maximum heart rate (205 beats per minute), and instructed to perform 20- to 30-min workouts at 80% of her target heart rate (164 beats per minute) (chapter 10).

PROGRESSION

One Week After Initial Examination

At the 1-week follow-up, prone active assisted flexion exercises through the full ROM—three sets of 15 repetitions twice a day (see Fig. 2-13)—were added to the athlete's program. She was also told to begin three sets of 30-sec straight-plane bilateral support efforts (leg press) on the Shuttle (Contemporary Design, Glacier WA) and to progress to three sets of 2-min efforts. Resistance was initiated at one cord and advanced to tolerance. Isotonic strengthening of the hip musculature in all planes was initiated (see Figs. 6-15 and 6-16). The athlete was allowed to begin full-weight-bearing ambulation in the immobilizer. Bilateral support activities consisting of reactive neuromuscular training using oscillating techniques for isometric stabilization were instituted in three sets of 1 min in straight-plane anterior, posterior, medial, and lateral weight shifts (see Figs. 14-3 to 14-6).

Conditioning efforts on the upper-extremity ergometer continued but were modified to also address anaerobic needs by encompassing two 20-min workouts with a 10-min rest between sessions. During each workout on the ergometer, the athlete was instructed to perform 15- to 30-sec all-out sprints every 2 min.

Because the patient was determined to be a candidate for a functional knee brace, a prescription was secured, and she was measured for a brace at that time.

Two Weeks After Initial Examination

At 2 weeks after the initial visit, prone active knee flexion was symmetrical and the athlete lacked less than 5° of seated knee extension. She was performing three sets of 2 min straight-plane unilateral leg press activities on the Shuttle with 125 lb of resistance. Functional progression activities were progressed to straight-plane bilateral nonsupport activities, which consisted of front-to-back line jumps (see Fig. 9-26). After the closed-chain activities, the athlete performed three sets of 15 repetitions of open-chain knee extension through the full ROM (see Fig. 6-18),

Three Weeks After Initial Examination

At the 3-week follow-up, active and passive ROM of the knee was full and symmetrical. Functional progression activities in the brace were advanced to include elastic cord resisted lateral stepping drills and stationary lateral bounding (see Figs. 14-17 to 14-19). The lateral stepping drills were performed in the functional brace and were gradually increased to a distance of 8 ft after initial resistance of the cord was encountered. In-place stationary bounding began at a distance slightly greater than shoulder width apart and was progressed to a distance of 3 ft. Both of these activities were performed for three sets of 1 min and were increased to three sets of 2 min. Straight-plane, unilateral nonsupport activities (excluding valgus loading) consisted of front-to-back lines hops for three sets of 15 sec and were progressed to 1 min. Multiplane bilateral nonsupport drills were also added.

It is at this point the athlete returned to the soccer field for early sport-related activities. Ball-handling skills and outside touch passing and kicking were allowed in the brace. She was also allowed to begin a straight-plane jogging program on level surfaces to address aerobic and anaerobic conditioning (Table 14-2). Open-chain knee extension through the full ROM continued to be performed three times a week after the closed-chain functional progression drills.

OUTCOME

As part of the formal exercise program, the athlete was ready for more strenuous unilateral support and nonsupport activities to stress valgus loading. Multiplane, unilateral nonsupport drills consisted of diagonal hopping (Table 14-6). Inside kicking, passing, and shooting were instituted at this point. Agility drills consisting of the figure-eight and cutting progressions were instituted (Table 14-7). When she completed the lateral power hop sequence, the athlete was allowed to return to competition 30 days after injury.

CASE STUDY 2

PATIENT INFORMATION

The patient was a 20-year-old college female cross-country runner with proximal lower left leg pain for 1 week. She was currently 2 weeks into the fall season and had run 3 to 4 mi daily during the summer. Training consisted of twice daily practices in which she ran 4 mi in the morning before school and 6 mi after school. The pain just below her left knee started as a dull ache after practice (3 on a 0 to 10 scale) the week before; but at the time of the appointment, it was much worse (8/10) with any weight-bearing activity. The patient did not remember a traumatic episode that triggered the pain; she denied sensory changes but noted that the previous two nights she had night pain. As per the coach's instructions, she decreased the mileage of her twice daily workouts to 2 mi in the morning and 4 mi after school.

Physical examination revealed a painful gait with no assistive device. Active ROM of both knees was normal. Passive hamstring flexibility was $-20°$ from neutral bilaterally with the hips flexed to 90°. Bilateral calf flexibility was $+5°$ of dorsiflexion bilaterally. The Ober test was negative; the Thomas test was positive at $-5°$ from neutral bilaterally. Rear foot to lower leg alignment was normal; the forefoot to rear foot relationship revealed approximately 8° of forefoot varus. She also demonstrated a dorsally mobile first ray and a slight amount of femoral anteversion. Ligamentous examination of the knee and the patellofemoral joint were unremarkable. The athlete was referred to a physician who ordered a bone scan. Results of the bone scan were positive for a proximal tibial stress fracture.

LINKS TO

Guide to Physical Therapist Practice and *Athletic Training Educational Competencies*

According to the *Guide*,[26] this patient falls in musculoskeletal practice pattern 4G. This pattern is described as "impaired joint mobility, muscle performance, and range of motion associated with fracture." Anticipated goals for this patient as they relate to functional progression include reducing the risk of secondary impairment; improving motor function, weight-bearing status, ventilation, respiration, circulation, and the patient's feeling of well-being; decreasing the loading of the involved body part; and protecting the healing injury.

The *Competencies*[27] refers to the ability to "revise goals and objectives and develop criteria for progression and return to competition based on level of function and patient outcomes." In addition, teaching objectives include "functional rehabilitation and reconditioning."

INTERVENTION

At the initial visit, the athlete was instructed in non-weight-bearing gait using axillary crutches. She was taught to maintain cardiovascular fitness using an upper-extremity ergometer (see Fig. 10-10) and was told to perform daily active ROM exercises of the knee and ankle joints (see Figs. 2-13, 2-14, and 2-16).

PROGRESSION

Three Weeks after Initial Examination

At the 3-week follow-up, the athlete was allowed to bear partial weight using the axillary crutches. Over the course of the following 2 weeks, she was told to gradually resume full weight bearing with the axillary crutches. During that time, cardiovascular conditioning efforts intensified to include swimming and pool running (see Fig. 13-30). Instead of traditional swimming strokes, initial efforts emphasized pool running, because the patient was not an avid swimmer. She performed the cardiovascular workouts in the deep end of the pool wearing a vest to minimize weight bearing. By week 4 after injury, the athlete was able to perform 30 min of pool running.

Four Weeks After Initial Examination

At the 4-week follow-up, the athlete was allowed to bear weight to tolerance on the affected lower extremity. During the following week, she used one crutch for ambulation; and during week 6, she transitioned to full weight bearing without an assistive device. Cardiovascular conditioning was then permitted on a stationary bicycle (see Fig. 10-5). She began by riding the bicycle for 20 min every other day during week 5. The days the athlete did not exercise on the bicycle, she continued her pool workouts. Over the course of the week, she gradually increased the conditioning time on the bike to a total of 30 min. During week 6, in an effort to begin the transition back into formal running, the athlete began a conditioning program on the stationary bike based on mileage instead of total time.

Six Weeks After Initial Examination

At 6 weeks, the patient was allowed to resume running up to one-quarter of the distance she used to run before the injury. The initial return to running program was performed every other day and took place on the track because of its level surface. A soft, full-length insert was placed in the shoe to aid shock absorption. She began the program by covering 2 mi, alternating 0.25-mi walks with 0.25-mi runs. The distance was increased 0.5 mi every other workout (Table 14-3).

OUTCOME

The athlete performed heel cord (see Figs. 3-17 and 3-18) and hamstring (see Figs. 3-7 and 3-8) stretching before and after her workouts. She progressed without incident to the point at which she was able to run 5 mi every other day. At that time, the patient was allowed to resume daily running (Table 14-4), and intervention was discontinued.

CASE STUDY 3

PATIENT INFORMATION

The patient was 10-year-old male soccer player who had been practicing and playing for 5 weeks during the fall season. He had "left foot/heel" pain for 1 week without having experienced a specific injury. The parent recalled the athlete sliding feet first into the goal upright several weeks earlier but could not recall if the patient hit with his left or right foot. The patient did not complain of foot problems after that incident and had been playing up until the previous week, when he stopped playing because of pain. The athlete was referred for examination and treatment and for advice concerning return to play.

The patient arrived for examination with the chief complaint of pain in the left heel when running during soccer games and in gym class at school; he reported minimal to no pain when walking. His goals were to return to playing soccer as soon as possible. The patient had been seen by the physician and was told to use heat and to wear an over-the-counter lace-up type ankle brace. Radiographs were negative for the left foot and ankle.

During the examination, the patient complained of pain in the heel with bilateral toe raises and had decreased push off on the left foot with jogging. Attempts to run faster or to perform cutting activities were difficult because of heel pain. Palpation indicated tenderness at the superior third of the posterior calcaneus and no pain in the Achilles tendon and bursa. ROM and strength were normal, except for pain when raising up on the toes. All ligament tests to the ankle were negative.

The patient was diagnosed with calcaneal apophysitis (Sever disease). This condition is relatively common in active, growing children.

LINKS TO

Guide to Physical Therapist Practice and *Athletic Training Educational Competencies*

According to the Guide,[26] calcaneal apophysitis is classified as musculoskeletal pattern 4E. This pattern is described as "impaired joint mobility, motor function, muscle performance, and range of motion associated with localized inflammation." Goals included coordinating care with the patient, parents, and volunteer soccer coach; reducing the disability associated with chronic irritation; enhancing physical function and sport participation; and improving sport-specific motor function and self-management of symptoms.

The *Competencies*[27] refers to the ability to "revise goals and objectives and develop criteria for progression and return to competition based on level of function and patient outcomes." In addition, teaching objectives include "functional rehabilitation and reconditioning."

INTERVENTION

Apophysitis is caused by musculotendinous traction forces on the immature epiphysis. Initial goals were to decrease inflammation, increase strength, and maintain muscle length. The child was instructed to discontinue use of the ankle brace and to stop all activities (running) that caused pain. Initial intervention consisted of the following:

1. Mild stretching to maintain length and motion of the gastrocnemius and soleus muscles (see Figs. 3-17 and 3-18).
2. Elastic tubing strengthening to the Achilles to maintain strength during the relative rest period from soccer.
3. Bicycle to maintain cardiovascular conditioning and lower-extremity endurance (see Fig. 10-5).
4. Ice for discomfort and irritation.

PROGRESSION

One Week After Initial Examination

One week after examination, the athlete demonstrated the ability to raise up on his toes without pain. Goals at this point were to increase strength with more advanced activities. Intervention was progressed as follows:

1. Toe raises and partial squats (see Fig. 9-10).
2. Continue lower-extremity bicycling.
3. Pain-free lunges (see Fig. 9-12).
4. Slide training for lateral movements (see Fig. 11-19).

Three Weeks After Initial Examination

At the 3-week follow-up, the patient had no complaints of pain when raising up on his toes, walking, or jogging. Goals were to advance the program to include functional progression activities to prepare the patient for return to sport. Intervention was as follows:

1. Low-velocity, low-vertical force plyometrics (see Fig. 9-27).
2. Lower-extremity functional progression, including running, cutting, changing directions, and low-level agility jumping (see Fig. 9-26).

OUTCOME

The patient returned to soccer without difficulty after 5 weeks. Clinicians should remember that the epiphyses and apophyses in young athletes are at risk for overuse and injury. The patient's injury may have been sparked by the collision into the goal post, but it really was the result of microtraumatic or repetitive use. Immobilization is not necessary for healing; instead, the athlete should decrease participation in activities that aggravate the symptoms.

CASE STUDY 4

PATIENT INFORMATION

The patient was a 64-year-old mildly obese male college professor who presented complaining of motor dysfunction, pain, and weakness associated with right knee arthroscopic surgery that occurred 8 weeks before the appointment. The patient related a history of right ankle sprain occurring approximately 2 months earlier when he stepped in a hole in his yard. He described right gastrocnemius soreness lasting for several days, which he self-treated by walking on a treadmill for 20 to 30 min per day. About 1 week after the ankle sprain, he reported slipping while walking on the treadmill, causing him to twist and forward fall onto his right knee. He indicated he felt a sharp pain just medial to the joint line, which remained constant for 2 weeks, and minimal swelling.

The orthopedic surgeon's report described a right arthroscopic surgery with removal of a loose body and abrasion chondroplasty of right medial condyle. The associated primary pathology was an osteochondral fracture of the right medial femoral condyle. The patient had been medically cleared to be full weight bearing and to begin rehabilitative therapy. During the 8 weeks postsurgery, the patient had been performing a daily self-designed home exercise regimen consisting of 20 to 25 min on a stationary bicycle, 10 min in a whirlpool bath, 20 to 25 repetitions of sitting knee flexion to extension with free weights of different poundages (heaviest, 10 lb), and 10 min on a treadmill at slow speed and no incline.

The patient appeared short of breath and flushed from the 500-yd walk into the building. He walked without an assistive device but with a pronounced left weight shift and right limp. Examination of the patient's knee indicated minimal joint swelling and calor. The arthroscopic entry portals were healed with little scarring. Palpation tenderness was noted along the medial right joint line and superior to the patella. Active ROM of the knee was 140° of flexion and −20° of extension. Passive ROM was painful toward the end range of flexion with soft end-feel. The patient's knee could be passively moved to −5° of full extension with no indication of pain. The left knee showed no limitations related to active or passive ROM.

Resisted right knee flexion was fairly strong (4/5 using a prone manual muscle test); resisted knee extension was weak (3/5 using a sitting manual muscle test) with mild suprapatellar pain. The left knee was considered strong (5/5 on all resisted manual muscle tests). Balance testing revealed a probable proprioceptive deficit in single-limb stance on either extremity and diminished postural responses to disturbances. He opted to use a compensatory hip strategy to recover balance when nudged in standing (see Fig. 11-24).

Gait analysis indicated a decreased step length on the right, limited knee flexion to extension excursion during the swing, a shortened stance phase on the right with a slight knee flexion at midstance, and decreased anterior to posterior oscillations of the pelvis. The resulting appearance was of a shuffling step on right with limited floor clearance and a hip hiking circumduction motion to advance the extremity.

LINK TO

Guide to Physical Therapist Practice

Pattern 4J of the Guide[26] describes the diagnosis of this patient. The pattern defines the specific patient/client diagnostic group as "impaired joint mobility, motor function, muscle performance, and range of motion associated with bony or soft tissue surgical procedures." Abrasion arthroplasty and bony débridement are included in this diagnostic category. Based on the examination and using the terminology of the Guide, the clinician made the more specific diagnosis of joint instability associated with impaired muscle performance and motor function related to right knee arthroplasty and removal of loose bodies.

The plan of care for this patient emphasized the following: coordinating care and instruction with the patient to develop a home program that would be acceptable and safe (given his past history of self-treatment); improving aerobic capacity, motor control, and strength through therapeutic exercise; and gait training to improve safety and efficiency of performance.

INTERVENTION

Initially, the goal of intervention was to decrease pain and associated inflammation, increase the pain-free range of the right knee in flexion, and increase flexion to extension excursion during the swing phase of gait. The patient was instructed to discontinue all self-designed home exercises because all of the exercises were stressing the suprapatellar soft tissue, resulting in inflammation and pain. In collaboration with the patient, a home program was developed as follows:

1. Ice before and after treatment and at regular intervals during the day for 15 min each application.
2. Stretching exercises with emphasis on knee flexion—patient lying prone and using a towel to apply gentle pressure toward flexion (see Fig. 3-9).
3. Isotonic exercises with patient lying supine using a 2-lb weight for short arc quads (see Fig. 6-17) and heel slides in the pain-free range (see Fig. 2-14).
4. Straight-leg raises in the supine position (see Fig. 6-14).
5. Bridging with forward and backward weight shift (Fig. 12-9)
6. Begin walking 0.5 mi at slow pace using an indoor track and being aware of the weight shift, foot placement, and knee flexion and extension.

PROGRESSION

One Week After Initial Examination

One week after the initial examination, the patient reported minimal pain with walking and with knee flexion. However, he continued to demonstrate a limp on the right, which became more pronounced with an increasing pace of walking. He was measured for a leg length discrepancy; the right leg was found to be approximately 0.5 in. longer than the left. Given this information, the clinician recommended that the patient consult the physician to be fitted with an appropriate custom heel lift to correct the discrepancy.

The home program was continued for 2 weeks more, with an emphasis on restoration of flexion range and strengthening (weight was increased to 3 lb) in non-weight-bearing gravity-controlled positions (see Fig. 6-18). The patient was instructed to return in 2 weeks.

Three Weeks After Initial Examination

The patient returned with a 0.5-in. heel lift added on to the left to correct for the leg length difference. He reported no pain in his right knee at the end range of full ROM for knee extension; the range increased to 155° degrees with the soft tissues of the thigh stopping the movement. Resisted right knee flexion was graded 4/5 on manual muscle test. Gait analysis revealed a more typical pattern of right knee excursion, and the limp was diminished. The patient walked with the weight more evenly distributed side to side. He continued to have limited pelvic mobility during gait, which was judged to be an age-related learned pattern the could indicate limited trunk mobility. Thus, diagonal patterns were included in the home program. The balance limitations were improved but were noted to be disturbed, especially when displaced toward the right. The home program was modified, with patient input, as follows:

1. Increased poundage on free weights to 5 lb for 3 sets of 10 repetitions per day.
2. Walk 1 mi at usual pace (patient tended to walk fast normally),

PEDIATRIC *Perspectives*

- Functional progression should be the culmination of a complete, well designed rehabilitation process for children, just as for adults. This progression provides the necessary link from treatment of impairments to functional return to activities of daily living or sport.
- Functional progression is particularly important in the return to sport of a child athlete. This progression can be used as described within the chapter to provide rehabilitation using various progressive skilled tasks related to specific sport movements or skills.
- Functional progression relates conceptually to Chapters 5, Principles of Resistance Training, and 9 Closed-Kinetic-Chain Exercise and Plyometric Activities. See pediatric insert boxes within those chapters for additional pediatric imformation, as well as safely considerations.

increasing 0.25 mi per week up to maximum of 3 mi three times a week on a variety of surfaces (grass, sidewalk, dirt).

3. Treadmill walking only if weather or time did not permit outdoor or track walking (see Fig. 10-8).
4. Quick stops and starts and turning while walking.
5. Lunges with right foot forward and then with left foot forward (see Fig. 9-12).
6. Mini-squats to a semi-squat position (only if pain-free)—5 repetitions twice a day (see Fig. 9-10).
7. Reaching forward and sideways within the limits of stability while standing on a foam cushion on the floor (chapter 11).
8. Continue ice as needed.

Furthermore, the patient was told to use pain as a guide for progression, and if pain occurred, back off the exercise.

OUTCOME

After 3 weeks of intervention, patient was discharged. He was cautioned against relying on self-treatment with no input from a trained professional.

SUMMARY

- No rehabilitation program is complete without a well-devised and thoroughly carried out functional progression program. This chapter provided the scientific and clinical basis of a functional progression program. The basic premise of the program is the need to address specific function.
- Functional progression is defined as a series of sport-specific, basic movement patterns that are graduated according to the difficulty of the skill and the client's tolerance. An intimate knowledge of the sport and, more important, the specific duties required of the athlete in his or her chosen sport are prerequisites for a successful functional progression program. Each program must be individualized, based on the injury and the demands placed on the athlete. The ideal functional program is developed by the clinician in conjunction with the individual and is based on the specific setting.
- If the client notes that pain persists for more than 2 hr after performing functional progression activities, the program should not be advanced.

REFERENCES

1. Tippett SR. Sports rehabilitation concepts. In: B Sanders, ed. Sports physical therapy. Norwalk, CT: Appleton & Lange, 1990: 9–14.
2. Tippett SR, Voight ML. Functional progressions for sport rehabilitation. Champaign, IL: Human Kinetics, 1995.
3. Yamamoto SK, Hartman CW, Feagin JA, Kimball G. Functional rehabilitation of knee: a preliminary study. Am J Sport Med 1975;3:288–291.
4. Kegerreis S. The construction and implementation of functional progression as a component of athletic rehabilitation. J Orthop Sport Phys Ther 1983;5:14–19.
5. Kegerreis S, Malone T, McCarroll J. Functional progression: an aid to athletic rehabilitation. Phys Sportsmed 1984:12:67–71.
6. Kaplan FS, Hayes WC, Keaveny TM, et al. Form and function of bone. In: SR Simon, ed. Orthopaedic basic science. Rosemont, IL: AAOS, 1994:127–184.
7. Cummings GS, Tillman LJ. Biologic mechanisms of connective tissue mutability. In: DP Currier, RM Nelson, eds. Dynamic of human biologic tissues. Philadelphia: Davis, 1992:1–44.
8. SL Woo, MA Gomez, TJ Sites, et al. The biomechanical and morphological changes in the medial collateral ligament of the rabbit after immobilization and remobilization. J Bone Joint Surg [Am] 1987;69:1200–1211.
9. Lechner CT, Dahners LE. Healing of the medial collateral ligament in unstable rat knees. Am J Sport Med 1991;19:508–512.
10. Gomez MA, Woo SL, Amiel D, et al. The effects of increased tension on healing medial collateral ligaments. Am J Sport Med 1991;19:347–354.
11. Indelicato PA, Hermansdorfer J, Huegel M. Nonoperative treatment of complete tears of the medial collateral ligament of the knee in intercollegiate football players. Clin Orthop 1990;256:174–177.

12. Anderson MA, Foreman TL. Return to competition: functional progression. In: JE Zachezewski, DJ Magee, WS Quillen, eds. Athletic injuries and rehabilitation. Philadelphia: Saunders, 1996:229–261.
13. Sandler-Goldstein T. Functional rehabilitation in orthopaedics. Gaithersburg, MD: Aspen, 1988.
14. Tippett SR. Closed chain exercise. Orthop Phys Ther Clin North Am 1992;1:253–268.
15. Bandy WD. Functional rehabilitation of the athlete. Orthop Phys Ther Clin North Am 1992;1:269–282.
16. Rivera JE. Open versus closed chain rehabilitation of the lower extremity: afunctional and biomechanical analysis. J Sport Rehab 1994;3:154–167.
17. Swanik CB, Lephart SM, Giannantonio FP, Fu, FH. Reestablishing proprioception and neuromuscular control in the ACL-injured athlete. J Sport Rehab 1997:6:182–206.
18. Voight ML, Cook G. Clinical application of closed kinetic chain exercise. J Sport Rehab 1996:5:25–44.
19. Cox RH. Sport psychology: concepts and applications. 3rd ed. Madison, WI: Brown & Benchmark, 1994.
20. Ievleva L, Orlick T. Mental links to enhanced healing. Sport Psychol 1991;5:25–40.
21. Duda JL, Smart AE, Tappe MK. Predictors of adherence in the rehabilitation of athletic injuries: an application of personal investment theory. J Sport Exer Psyiol 1989;11:265–275.
22. Dye SF. The knee as a biologic transmission with an envelope of function: a theory. Clin Orthop 1996;323:10–18.
23. O'Connor FG, Sobel JR, Nirschl RP. Five-step treatment for overuse injuries. Phys Sportsmed 1992;20:128–142.
24. Fyfe I, Stanish WD. The use of eccentric training and stretching in the treatment and prevention of tendon injuries. Clin Sports Med 1992;11:601–624.
25. Xethalis JL, Boiardo RA. Soccer injuries. In: JA Nicholas, EB Hershman, eds. The lower extremity and spine in sports medicine. St, Louis: Mosby, 1986:1580–1667.
26. American Physical Therapy Association. Guide to physical therapist practice, second edition. Phys Ther 2001;81:1–768.
27. National Athletic Trainers' Association. Athletic training educational competencies. 3rd ed. Dallas: NATA, 1999.

CHAPTER 15

Functional Progression: Upper Extremity

Kevin E. Wilk, PT

William D. Bandy, PhD, PT, SCS, ATC (Case Study 1)
Barbara Hoogenboom, PT, SCS, ATC (Case Study 2)
Reta Zabel, PhD, PT, GCS (Case Study 3)

Functional progression is a planned sequence of activities designed to progressively stress the injured client in a controlled environment to return him or her to as high a level of activity (competition) as possible without reinjury.[1] Functional progression depends on the specific work and leisure activities in which the individual participates or wants to participate. Based on the demands imposed, the clinician must design a rehabilitation program that stimulates and replicates functional activities that are tailored to the client's goals. If the program does not result in the unrestricted return to participation in work and leisure activities, it cannot be considered complete or successful.

When performing the initial examination, the clinician should consider the patient's functional goals. The clinician then designs the intervention program to progress the patient from the current level of function to the ultimate goal of function. To reach the goal, the patient is advanced along a continuum of functional skills, trying more advanced activities as each set of exercises is mastered. The clinician must carefully monitor the patient's tolerance to the new, more aggressive exercises to ensure a safe return to work or leisure activities.

■ *Scientific Basis*

Whether the treatment is conservative or surgical, intervention plays a vital role in achieving a successful outcome. The process must be sequential and progressive in nature, with the ultimate goal of a rapid return to pain-free function. A reliable functional progression program is based on six basic principles, presented in Table 15-1.

The patient's goal is usually to return to participating in unrestricted, symptom-free competitive or recreational activity. Patients with upper extremity dysfunction generally want to participate in a wide range of pain-free activities including working overhead, painting, combing one's hair, and throwing a ball. The rehabilitative program must be designed to progress the patient to his or her ultimate level of desired function. The functional approach to treatment suggests that patients with upper extremity dysfunction must exhibit dynamic joint stability before any functional sport-type movement can be safely and effectively initiated. For example, because the function of the rotator cuff and biceps brachii is to stabilize the humeral head within the glenoid, rehabilitation of these muscles must be emphasized early in the rehabilitative program to enable dynamic motion to occur at the glenohumeral joint without complications.

In addition, the concept of proximal stability for distal mobility must be addressed. For example, for overhead sport movements to occur without complications, proximal stability should be accomplished via the scapulothoracic joint, thereby enabling the arm to move effectively through space. Last, the rehabilitation program should be progressive, and isometric stability should be accomplished before attempting isotonic (concentric and eccentric) strengthening (chapters 5 and 6).

TABLE 15-1 Six Principles of a Reliable Functional Progression Program

Successful treatment is based on a team approach; the physician, patient, and clinician work together toward a common goal.
The effects of immobilization must be minimized; early motion and strengthening are preferred whenever possible.
Healing tissue should never be overstressed.
The patient must fulfill specific objective criteria before progressing to the next rehabilitative stage.
The rehabilitation program must be based on sound, current clinical, and scientific research.
The rehabilitation program must be individualized to the patient's specific work- and leisure-related activities.

Clinical Guidelines

Information on the basic science for functional return was introduced in Chapter 14, which focused on the lower extremity. Thus, rather than repeat that information, this chapter will introduce a criterion-based program for progressing the patient with upper extremity dysfunction. Of course, the information presented in Chapter 14 can be used to treat patients with upper extremity dysfunction, just as information presented in this chapter can be used to treat patients with lower extremity dysfunction. Furthermore, all patients are best served by a program that incorporates the principles of both a functional progression and a criterion-based program.

CRITERION-BASED INTERVENTION

The key to a criterion-based program is the interdependent, four-phased rehabilitative approach that is linked to a variety of exercises that guide the patient through a sequential progression of functional activities.[2] For each phase of the rehabilitation program, the clinician establishes objective and functional criteria that are used to guide the patient's advancement and ensure the appropriate rate of progression. This type of program requires the patient to fulfill minimal objective criteria before attempting more advanced levels of exercise and function. This basic rehabilitative approach can be adapted for a wide variety of surgical and nonsurgical conditions.

By ensuring strict adherence to the fulfillment of the predetermined objective criteria before advancing the patient to the next phase, the clinician is able to individualize the pace of the program based on the patient's age, injury, affected tissue type, activity level, sport or position, and surgical procedure. It is imperative to remember that the specific exercises, positions, and progression used depend on the extent of the injury, type of surgical procedure performed, healing constraints, and tissues stressed during rehabilitation. This chapter provides an overview of a multiphased, criterion-based rehabilitation program for the patient with upper extremity dysfunction. This type of program can be adapted to a variety of situations as long as strict adherence to the fulfillment of the criteria before advancing the patient is maintained.

THE PHASES

I: Immediate Motion Phase

The three primary goals for the initial rehabilitative phase are to re-establish nonpainful range of motion (ROM), to retard muscular atrophy, and to decrease pain and inflammation. It is imperative to re-establish "normal" motion. Immediately after any upper-extremity injury or surgery, motion is allowed in a safe, protected, and relatively nonpainful arc. This motion helps minimize or eliminate the potentially deleterious effects of immobilization, which include articular cartilage degeneration and muscular atrophy.[2–4] In addition, early motion assists in aligning healing collagen fibers along appropriate stress patterns, thereby avoiding adverse collagen tissue formation.[3] Active-assistive ROM exercises are used to accomplish immediate early motion activities (see Chapter 2).

Passive joint mobilization techniques to assess and restore normal joint mobility through the movement of one joint surface on another are also incorporated early in the rehabilitative process.[5,6] The direction and magnitude of displacement are determined by the capsuloligamentous integrity. The magnitude of the glide is determined by the amount of stretch desired on the capsule and is referred to in grades, which range from 1 to 5 (Chapter 4).

Immediate motion exercises are also beneficial in decreasing the client's perception of pain. By allowing controlled movement, type 1 and 2 joint mechanoreceptors are stimulated, which presynaptically inhibit pain fiber transmission at the spinal cord level. Therefore, by allowing immediate motion, patients feel better and achieve control of the extremity sooner.

Functional decrease in the strength of musculature secondary to pain and swelling is common after injury or surgery. Frequently, the pain patients experience with ROM exercises occurs secondary to poor strength. Pain-free, submaximal isometric muscular contractions performed at multiple angles are used initially[7] (Chapter 6). Each isometric contraction should be held for 6 to 8 sec and progressed from one or two sets of 10 to 15 repetitions to four or five sets of 10 to 15 repetitions, as tolerated. These exercises should be performed two to three times daily in conjunction with the active-assisted ROM exercises previously described.

After incorporation of submaximal isometrics, the exercise program should be progressed to short-arc isotonic activities. In addition, closed-chain, weight-bearing exercises are added during phase I to facilitate co-contractions of the muscles of the upper extremity (Chapter 9).

Before progressing to phase II, specific objective criteria must be exhibited by the patient on physical examination. The criteria are full, nonpainful passive ROM; minimal, palpable tenderness and pain; and good strength (4/5 on a manual muscle test).

II: Intermediate Phase

The goals of the second rehabilitative phase are to improve muscular strength, endurance, and neuromuscular control. During this phase, strengthening exercises are advanced to isotonic and isokinetic activities (Chapter 6). The exercises incorporated during the first portion of the phase are low-weight, submaximal isotonic contractions. Usually, the program is advanced in 1- to 2-lb intervals working up to five sets of 10 repetitions for each exercise using 5 to 10 lb of resistance.[7,8]

Submaximal isokinetic exercises can be initiated as the patient progresses during this rehabilitative phase (Chapter 6). Isokinetic exercise allows for high-speed, high-energy activities, beginning in a relatively safe and stable position.

Single-plane, submaximal isotonic and isokinetic strengthening exercises should be combined with multiplane diagonal pattern activities using synergic movements, such as proprioceptive neuromuscular facilitation (PNF) exercises (Chapter 8). The exercise progression thus moves from basic concepts and exercises to more complex and difficult levels of physical activity. The clinician should incorporate PNF patterns in a range of positions (e.g., side lying, seated, standing, and supine) to vary the neuromuscular input and maximally challenge the ability of the dynamic stabilizers to control the upper extremity muscles.

To progress from phase II to phase III, the patient must exhibit full, nonpainful active ROM, no pain or palpable tenderness on clinical examination, and at least 70% of the strength of the contralateral uninjured extremity. The client must exhibit these specific criteria before any attempt at performing the phase III exercise drills are done. The drills, activities, and exercises used in the advanced rehabilitative phase require greater strength, power, and endurance and prepare the patient for return to strenuous, unrestricted athletic activities.

III: Advanced Strengthening Phase

Phase III exercises are considered dynamic strengthening exercises and drills. The goals of this phase are to increase strength, power, and muscular endurance; improve neuromuscular control; and prepare the patient for a gradual, controlled return to functional activities. These exercises include high-speed, high-energy strengthening drills, eccentric muscular contractions, diagonal movements in functional positions, isotonic dumbbell movements, resistive exercise tubing movements with concentric and eccentric contractions, isokinetic exercises, and plyometric activities.

Plyometric drills provide the patient with a functional progression to unrestricted, sport-specific movements such as throwing, swinging, and catching. These dynamic, high-energy exercises prepare the upper-extremity musculature for the microtraumatic stresses experienced during most sports activities (see Chapter 9).

The patient must meet the following four specific criteria to progress to the final phase of rehabilitation: full, nonpainful active and passive ROM; no pain or palpable tenderness on clinical examination; satisfactory muscular strength, power, and endurance based on functional demands; and satisfactory clinical examination.

IV: Return to Activity

Phase IV is a transitional phase directed toward returning the patient to unrestricted, symptom-free athletic activity. During this phase, the patient is encouraged to continue specific exercises to address any remaining strength deficits and to improve upper extremity muscular strength as it relates to the functional demands of the sport. In addition, the patient begins a progressive and gradual return to athletics, using a controlled program that specifically meets the patient's individual needs.

The purpose of an interval sports program is to progressively and systematically increase the demands placed on the upper extremity while the athlete performs a sport-specific activity.[9] A progressive program can be adapted for any functional athletic rehabilitation program. Tables 15-2 to 15-5 provide examples of interval programs for throwers, golfers, and tennis players. The interval program presented in the tables are intended to be used as guidelines; the clinician should make modifications based on the individual response of the patient.

TABLE 15-2 Phase I Interval Throwing Program

45-ft throwing distance
Step 1: 50 throws with 15-min rest[a]
Step 2: 75 throws with 20-min rest[b]
60-ft throwing distance
Step 3: 50 throws with 15-min rest[a]
Step 4: 75 throws with 20-min rest[b]
90-ft throwing distance
Step 5: 50 throws with 15-min rest[a]
Step 6: 75 throws with 20-min rest[b]
120-ft throwing distance
Step 7: 50 throws with 15-min rest[a]
Step 8: 75 throws with 20-min rest[b]
150-ft throwing distance
Step 9: 50 throws with 15-min rest[a]
Step 10: 75 throws with 20-min rest[b]
180-ft throwing distance
Step 11: 50 throws with 15-min rest[a]
Step 12: 75 throws with 20-min rest[b]
Following step 12, begin throwing off mound or return to respective position.

[a]Part A consists of (1) warm-up throwing, (2) 25 throws at distance, (3) 15-min rest, (4) warm-up throwing, and (5) 25 throws at distance.
[b]Part B consists of (1) warm-up throwing, (2) 25 throws at distance, (3) 10-min rest, (4) warm-up throwing, (5) 25 throws at distance, (6) 10-min rest, (7) warm-up throwing, and (8) 25 throws at distance.

TABLE 15-3 Phase II Interval Throwing Program[a]

Stage 1 (fastball only)
Step 1: 15 throws off mound at 50% speed
Step 2: 30 throws off mound at 50% speed
Step 3: 45 throws off mound at 50% speed
Step 4: 60 throws off mound at 50% speed
Step 5: 30 throws off mound at 75% speed
Step 6: 30 throws off mound at 75% speed; 45 throws off mound at 50% speed
Step 7: 45 throws off mound at 75% speed; 15 throws off mound at 50% speed
Step 8: 60 throws off mound at 75% speed
Stage 2 (fastball only)
Step 9: 45 throws off mound at 75% speed; 15 throws in batting practice
Step 10: 45 throws off mound at 75% speed; 30 throws in batting practice
Step 11: 45 throws off mound at 75% speed; 45 throws in batting practice
Stage 3 (variety of pitches)
Step 12: 30 fastballs off mound at 75% speed; 15 breaking balls off mound at 50% speed; 45 to 60 fastballs in batting practice
Step 13: 30 fastballs off mound at 75% speed; 30 breaking balls at 75% speed; 30 throws in batting practice
Step 14: 30 fastballs off mound at 75% speed; 60 to 90 breaking balls in batting practice at 25% speed
Step 15: Simulated game, progressing by 15 throws per workout

[a]All throwing off the mound should be done in the presence of the pitching coach, who should stress proper throwing mechanics. The use of a speed gun may help pitcher control intensity.

Case Studies

Several case studies are presented in this chapter to demonstrate the integration of information from all previous chapters in the text.

CASE STUDY 1

PATIENT INFORMATION

The patient was a 23-year-old collegiate volleyball player. In the initial examination, the patient complained of right shoulder pain and popping when serving and hitting. The athlete stated that she played through the pain and had not cut down on practice or competition. She also noted that the volleyball season was over and her goals were to play and practice pain free during the following season.

The patient's history indicated surgery (arthroscopic capsular shift of the anterior and inferior glenohumeral ligaments secondary to impingement) 1 year earlier on the same shoulder. The athlete was unable to remember any rehabilitation after surgery. She also reported a shoulder injection secondary to pain about 2 months earlier, which relieved her symptoms for 1 week.

Examination of the right shoulder indicated a painful arc during active shoulder abduction and severe pain during pas-

TABLE 15-4 Interval Golf Program

Week	Monday	Wednesday	Friday
1	Stretch 10 putts 10 chips 5-min rest 15 chips Use ice	Stretch 15 putts 15 chips 5-min rest 25 chips Use ice	Stretch 20 putts 20 chips 5-min rest 20 putts 20 chips 5-min rest 10 chips 10 short irons Use ice
2	Stretch 20 chips 10 short irons 5-min rest 10 short irons Use ice	Stretch 20 chips 15 short irons 10-min rest 15 chips Use ice	Stretch 15 short irons 10 medium irons 10-min rest 15 chips Use ice
3	Stretch 15 short irons 15 medium irons 10-min rest 5 long irons 15 short irons 15 medium irons 10-min rest 20 chips Use ice	Stretch 15 short irons 10 medium irons 10 long irons 10-min rest 10 short irons 10 medium irons 5 long irons 5 woods Use ice	Stretch 15 short irons 10 medium irons 10 long irons 10-min rest 10 short irons 10 medium irons 10 long irons 10 woods Use ice
4	Stretch 15 short irons 10 medium irons 10 long irons 10 drives 15-min rest Repeat Use ice	Stretch Play 9 holes Use ice	Stretch Play 9 holes Use ice
5	Stretch Play 9 holes Use ice	Stretch Play 9 holes Use ice	Stretch Play 18 holes Use ice

Putts, putter; *chips,* pitching wedge; *short irons,* W, 9, 8; *medium irons,* 7, 6, 5; *long irons,* 4, 3, 2; *woods,* 3, 5; *drives,* driver.

TABLE 15-5 Interval Tennis Program

Week	Monday	Wednesday	Friday
1	12 FH 8 BH 10-min rest 13 FH 7 BH Use ice	15 FH 8 BH 10-min rest 15 FH 7 BH Use ice	15 FH 10 BH 10-min rest 15 FH 10 BH Use ice
2	25 FH 15 BH 10-min rest 25 FH 15 BH Use Ice	30 FH 20 BH 10-min rest 30 FH 20 BH Use Ice	30 FH 25 BH 10-min rest 30 FH 15 FH 10 OH Use Ice
3	30 FH 25 BH 10 OH 10-min rest 30 FH 25 BH Use ice	30 FH 25 BH 15 OH 10-min rest 30 FH 25 BH 15 OH Use ice	30 FH 30 BH 10-min rest 30 FH 15 OH 10-min rest 30 FH 30 BH 15 OH Use ice
4	30 FH 30 BH 10 OH 10-min rest Play 3 games 10 FH 10 BH 5 OH Use ice	30 FH 30 BH 10 OH 10-min rest Play set 10 FH 10 BH 5 OH Use ice	30 FH 30 BH 10 OH 10-min rest Play 1.5 sets 10 FH 10 BH 10 OH Use ice

FH, forehand ground stroke; *BH,* backhand ground stroke; *OH,* overhead shot.

sive overpressure of shoulder flexion and internal rotation (positive impingement signs). Resisted movement of the shoulder caused pain during abduction and external rotation, and weakness of those muscles (3/5). Palpation indicated pain at the anterior portion of the greater tuberosity and slight discomfort at the bicipital groove. Tests for shoulder instability were negative. The ROM of the right shoulder was equal to that of the left.

The diagnosis was consistent with shoulder impingement. Examination also suggested involvement of the rotator cuff muscles, specifically the supraspinatus muscle.

LINKS TO

Guide to Physical Therapist Practice and *Athletic Training Educational Competencies*

According to the *Guide,*[10] the patient's diagnosis was included in musculoskeletal practice pattern 4D. This pattern is described as "impaired joint mobility, motor function, muscle performance, and range of motion associated with connective tissue dysfunction". The anticipated goals for this patient as related to functional progression included increasing motor function; improving joint mobility; improving weight-bearing status; improving strength, power, and endurance; protecting the injured body part; and minimizing the risk of recurrent injury.

The therapeutic exercise domain in the *Competencies*[11] refers to the ability to "revise goals and objectives and develop criteria for progression and return to competition based on level of function and patient outcomes." The teaching objectives include "functional rehabilitation and reconditioning."

INTERVENTION

Given the irritability of the athlete's shoulder, the initial goals were to decrease pain and inflammation, maintain ROM with pain-free intervention, and initiate gentle strengthening activities (phase I of a criterion-based program). The athlete was instructed to discontinue all overhead activities. Given that the volleyball season was complete, these directions were met with no resistance. She was seen three times a week in the clinic, and treatment consisted of the following:

1. Ice before treatment.
2. Codman exercise.
3. Active assistive abduction, internal and external rotation in pain-free range (see Fig. 2-22).
4. Isometric external rotation and abduction, performed with athlete's arm at the side.
5. Isometric elbow flexion in two parts of the ROM (see Fig. 6-6).
6. Ice after treatment.

The athlete was instructed to perform the following home exercise program:

1. Codman exercise.
2. Wall walking within the pain-free ROM: stand near a wall, walk fingers up wall, elevating shoulder.
3. Ice after treatment.

PROGRESSION

Two Weeks After Initial Examination

The initial treatment program was prescribed for 1 week. However, at the 1-week follow-up, the athlete, although improved, still had significant pain and inflammation. Thus the program was continued for another week. The difficulty in decreasing the inflammation was attributed to the fact that the athlete had played through her pain for more than 2 months, which caused a severe inflammatory process that required 2 weeks to subside.

At the 2-week follow-up the strength of the abductors were equal bilaterally, but the external rotators on the right were still weak (4/5). The athlete could actively abduct through the full ROM with no pain, and no painful arc was present. The athlete still complained of pain with overpressure into full flexion and internal rotation, but the pain was not as severe as during the initial examination. The goals for the patient were advanced to increase strength of the muscles surrounding the shoulder (phase II of a criterion-based program). The patient continued to be seen in the clinic three times a week; the exercise program was progressed as follows:

1. Abduction from 0 to 90° in plane of scapula with shoulder held in internal rotation using dumbbells (see Fig. 6-11).
2. Internal and external rotation with the upper arm held against body (stable position) using elastic band (see Fig. 6-13A).
3. Axial compression against table and isometric push-ups (see Figs. 9-3 and 9-4).
4. Biceps curls using dumbbells.
5. Ice after treatment.

Patient was instructed to continue with the home program adding isometric internal and external rotation exercises. This stage of the intervention was performed for 2 weeks.

Four Weeks After Initial Examination

Examination at the 4-week follow-up indicated ROM of the right shoulder equal to the left and no pain on overpressure into full flexion and internal rotation (negative impingement sign). Isokinetic examination indicated a 50% deficit in the shoulder external rotators of the right compared to the left.

Goals now were to increase muscular strength in preparation for a gradual return to functional activities (phase III of a criterion-based program). The treatment program was progressed by increasing the amount of weight used for each exercise. Internal and external rotation using the elastic band was progressed by moving the upper arm (previously held close to the body) into 45°. The following exercises were added to the in-clinic program:

1. D2 upper-extremity PNF pattern with manual resistance (see Figs. 8-7 and 8-8).
2. Resisted axial load side to side on sliding board (see Fig. 12-20).
3. Initiation of a 1-mi jogging program (see Table 14-2).

Six Week After Initial Examination

Isokinetic examination after 6 weeks of intervention indicated a 25% deficit in external rotation. The patient was deemed ready for a functional progression program (phase IV of a criterion-based program). The patient was instructed to complete the following program 3 days a week:

1. Internal and external rotation using elastic band in 90° of shoulder abduction (see Fig. 6-13B).
2. Jogging 1 mile.
3. Balance activities (see Figs. 11-16 to 11-18).
4. Push-up activities (see Figs. 9-4, 9-6, and 9-8).
5. Overhead throwing of volleyball (standing on two feet and progressing to one foot).
6. Serving volleyball over net at half intensity but not hitting the ball inside the baseline.

Eight Weeks After Initial Examination

At the 8-week examination, the patient reported no pain with the activities performed the previous week. Her program was progressed as follows:

1. Continuation of elastic band, jogging, balance, and push-up exercises two times per week.
2. Serving inside the baseline, progressing to three quarters and then full intensity three times per week.
3. Outside hitting drills with her coach two times per week.

OUTCOMES

Ten weeks after the initial examination, the athlete participated in supervised off-season volleyball practice with no return of symptoms. She was discharged from formal intervention. The athlete was able to participate in a full season of play the following year with no complaints or return of symptoms.

CASE STUDY 2

PATIENT INFORMATION

A 12-year-old U.S. Gymnastics Association elite-level gymnast presented with left upper extremity pain and dysfunction related to an injury sustained 3 days before her appointment. While working on her bar routine she missed a catch (after a release move) with her right upper extremity and was left hanging and swinging by the left upper extremity on the higher bar. She lost her grasp and fell to the mat onto her buttocks. She was able to continue practicing that day, but the next morning she woke up with significant medial scapular pain and general upper extremity pain. Her mother initiated an orthopedic examination, which occurred a day later. She was referred by the orthopedist for intervention 3 days after injury. Radiographs indicated no fracture, and the orthopedist had diagnosed a shoulder strain.

The athlete arrived at the clinic wearing a sling. During the initial visit, the athlete reported sharp aching pain (5/10) in the posterior medial scapula and glenohumeral joint, a sensation of a muscle pull with pain (3/10) into the left side of the neck and entire left upper extremity, and stiffness of entire left upper extremity when attempting activities of daily living (dressing, grooming). The patient was tender to palpation to the rhomboids, levator scapulae, all parts of the trapezius, and posterior rotator cuff muscles. She was mildly tender to palpation in teres major and pectoralis major and minor muscles. Examination indicated multiple trigger points in the upper trapezius and medial scapular region.

Examination of active ROM of the left shoulder indicated flexion of 95°, abduction of 85°, external rotation of 70°, and internal rotation of 60°. All ROM was limited by pain in the scapular region. Cervical ROM was within normal limits in all motions, except right side bending was decreased and caused pain in left upper trapezius muscle.

Manual muscle test of the left upper extremity indicated the following strengths: external rotation at 3/5 with pain, internal rotation at 4/5 with no pain, middle trapezius at 3/5 with pain, lower trapezius at 2/5 with pain, and serratus anterior at 3/5 with pain. The elbow, wrist, hand, and cervical musculatures were full strength (5/5) and pain free. In addition, all special tests for laxity and impingement were negative.

The examination revealed strain of the left scapular and posterior rotator cuff musculature owing to a traction-type injury. The athlete had no increase in laxity of the injured (left) shoulder compared to the uninjured side.

LINKS TO

Guide to Physical Therapist Practice and *Athletic Training Educational Competencies*

According to the *Guide*,[10] the patient's diagnosis was classified into musculoskeletal practice pattern 4D. This pattern is described as "impaired joint mobility, muscle performance, and range of motion associated with connective tissue dysfunction." The goals of this patient as related to functional progression and return to sport participation were coordinating care among patient, family, coach, and all concerned medical professionals; preventing chronic or prolonged disability; improving performance of activities of daily living, recreation, school, and sport; reducing risk of reinjury; reducing risk of secondary impairment (e.g., neck dysfunction); and returning to high-level competitive gymnastics within 3 to 4 months.

The therapeutic exercise domain in the *Competencies*[11] refers to the ability to "revise goals and objectives and develop criteria for progression and return to competition based on level of function and patient outcomes." The teaching objectives include "functional rehabilitation and reconditioning."

INTERVENTION

The initial goals for the athlete were to minimize the inflammatory response caused by the injury and initiate gentle ROM activities (phase I of a criterion-based program). Intervention included the following:

1. Instruction in active assistive ROM with support for the left upper extremity provided by the right upper extremity.
2. Low-level weight bearing through bilateral upper extremities with medial lateral shifting and anterior-posterior shifting when standing at plinth.
3. Isometric exercises for shoulder abduction in the plane of the scapula (see Fig. 6-7).
4. Active ROM for scapular protraction and retraction, abduction and adduction (see Fig. 2-21), elevation, and depression.
5. Removal of sling for activities of daily living at waist to chest level, avoiding abnormal scapular mechanics for overhead work.
6. Manual therapy for trigger-point treatment.
7. Scapular PNF patterns using mild manual resistance (see Figs. 8-1 to 8-4).
8. Use of an exercise bicycle for maintenance of cardiovascular conditioning (see Fig. 10-5).
9. Ice applied to the posterior scapula for pain management.

PROGRESSION

Two Weeks After Initial Examination

The 2-week examination indicated that the patient had regained normal ROM but still had general weakness in the shoulder muscles. The goals were progressed to increase strength (phase II of a criterion-based program) as follows:

1. Isotonic external rotation (see Fig. 6-12).
2. Supine punches for serratus anterior (see Fig. 9-7).
3. Isolated internal and external rotation using elastic tubing with arm close to side (see Fig. 6-13A).
4. PNF diagonals with manual resistance (see Figs. 8-5 to 8-8).
5. Closed-kinetic-chain push-ups while standing with upper extremities 90° against wall (see Fig. 9-3).
6. Continue exercise bicycle.
7. Begin dance routines.

Four Weeks After Initial Examination

At the 4-week follow-up, the patient demonstrated normal active ROM with excellent scapular control. Manual muscle tests of the rotators and scapular stabilizers were all 4+/5 to 5/5. No trigger points or tenderness were noted on palpation. The goals at this stage were to continue to increase strength, while progressively increasing the athlete's gymnastic activities (phase III of a criterion-based program). Intervention included the following:

1. Progressive increased isotonic exercises in more elevated positions (90° and 90°) for external rotation and internal rotation (see Fig. 6-13B).
2. PNF diagonals progressing to standing with elastic tubing (see Fig. 8-20).
3. Closed-kinetic-chain training in the push up position (see Fig. 9-8).
4. Initiation of a quadriped program, stressing neutral position of the spine (see Figs. 12-13 and 12-14).

Six Weeks After Initial Examination

After 6 weeks, the patient showed no signs of adverse effects of the previous 2 weeks of training; in fact, she indicated a desire to do more. The goals were now to monitor the functional progression program to full participation (phase IV of a criterion-based program). The athlete was progressed to the following activities:

1. Progression in quadruped program (see Figs. 12-17, 12-18, 12-27).
2. Initiation of a plyometric upper-extremity program using push-ups (see Fig. 9-21).
3. Progression to low-level, upper-extremity, closed-chain tumbling activities (e.g., cartwheels).
4. Swinging from the upper extremity (e.g., chin-ups, swinging from upper bar) with progression to light release and catch skills (low velocity and distance).
5. Initiation of return to sport-specific progression for other activities, including running, jumping, and lower-extremity landing tasks (see Figs. 9-27 to 9-29 and Table 14-6).

OUTCOMES

At 8 weeks postinjury, the clinician monitored the patient during a minimal workout in the gym. The athlete participated in supervised, gradual return to full activity over the following 4 weeks. Close communication with her parents and coach helped with the successful return to sport in this case. More caution and time were taken with this young athlete than may have been taken with an adult. But it was important to be sure that the athlete had excellent return of strength and endurance of musculature before she returned to her sport. The patient was released from intervention at 12 weeks and was allowed to participate in full gymnastic activities.

CASE STUDY 3

PATIENT INFORMATION

The patient, a 66-year-old woman, was a secretary in a busy office. She was referred for ROM and strengthening after 8 weeks of immobilization and restricted use of left upper extremity. The patient reported falling in a dark hallway in her home and hitting the door frame, resulting in a midshaft humeral fracture. The fracture was classified as a closed transverse fracture, sparing the radial nerve and brachial artery. The extremity had been immobilized using an external coaptation splint followed by functional bracing with a molded sleeve applied proximal to the elbow at approximately 4 weeks postinjury.

The patient had been performing active ROM exercises of her wrists and fingers. All activity, including range of the shoulder and elbow, weight bearing, and the use of the arm, had been restricted during the period of immobilization. The patient had been directed to use her noninvolved extremity for self-care and work duties. Reciprocal arm swing during gait had been limited by pain. At 6 weeks postinjury, she began to use her left extremity in self-care and had initiated self-directed pendulum exercises twice a day.

At this point, the bone was considered healed and the orthopedic surgeon released the patient to perform full weight bearing, ROM, and progressive strengthening exercises for the elbow and shoulder. However, the patient had been cautioned to perform only light lifting activities for the first 4 weeks.

The initial examination revealed

Palpation tenderness over the fracture site.

Active left shoulder ROM: abduction 110°, adduction 40°, flexion 110°, extension 50°, internal rotation 40° with pain, and external rotation 15° with pain.

Active right shoulder ROM: abduction 125°, adduction 40°, flexion 160°, extension 50°, internal rotation 70°, and external rotation 50°.

Elbow ROM equal on both sides.

Manual muscle test of left shoulder: pectoralis major 4/5, deltoid 3/5, biceps 4/5, triceps 5/5.

Manual muscle test of right shoulder: 4/5 overall.

The patient had no symptoms of reflex sympathetic dystrophy (pain with passive motion, burning pain, pallor, swelling, coldness, hypersensitivity to contractual stimuli, clothing, changes in ambient airflow, or air temperature). Observation of her gait revealed a decreased left arm swing during right stepping.

LINK TO

Guide to Physical Therapist Practice

Pattern 4G of the *Guide*[10] is appropriate for this patient: "Impaired joint mobility, muscle performance, and range of motion associated with fracture." The goals for this patient emphasized initiating a home program that could be integrated into her daily routine at work and home; performing therapeutic exercises to improve ROM, increase strength, and promote functional use of the involved extremity; and undergoing functional gait training to reintegrate left arm swing.

PEDIATRIC *Perspectives*

- Functional progression should be the culmination of a complete, well-designed rehabilitation process for children, just as for adults. This progression provides the necessary link from treatment of impairments to functional return to activities of daily living or sport.
- Functional progression is particularly important in the return to sport of a child athlete. The program should provide rehabilitation by using a variety of progressive tasks related to specific sport movements or skills.
- Depending on the chosen activity to which the child must return, the upper-extremity functional progression may involve more open-kinetic-chain activities (throwing) than a program for the lower extremity. However, incorporation of closed-kinetic-chain and plyometric activities in an upper-extremity functional progression is common for children, as for adults.
- Functional progression relates conceptually to muscular training, closed-kinetic chain and plyometric activities, and reactive neuromuscular straining. See "Pediatric Perspectives" in Chapters 5, 6, and 9.

INTERVENTION

Initially, the patient was instructed to perform a home program to initiate ROM activities (phase I of a criterion-based program) involving pendulum exercises, wall presses, and internal to external rotation (placing the dorsum of the left hand on the low back and then placing the palm of the same hand on the back of the head) (see Figs. 2-24 and 2-25). She was told to repeat the exercises for 10 repetitions twice a day for 1 week and then to return to the clinic for progression. In addition, she was instructed to move slowly, to use warmth before exercising, and to use ice after exercise. For home and work, she was told to support her left arm on a pillow if sitting for long periods in a chair without armrests and to functionally use her arm as much as possible without causing undue pain (5/10).

PROGRESSION

One Week After Initial Examination

Upon return to the clinic, the patient reported minimal discomfort when using the left arm in weight-bearing activities but continued difficulty using the arm for functional activities, such as reaching into an overhead cabinet or washing and drying her back. At the clinic she performed PNF techniques of repeated contraction, and hold-relax-contract exercises were incorporated in the D1 pattern to address weakness and loss of active ROM (see Figs. 8-5 and 8-6). The home program was progressed to include cane exercises for shoulder flexion, abduction and adduction (see Fig. 2-30), and rotation (see Fig. 2-31). The patient was asked to return after 1 week.

Two Weeks After Initial Examination

At the 2-week follow-up, the patient reported increased functional use of her left arm when lifting light objects to and from overhead cabinets but continued limitation with activities like drying her back. The pain at end range had decreased to a level that allowed some passive mobilization of the shoulder and scapula (see Figs. 4-14 to 4-16). The active ROM gained 5° in flexion and abduction; but internal and external rotation continued to be limited.

Progressive resistive exercise was added to the program to initiate strengthening activities (phase II of a criterion-based program). In the clinic, the patient performed isometric shoulder abduction in the plane of the scapula (see Fig. 6-7) and external rotation exercises in side lying using a 1-lb weight. The home program was continued, and the patient was instructed to increase the functional use of her left arm while performing activities of daily living and working.

Three Weeks After Initial Examination

After 3 weeks, the patient reported fair tolerance of activities requiring left upper-extremity internal and external rotation, as in dressing. She was able to bring her left fingertips to within 1 in. of the right fingertips behind her back (right external rotation and left internal rotation). Active left shoulder ROM was as follows: abduction 125°, adduction 40°, flexion 115°, internal rotation 45°, and external rotation 35°. Her right shoulder range remained unchanged from the initial examination. Likewise, manual muscle testing showed no change.

The treatment session was used to functionally reintegrate the left upper extremity during performance of bimanual tasks, e.g., stirring food in a bowl, folding bed linens, and rubbing lotion on the hands. In addition, two 6-ft. × 2-in. dowel rods were used as mobile parallel bars to facilitate reciprocal arm swing during gait. The swing movement of the left upper extremity was exaggerated during stepping with right lower extremity to promote reacquisition of reciprocal gait.

OUTCOMES

Examination of the ROM and strength at the 3-week follow-up indicated that the patient was functional. She was disharged with instructions to continue the home program, to use ice as needed, and to functionally use the left upper extremity during activities.

SUMMARY

- The functional progression of an athlete with upper-extremity dysfunction should consist of a well-designed criterion-based intervention program that progresses from an initial program to a specific interval sports program to a return to the sport.
- Sport-specific training drills performed in the latter phases of rehabilitation can be successfully initiated only when the building blocks of the rehabilitation program have been firmly established.
- This chapter offers the clinician a criteria-based, functionally progressive, rehabilitation program that can be incorporated into the treatment of patients with upper-extremity dysfunction.

REFERENCES

1. Keggereis S, Malone T, McCarroll J. Functional progression: an aid to athletic rehabilitation. Phys Sports Med 1984;12:67–71.
2. Arrigo CA, Wilk KE. Shoulder exercises: criteria based approach to rehabilitation. In: MJ Kelly, WA Clark, eds. Orthopaedic therapy of the shoulder. Philadelphia: Lippincott, 1994: 337–361.
3. Akeson WH, Woo SLY, Amiel D. The connective tissue response to immobility: biomechanical changes in periarticular connective tissue of the immobilized rabbit knee. Clin Orthop 1973;93: 356–362.
4. Dehne E, Tory R. Treatment of joint injuries by immediate mobilization, based upon the spinal adaption concept. Clin Orthop 1971;77:218–232.
5. Maitland G. Peripheral manipulation. 2nd ed. Boston: Butterworth, 1977.
6. Kaltenborn F. Manual therapy of the extremity joints. Oslo: Borkhandel, 1973.
7. Wilk KE, Arrigo CA. An integrated approach to upper extremity exercises. Orthop Phys Ther Clin North Am 1992;1:337–360.
8. Wilk KE, Arrigo CA. Current concepts in the rehabilitation of the athletic shoulder. J Orthop Sports Phys Ther 1993;18: 365–378.
9. Wilk WE, Arrigo CA. Interval sport program for the shoulder. In JR Andrews, KE Wilk, eds. The athlete's shoulder. New York: Churchill Livingstone, 1994:569–628.
10. American Physical Therapy Association. Guide to physical therapist practice, second edition. Phys Ther 2001;81:1–768.
11. National Athletic Trainers' Association. Athletic training educational competencies. 3rd ed. Dallas: NATA, 1999.

SUBJECT INDEX

Page numbers in *italics* indicate figures. Page numbers followed by "t" indicate tables.